Management of Acute Stroke

NEUROLOGICAL DISEASE AND THERAPY

Series Editor

WILLIAM C. KOLLER

Department of Neurology
University of Kansas Medical Center
Kansas City, Kansas

1. Handbook of Parkinson's Disease, *edited by William C. Koller*
2. Medical Therapy of Acute Stroke, *edited by Mark Fisher*
3. Familial Alzheimer's Disease: Molecular Genetics and Clinical Perspectives, *edited by Gary D. Miner, Ralph W. Richter, John P. Blass, Jimmie L. Valentine, and Linda A. Winters-Miner*
4. Alzheimer's Disease: Treatment and Long-Term Management, *edited by Jeffrey L. Cummings and Bruce L. Miller*
5. Therapy of Parkinson's Disease, *edited by William C. Koller and George Paulson*
6. Handbook of Sleep Disorders, *edited by Michael J. Thorpy*
7. Epilepsy and Sudden Death, *edited by Claire M. Lathers and Paul L. Schraeder*
8. Handbook of Multiple Sclerosis, *edited by Stuart D. Cook*
9. Memory Disorders: Research and Clinical Practice, *edited by Takehiko Yanagihara and Ronald C. Petersen*
10. The Medical Treatment of Epilepsy, *edited by Stanley R. Resor, Jr., and Henn Kutt*
11. Cognitive Disorders: Pathophysiology and Treatment, *edited by Leon J. Thal, Walter H. Moos, and Elkan R. Gamzu*
12. Handbook of Amyotrophic Lateral Sclerosis, *edited by Richard Alan Smith*
13. Handbook of Parkinson's Disease: Second Edition, Revised and Expanded, *edited by William C. Koller*
14. Handbook of Pediatric Epilepsy, *edited by Jerome V. Murphy and Fereydoun Dehkharghani*
15. Handbook of Tourette's Syndrome and Related Tic and Behavioral Disorders, *edited by Roger Kurlan*
16. Handbook of Cerebellar Diseases, *edited by Richard Lechtenberg*
17. Handbook of Cerebrovascular Diseases, *edited by Harold P. Adams, Jr.*
18. Parkinsonian Syndromes, *edited by Matthew B. Stern and William C. Koller*
19. Handbook of Head and Spine Trauma, *edited by Jonathan Greenberg*
20. Brain Tumors: A Comprehensive Text, *edited by Robert A. Morantz and John W. Walsh*

21. Monoamine Oxidase Inhibitors in Neurological Diseases, *edited by Abraham Lieberman, C. Warren Olanow, Moussa B. H. Youdim, and Keith Tipton*
22. Handbook of Dementing Illnesses, *edited by John C. Morris*
23. Handbook of Myasthenia Gravis and Myasthenic Syndromes, *edited by Robert P. Lisak*
24. Handbook of Neurorehabilitation, *edited by David C. Good and James R. Couch, Jr.*
25. Therapy with Botulinum Toxin, *edited by Joseph Jankovic and Mark Hallett*
26. Principles of Neurotoxicology, *edited by Louis W. Chang*
27. Handbook of Neurovirology, *edited by Robert R. McKendall and William G. Stroop*
28. Handbook of Neuro-Urology, *edited by David N. Rushton*
29. Handbook of Neuroepidemiology, *edited by Philip B. Gorelick and Milton Alter*
30. Handbook of Tremor Disorders, *edited by Leslie J. Findley and William C. Koller*
31. Neuro-Ophthalmological Disorders: Diagnostic Work-Up and Management, *edited by Ronald J. Tusa and Steven A. Newman*
32. Handbook of Olfaction and Gustation, *edited by Richard L. Doty*
33. Handbook of Neurological Speech and Language Disorders, *edited by Howard S. Kirshner*
34. Therapy of Parkinson's Disease: Second Edition, Revised and Expanded, *edited by William C. Koller and George Paulson*
35. Evaluation and Management of Gait Disorders, *edited by Barney S. Spivack*
36. Handbook of Neurotoxicology, *edited by Louis W. Chang and Robert S. Dyer*
37. Neurological Complications of Cancer, *edited by Ronald G. Wiley*
38. Handbook of Autonomic Nervous System Dysfunction, *edited by Amos D. Korczyn*
39. Handbook of Dystonia, *edited by Joseph King Ching Tsui and Donald B. Calne*
40. Etiology of Parkinson's Disease, *edited by Jonas H. Ellenberg, William C. Koller, and J. William Langston*
41. Practical Neurology of the Elderly, *edited by Jacob I. Sage and Margery H. Mark*
42. Handbook of Muscle Disease, *edited by Russell J. M. Lane*
43. Handbook of Multiple Sclerosis: Second Edition, Revised and Expanded, *edited by Stuart D. Cook*
44. Central Nervous System Infectious Diseases and Therapy, *edited by Karen L. Roos*
45. Subarachnoid Hemorrhage: Clinical Management, *edited by Takehiko Yanagihara, David G. Piepgras, and John L. D. Atkinson*

46. Neurology Practice Guidelines, *edited by Richard Lechtenberg and Henry S. Schutta*
47. Spinal Cord Diseases: Diagnosis and Treatment, *edited by Gordon L. Engler, Jonathan Cole, and W. Louis Merton*
48. Management of Acute Stroke, *edited by Ashfaq Shuaib and Larry B. Goldstein*

Additional Volumes in Preparation

Sleep Disorders and Neurological Disease, *edited by Antonio Culebras*

Management of Acute Stroke

edited by

Ashfaq Shuaib

University of Alberta Hospital
Edmonton, Alberta, Canada

Larry B. Goldstein

Duke University Medical Center and
Durham VA Medical Center
Durham, North Carolina

MARCEL DEKKER, INC. NEW YORK • BASEL

Library of Congress Cataloging-in-Publication

Management of acute stroke / edited by Ashfaq Shuaib, Larry B. Goldstein.
p. cm. — (Neurological disease and therapy; v. 48)
Includes bibliographical references and index.
ISBN 0-8247-7092-7 (alk. paper)
1. Cerebrovascular disease—Treatment. I. Shuaib, Ashfaq. II. Goldstein, Larry B. III. Series.
[DNLM: 1. Cerebrovascular Disorders—therapy. 2. Acute Disease. WL 355 M265 1999]
RC388.5.M3345 1999
616.8'1—dc21
DNLM/DLC
for Library of Congress 99-35713
CIP

This book is printed on acid-free paper.

Headquarters
Marcel Dekker, Inc.
270 Madison Avenue, New York, NY 10016
tel: 212-696-9000; fax: 212-685-4540

Eastern Hemisphere Distribution
Marcel Dekker AG
Hutgasse 4, Postfach 812, CH-4001 Basel, Switzerland
tel: 41-61-261-8482; fax: 41-61-261-8896

World Wide Web
http://www.dekker.com

The publisher offers discounts on this book when ordered in bulk quantities. For more information, write to Special Sales/Professional Marketing at the headquarters address above.

Current printing (last digit)
10 9 8 7 6 5 4 3 2 1

PRINTED IN THE UNITED STATES OF AMERICA

Series Introduction

This book addresses cerebrovascular disease, focusing on the initial events in stroke. With proper diagnosis and treatment it is possible that neurological deficits in many patients with cerebrovascular disease can be prevented. *Management of Acute Stroke* is a book that is clearly needed for all physicians and healthcare providers who deal with patients presenting with acute neurological deficits.

The treatment of acute stroke has changed dramatically with the advent of drugs that may prevent progression of neurological deficit if given very early in the course of the stroke. This book presents a concise accounting of the advances in the evaluation and management of patients presenting with acute stroke. The volume is divided into two sections: (1) Evaluation and Diagnosis, with 13 chapters, and (2) Therapy: Managing the Acute Insult and Preventing Recurrences, also with 13 chapters.

This book is clearly a timely treatise and will be a reference for all healthcare providers who take care of stroke victims.

William C. Koller, M.D., Ph.D.

Preface

Until recently, patients who presented to the emergency room with acute ischemic stroke were admitted to the medical or neurology service and treated symptomatically to prevent complications, reduce the chances of recurrence, and begin the process of rehabilitation. In December 1995, the results of the U.S. National Institutes of Health-sponsored study of tissue plasminogen activator therapy of acute ischemic stroke were published. For the first time, a treatment was shown to improve outcome if used very early in patients arriving at the hospital with this disease. Other studies presented at the 1999 American Heart Association Stroke Meeting revealed that intra-arterial thrombolysis could significantly improve outcome in patients with large middle cerebral artery occlusion-related stroke and that another fibrolytic agent is efficacious when given soon after ischemic stroke. It was also shown that patients who have fever or hyperglycemia at onset of stroke or who develop aspiration pneumonia in the days after acute stroke may exhibit delayed recovery and require prolonged hospitalization.

It may soon be possible to differentiate the tissue at risk for damage from a completed infarction by magnetic resonance imaging techniques. The development of special acute stroke units and stroke critical pathways is facilitating the rapid evaluation and treatment of patients. The use of thrombolytics in selected patients and the potential advent of neuroprotective therapies offer the hope of changing attitudes concerning the management of patients with acute ischemic stroke.

Although there are many books on cerebrovascular diseases aimed at neurologists and stroke specialists, very little effort has been made to assemble a monograph especially intended for non-neurologists (who treat the vast majority of stroke patients). One of the main goals of this book is to provide the physician who is not a stroke specialist with a concise volume on the advances in evaluation and management of acute stroke that have occurred over the last decade. We wish to keep clinical maangement of acute stroke the major focus of this work. Thus, the reader will find that after an introductory chapter on the burden of stroke, the next several chapters feature various stages in the care of stroke patients. Rapid assessment, care of the patient prior to coming to hospital, and emergency evaluation are the only means available to use to increase the number of patients who benefit from thrombolysis or prevention of complications. Although a number of stroke centers have implemented programs to rapidly assess patients with acute stroke, unfortunately, the majority of stroke patients still have the nihilistic attitude that there is nothing to be offered them.

We have included a number of chapters that specifically address the questions of the neurological examination, the use of laboratory tests, and potential complications that may arise after stroke, followed by a section on thrombolysis and neuroprotection, to bring the reader up to date on recent advances. Prevention of subsequent stroke requires that appropriate therapy be offered for the underlying etiology, and this topic is reviewed. In other chapters, we provide current evidence on the use of aspirin and other antiplatelet agents, heparin, and oral anticoagulant therapy in the prevention of recurrence. Additionally, we review information on the use of carotid endarterectomy in patients with carotid stenosis. Our objective in the second part of the book is to provide new information that may change the way practitioners manage cerebrovascular disease.

We believe this book will be useful for all physicians who care for stroke patients, including internists, family practitioners, emergency room physicians, neurologists, rehabilitation specialists, and geriatricians. These are truly exciting and hopeful times for the treatment of patients with acute stroke.

It has been a pleasure to work with the editorial staff of Marcel Dekker, Inc. Their assistance and suggestions were most valuable in the planning and development of this volume. Special appreciation is extended to Mrs. Doris Kanigan, University of Saskatchewan, who provided editorial support and encouragement. The book would not be the same without her invaluable help. She devoted countless hours to ensure that every manuscript was handled on time and she personally reviewed all the materials submitted to us with utmost care and diligence.

Ashfaq Shuaib
Larry B. Goldstein

Contents

Contributors

Paul Abrahamse, M.A. Research Associate, Department of Internal Medicine, University of Michigan, Ann Arbor, Michigan

Harold P. Adams, Jr., M.D. Professor, Department of Neurology, University of Iowa, College of Medicine, Iowa City, Iowa

Mark J. Alberts, M.D. Associate Professor, Division of Neurology, Department of Medicine, and Director, Stroke Acute Care Unit, Duke University Medical Center, Durham, North Carolina

Henry J. M. Barnett, O.C., M.D., F.R.C.P.(C) Professor Emeritus, Department of Clinical Neurological Sciences, The John P. Roberts Research Institute, London, Ontario, Canada

Oscar Benavente, M.D., F.R.C.P.(C) Assistant Professor, Division of Neurology, Department of Medicine, University of Texas Health Science Center, San Antonio, Texas

Alastair M. Buchan, M.D., F.R.C.P. Professor of Stroke Research, Department of Clinical Neurosciences, University of Calgary, Calgary, Alberta, Canada

Ahmar Aziz Butt, M.D. Co-Chief, General Internal Medicine, The Brooklyn Hospital Center, and Clinical Assistant Professor, New York University School of Medicine, Brooklyn, New York

Marc I. Chimowitz, M.B., Ch.B. Associate Professor, Department of Neurology, Emory University, Atlanta, Georgia

Robert Côté, M.D., F.R.C.P.(C) Associate Professor, Department of Neurology and Neurosurgery, McGill University, Montreal, Quebec, Canada

Kevin M. Curtis, M.D. Adjunct Instructor, Department of Emergency Medicine, George Washington University Medical Center, Washington, D.C.

Larry B. Goldstein, M.D. Associate Professor, Division of Neurology, Department of Medicine, Director, Duke Center for Cerebrovascular Disease, Head, Stroke Policy Program, Center for Clinical Health Policy Research, Duke University Medical Center, and Attending Neurologist, Durham VA Medical Center, Durham, North Carolina

David C. Good, M.D. Professor, Department of Neurology, and Director of Rehabilitation, Wake Forest University School of Medicine, Winston-Salem, North Carolina

Carmelo Graffagnino, M.D., F.R.C.P.(C) Assistant Professor, Division of Neurology, Department of Medicine, and Co-Director, Neuro-Intensive Care Unit, Duke University Medical Center, Durham, North Carolina

E. Clarke Haley, Jr., M.D. Professor, Departments of Neurology and Neurosurgery, University of Virginia Health System, Charlottesville, Virginia

Robert G. Hart, M.D. Professor, Division of Neurology, Department of Medicine, University of Texas Health Science Center, San Antonio, Texas

Edmond A. Hooker, M.D. Assistant Clinical Professor, Department of Emergency Medicine, University of Louisville, Louisville, Kentucky

Tom Jeerakathil, M.D. Chief Resident, Division of Neurology, University of Alberta Hospital, Edmonton, Alberta, Canada

Mark Johnson, M.D. Stroke Fellow, Department of Neurology, George Washington University Medical Center, Washington, D.C.

Richard Kay, M.D., F.R.C.P. Professor, Department of Medicine and Therapeutics, The Chinese University of Hong Kong, Shatin, Hong Kong, China

Derk W. Krieger, M.D. Associate Professor and Staff Physician, Section of Adult Neurology, Department of Neurology, Cerebrovascular Center, The Cleveland Clinic Foundation, Cleveland, Ohio

Daniel Laskowitz, M.D. Assistant Professor, Division of Neurology, Department of Medicine, Duke University Medical Center, Durham, North Carolina

Enrique C. Leira, M.D. Division of Cerebrovascular Diseases, Department of Neurology, University of Iowa College of Medicine, Iowa City, Iowa

Zachary T. Levine, M.D. Chief Resident, Department of Neurological Surgery, George Washington University, Washington, D.C.

Joseph Lipscomb, Ph.D. Associate Professor, Sanford Institute of Public Policy, Duke University, Durham, North Carolina

Betsy B. Love, M.D. Clinical Assistant Professor, Department of Neurology, Indiana University College of Medicine, Indianapolis, Indiana

Brian J. Maguire, M.S.A., M.R.E.M.T.-P. Assistant Professor, Department of Emergency Medicine, George Washington University, Washington, D.C.

David B. Matchar, M.D., F.A.C.P. Professor, Department of Medicine, Duke University Medical Center, and Durham Veterans Affairs Medical Center, Durham, North Carolina

Jeffrey Minuk, M.D., F.R.C.P.(C) Assistant Professor, Department of Neurology and Neurosurgery, McGill University, Montreal, Quebec, Canada

Lewis B. Morgenstern, M.D. Assistant Professor and Co-Director, Stroke Program, Department of Neurology, University of Texas, Houston, Texas

Paul Morley, Ph.D. Senior Research Officer, Institute for Biological Sciences, National Research Council of Canada, Ottawa, Ontario, Canada

Anil Narang, M.D. Department of Radiology, Neuroradiology, George Washington University Medical Center, Washington, D.C.

Gregory P. Samsa, Ph.D. Assistant Professor, Department of Community and Family Medicine, Duke University Medical Center, Durham, North Carolina

Shiva Sarraf-Yazdi, M.D. Duke University School of Medicine, Durham, North Carolina

Gregory Scott, M.D. Fellow, Department of Neurology, Wake Forest University School of Medicine, Winston-Salem, North Carolina

Laligam Sekhar, M.D., F.A.C.S. Professor, Department of Neurosurgery, George Washington University, Washington, D.C.

Robert Shesser, M.D., M.P.H. Professor, Department of Emergency Medicine, George Washington University, Washington, D.C.

Ashfaq Shuaib, M.D., F.R.C.P.(C) Professor of Medicine and Director of Neurology, University of Alberta Hospital, Edmonton, Alberta, Canada

Muzaffar Mustafa Siddiqui, M.D. Research Fellow, Stroke Research Unit, University of Alberta Hospital, Edmonton, Alberta, Canada

Daniel L. Small, Ph.D. Research Officer, Institute for Biological Sciences, National Research Council of Canada, Ottawa, Ontario, Canada

Alexander G. G. Turpie, M.D., F.R.C.P.(C) Professor of Medicine, McMaster University, Hamilton, Ontario, Canada

David S. Warner, M.D. Professor, Departments of Anesthesiology, Neurobiology, and Surgery, Duke University Medical Center, Durham, North Carolina

Ka Sing Wong, M.B., M.R.C.P.(UK) Associate Professor, Department of Medicine and Therapeutics, The Chinese University of Hong Kong, Shatin, Hong Kong, China

Jerome Y. Yager, M.D., F.R.C.P.(C) Associate Professor, Department of Pediatrics (Neurology), University of Saskatchewan, Saskatoon, Saskatchewan, Canada

1

Policy Perspective on Acute Stroke Treatment

David B. Matchar
Duke University Medical Center, Durham, North Carolina, and Durham Veterans Affairs Medical Center, Durham, North Carolina

Paul Abrahamse
University of Michigan, Ann Arbor, Michigan

Joseph Lipscomb
Sanford Institute of Public Policy, Duke University, Durham, North Carolina

Gregory P. Samsa
Duke University Medical Center, Durham, North Carolina

By any measure, stroke is a massive public health problem. Stroke is the third leading cause of death in the United States and the most common cause of disability among adults. In addition to the mortality and morbidity due to stroke, the aggregate cost of the disease exceeds $30 billion per year.[1,2]

In comparison with heart disease and cancer, attention to stroke as a public health problem has been limited. In part this has been due to the limited range of proven options for preventing and treating stroke. However, in the past two decades the picture for stroke prevention and treatment has brightened substantially. Several medical therapies have been demonstrated in clinical trials to reduce stroke risk, including the use of warfarin for individuals with atrial fibrillation (AF), aspirin for people with stroke or transient ischemic attack (TIA), and antihypertensive treatment.[3,4,5]

Evidence is also emerging that HMGCoA reductase inhibitors for hypercholesterolemia can also reduce stroke risk.[6] The surgical intervention carotid endarterectomy has been shown to have a clinically substantial benefit in patients with stroke or TIA who also have >70% stenosis of their carotid artery on the symptomatic side.[7] Appreciation of the magnitude of the problem and the potential for prevention has led to a variety of public responses. These include new prevention trials funded both by the National Institutes of Health (NIH) and industry, significant public education and screening efforts (e.g., American Heart Association, National Stroke Association), and the initiation of several research efforts to promote informed stroke policy decision making, including the Stroke Prevention Patient Outcomes Research Team (PORT) , funded by the federal Agency for Health Care Policy and Research (AHCPR).[8]

In 1995, the National Institute for Neurological Diseases and Stroke of the NIH announced, prior to later formal publication, the preliminary results of the U. S. tissue plasminogen activator (tPA) study, indicating that a treatment had been found that can diminish the mortality and morbidity of stroke.[9] Even more than the emergence of stroke prevention strategies, this announcement has stimulated substantial public interest. This greater interest, in part, relates to natural enthusiasm for the drama of acute interventions. It is also based on an appreciation that even if prevention leads to a more efficient use of resources than does acute treatment (and it often does[10]), equity considerations dictate that those who have a stroke deserve our best efforts as well. And, whether aimed at prevention or acute treatment, our efforts to improve care must occur at the clinical *and* policy levels

A dominant issue in improving stroke care is the development and implementation of new therapies. In general, new medical interventions, whether diagnostic or therapeutic, present two sets of questions. The first set is related to whether and when a new treatment works. Subsidiary questions here include (1) is there is a biological effect? and (2) is the effect clinically meaningful? The second set of questions—those that require a public policy response—relate to the implications of treatment beyond the isolated clinical encounter. Subsidiary questions here include (1) is the treatment a reasonable use of public resources? and (2) what are the practical implications of making changes in established patterns of care required by new therapies?

In this chapter, we highlight the public policy questions related to stroke care. First, we describe briefly the framework for examining whether a new therapy is a reasonable use of public resources and provide a simple example of a hypothetical new stroke treatment. Second, we consider policy questions related to patterns of care. Here we consider policy options in light of an example of care for myocardial infarction (MI). In closing, we will suggest a model for how to construct a sensible stroke policy that simultaneously accounts for scientific evidence and the realities of providing medical care.

TWO PUBLIC POLICY QUESTIONS

Is Stroke Treatment a Reasonable Use of Public Resources?

Background

The accelerating increase in health care expenditures in the late 1980s and early 1990s has led to concern that these costs could overwhelm other important public needs. In 1994, 14% of the gross domestic product was spent on health care.[11] With the rapid growth of new medical technologies, the aging of the population, and the lack of significant "brakes" on health care utilization, there has been little reason to believe that the increase in costs would abate without aggressive intervention. Consequently, "cost containment" measures were initiated, taking the form of administrative restrictions on services (usually by limiting insurance coverage) and the use of capitation payment schemes. The presumption in cost containment efforts is that health care providers will respond to constrained resources by eliminating the use of unnecessary services. Although these efforts have had some success in checking the acceleration of health costs, cost containment can have a nonspecific effect on the use of services; it could lead to a decrease in both necessary and unnecessary care.[12]

Cost-Effectiveness: A Measure of Value

To help address the problem of how to contain costs while not significantly impairing the quality of care—indeed, while perhaps improving the quality of care—there has been an expanded focus on economic analyses for establishing priorities among competing interventions.[13,14] The most prominent economic approach found in the clinical literature to date is cost-effectiveness analysis (CEA), in which interventions are compared in terms of the amount of health outcome improvement offered per dollar spent (i.e., "bang for the buck")

Operationally, in CEA one measures the relative value of competing interventions by calculating for each its incremental cost-effectiveness ratio (ICER). The ICER is the gain in "effectiveness" achieved per dollar of extra cost incurred, where the comparison is made with the next most expensive intervention. Assuming there is a set of mutually exclusive competing interventions aimed at some health problem (e.g., stroke), one first eliminates from consideration any intervention X that is "dominated" by another intervention, Y; typically, this will mean that X is at least as expensive as Y, but yields a lower health benefit. Then one rank orders the remaining interventions in terms of their ICERs. The intervention with the lowest ICER is the most cost-effective option—and should be adopted if the decision maker concludes that the value for money offered by this option compares favorably with alternative possible uses for these same resources (e.g., interventions to prevent heart attacks). The ICER can be condition-specific, e.g., dollars spent per stroke averted, or more generic, e.g., dollars spent per life-year saved. An illustrative calculation of an ICER for stroke prevention is presented below.

Consider a hypothetical new stroke treatment for which we wish to assess the "value" in the form of the ICER. To do this, we must first measure its cost and effectiveness in relation to conventional treatment.

Analyzing the cost of a new stroke treatment involves comparing the total cost of treating one stroke patient, using the new treatment, with the cost of treating a patient using conventional means. The cost of the new treatment is the total economic burden of treating a stroke patient, measured in dollar terms. This includes the cost of the new treatment itself; all costs associated with initial and subsequent hospitalizations; and the costs of outpatient care, drugs, rehabilitation, home health care, and long-term care. Similarly, the cost of conventional stroke treatment includes all these items, without the cost of the new therapy. Because stroke is a very expensive disease, both in the initial hospitalization and in long-term costs,[1,2] both of these total cost estimates can be quite high. In this example, we will assume that treating stroke with conventional methods has a total cost of $50,000, and treating a patient with the new therapy has a total cost of $56,000. The *incremental* cost of the new treatment is the difference between these two costs—in this case, $6,000. Throughout, we assume that costs are defined from a "societal" perspective. That is, the cost of each good or service is measured in terms of the economic opportunity costs of the resources consumed; the distribution of these costs among payers is not at issue. Although this is the most common perspective taken in the clinical-decision literature, it is not the only one relevant for clinical decision making in practice (as noted below).

Effectiveness, like cost, is analyzed by comparing the outcome of the new treatment with that of traditional therapy. There are many methods of measuring effectiveness. For a stroke treatment, we could use such measures as mortality rates, life expectancy after stroke, or a measure that incorporates quality of life with life expectancy. Because stroke can have a major impact on quality of life, we will use the third type of measure in this example. The standard metric for this type of effectiveness measure is the quality-adjusted life-year (QALY). The QALY incorporates quantity of life and quality of life into one measure. A treatment outcome that resulted in a patient living 1 year in perfect health would be valued as 1 QALY. If the patient lived 1 year in a state with a lower quality of life, the QALY value of the outcome would be 1 times some value reflecting the desirability of that state to the patient. For example, if the current state of health was deemed to offer only half as much quality of life as perfect health, then a year spent in the former would be assigned a value of 0.5 QALY. These QALY values can be obtained from previous survey studies reported in the literature, or they can be derived by the investigator who wants to better tailor his outcome measures to the matter at hand.

Studies of patient quality of life after stroke show very low QALYs associated with severe strokes.[15] A treatment that reduces the severity of a stroke, while not greatly affecting life expectancy, can thus have a major effect on quality-adjusted life expectancy. Based on preliminary simulation modeling, we have estimated that the early benefits of a modestly effective hypothetical stroke treatment can, over the life span, translate into an average of 2.5–2.8 QALYs, while traditional therapy results in only 2.4 QALYs. The *incremental effectiveness* of the new treatment is the difference between these two values—0.1 to 0.4 QALYs, depending upon the exact specification of the efficacy of the new treatment.[16]

Once the cost and effectiveness of the new and traditional therapies have been estimated, the ICER can be calculated. This is simply the ratio of the incremental cost to the incremental effectiveness. In this example, it is $6,000/0.4 QALYs, or $15,000/QALY. In fact, an intervention with an ICER in this range can compare quite favorably with a number of other interventions already in common practice.[17] This calculation is used for purposes of illustration only. The denominator would range from 0.1 to 0.4 QALYs, depending upon the precise specification of the efficacy of the intervention. The numerator should also reflect the long-term cost savings associated with any reductions in disability. When these savings are considered, an acute stroke treatment which is even modestly effective may well save both lives and money.[16]

How Do We Improve Patterns of Stroke Care?

Although cost-effectiveness analysis serves to shed light on the most highly valued health care practices, an "acceptably low" ICER is a necessary but not sufficient condition for allocating resources to stroke prevention and treatment. One reason is that an ICER computed from a "societal" perspective may not be compelling to the relevant decision maker—for example, an administrator in a managed care organization. Furthermore, we have a pluralistic society in which there are many decision makers, and any one of them may resist cost-effectiveness arguments for resource allocation.

Another reason cost-effectiveness is not sufficient is that an ICER does not tell the whole story about what it will take to implement a treatment in a real-world setting. The issue is not just generalizability (can the treatment be provided as well and as efficiently as in the research environment?), but also feasibility (can it be provided at all, given local resource constraints?). Thus, if stroke policy is to have an impact on practices, it is not only important that it be based on basic principles of efficient resource allocation, but it must also address the barriers to optimal practice in typical care settings.

A Case Study: The Evolution of New Practice Patterns in MI

Care of MI patients provides a useful illustration of a condition whose management has undergone major changes over time. To some extent, these changes have been due to the development of new tests and treatments. However, the translation of new treatments to improved care has involved an ongoing series of system-level changes.

Historically, MI was treated "expectantly" with pain medication and rest. Those lucky enough to survive were kept in the hospital for weeks before beginning a prolonged, and typically incomplete, recovery.[18] In recent decades, the treatment of MI has changed substantially with the advent in the 1960s of coronary care units (CCUs) and in the 1980s of thrombolytic agents. CCUs were touted as a strategy for maintaining constant monitoring of heart rhythm to permit immediate intervention if "malignant arrhythmias" or cardiac arrest occurred. Despite controversy about the merits of CCUs, they have become a standard fixture in the modern hospital. Thrombolytics have been shown in multiple studies to be of benefit to some MI patients when provided soon after the onset of ischemia.[19–24] Both CCUs, where early, dangerous cardiac arrhythmias could be detected and hopefully treated, and thrombolytics, which required prompt administration, made time "of the essence."

The response to these treatments by professional societies, patient advocacy groups, and pharmaceutical companies was to create a vast change in the way chest pain was viewed by the public and a realignment of medical services to accommodate hyperacute MI care. The use of these therapies has been clarified through clinical guidelines promulgated by professional societies and the AHCPR.[25,26] However, studies of clinical practices have documented suboptimal practices even for relatively noncontroversial interventions such as the use of aspirin and beta blockers.[27–30] As we will note, a similar evolution has been occurring for stroke care.

Stroke Experience to Date

Until recently, stroke care was much like MI care in the 1960s. Stroke was treated supportively and, by the description of some experts, "nihilistically."[31] Until the advent of tPA, there had been little obvious incentive for a hyperacute response to stroke. Nevertheless, as clinical trials for acute stroke treatments have proceeded, it has become increasingly apparent that stroke patients often delay seeking medical attention. Once in the medical system, such patients were generally not rapidly identified.[32] This led to concern that even in the absence of specific treatment, stroke patients were losing the opportunity for prompt supportive care and institution of secondary prevention strategies.[33] In addition, delays in presentation and identification of stroke patients limited subject accrual in clinical trials.[34] This has led to efforts on the part of pharmaceutical companies, the

American Heart Association, and the National Stroke Association to promote greater public awareness of stroke in the hope that patients will present earlier. These efforts, which have accelerated since the Food and Drug Administration's approval of tPA in 1995, include educational campaigns aimed at physicians, emergency medical technicians, and the general public (through the "Brain Attack" and "Time Is Brain" campaigns).

Similarities and Differences Between Stroke and MI

Despite apparent similarities between MI and stroke—in particular, both involve sudden loss of blood supply leading to tissue death—stroke care is notably different.[35] Stroke victims tend to disregard symptoms, typically arriving in the hospital long past the time drug treatment would be expected to be useful. Significant delays often occur once the patient presents for care.

Is a public policy aimed at shifting the view of stroke to a "brain attack," akin to a "heart attack," appropriate? The answer depends not only on the emerging trial data about the value of hyperacute stroke treatments, but also on an understanding of the magnitude and cost of the effort to decrease the time delay from stroke onset to medical attention. In highly motivated academic centers involved in acute stroke clinical trials, it is possible to make substantial progress. The question is whether this sort of effort is feasible in more typical clinical settings. Furthermore, treatment in the period immediately following the onset of neurological symptoms is not the only (or perhaps even the most important) question. As in the case of MI management, there is also a need to consider the entire continuum of care, including acute hospitalization and rehabilitation.

DO WE NEED TO IMPROVE PATTERNS OF STROKE CARE?

Pattern-of-care studies in acute stroke make it clear that there is no "typical" model for stroke care. There are substantial variations in care, relating to geographical region, availability of specialists, and organization of health services.[36] This raises the question of whether there is an optimal pattern of care.[37] In considering patterns of care, we focus here on three issues: (1) What sorts of services should be provided? (2) Who should provide stroke care? and (3) Where should stroke care be provided?

What Sorts of Services?

This is a value question: of potential investigations and interventions available for the care of the acute stroke patient, which are effective and cost-effective? This issue is addressed generically in the previous discussion of cost-effectiveness. However, as indicated by the American Heart Association guidelines for acute stroke regarding potential investigations and interventions available for care,[34] there is scant empirical support for most specific interventions. What we do know is that not only is there substantial practice variation in stroke care, there is also substantial variation in outcomes. More detailed investigation will be needed to support whether the variations in outcome can be directly attributed to specific patterns of care, particularly patterns of care that are supported by scientific evidence (such as use of tPA) and those with strong consensus support (such as measures to prevent aspiration, restrained blood pressure control in the acute phase, and rapid mobilization of the patient).

Who Should Provide Services: Neurologists Versus Nonneurologists

Unlike MI patients, who are quickly attended by a cardiologist and monitored in a CCU, patients with stroke are usually treated by generalists in a nonintensive setting. According to studies performed as part of the Stroke PORT, 47% of Medicare-covered stroke patients are managed solely by a nonneurologist, without a consultation by a neurologist, while only 11% are cared for primarily by a neurologist.[38] Most stroke patients are cared for in a nonintensive setting, usually a medical service without cardiac monitoring.

A series of studies have demonstrated that patients cared for by a neurologist are more likely to survive the acute event and more likely to be discharged home.[37] These findings have led to a lively debate about the reasons for the difference and the appropriate policy response. Should all stroke patients be cared for by a neurologist, or can the provider be a "stroke-knowledgeable" physician? Whatever type of physician provides care, how do we assure their competency?

The answers to these questions depend on the reasons for the differences in outcomes between patients cared for by neurologists and nonneurologists. One possible explanation that has not been entirely excluded for improved outcomes observed is that the relationship between care by a neurologist and outcome is due to confounding by factors unrelated to the neurologist's care (such as severity of stroke or presence of comorbidity). A second potential explanation is that the improvement is due to a "specific" neurologist effect (i.e., the ability of a neurologist to make a precise assessment and treatment plan—an ability requiring substantial training reflected in specialty board recognition). The third explanation is that the improvement associated with care by a neurologist is due to a "general" effect (i.e., associated with a better understanding of how to efficiently provide supportive in-hospital care and to arrange appropriate rehabilitation care after discharge).

If the observed relationship between provider type and outcome is due to confounding factors, then we must look elsewhere for guidance on ways to improve stroke care. If the effect is specific to neurologists' training, then the policy question is how to provide timely access to neurologists. If the effect is general, then the policy question is how to train nonneurologists to have adequate stroke expertise. Although there are no definitive answers to these questions, it has been suggested by those who promote improved stroke care that new therapies require a cadre of physicians with stroke expertise, including a core foundation in neurology and an understanding of the criteria for the use of thrombolytics, including skill in reading a CT scan at least sufficient to distinguish hemorrhage.[35]

Where Should Care Be Provided? Medical Service Versus Stroke Service

Since the 1970s, there have been various efforts to promote acute stroke units.[26] The arguments favoring such units are similar to those favoring CCUs: support services specific to stroke, such as aspiration prevention and rapid return to mobility, and cardiac monitoring to facilitate quick treatment of dangerous arrhythmias. Several clinical trials taken together appear to support the idea of an acute stroke service.[39] In terms of numbers needed to treat, between 10 and 20 patients may need to be managed in an acute stroke unit to achieve the saving of one life.

As for the question of neurologists versus nonneurologists, the apparently simple question of whether a stroke unit is better than a general medical ward is actually quite subtle. Since it does appear that stroke services lead to improved outcomes, the policy questions relate to whether the effect of a stroke unit is "specific" or "general." Perhaps it would be possible to assess the essential elements of what a stroke service accomplishes. This leads to the issue of how to proceed with developing a rational and feasible stroke policy.

DEVELOPING A RATIONAL AND FEASIBLE STROKE POLICY: A MODEL

Substantial variation in prevention and management of stroke has existed for some time. However, new therapies have raised the stakes. Not only do new treatments offer opportunities for improving stroke outcomes directly, but the system-level changes involved in making such therapies available may result in improved outcomes by inducing providers to attend to the otherwise seemingly minor details of care.

Policy decisions are complex, and to make the issues tractable there is a natural tendency to frame the discussion in overly simplistic terms by asking questions such as the following: Does the drug treatment cost too much to include on the hospital or HMO formulary? Should neurologists see all stroke patients? Should all hospitals have an acute stroke unit? A more useful approach is to start with the objectives of stroke care and to define optimal care functionally by asking, *Based on the best evidence, what do we want to accomplish in stroke care*? Once the functions of optimal stroke care are defined, we can then ask, *How can the functions defining optimal stroke care be best accomplished*? This "functional specification" should not be limited to hyperacute care but should include the range of issues ranging from primary prevention to hyperacute management to rehabilitation to secondary prevention and, finally, to long-term care.

As an example of functional specifications, the objectives of stroke prevention might include appropriate and high-quality use of anticoagulants for individuals with high embolic risk (e.g., AF) and evaluation of the carotid arteries of symptomatic patients. The objectives of hyperacute management might include rapid evaluation for thrombolysis and moderation in use of antihypertensives. The objectives of postacute management might include attention to secondary prevention, rehabilitation, and general coordination of outpatient social support.

Having defined the objectives of care, the next step is to examine current practice patterns to identify discordance between what we are currently accomplishing and what we would like to accomplish. Examples include undesirable delays in initial evaluation and treatment, not using appropriate specific therapies, excessive treatment of hypertension, lack of swallowing evaluation and management, delayed mobilization and rehabilitation referral, failure to evaluate and treat risk factors for recurrent stroke, and inadequate discharge planning. Note that although some of these issues are controversial (usually because the scientific evidence is limited or otherwise unconvincing), most are not.

The crucial step is to develop a program to improve clinical practice. Substantial efforts in practice improvement have yielded several lessons. First, education alone, including the dissemination of specific guidelines, is not effective for improving practice.[40] Second, effective interventions require system change; in particular, the problem is seldom with the motivation of busy providers to improve practice, but rather that the system of care must be modified in order to give providers the necessary tools to successfully act. Third, barriers to practice improvement (e.g., antiquated medical record systems, inadequate training, financial disincentives) must be explicitly considered when developing practice improvement initiatives.[7,41] Fourth, the greatest benefit is likely to be achieved by local efforts, particularly if they are associated with the participation of local opinion leaders and performance feedback.[42–46] Fifth, practice improvement efforts require at least a rough consensus about the correct management strategy; accordingly, there is much to be gained by initially focusing on topics that are not controversial.

A final lesson is that since health service provider units (e.g., group practice, hospital, managed care organization) are often different in fundamental ways, no single intervention is likely to work for all sites. Thus, it becomes particularly useful to accompany the functional specification of the objectives with a "toolbox" of management strategies.[30] For example, in addressing the goal of ensuring adherence with practice guidelines for the acute management of stroke patients, the toolbox would contain options such as mandating neurologist involvement in triage, designating an appropriately trained "stroke MD," creating stroke teams or acute stroke units, implementing critical pathways, or installing computerized decision support systems. The site would then select the option(s) that make most sense for them, given their current system, potential staffing, barriers to improved practice, and so forth.

Samsa[47] illustrates the application of the above principles to improving of stroke prevention among patients with atrial fibrillation. A similar framework is applicable to stroke management and rehabilitation and, indeed, to the development of practice improvement initiatives in general.

CONCLUSION

The availability of new treatments makes this an exciting time for those involved in preventing and treating stroke. Naturally, with the expense and complexity of providing treatment advances comes a challenge to assure that these treatments are both cost-effective and feasible in typical practice settings. Health policy analysis serves to address these issues: Is the treatment worth it if we can provide it well? Can we provide it well?

The evolution of MI care provides a useful guide to how we can proceed with improving stroke care in light of new therapies. To do this, we propose a model of practice improvement that builds on a functional definition of good stroke care. This functional definition provides guideposts for determining optimal organization of care—first by allowing us to identify areas of practice that need improvement, and then by focusing our attention on providing optimal service subject to local constraints and resources. In this way, we can more effectively negotiate areas of scientific controversy and political sensitivities and attend to the ultimate goal of stroke policy: to decrease the risk of stroke and, for individuals with stroke, to minimize its impact.

REFERENCES

1. Matchar DB, Duncan PW. Cost of stroke. Stroke Clin Updates 1994; 5:9–12.
2. Taylor TN, Davis PH, Torner JC, Holmes J, Meyer JW, Jacobson MF. Lifetime cost of stroke in the United States. Stroke 1996; 27(9):1459–1466.

3. Collins R, Peto R, MacMahon S, et al. Blood pressure, stroke, and coronary heart disease. Part 2. Short-term reductions in blood pressure: overview of randomised drug trials in their epidemiological context. Lancet 1990; 335:827–838.
4. Matchar DB, McCrory DC, Barnett HJ, Feussner JR. Medical treatment for stroke prevention. Ann Intern Med 1994; 121(1):41–53.
5. Laupacis A, Albers G, Dalen J, Dunn M, Feinberg W, Jacobson A. Antithrombotic therapy in atrial fibrillation. Chest 1995; 104:352S–359S.
6. Crouse JR 3d, Byington RP, Hoen HM, Furberg CD. Reductase inhibitor monotherapy and stroke prevention. Arch Intern Med 1997; 157:1305–1310.
7. Goldstein LB, Hasselblad V, Matchar DB, McCrory DC. Comparison and meta-analysis of randomized trials of endarterectomy for symptomatic carotid artery stenosis. Neurology 1995; 45(11):1965–1970.
8. Matchar DB, Duncan PW, Samsa GP, Whisnant JP, DeFriese GH, Ballard DJ, Paul JE, Witter DM Jr., Mitchell JP. The Stroke Prevention Patient Outcomes Research Team. Goals and methods. Stroke 1993; 24(12):2135–2142.
9. The National Institute of Neurological Disorders and Stroke t-PA Stroke Study Group. Tissue plasminogen activator for acute ischemic stroke. N Engl J Med 1995; 333(24):1581–1587.
10. Tengs TO, Adams ME, Pliskin JS, Safran DG, Siegel JE, Weinstein MC, Graham JD. Five-hundred life-saving interventions and their cost-effectiveness. Risk Anal 1995; 15(3):369–390.
11. Office of National Health Statistics, Office of the Actuary. National Health Expenditures, 1994. Health Care Financing Review 17(3). HCFA Pub. No. 03373. Washington: Health Care Financing Administration, 1996.
12. Chassin MR, Brook RH, Park RE, Keesey J, Fink A, et al. Variations in the use of medical and surgical services by the Medicare population. N Engl J Med 1986; 314:285–290.
13. Gold MR, Siegel JE, Russell JB, Weinstein MC, eds. Cost-Effectiveness in Health and Medicine. New York: Oxford University Press, 1996.
14. Kamlet M. A Framework for Cost-Utility Analysis of Government Health Care Programs. Washington, DC: Public Health Service, U.S. Dept. of Health and Human Services, 1992.
15. Samsa GP, Matchar DB, Bonito A, Duncan PW, Lipscomb J, Enarson C, Witter D, Venus P, Paul JE, Weinberger M. Utilities for major stroke: results from a survey of preferences among persons at increased risk for stroke. Am Heart J 1998; 136(Pt 1):703–713.
16. Samsa GP, Reutter RA, Parmigiani G, Ancukiewicz M, Abrahamse P, Lipscomb J, Matchar DB. Performing cost-effectiveness analysis by integrating randomized trial data with a comprehensive decision model: application to treatment of acute ischemic stroke. J Clin Epidemiol. 1999; 52:259–271.
17 Mason J, Drummond M, Torrance G. Some guidelines on the use of cost effectiveness league tables. BMJ 1993; 306:570–572.
18. Meltzer LE. The concept and system for intensive coronary care. Bull Acad Med NJ 1964; 10:304.

19. Gruppo Italiano per lo Studio della Streptochinasi nell' Infarto Miocardico (GISSI). Effectiveness of intravenous thrombolytic treatment in acute myocardial infarction. Lancet 1986; 1:397–402.
20. ISIS-2 (Second International Study of Infarct Survival) Collaborative Group. Randomised trial of intravenous streptokinase, oral aspirin, both, or neither among 17,187 cases of suspected acute myocardial infarction: ISIS-2. Lancet 1988; 2:349–360.
21. Wilcox RG, von der Lippe G, Olsson CG, Skene AM, et al. Trial of tissue plasminogen activator for mortality reduction in acute myocardial infarction: Anglo-Scandinavian Study of Early Thrombolysis (ASSET). Lancet 1988; 2:525–530.
22. AIMS Trial Study Group. Effect of intravenous APSAC on mortality after acute myocardial infarction: preliminary report of a placebo-controlled clinical trial. Lancet 1988; 1:545–549.
23. Tiefenbrunn AJ, Sobel BE. Timing of coronary recanalization: paradigms, paradoxes, and pertinence. Circulation 1992; 85:2311–2315.
24. Weaver DW, Cercueira M, Hallstrom AP, Litwin PE, et al. Prehospital-initiated vs. hospital-initiated thrombolyic therapy. The Myocardial Infarction Triage and Intervention Trial. JAMA 1993; 270:1211–1216.
25. National Heart Attack Alert Program Coordinating Committee, 60 Minutes to Treatment Working Group. Emergency department: rapid identification and treatment of patients with acute myocardial infarction. Ann Emerg Med 1994; 23(2):311–329.
26. Ryan TJ, Anderson JL, Antman EM, et al. ACC/AHA guidelines for the management of patients with acute myocardial infarction. A report of the American College of Cardiology/American Heart Association Task Force on Practice Guidelines (Committee on Management of Acute Myocardial Infarction). J Am Coll Cardiol 1996; 28(5):1328–1428.
27. Braunwald E, Mark D, Jones R, et al. Unstable angina: diagnosis and management. Guideline overview. Agency for Health Care Policy and Research. JAMA 1994; 86(9):649, 710–712.
28. Jollis JG, DeLong ER, Peterson ED, Muhlbaier LH, Fortin DF, et al. Outcome of acute myocardial infarction according to the specialty of the admitting physician. N Engl J Med 1996; 335:1880–1887.
29. Nash IS, Nash DB, Fuster V. Do cardiologists do it better? J Am Coll Cardiol 1997; 29:475–478.
30. Ayanian JZ, Hauptman PJ, Guadagnoli E, Antman EM, Pashos CL, et al. Knowledge and practices of generalist and specialist physicians regarding drug therapy for acute myocardial infarction. N Engl J Med 1994; 331:1136–1142.
31. Hachinski V, Norris JW. The Acute Stroke. Philadelphia: Davis, 1985.
32. Bratina P, Greenberg L, Pasteur W, Grotta JC. Current emergency department management of stroke in Houston, Texas. Stroke 1995; 26:409–414.
33. Camarata PJ, Heros RC, Latchaw RE. "Brain attack": the rationale for treating stroke as a medical emergency. Neurosurgery 1994; 34:144–158.
34. Adams HP Jr, Brott TG, Crowell RM, et al. Guidelines for the management of patients with acute ischemic stroke. A statement for healthcare professionals from a

special writing group of the Stroke Council, American Heart Association. Stroke 1994; 25(9):1901–1914.
35. Marler JR, Jones PW, Emr M, eds. Setting new directions for stroke care. Proceedings of a National Symposium on Rapid Identification and Treatment of Acute Stroke. Bethesda, MD: National Institute of Neurological Disorders and Stroke, National Institutes of Health, 1997.
36. Hopkins A, Menken M, DeFriese GH, Feldman RG. Differences in strategies for the diagnosis and treatment of neurologic disease among British and American neurologists. Arch Neurol 1989; 46(10):1142–1148.
37. Horner RD, Matchar DB, Divine GW, Feussner JR. Relationship between physician specialty and the selection and outcome of ischemic stroke patients. HSR 1995; 30:275–287.
38. Mitchell JB, Ballard DJ, Whisnant JP, Ammering CJ, Samsa GP, Matchar DB. What role do neurologists play in determining the costs and outcomes of stroke patients? Stroke 1996; 27:1937–1943.
39. Stroke Unit Trialists' Collaboration. Collaborative systematic review of the randomised trials of organised inpatient (stroke unit) care after stroke. BMJ 1997; 314(7088):1151–1159.
40. Davis DA, Thomson MA, Oxman AD, Haynes RB. Changing physician performance. A systematic review of the effect of continuing medical education strategies. JAMA 1995; 274:700–705.
41. Goldstein LB, Matchar DB. The Stroke PORT: secondary and tertiary prevention of ischemic stroke. Stroke Prevention Patient Outcomes Research Team. Health Rep 1994; 6(1):154–159.
42. Eisenberg JM. Doctors' Decisions and the Cost of Medical Care: The Reasons for Doctors' Practice Patterns and Ways to Change Them. Ann Arbor, MI: Health Administration Press, 1986.
43. Schroeder SA. Strategies for reducing medical costs by changing physicians' behavior: efficacy and impact on quality of care. Int J Technol Assess Health Care 1987;3:39–50.
44. Lomas J, Enkin M, Anderson GM, Hannah WJ, Vayda E, Singer J. Opinion leaders vs. audit and feedback to implement practice guidelines. Delivery after previous cesarean section. JAMA 1991; 265:2202–2207.
45. Lomas J, Haynes RB. A taxonomy and critical review of tested strategies for the application of clinical practice recommendations: from "official" to "individual" clinical policy. Am J Prev Med 1988; 4(Suppl):77–94.
46. Soumerai SB, McLaughlin TJ, Avorn J. Improved drug prescribing in primary care: a critical analysis of the experimental literature. Milbank Q 1989: 67:268–317.
47. Samsa GP, Matchar DB, Cohen SJ, Lipscomb J, Abrahamse P, McCormack M. A seven-step model for practice improvement research: description and application to the Managing Anticoagulation Services Trial. New Med 1998; 2:139–146.

2

Management of Acute Stroke Prior to the Emergency Room

Kevin M. Curtis, Robert Shesser, and Brian J. Maguire
George Washington University Medical Center, Washington, D.C.

INTRODUCTION

Prehospital management of the acute stroke is a multifaceted task requiring a paradigm shift in the overall perception of the stroke patient. With the advent of new therapeutic interventions, it is no longer appropriate to treat these patients in a nonurgent and observant manner. Instead, the public as well as the medical community must be educated in the importance of early symptom recognition, prompt notification of the Emergency Medical System (EMS), and rapid evaluation and transport. The seven essential components of an effective pre-hospital stroke management system are:

1. An extensive public education campaign
2. Early involvement of the EMS
3. Priority dispatch of a paramedic team
4. Rapid and effective field evaluation
5. Prompt notification of a hospital with a stroke team
6. Prearrival hospital preparation
7. Rapid transport

PREHOSPITAL MANAGEMENT OF MYOCARDIAL INFARCTION

This conceptual approach is very similar to that currently taken with the acute myocardial infarction (AMI) patient, and in many aspects the evolution of the treatment of AMI parallels that of the stroke patient. For many years, there was a somewhat reduced sense of urgency among patients and providers with respect to AMI. This was at least partly due to the historically supportive and non-emergent nature of the hospital treatment of myocardial infarction. However, with the advent of thrombolytic therapy, both the treatment and the approach to AMI patients were revolutionized. Not only was there potential for myocardial salvage, but in both the GISSI[1] and ISIS-2 studies,[2] a clear relationship was shown between time to therapy and subsequent myocardial function and mortality.

SOURCE OF PREHOSPITAL DELAYS

With time as a critical factor, a new emphasis was placed on the prehospital setting. One of the first steps was to analyze the source of delays in obtaining medical care. Prior to 1988, it had been noted that 26% to 44% of AMI patients waited over 4 hours to seek medical care.[3–5] When combined with the time for EMS response, field evaluation, stabilization, transportation, and definitive hospital diagnosis, the majority of potential thrombolysis candidates had missed the window of opportunity for significant intervention. These pretreatment delays were divided into those that affected the time to seek medical care, those of prehospital evaluation and treatment, and in-hospital delays. The first two specifically relate to the prehospital environment. Factors that increased the time for patients with AMI to seek medical care included a past history of hypertension, diabetes mellitus, or angina; older age; consultation with the patient's private physician; attempts at self-treatment; having a smaller infarct with hemodynamic stability; and attributing symptoms to a noncardiac cause.[6,7] Two underlying factors in these sources of delay are patient denial and a lack of recognition of the cause or severity of symptoms. These initial delays were further compounded by the fact that when medical care was sought, only half of patients used emergency medical services.[8] In the case of patients with acute stroke, there has been relatively little emphasis in the past on early identification and treatment. Even in the majority of past stroke trials, the average treatment time has been between 24 and 48 hours from the onset of symptoms, and as long as 10 days.[9,10] As part of the National Institute of Neurologic Disorders and Stroke Tissue-Type Plasminogen Activator Pilot Study, Barsan evaluated over 1100 stroke patients to determine the factors that affected the time from symptom onset to arrival at the hospital.[11] The most significant factor was the type of first medical contact, with a marked decrease in time to arrival in cases in which 911 was used versus contact with a personal physician or with one of the study hospitals. Forty-seven percent of all patients evaluated used 911 as the first medical contact, and 65% of those arriving within 90 minutes. Other factors which increased delay included symptoms occurring at work (vs. home), older age groups, and strokes occurring at night (vs. morning or evening).

No effect was shown for gender, race, or presence of blood on CT. Of all the patients studied, 39% presented with 90 minutes, 59% within 3 hours, and 66% within 4 hours. Therefore although a significant percentage of patients presented within the "3 hour window" of thrombolyties a minority would still be eligible after basic interventions and head CT. Of note is the fact that public education efforts were ongoing throughout the study including radio, television, and newspaper advertisements as well as medical education to nurses, paramedics, and physicians. In addition to prolonged entry into the medical system, a second potential source of prehospital delay is that of ambulance response, evaluation, stabilization, and transport. A report from the Pre-hospital Study Group and the Cincinnati Heart Project evaluating these delays in the case of AMI found the average time from the EMS notification to hospital arrival to be 46 minutes[12] (and from hospital arrival to thrombolysis 83.8 minutes). Similar results were obtained from the Thrombolysis in Myocardial Infarction (TIMI) II trial.[13] The first component of EMS response is obviously notification. To maximize the ease of system access, the 911 telephone number is implemented, which also allows for regional centralization of dispatch and more rapid and appropriate emergency response. However, although 911 is used in the majority of U S. cities, it serves a minority of the rural population (75% of the population is covered, but only 25% geographically)[14]. A relatively new form of 911 is that of enhanced 911. When a call is received a computer displays the caller's telephone number and address. This could prove invaluable for those acute stroke patients with difficulty communicating. Fortunately, 95% of areas with 911 have the enhanced mode. Further expansion of this system will improve access and enhance response time. In the Cincinnati Heart Project study, it was shown that once 911 is activated in an urban setting, the average time to ambulance arrival is actually quite low, averaging 7.7 minutes.[12] For the system to be effective for acute stroke patients, EMS dispatchers must be educated with respect to the basic symptoms, and should make every effort to activate a paramedic unit rather than an EMT unit. (Paramedic training typically consists of 700 to 1900 hours of training including Advanced Cardiac Life Support, intravenous access, intubation, etc. Basic Emergency Medical Technician (EMT) training is 120 hours and is First Responder Level instruction.) Both the dispatchers and EMS personnel must be aware of the hospitals in their region that offer thrombolysis for the stroke patient, and all potential candidates brought to those facilities whenever practical.

The majority of the paramedic response time for the AMI patient was in field evaluation and treatment, which typically took 25.8 minutes.[12] In the case of the acute stroke, there are at least three areas with the potential for considerable time savings. The first is in the education of the paramedics in terms of the "new urgency" of the stroke patient and the need for rapid evaluation. Interestingly, in the Cincinnati study, although the paramedics often felt that they were "scooping and running" with AMI patients, the actual prehospital time from notification to hospital arrival was 60% longer than what they perceived.[12] An example of the information provided to Washington, DC, paramedics is provided as Figure 1. It briefly discusses the rationale, emphasizes the urgency, and highlights the most important aspects of the EMS approach.

Prehospital evaluation, treatment, and transport can also be expedited through the use of a protocol-driven prehospital evaluation. The current paramedic training in stroke is relatively scant, and EMS education should be improved to

WHAT IS A BRAIN ATTACK TEAM?

Studies have shown that if the patient can get to a facility that has the personnel trained in the acute treatment of strokes, quick access to CT scanners, and the tools to treat these patients, chances for recovery are good.

WHY?

Recent scientific evidence has shown that in the event of stroke from an infarction, good long term results for recovery can be obtained if the signs and symptoms can be recognized and treated in time. This is why the "EMS Response Team" is so important. It is you the pre-hospital care provider who must recognize this event and ensure that the patient is sent to the appropriate facility.

WHAT CAN I DO?

Some of the most critical aspects of stroke intervention are time and recognition. It is of extreme importance that a patient presenting with stroke like symptoms be seen within 3 hours. It is this window of opportunity that holds the greatest chance of recovery. This is why you, the pre-hospital care provider, has to be able to recognize and assess patients with stroke like symptoms, perform interventions and transport rapidly to the appropriate facility.

WHAT'S NEW THAT WORKS

One of the new advances in stroke therapy include the use of thrombolytics in essentially the same way as they are used for heart attacks. Newer advances in research show promise in the field of brain resuscitation therapy and surgical interventions.

WHAT DO I NEED TO KNOW?

The second page of this handout is a pre-hospital assessment form. This will help you assess the severity of the stroke and let us know what the patient's status was prior to the stroke and before arrival at the hospital. The following is a checklist of things to know and do.

1. Gather all medications and bring them.
2. Bring any family member and friend available.
3. Notify the hospital as soon as possible.
4. Fill out the assessment sheet.
5. Consult med. control if patient is hypertensive.
6. Do not violate your protocols.

Along with your already excellent EMS training and reading about the latest advancements in stroke therapy, it is your participation in training sessions such as these that will ensure the citizens of this city will receive the best care possible by the best educated provider.

Figure 1 EMS approach to stroke

include both an increase in general didactic training as well as specific education with respect to their role as a member of the acute stroke team. Specifically, implementation should consist of:

1. Didactic training of current prehospital personnel, including
   a. basic neurological examination and assessment
   b. new approaches to acute stroke patients
   c. importance of prehospital providers as members of the acture stroke team
   d. emphasis on early hospital notification and minimizing time to hospital arrival
   e. review of pertinent interventions
2. List of local hospitals offering acute interventions for stroke patients
3. Formal system of quality assurance review and system improvement
4. Periodic refresher courses
5. Extension and update of the future EMS curriculum with respect to the acute stroke patient.

In addition to improved didactic training, evaluation can be enhanced by specific protocols as listed in Table 1.

Table 1 Specific Protocols for Evaluation of Acute Stroke

1. ABCs, vital signs
   a. ensure adequate airway
      (1) use of nasopharngeal airways, ventilatory assistance, intubation as appropriate
   b. oxygen 4L by nasal cannula
      (1) adjustment based on pulse oximeter and/or symptoms
   c. implementation of ACLS protocols as appropriate
2. Cardiac monitor
3. IV access (NS or LR at KVO)
4. Check of blood glucose for altered mental status
   a. D50 per protocol
5. Targeted history and physical (Fig. 2)
6. Early hospital notification
7. Past medical history
   a. baseline function
   b. history of strokes, hypertension, diabetes, cardiac disease
   c. medications
   d. exclusion criteria for thrombolysis (optional)
8. Other medical interventions per standard protocols and/or online medical direction
   a. anticonvulsants
   b. hyperventilation for herniation syndromes

PRE-HOSPITAL
STROKE ASSESSMENT FORM

1. ONSET OF SYMPTOMS:
   TIME:____________________
   WITNESSED:____________________

2. PRESENCE OF HEADACHE:
   YES____________NO____________

3. LEVEL OF CONSCIOUSNESS:
   AWAKE__________DROWSY__________COMA__________

4. ARM/LEG WEAKNESS_______PARTIAL WEAKNESS_____ NO MOVEMENT___

5. SPEECH:
   NORMAL______________ABNORMAL______________

6. VITAL SIGNS:
   PULSE_________BLOOD PRESSURE_________RESPIRATION_________

7. FACIAL DROOP:
   YES________NO________

UNIT:__________DATE:__________________TIME:____________

INCIDENT NUMBER:_____________MEDICAL RECORD NUMBER:_____________

ALS:___________BLS:____________

Figure 2 Targeted pre-hospital history and physical exam

PUBLIC EDUCATION

Since early recognition and implementation of EMS is an essential component of the prehospital management of the acute stroke patient, the community must be educated in the importance of involving 911 as soon as symptoms are suspected. In the case of AMI, efforts to decrease the delay in seeking care included a variety of public education campaigns with mixed success. In King County, Washington, a 2-month public education campaign was instituted involving newspapers, radio stations, and television, and designed to target people over 35 years of age.[4] Education included identifying the symptoms of AMI and the importance of calling 911 quickly. However, although the campaign resulted in a increase in the public awareness of AMI and its symptoms, there was no decrease in delay to seeking care or in the use of EMS. A public education campaign performed in Jacksonville, Illinois, consisted of 2 years of television, radio, and newspaper advertisements, public talks, brochures, and posters.[15] AMI symptoms were included as well as the need to seek medical care rapidly. Unfortunately, results showed no decrease in delays. Other campaigns have been somewhat more successful. Radio and television public announcements over an 8-week period in Halifax, Nova Scotia, resulted in a significant increase in the percentage of people presenting to the emergency ward within 2 hours of symptoms (31.5% vs. 15.8%).[16] A similar 4-month program in Goteborg, Sweden, found a 15% increase in the number of patients presenting to the emergency ward within 2 hours of the onset of chest pain.[17] Programs in West Germany and in Switzerland also showed evidence of positive effects.[18,19]

Although several of these AMI public education campaigns were unsuccessful, this is an essential component of effective treatment of the acute stroke patient and an areas where methods must be improved and efforts increased. The campaign should include the use of radio, television, newspaper, and the Internet, as well as public displays and discussions. In addition, unlike much of the work done in the area of AMI, the target population for stroke education campaigns should not only include the high-risk population itself, but be extended to family members and to the general public. This is particularly important since many stroke patients are either asymptomatic, unable to communicate effectively, or unaware of their symptoms. Table 2 gives essential components of a public education campaign. These efforts should originate at the national level, with a commitment equivalent to that taken in the area of myocardial infarction. Although public education programs may not result in an immediate change in patient behavior, they should prove beneficial over the long term.

HOSPITAL NOTIFICATION AND PREPARATION

The other crucial component of an effective prehospital management system is early hospital notification and preparation for the incoming stroke patient. At the time of patient arrival, the stroke team and equipment should have already been assembled and waiting. This can be achieved through field notification by the paramedics, including a protocol driven evaluation, as described above; a checklist of inclusion and exclusion criteria for thrombolysis; and a prehospital evalu-

Table 2 Components of a Public Education Program in Acute Stroke

1. Provide information on risk factors, signs, and symptoms of stroke
2. Accentuate the need for immediate notification of EMS
3. Discuss the potential benefit of early intervention
4. Discourage attempts at:
   a. self-treatment
   b. repeated efforts to contact a private physician
   c. waiting for symptoms to resolve

ation of baseline function prior to the current event (Fig. 3). In the Cincinnati study of AMI patients,[12] the combination of a checklist, a transmitted EKG, and early hospital notification resulted in a 25% reduction in time from hospital arrival to thrombolysis.

With the importance of minimizing the time from onset of symptoms to treatment, the potential role of prehospital thrombolytic administration in AMI has undergone evaluation. Although the need to obtain a CT scan prior to treatment appears to preclude paramedic thrombolytic treatment in acute stroke, it is worth reviewing as it could become an issue in the future. Early studies in other countries, including Belgium[20] and Israel,[21] found the use of prehospital

BASELINE
MODIFIED RANKIN SCALE

Patient Name [ ] **Date** [/ /] dd mm yy

PIN [ ]

Time of exam [ ]

DESCRIPTION	GRADE	SCORE
No symptoms at all	0	
No significant disability despite symptoms: able to carry out all usual duties and activities	1	
Slight disability: unable to carry out all previous activities but able to look after own affairs without assistance	2	
Moderate disability: requiring some help but able to walk without assistance	3	
Moderately severe disability: unable to walk without assistance and unable to attend to own bodily needs without assistance	4	
Severe disability: bedridden, incontinent, and requiring constant nursing care and attention	5	
Death	6	
	TOTAL SCORE	

Figure 3 Assessment of preceding functional ability

thrombolytics to be safe, fast, and associated with improved outcome. However, administration was by way of ambulances and mobile ICUs staffed by physicians and nurses, which is an unrealistic scenario in the United States. In the Myocardial Infraction Triage and Intervention Project (MITI),[22] an evaluation was done of the feasibility and potential time savings of prehospital administration of thrombolytics in patients with AMI. A prehospital checklist was used that included signs and symptoms as well as inclusion and exclusion criteria. For potential qualifiers, an EKG was transmitted to the hospital for review by an emergency physician, followed by discussion between the paramedics and physician. The European Myocardial Infarction Project (EMIP) compared prehospital and inhospital use of anisoylated plasminogen-streptokinase activator complex (APSAC).[23] Prehospital administration resulted in a 1-hour reduction in time to treatment, and comparison at 1 month showed a 13% reduction in mortality. In contrast, Phase II of MITI, which also involved the actual administration of prehospital thrombolytics, did not show an advantage in the majority of patients.[24] In addition, at a minimum, prehospital thrombolysis carries the same risks as hospital administration, and one clinical decision model using a 5% major bleed rate predicted that >11,000 major bleeds would occur in the field per year.[25] In combination with increased costs, the need for prehospital refrigeration, and the potential for considerable litigation, the practicality becomes questionable.

However, probably the most important result of Phase II, particularly as it applies to acute stroke patients, is that paramedic identification of patients eligible for thrombolysis decreased the hospital treatment time from 60 minutes to 20 minutes; that is, as stated previously, the greatest benefit appeared to be in the evaluation of patients by paramedics as potential candidates for thrombolysis and the subsequent preparation by the hospital team. Therefore, paramedics can have an essential role in the diagnosis, evaluation of inclusion and exclusion criteria for thrombolysis, and early hospital notification.

PARAMEDIC EVALUATION, DIAGNOSIS, AND TREATMENT

For the prehospital evaluation to be effective, it is critical that paramedics have the capability to perform an accurate evaluation in these potentially critical patients. The ability of paramedics to accurately diagnose patients with critical conditions has been verified in multiple studies. For example, in the case of pulmonary edema, paramedic diagnosis was confirmed in 89% of patients.[26] In a study of AMI patients, through the use of a checklist and independent ECG reading, paramedics and nurses diagnosed a myocardial infarction definitively with 94% accuracy, and either recognized AMI or had a high index of suspicion in 100% of cases.[27] Similarly, in patients with head trauma, paramedics have shown the ability to accurately apply clinical criteria to patients with altered mental status, specifically as it relates to use of the Glasgow coma scale.[28] Finally, a study performed in the Cincinnati area looked at the frequency and accuracy of prehospital personnel to accurately diagnose stroke.[29] Of 86 patients initially diagnosed by an EMT or paramedic as having a stroke or a transient ischemic attack (TIA), 72% received a subsequent hospital diagnosis of TIA, ischemic stroke, intracerebral hemorrhage, or subarachnoid hemorrhage. These prehospital assessments were in the abscence of any published guidelines for stroke and only a small amount of paramedic training dedicated to stroke. Of the 28% incorrectly diagnosed, 1/3 had infectious etiologies, 1/3 myocardial ischemia or syncope, and 1/3 other diagnoses. Other notable findings from the same study were that 26% of the 86 patients needed paramedic level interventions including three intubations, four nasopharyngeal airways, and two incidences requiring intravenous anticonvulsants.

Since airway protection is always a concern in the acute setting, but particularly as it applies to acute stroke patients, intubation is an important potential intervention for prehospital providers. Although paramedics have an extensive history of successful intubations of apneic patients, many of the intubations in stroke patients may require the use of paralytics. In reviews of both ambulance-based paramedics and aeromedical prehospital teams, it was shown that neuromuscular blockade could be administered and subsequent intubation performed in a safe and effective manner.[30,31] Specifically, a study of paramedics in Cincinnati who used succinylcholine in 95 critically ill patients found a 96% success rate, and no incidences of esophageal intubations or need for emergent cricothyrotomy. The use of neuromuscular blockade and intubation by aeromedical nurse/paramedic teams in Illinois resulted in outcomes comparable to in-hospital intubation. There are two caveats to these results. The former study involved paramedics who had performing succinylcholine-assisted intubations for 10 years and therefore may not be indicative of other EMS systems. Also, many EMS systems do not allow the prehospital use of paralyzing agents.

The success of these prehospital diagnoses of critical conditions and the use of advanced-level interventions obviously require that the responding prehospital team is an advanced life support unit staffed by paramedics. Although this is likely in most urban settings, it is variable in rural areas. In fact, most of the ambulances in the United States are staffed by EMTs. Certainly, for the potential acute stroke patient, paramedics should be used whenever possible.

CONCLUSION

Without effective prehospital management of the acute stroke patient, the opportunity for implementation of new therapeutic interventions will be lost. With a long history of a nonemergent approach to patients with symptoms of stroke, both the public and the medical community must be educated in the new importance of early evaluation and treatment. The first step is a national public campaign and requires a long-term commitment, as benefits may not be immediately apparent. Education of the health care providers should not only include paramedics, emergency department staff, and neurologists, but be extended to all physicians since consultation with one's private doctor has been shown to be a source of delay in time to hospital presentation. Although this new approach to the stroke patient is a complete change from that previously taken, the relatively recent developments in the acute treatment of myocardial infarction provide a basic template on which to design a prehospital strategy for stroke. Finally, the essential components of the prehospital management of the acute stroke patient should include:

1. Public education campaigns
2. Extended 911 system, particularly enhanced 911
3. Updated EMS education
4. Expansion of paramedic units
5. Protocol-driven EMS evaluations
6. Triage plan for potential stroke patients with respect to brain attack centers
7. Early hospital notification
8. Hospital education
9. General physician and health care provider education

REFERENCES

1. Gruppo Italiano per lo Studio della Streptochinasi nell'Infartc Miocardico (GISSI). Effectiveness of intravenous thrombolytic treatment in acute myocardial infarction. Lancet 1986; 1:397–402.
2. ISIS (Second International Study of Infarct Survival) Collaborative Group. Randomized trial of intravenous streptokinase, oral aspirin, both or neither amount 17,187 cases of suspected acute myocardial infarction. ISIS-2. Lancet 1988; 2:349–360.
3. Wioelgosz ATJ, Nolan RP, Earp JA, Biro E. Reasons for patients' delay in response to symptoms of acute myocardial infarction. Can Med Assoc J 1988; 139:853–857.
4. Ho MT, Eisenberg MS, Litwin PE, Schaeffer SM, Damon S Delay between onset of chest pain and seeking medical care: the effect of public education. Ann Emerg Med 1989; 18:727–731.
5. Leitch JW, Birbara T, Freedman B, Wilcox I, Harris PJ. Factors influencing the timme from onset of chest pain to arrival at the hospital. Med J Aust 1989; 150:6–8.
6. Dracup K, Moser D. Treatment-seeking behavior among those with symptoms and signs of acute myocardial infarction. Proceedings of the National Heart, Lung, and

Blood Institute Symposium on Rapid Identification and Treatment of Acute Myocardial Infarction. September 1991.
7. Ornato J, Peberdy M. Delays to thrombolytic therapy in patients with acute myocardial infarction. Challenges of Thrombolytic Therapy Part II. New York: Cahners Health Care Communications and American Journal of Cardiology, 1993.
8. Hackett TP, Cassem NH. Factors contributing to delay in responding to the signs and symptoms of acute myocardial infarction. Am J Cardiol 1969; 24:651–658.
9. Capildeo R, Haberman S, Rose FC. Stroke trials: the facts. In: Rose FC, ed. Advances in Stroke Therapy. New York: Raven Press, 1987.
10. Barsan WG, Brott TG, Olinger CP, et al. Identification and entry of the patient with acute cerebral infarction. Ann Emerg Med 1988; 17:1192–1195.
11. Barsan WG, Brott TG, Broderick JP, et al. Time of hospital presentation in patients with acute stroke. Arch Intern Med 1993; 153:2558–2561.
12. Kereiakes DJ, Weaver WD, Anderson JL, et al. Time delays in the diagnosis and treatment of acute myocardial infarction: a tale of eight cities. A report from the pre-hospital group and the Cincinnati heart project. Am Heart J 1990; 120:773–779.
13. Passamani E, Hodges M, Herman M, et al. The thrombolysis in myocardial infarction (TIMI) phase II pilot study: tissue-plasminogen activator followed by percutaneous transluminal coronary angioplasty. J Am Coll Cardiol 1987; 10(suppl):51B–64B.
14. Roush WR. Principles of EMS Systems. Dallas: American College of Emergency Physicians, 1984.
15. Moses HW, Engelking N, Taylor GJ, et al. Effect of a two-year public education campaign on reducing response time of patients with symptoms of acute myocardial infarction. Am J Cardiol 1991; 68:249–251.
16. Mitic WR, Perkins J. The effect of a media campaign on heart attack delay and decision times. Can J Public Health 1984; 75:414–418.
17. Herlitz J, Blohm M, Hartford M, Hjalmarsson A, Holmberg S, Karlson BW. Delay time is suspected acute myocardial infarction and the importance of its modification. Clin Cardiol 1989; 12:370–374.
18. Rustige JM, Burczk U, Schiele R, et al. Media campaign on delay times in suspected myocardial infarction. The Ludwigshafen community project. Eur Heart J 1990; 11(suppl):171. Abstract.
19. Gazpos J-M, Unger P-F, Urban P, et al. Impact of a public campaign on pre-hospital time delays in suspected acute myocardial infarction. Circulation 1993; 88(4 suppl 12):1–13. Abstract.
20. Bossaert LL, Demey HE, Colemont LJ, et al. Prehospital thrombolytic treatment of acute myocardial infarction with anisoylated plasminogen streptokinase activator complex. Crit Care Med 1988; 16:823–830.
21. Barbash GI, Roth A, Hod H, et al. Improved survival but not left ventricular function with early and prehospital treatment with tissue plasminogen activator in acute myocardial infarction. Am J Cardiol 1990; 66:261–266.
22. Weaver WD, Eisenberg MS, Martin J, et al. Myocardial Infarction Triage and Intervention Project—Phase I: Patient characteristics and feasibility of prehospital initiation of thrombolytic therapy. J Am Coll Cardiol 1990; 15:925–931.

23. European Myocardial Infarction Project (EMIP). Time intervals for prehospital intervention in acute myocardial infarction. The EMIP experience. Circulation 1992; 86(suppl 1):1–15. Abstract.
24. Weaver WD, Cerqueira M, Hallstrom AP, et al. Prehospital-initiated vs hospital initiated thrombolytic therapy. The Myocardial Infarction Triage and Intervention Trial. JAMA 1993; 270:1211–1216.
25. Ornato JP. The earliest thrombolytic treatment of acute myocardial infarction: ambulance or emergency department? Clin Cardiol 1990; 13:VIII:27–31.
26. Tresch DD, Dabrowski RC, Fioretti GP, Darin JC, Brodis HL. Out of hospital pulmonary edema: diagnosis and treatment. Ann Emerg Med 1983; 12:533–537.
27. Foster DB, Dufendach JH, Barkdoll CM, Mitchell BK. Prehospital recognition of AMI using independent nurse/paramedic 12-lead ECG evaluation: impact on inhospital times of thrombolysis in a rural community hospital. Am J Emerg Med 1994; 12:25–31.
28. Menegazzi JJ, Davis EA, Sucov AN, Paris PM. Reliability of the Glasgow coma scale when used by emergency physicians and paramedics. J Trauma 1993; 34:46–48.
29. Kothari R, Barsan W, Brott T, Broderick J, Ashbrock S. Frequency and accuracy of prehospital diagnosis of stroke. Stroke 1995; 26:937–941.
30. Hedges JR, Dronen SC, Feero S, et al. Succinlycholine-assisted intubations in prehospital care. Ann Emerg Med 1988; 17:469–472.
31. Murphy-Macabobby M, Marshall WJ, Schneider C, Dries D. Neuromuscular blockade in aeromedical airway management. Ann Emerg Med 1992; 21:664–668.

3

Emergency Department Management of Acute Stroke

Edmond A. Hooker
University of Louisville, Louisville, Kentucky

INTRODUCTION

The treatment of patients suffering cerebral ischemia in the emergency department (ED) starts long before the arrival of the patient. Although it would be optimal to have all EDs staffed by board-certified emergency physicians who appreciate the importance of rapid and accurate diagnosis of stroke, the staffing of emergency departments is quite variable. All emergency physicians must be able to confidently identify and manage the patient during the first few minutes until the stroke team, if available, can be mobilized.

Rapid recognition is the first and most important part of the treatment of stroke.[1] Nurses and the emergency medical services(EMS) must be trained to identify patients who may have had a stroke or who are at risk for impending stroke. (See Chap. 2 on prehospital management.) A list of presenting symptoms that could indicate a stroke should be made available to all EMS personnel and nurses as a pocket card (Table 1).

Especially in small hospitals and areas with long transport times, rapid identification of a stroke victim and mobilization of resources prior to ED presentation may be necessary. Since current clinical practice allows for thrombolytics to be given only within 3 hours of symptom onset, it is vital that necessary resources be available as quickly as possible. Computerized tomography (CT) scanners may need to be prepared, or a CT technician may need to be called.

Once a stroke victim is identified, these patients must be quickly brought to the treatment area and the physician must be immediately notified. While the term "brain attack" may never be popularized, nurses must understand how simi-

Table 1 Clinical Presentations of Acute Stroke

Alteration in consciousness (coma, stupor, confusion, seizures, delirium)
Intense or unusually severe headache of sudden onset or any headache associated with decreased level of consciousness or neurological deficit; unusual or severe neck or facial pain
Aphasia (incoherent speech or difficulty understanding speech)
Facial weakness or asymmetry (paralysis of the facial muscles, usually noted when the patient speaks or smiles); may be on the same side or on the opposite side from the limb paralysis
Incoordination, weakness, paralysis, or sensory loss of one or more limbs; usually involves on half of body and in particular the hand
Ataxia (poor balance, clumsiness, or difficulty walking)
Visual loss (monocular or binocular); may be partial loss of visual field
Dysarthria (slurred or indistinct speech)
Intense vertigo, double vision, unilateral hearing loss, nausea, vomiting, photophobia or phonophobia

Source: Ref. 40.

lar a stroke is to a heart attack. Physicians must take time to give in-service training to the nurses. This training should include education about stroke, the planned therapies at the particular institution, and the appropriate management of the expected complications. Delays in triage and registration could cause some patients who would otherwise have been candidates for aggressive therapy to be managed with only supportive care. The potential ramifications of failure to treat a stroke patient who could have been a candidate for thrombolytics are obvious.

WORKUP OF PATIENTS WITH SUSPECTED STROKE

The emergency physician should be notified as soon as a possible stroke patient is identified. There is a minimum baseline evaluation that should be done on all patients suspected of having a stroke, preferably by a written protocol or standing orders. (Fig. 1; Table 2).

The first priority is securing an airway and obtaining a complete set of vital signs. While most patients with acute ischemic stroke will not require aggressive airway management, even mild hypoxia should be treated. Oxygen saturation should be measured by noninvasive techniques, and supplemental oxygen should be given to any patient with evidence of hypoxia. The decision to obtain an arterial blood gas if the oxygen saturation is decreased depends of the suspicion for hypercarbia or acidosis. However, some patients will be candidates for thrombolytics, and arterial punctures should be avoided if possible. Currently,

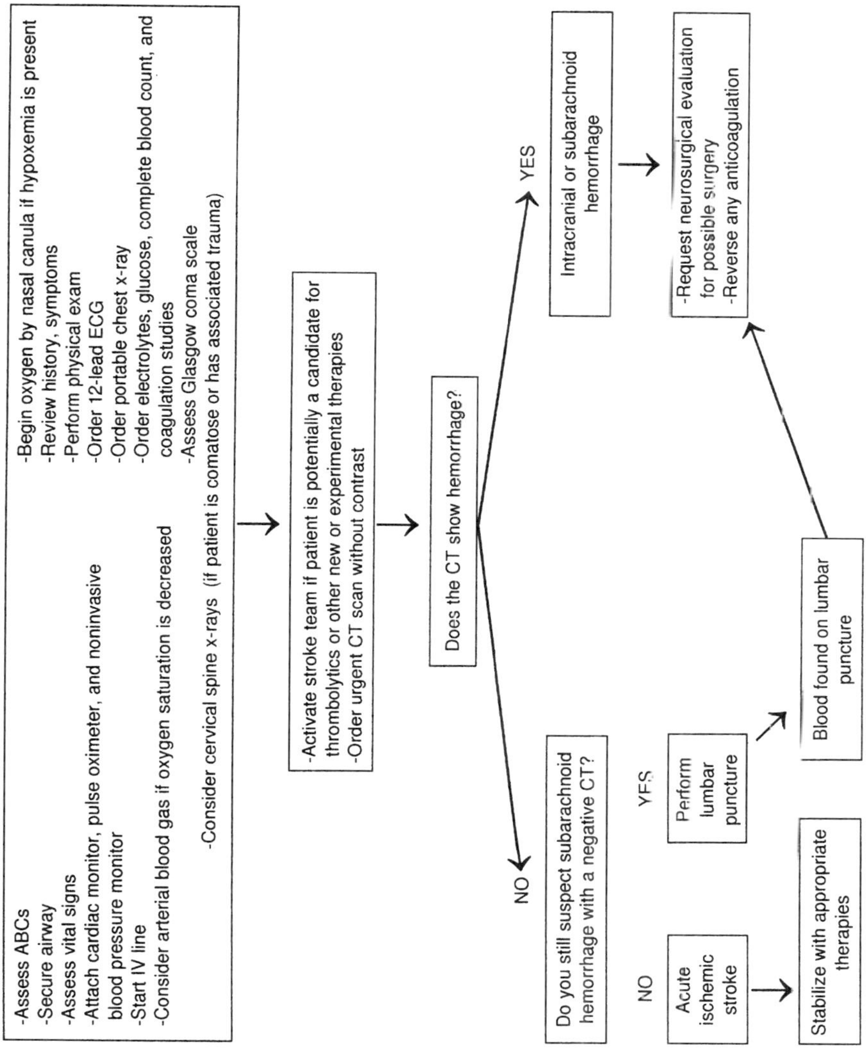

Figure 1 Algorithm for the initial management of suspected stroke. (From Ref. 40.)

Table 2 Work-up for All Patients with Suspected Stroke

CT of the brain without contrast
Electrocardiogram
Chest x-ray
Complete blood count
Platelet count
Prothrombin time
Partial thromboplastin time
Serum electrolytes
Serum glucose
Renal and hepatic chemical analysis
Oxygen saturation
Consider arterial blood gas if oxygen saturation decreased.*
Consider cervical spine x-rays (in patients who are comatose or who have cervical spine pain or tenderness).

*Arterial puncture will exclude subsequent use of rt-PA.
Source: Ref. 40.

routine supplemental oxygen is not recommended in all patients with acute ischemic stroke.[1]

Fever has been found to accompany about 44% of acute ischemic strokes and correlates with clinical severity.[2] It is important to identify patients with fever because it may indicate the patient has an infectious process. However, no matter what the cause, fever must be treated, because even mild hyperthermia may increase ischemic damage.

Blood pressure should be measured immediately and repeated at least every 10 minutes. The treatment of hypertension associated with acute stroke is controversial; this will be discussed later is the chapter.

After obtaining vital signs and assuring an adequate airway, the emergency physician must obtain a history and perform a physical examination. This examination should help to identify possible stroke mimics (Table 3). Certain clinical features affect the chances of an etiology other than stroke. Decreased level of consciousness has been shown to independently predict the presence of a stroke mimic.[3] Items that increase the chances of a stroke include abnormal visual fields, initial diastolic pressure >90 mm Hg, atrial fibrillation, or a history of angina. However, these features do not have sufficient predictive value to obviate the need for neuroimaging studies.

Blood glucose testing is necessary to exclude hyperglycemia, or hypoglycemia and should be performed at the bedside as part of the initial evaluation of all patients with suspected stroke, particularly those with altered mental status. The glucose level should subsequently be confirmed in the laboratory. Signifi-

Table 3 Conditions That Mimic Stroke

Seizure
Systemic infections
Brain tumor
Toxic-metabolic
Positional vertigo
Cardiac
Syncope
Trauma
Subdural hematoma
Herpes encephalitis
Transient global amnesia
Dementia
Demyelinating disease
Cervical spine fracture
Myasthenia gravis
Parkinsonism
Hypertensive encephalopathy
Conversion disorder

**Source*: Libman.

cant alterations in the blood glucose must be identified, because they mimic stroke. Further, hyperglycemia is associated with higher mortality because it may increase ischemic damage.[4,5] Renal and hepatic chemistries should be drawn, because renal or hepatic failure can result in stroke like symptoms.

Obtaining a CT scan in a patient with suspected stroke must have the same urgency as obtaining an EKG in a patient with chest pain. Delays in obtaining the CT could prevent a patient from being considered for r-TPA or other hyperacute therapies. Differentiation between an intracranial hemorrhage (ICH), subarachnoid hemorrhage (SAH), subdural hematomas, or other conditions, and an acute ischemic stroke is an important priority. However, identification of extensive ischemic injury including hypodensity and edema is also of critical importance.[1] The CT should be interpreted by physicians with "expertise in reading this imaging study."[6] The signs of SAH or ICH can be very subtle and easily missed by even experienced physicians. The negative consequences of giving thrombolytics or heparin to these patients makes accurate interpretation mandatory. Currently guidelines do not recommend emergent magnetic resonance imaging (MRI) in acute stroke because it does not offer any real advantage over CT for most acute management decisions.[1,6,7]

A normal CT of the head is not sufficient to rule out SAH.[8] In patients in whom this diagnosis is strongly suspected, a lumbar puncture may need to be performed because even the newest generation of CT scanners may not detect some patients with SAH.[9] One recent study found these "newer generation scanners" to be 100% sensitive for SAH if done during the first 12 hours after the onset of symptoms, and 81.7% sensitive after 12 hours.[10] Whether this finding will be confirmed with subsequent studies has yet to be determined. If a lumbar puncture is performed, the patient cannot receive a thrombolytic. Therefore, the decision to perform a lumbar puncture should be left to the neurologist, and early consultation should be obtained.

An electrocardiogram is important to exclude coexisting myocardial ischemia or infarction as well as to evaluate for cardiac dysrhythmias such as atrial fibrillation. Prolonged cardiac monitoring should be continued to help detect any potentially life-threatening dysrythmias or atrial fibrillation.[1,11]

ANTITHROMBOTIC THERAPIES AND ANTIPLATELET-AGGREGATING DRUGS

Because of the general lack of prospective randomized data, the use of heparin in patients with acute ischemic stroke is controversial.[1] The use of heparin has been shown to decrease the rate of recurrent events in patients with acute cardioembolic stroke.[12] The value of heparin in thrombotic stroke is not so clear. The concerns over hemorrhagic transformation of the ischemic stroke because of the use of heparin appear unfounded.[9,13] Hemorrhagic transformation is associated with large infarct volume, midline shift, and increasing age. The incidence of hemorrhagic transformation appears to be unrelated to the use of heparin or the level of hypertension. The use of heparin at the present time is a matter of preference until more data are available. However, the International Stroke Trial found no benefit from acute heparin therapy at a dose of 12,500 units twice daily or 5000 units twice daily.14

The use of aspirin in acute ischemic stroke is generally accepted by most clinicians. The Chinese Acute Stroke Trial (CAST) found improved outcomes for those treated with aspirin.[15] Although the exact dose that should be given is uncertain, based on the CAST, 325 mg aspirin a day is probably adequate.

Treatment with Thrombolytics

The findings of the National Institute of Neurological Disorders and Stroke (NINDS) study show that intravenous recombinant tissue plasminogen activator (r-TPA) improves outcome after ischemic stroke if given within 3 hours of symptom onset.[6] The use of this therapy requires a well-thought-out team approach and the establishment of a system to facilitate its administration. The inclusion and exclusion criteria must be carefully evaluated (Table 4). It is important that patients and patient's families be aware of the potential complications of the therapy. Also, caution should be used before giving r-TPA to persons with severe stroke (National Institutes of Health Stroke scale >22) and in those with significant ealy changes on CT scan.[16]

As more data become available, thrombolytics may be used on a wider range of patients. The current guidelines do not allow for the use of r-TPA outside the 3-hour window or for the use of thrombolytics other than r-TPA.[6] It is critical that the time of symptom onset be accurately established. Details of the use of thrombolytics and its complications are reviewed in Chapter XX.

Table 4 Management of Hypertension in Patients with Acute Ischemic Stroke

Monitor arterial blood pressure during the first 24 hours
—Every 15 minutes for the first 2 hours, then
—Every 30 minutes for 8 hours, then
—Every 60 minutes until 24 hours

If systolic blood pressure is 180 to 230 mm Hg or if diastolic blood pressure is 105 to 120 mm Hg for two or more readings 5 to 10 minutes apart:
—No therapy unless patient has received a thrombolytic agent
—If patient has been treated with a thrombolytic agent:
1. Give intravenous labetalol 10 mg over 1 to 2 minutes. The dose may be repeated and doubled every 10 minutes up to a total dose of 150 mg.
2. Monitor the blood pressure every 15 minutes during the labetalol treatment and observe for development of hypotension.

If systolic blood pressure is >230 mm Hg or if diastolic blood pressure is 121 to 140 mm Hg for two or more readings 5 to 10 minutes apart:
—Give intravenous labetalol 10 mg over 1 to 2 minutes. The dose may be repeated and doubled every 10 minutes up to a total dose of 150 mg.
—Monitor the blood pressure every 15 minutes during the labetalol treatment and observe for development of hypotension.
—If no satisfactory response, infuse sodium nitroprusside (0.5 to 10 μg/kg/min)*
—Continue monitoring blood pressure

If diastolic blood pressure is >140 mm Hg for two or more readings 5 to 10 minutes apart:
—Infuse sodium nitroprusside (0.5-10 æg/kg per minute)*
—Monitor blood pressure at least every 15 minutes during infusion of sodium nitroprusside and observe for the development of hypotension.

*Continuous arterial monitoring is advised if sodium nitroprusside is used. The risk of bleeding secondary to an arterial puncture should be weighed against the possibility of missing dramatic changes in the blood pressure during infusion.

TREATMENT OF COMPLICATIONS OF ACUTE STROKE

Treatment of Hypertension

Background

Arterial hypertension has been shown to be one of the most important modifiable risk factorsr for stroke.[17,18] There has been a well demonstrated decrease in the occurrence of first stroke for patients in whom prolonged pharmacological reduction in blood pressure was achieved.[19] Antihypertensive therapy has become the cornerstone to reducing risk of all cardiovascular disease, including stroke.

Management of hypertension in the setting of an acute ischemic stroke has been controversial.[20,21]1 Blood pressure has been shown to increase immediately following an acute stroke.[22] This increased blood pressure naturally improves without any therapy over the next 10 days.[23] While there is an increased risk of death in patients with higher blood pressures, it is not clear if the hypertension is the cause or merely a marker of a more severe stroke.[24] Currently, there is no evidence that has shown an improvement in morbidity or mortality from acute lowering of blood pressure in patients suffering an acute ischemic stroke.

The presence of severely elevated blood pressure in the setting of an ischemic stroke has been considered by some authors to represent an hypertensive emergency.[25] However, aside from hypertensive encephalopathy, and possibly the presence of an ICH or SAH, aggressive treatment of acute hypertension may be hazardous.[26] The diagnosis of hypertensive encephalopathy requires the presence of global cerebral dysfunction (headache, lethargy). Papilledema is often, but not invariably, present on exam.[27]

Pathophysiology

Before treating patients with hypertension associated with acute stroke, the physician must understand the neurophysiology of cerebral perfusion. Cerebral perfusion is determined by cerebral blood flow (CBF). The determinates of cerebral blood flow are cerebral perfusion pressure (CPP) and cerebrovascular resistance (CVR)(Fig. 2).[27] In normal individuals, cerebral autoregulation maintains optimal blood flow over a wide range of blood pressures. In normotensive adults it is probably maintained over the range of 60 to 120 mm Hg; however, in hypertensive adults this range is higher (approximately 120 to 160 mm Hg).[28] In fact, patients have suffered focal cerebral ischemia after being treated for their hypertension.[29]

During an acute stroke there is impaired autoregulation, and CBF is passively dependent on arterial pressure. The marginal ischemic penumbrum can be expected to suffer a reduction in blood flow if the systemic blood pressure is lowered.[21] While there are conflicting recommendations in the literature, most authors are recommending no therapy for most patients and only minimal therapy for those with the most severely elevated blood pressures.[1,27,30–32]

$$\text{cerebral blood flow (CBF)} = \frac{\text{cerebral perfusion pressure (CPP)}}{\text{cerebrovascular resistance (CVR)}}$$

$$\text{CPB} = \text{arterial blood pressure–venous backpressure}$$

Treatment

Treatment of hypertension associated with acute ischemic stroke should start with simple, nonpharmacologic measures. The patient should be placed in a quiet room, the bladder emptied, pain controlled, and the patient allowed to rest.[1,33] Multiple readings must be taken 5-10 minutes apart. If the patient continues to have sustained hypertension on repeated measurements, then consideration of pharmacologic therapy should be made.

The exact level of blood pressure above which antihypertensive therapy should be considered is controversial. Recently published reviews of hypertension associated with acute ischemic stroke vary considerably. One author and the current published national guidelines recommend no therapy for blood pressure unless the mean blood pressure (systolic + (2× dyastolic)/3) is >130 mm Hg or the systolic blood pressure is >220 mm Hg.[1,31] Other authors recommend no therapy at all unless there is other evidence of end organ damage to the heart or kidney, or there is evidence of encephalopathy or intracranial bleeding.[32]

We have developed a treatment protocol modeled after the NINDS Study Group (Table 4).[6] This approach does not require calculations of mean arterial pressures to be made by the nursing staff. Unless there is evidence of other end-organ damage, intracranial bleeding, or the patient has received intravenous thrombolytics, we do not treat SBP <230 mm Hg or DBP <120 mm Hg. More aggressive control is required if the patient has received thrombolytics (Table 4). In any case the blood pressure should be cautiously lowered, never more than 16% below the baseline.[34]

Drug Choice

The parenteral antihypertensive agent to be used for the treatment of severely elevated blood pressure associated with stroke should be easily titrated and have a minimal effect on cerebral blood vessels. Labetalol is recommended in both recent guidelines published by the American Heart Association (AHA) and the new Advanced Cardiac Life Support textbook.[1,31,35] It has a relatively quick time to maximal decreases in blood pressure (5 to 30 minutes).[36] However, it must be

Table 5 Drugs that should be avoided when treating hypertension associated with acute ischemic stroke

Drug	Reason
Oral or sublingual calcium channel blockers (nifedipine, nicardipine, etc.)	Precipitous drops in blood pressure
Hydralazine	Causes cerebral vasodilation and may further impair autoregulation
Clonidine	Depresses global cerebral function
Methyldopa	Depresses global cerebral function
Diuretics	May cause dehydration and hypovolemia

remembered that its effects can last for up to 24 hours. Early use of the drug was associated with more hypotension because of the use of higher starting doses, 20 to 80 mg. Newer protocols start with 10 mg. We consider this the first-line therapy in all but the most severely elevated blood pressures.

In patients who are not responding to labetalol or in whom the blood pressure reaches very high levels (SBP> 230 mm Hg. or DBP >140 mm Hg), consideration must be given to using intravenous sodium nitroprusside (SNP). SNP has almost immediate onset of action and can be titrated. It is very potent and requires very close monitoring, preferably by continuous intra-arterial measurement. However, SNP causes an increase in ICP and a decrease in CPP, which may be detrimental to stroke patients.[37] Other drugs may become available in the future to treat hypertension associated with stroke. Certain drugs should be avoided in patients with acute ischemic stroke (Table 5).

Sublingual or oral nifedipine should be avoided because of the potential for precipitous decline of the blood pressure and the rapid onset.[1,31] Likewise, nicardipine can cause precipitous drops in blood pressure.[34] It is probably prudent to avoid the entire class of calcium channel blockers, including enalapril, until controlled trials can document their safety for emergent treatment of hypertension associated with stroke. Hydralazine should be avoided because it is associated with cerebral vasodilation and may further impair autoregulation.[32] Clonidine and methyldopa should be avoided because of their depressive effect on global cerebral function.[38]

Treatment of Cerebral Edema

Clinically significant cerebral edema can be expected to develops in 10% to 20% of patients who suffer an ischemic stroke.[1] Most patients will not have clinically significant edema in the first 24 hours. However, edema may cause brainstem compression or acute hydrocephalus in patients with large cerebellar infarcts.

Clinically significant cerebral edema should be treated with hyperventilation and osmotherapy.[1] Surgical drainage of hydrocephalus and, in the case of cerebellar infarction, possible craniotomy should be considered. There are no indications for corticosteroids.

Treatment of Seizures

The exact incidence of seizures after an acute ischemic stroke is not clear.[39] There is no evidence to support the routine use of prophylactic anticonvulsants in patients suffering an acute stroke.[1] Anticonvulsants are indicated in patients who have a seizure, because recurrent seizures are seen in up to 80% of cases. Most seizures can be controlled with a single medication, either carbamazepine or phenytoin. Status epilepticus should be treated as a medical emergency.

REFERENCES

1. Adams HP, Brott TG, Crowell RM, et al. Guidelines for the management of patients with acute ischemic stroke: a statement for healthcare professionals from a special writing group of the Stoke Council, American Heart Association. Stroke 1994; 25:1901–1914.
2. Hindfelt B. The prognostic significance of subfebrility and fever in ischemic cerebral infarction. Acta Neurol Scand 1976; 53:72–79.
3. Libman RB, Wirkowski E, Alvir J, Rao TH. Conditions that mimic stroke in the emergency department. Arch Neurol 1995; 52:1119–1122.
4. Candelise L, Landi G, Orazio EN, Boccardi E. Prognostic significance of hyperglycemia in acute stroke. Arch Neurol 1985; 42:661–663.
5. Pulsinelli WA, Waldman S, Rawlinson D, Plum F. Moderate hyperglycemia augments ischemic brain damage: a neuropathologic study in the rat. Neurology 1982; 32:1239–1246.
6. Adams HP, Brott TG, Furlan AJ, et al. Guidelines for thrombolytic therapy for acute stroke: a supplement to the guidelines for the management of patients with acute ischemic stroke: a special statement for healthcare professionals from a special writing group of the Stroke Council, American Heart Association. Circulation 1996; 94:1167–1174.
7. Mohr JP, Biller J, Hilal SK, et al. Magnetic resonance versus computed tomography imaging in acute stroke. Stroke 1995; 26:807–812.
8. Mayberg MR, Batjer HH, Dacey R, et al. Guidelines for the management of aneurysmal subarachnoid hemorrhage: a statement for healthcare professionals from a special writing group of the Stroke COuncil, American Heart Association. Circulation 1994; 90:2592–2605.
9. Sames TA, Storrow AB, Finkelstein JA, Magoon MR. Sensitivity of new-generation computed tomography in subarachnoid hemorrhage. Acad Emerg Med 1996; 3:16–20.

10. Sidman R, Connolly E, Lemke T. Subarachnoid hemorrhage diagnosis: lumbar puncture is still needed when the computed tomography scan is normal. Acad Emerg Med 1996; 3:827–831.
11. Oppenheimer S, Hachinski V. Complications of stroke. Lancet 1992; 339:721–727.
12. Furlan AJ, Cavalier SJ, Hobbs RE. Hemorrhage and anticoagulation after nonseptic embolic brain infarction. Neurology 1982; 32:280–282.
13. Toni D, Fiorelli M, Bastianello S, et al. Hemorrhagic transformation of brain infarct: Predictability in the first 5 hours from stroke onset and influence on clinical outcome. Neurology 1996; 46:341–345.
14. International Stroke Trial Collaborative Group. The International Stroke Trial (IST): a randomized trial of aspirin, subcutaneous heparin, both, or neither among 19,434 patients with acute ischemic stroke. Lancet 1997; 349:1569–1581.
15. CAST (Chinese Acute Stroke Trail) Collaborative Group. CAST: randomized placebo-controlled trial of early aspirin use in 20,000 patients with acute ischaemic stroke. Lancet 1997; 349:1641–49.
16. Allexandrov AV, Masdeu JC, Devous MD, Black SE, Grotta JC. Brain single-photon emission CT with HMPAO and safety of thrombolytic therapy in acute ischemic stroke. Proceedings of the Meeting of the SPECT Safe Thrombolysis Study Collaborators and the Members of the Brain Imaging Council of the Society of Nuclear Medicine. Stroke 1997; 28:1830–1834.
17. Gueyffier F, Froment A, Gouton M. New meta-analysis of treatment trials of hypertension: improving the estimate of therapeutic benefit. J Hum Hypertens 1996; 10:1–8.
18. MacMahon S, Peto R, Culter J, et al. Blood Pressure, stroke, and coronary heart disease. Part 1. Prolonged differences in blood pressure: prospective observational studies corrected for the regression dilution bias. Lancet 1990; 335:765–774.
19. Collins R, Peto R, MacMahon S, et al. Blood pressure, stroke, and coronary heart disease. Part 2. Short-term reductions in blood pressure: overview of randomized drug trials in their epidemiological context. Lancet 1990; 335:827–838.
20. Spence JD, Del Maestro RF. Hypertension in acute ischemic strokes: Treat. Arch Neurol 1985; 42:1000–1002.
21. Yatsu FM, Zivin J. Hypertension in acute ischemic strokes: not to treat. Arch Neurol 1985; 42:999–1000.
22. Broderick J, Brott T, Barsan W, et al. Blood pressure during the first minutes of focal cerebral ischemia. Ann Emerg Med 1993; 22:1438–1443.
23. Wallace JD, Levy LL. Blood pressure after stroke. JAMA 1981; 246:2177–2180.
24. Britton M, Carlsson A, de Faire U. Blood pressure course in patients with acute stroke and matched controls. Stroke 1986; 17:861–864.
25. Houston MC. Pathophysiology, clinical aspects, and treatment of hypertensive crises. Prog Cardiovasc Dis 1989; 32:99–148.
26. Brott T, Reed RL. Intensive care for acute stroke in the community hospital setting: The first 24 hours. Stroke 1989; 24:1–5.
27. Powers WJ. Acute hypertension after stroke: the scientific basis for treatment decisions. Neurology 1993; 43:461–467.
28. Strandgaard S, Oleses J, Skinhoj E, Lassen NA. Autoregulation of brain circulation in severe arterial hypertension. Br Med J 1973; 1:507–510.

29. Hankey GJ, Gubbay SS. Focal cerebral ischaemia and infarction due to antihypertensive therapy. Med J Aust 1987; 146:412–414.
30. Lavin P. Management of hypertension in patients with acute stroke. Arch Intern Med 1986; 146:66–68.
31. Kenton EJ. Diagnosis and treatment of concomitant hypertension and stroke. J Natl Med Assoc 1996; 88:364–368.
32. O'Connell JE, Gray CS. Treatment of post-stroke hypertension: a practical guide. Drugs Aging 1996; 6:408–415.
33. Carlberg B, Asplund K, Hagg E. Factors influencing admission blood pressure levels in patients with acute stroke. Stroke 1991; 22:527–530.
34. Lisk DR, Grotta JC, Lamki LM, et al. Should hypertension be treated after acute stroke: a randomized controlled trial using single photon emission computed tomography. Arch Neurol 1993; 50:855–862.
35. American Heart Association. Acute stroke. In: Cummins RO, ed. Advanced Cardiac Life Support. Dallas: American Heart Association, 1997: 10:1–10:28.
36. Goa KL, Benfield P, Sorkin EM. Labetalol. A reappraisal of its pharmacology, pharmacokinetics and therapeutic use in hypertension and ischemic heart disease. Drugs 1989; 37:583–627.
37. Cottrell JE, Patel K, Turndorf H, Ransohoff J. Intracranial pressure changes induced by sodium nitroprusside in patients with intracranial mass lesions. J Neurosurg 1978; 48:329–331.
38. Phillips SJ. Pathophysiology and management of hypertension in acute ischemic stroke. Hypertension 1994; 23:131–136.
39. Kilpatrick CJ, Davis SM, Tress BM, Rossiter SC, Hopper JL, Vandendriesen ML. Epileptic seizures in acute stroke. Arch Neurol 1990; 47:157–160.
40. Emergency Cardiac Care Committee and Subcommittees, American Heart Association. Guidelines for cardiopulmonary resuscitation and emergency care. IV. Special resuscitation situations. JAMA 1992; 268:2242–2250.

4

Early Recognition and Assessment of Acute Stroke

Larry B. Goldstein
Duke University Medical Center and Durham VA Medical Center, Durham, North Carolina

INTRODUCTION

With the advent of new therapies such as rt-PA and neuroprotective agents, the rapid diagnosis and clinical assessment of patients suspected of having an acute stroke is becoming increasingly important. An organized approach is essential as even in patients who might not be candidates for hyperacute interventions, the data collected at the time of the initial assessment may be critical for the patient's subsequent management (Fig. 1). The availability of neuroimaging studies does not obviate the need for careful clinical assessment. Computed tomographic (CT) scans are frequently negative during the first hours after ischemic stroke, and technical limitations often impair CT imaging of the posterior fossa.[1,2] Furthermore, abnormalities found on neuroimaging studies may be unrelated to the patient's acute problem. The clinical evaluation is crucial both to properly respond to progression or improvement of the patient's deficits and to classify a stroke with respect to the area of damaged brain. The purpose of this chapter is to provide a logical approach to the initial assessment of the stroke patient for the nonneurologist in a way that helps guide acute and later management.

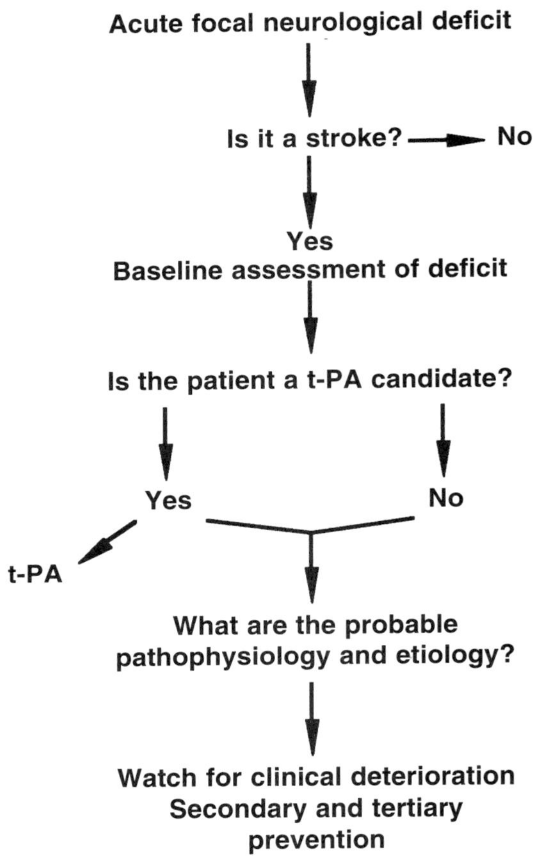

Figure 1 Clinical Evaluation of the Stroke Patient

INITIAL HISTORY

Stroke

The first step in the clinical assessment of patients presenting with a new focal neurological deficit is to carefully consider the differential diagnosis and to gather data to help rapidly exclude other conditions that may mimic stroke. In one study, patients with a history of a persistent focal neurological deficit of acute onset during the prior week (but no history of head trauma) were considered to have had a stroke.[3] Using this rule, emergency room physicians correctly identified 152 of 176 consecutive patients with stroke (sensitivity, 86.4%) and 1,818 of 1,835 patients without stroke (specificity, 99.1%). However, in other series, 13%

to 19% of patients initially diagnosed with stroke were finally determined to have other conditions.[4,5] The most frequent causes of misdiagnosis were unrecognized seizures, confusional states, syncope, toxic and metabolic abnormalities, systemic infections, neoplasms, and subdural hematomas. With time being of the essence in patients presenting soon after the onset of a focal neurological deficit, the medical history should be directed at identifying any factors which may place them at increased risk for any of these other conditions. In addition, for those presenting soon after the onset of the neurological deficit, the history should also focus on establishing whether the patient may be a candidate for thrombolytic therapy (Table 1; see Chap. 16).

After this basic historical information is obtained, patients who remain candidates for thrombolytic therapy should have a rapid, directed general physical and neurological examination and selected laboratory studies as described in the sections below. With these tasks and a decision with regard to the use of thrombolytic therapy accomplished, additional historic details should be sought to help in the diagnosis of stroke subtype and potential etiology and to identify stroke risk factors for later management. In this regard, it is important to recognize that stroke is not a single disease. It has varying etiologies and pathophysiologies that impact on both treatment and outcomes (Table 2). Stroke may result from either hemorrhage or ischemia. Each is heterogeneous with a variety of causes. About 15% of strokes are due to hemorrhage within or around the brain.[6] Parenchymal brain hemorrhage can be associated with several conditions including hypertension, vascular malformations, coagulopathies, and angiopathies. Ischemic stroke may be the result of emboli from another blood vessel or from the heart. It can also be caused by local narrowing of extracranial or intracranial blood vessels. Intracranially, either small penetrating vessels or larger vessels supplying an entire region of brain parenchyma can be affected. Although most commonly related to atherosclerosis (atherothrombosis), nonembolic is-

Table 1 t-PA for Ischemic Stroke—History

1. Established time of symptom onset (based on the last time the patient was known to be well)
2. No history of stroke or head trauma within 3 months
3. No history of major surgery or invasive procedures within 14 days
4. No history of intracranial hemorrhage
5. No history of noncompressible arterial puncture or internal biopsy within 7 days
6. No history of seizure preceding or during the current stroke
7. No history of pericarditis, endocarditis, septic emboli, recent pregnancy, or inflammatory bowel disease (active)
8. No history of active alcohol or drug abuse

Source: Ref. 64.

Table 2 Stroke Subtypes

1. Hemorrhage
Intraparenchymal hemorrhage
Subarachnoid hemorrhage
2. Ischemia*
Large-vessel atherothrombosis
Small-vessel occlusive
Cardioembolic
Other defined etiology
Multiple defined etiologies
Undetermined etiology

*See Ref. 65 for details of diagnostic criteria.

chemic stroke can be caused by other mechanisms including arterial dissection, fibromuscular dysplasia, inflammatory arteritidies, and coagulopathies.

Studies have identified certain historic features that increase the likelihood that the patient has had an intracranial hemorrhage. For example, a very severe, acute headache accompanied by meningismus and photophobia suggests subarachnoid hemorrhage.[7] A headache in association with the stroke and a history of hypertension may increase the likelihood of intracerebral hemorrhage.[8] However, as discussed below, the history alone or in combination with findings on physical and neurological examinations does not allow the clinician to reliably determine whether an individual patient has had a parenchymal hemorrhage or an ischemic stroke. This distinction can only be made with a neuroimaging study such as CT.

An additional goal of the history is to provide data to help in the diagnosis of ischemic stroke mechanism. After hemorrhage has been excluded and a decision with regard to thrombolytic therapy has been made, further management may depend on whether the patient is believed to have had a large-vessel atherothrombotic, cardioembolic, or small-vessel stroke (Table 2). For example, the distinction between ischemic stroke subtypes can be an important guide for specific therapy such as the use of anticoagulants.[9] Simple clinical features useful at the bedside can help with this distinction. The acute onset of a focal neurologic deficit in a patient with an embolic source increases the odds of embolic stroke 11-fold whereas the absence of these features drops the odds of embolic stroke by one-third to one-half.[3,10]

TIA

Some patients presenting with *focal* symptoms suggesting an acute stroke may return completely to normal within 24 hours. The most common symptoms of carotid distribution TIA are an ipsilateral monocular visual distrubance and contralateral weakness or sensory complaints in either carotid system and language disturbances if the dominant hemisphere was affected.[11] In the vertebrobasilar system, the most common symptoms were bilateral visual blurring, diplopia, and ataxia and dizziness.[11] By definition, if these transient symptoms are due to ischemia, the patient is diagnosed with a transient ischemic attack (TIA). These patients may actually have had either a TIA (without any permanent brain damage) or cerebral infarction with transient symptoms.[12,13] One study found that only 14% of patients with symptoms lasting more than 60 minutes had transient ischemia without radiographic or clinical evidence of stroke.[14]

Because most TIAs last <4 hours,[15] the diagnosis is usually based on history rather than findings on examination. The diagnosis of TIA has gained increased importance because carotid endarterectomy,[16–18] aspirin,[19] ticlopidine clopidogral[21a] and aspiring/sustained release dipyridamole[21b] have been shown to be efficacious for selected patients with TIA or minor stroke. Despite its clinical importance, it should be recognized that the diagnosis of TIA can be unreliable. For example, in one study, histories were obtained from 28 patients by pairs of neurologists.[22] Agreement in the number of TIAs was observed in about one-half of the cases. There was agreement in the time of the first TIA and the duration of the episode in about two-thirds of the cases, and frequency and type of symptoms in less than half of cases. Two examiners agreed on vascular territory in only two-thirds of cases. Another study similarly found poor agreement in the diagnosis of the vascular territory of the TIA.[23] This distinction has obvious clinical importance. For example, patients with vertebrobasilar distribution TIA would not be expected to benefit from carotid endarterectomy. The ultimate diagnosis in patients with an initial diagnosis of TIA is "something else" in about one-third of cases and "definitely not established" in an additional third.[24] With these potential difficulties in mind, any patient with suspected TIA should be rapidly evaluated both to exclude other potential causes and to determine whether surgical (carotid endarterectomy) and/or medical (aspirin, ticlopidine) therapy is appropriate.

INITIAL GENERAL PHYSICAL EXAMINATION

The initial general physical examination is aimed at assuring that the patient is medically stable and at the identification of findings that may be relevant for the initial differential diagnosis and treatment. This evaluation begins with the assessment of airway patency, breathing, the circulatory system, and temperature. In patients who are obtunded, particular attention must be given to protection of the airway to prevent aspiration pneumonia. Hypotension in the setting of acute ischemic stroke should be avoided as this may increase the amount of ischemic damage. An irregular heart rhythm may indicate atrial fibrillation. Fever may indicate systemic infection and is also important to recognize and treat early as even mild hyperthermia may significantly affect the potential viability of ischemic neurons.[25–27]

With the assessment of vital signs completed, a brief general physical examination should next focus on other signs that could influence acute management. The patient should be inspected for signs of trauma and for ecchymoses or petechia that could indicate a bleeding diathesis. Palpation of the temporal arteries may hold clues to the mechanism of stroke in patients with hemispheric symptoms. A decreased ipsilateral temporal artery pulse may suggest common carotid stenosis or occlusion. An augmented ipsilateral temporal artery pulse may suggest internal carotid disease. Chest auscultation should be performed for signs of pneumonia or congestive heart failure. Cardiac auscultation should be performed to detect a heart murmur that could reflect a potential source of cardiogenic embolism. Hepatic or splenic enlargement is evaluated as part of the abdominal examination. The distal limbs should be examined for evidence of local cyanosis that may suggest recent embolism as well as for splinter hemorrhages that can be found in patients with septic emboli. This brief general physical examination can be completed in just a few minutes.

INITIAL NEUROLOGICAL EXAMINATION

There are several goals of the neurological examination. The first is to assess the patient's level of consciousness. As indicated above, obtunded patients are at particularly high risk of aspiration pneumonia. In addition, obtundation may exclude a patient from receiving thrombolytic therapy (see Chap. 16). To affect consciousness, the stroke must either disturb the normal relationship between the reticular activating system in the tectum of the midbrain and pons and the cerebral hemispheres, or affect both cerebral hemispheres. This occurs when a discrete infratentorial lesion disturbs the reticular activating system, when there are diffuse or bilateral supratentorial lesions, or when a unilateral supratentorial lesion results in a shift of midline structures. Thus, obtundation in a patient with signs of a unilateral hemispheric stroke may suggest edema with raised intracranial pressure that could require emergent management. Obtundation in a patient with other signs of a cerebellar lesion could indicate brainstem compression that could necessitate rapid medical management and acute neurosurgical intervention. Finally, the initial level of consciousness is the single most important finding on examination predictive of mortality (provided the obtundation is not due to a metabolic or other systemic cause). For example, one study found that no patient who was alert, but 37% of those whose consciousness was initially impaired, died within the first 3 weeks of stroke.[28]

Another important goal of the initial neurological examination is to provide baseline data with regard to the nature and severity of the patient's neurological deficits. Patients with presumed acute atherothrombotic stroke are at risk for clinical worsening. In patients with carotid distribution stroke, the greatest risk of further deterioration is over the first 24 to 48 hours[29]; in the setting of vertebrobasilar distribution stroke, the greatest risk of further clinical worsening is over the first 96 hours.[30] Stroke patients may deteriorate for a variety of reasons, and rapid identification of a change in neurological status may result in a change in therapy such as a decision to use an anticoagulant. As several physicians may be involved in the patient's care, accurate documentation of the neurological deficit is essential.

The third goal of the neurological examination is to determine the area of brain affected by the stroke. Localization in the setting of acute stroke is not an academic exercise, but can be an important guide for further management. Current neuroimaging studies cannot replace this portion of the clinical assessment. Many brain CT scans are unrevealing in the first several hours after acute ischemic stroke. CT imaging of structures in the posterior fossa are particularly subject to technical limitations. MRI, with a better capacity to image an area of acute ischemia and better resolution of structures in the posterior fossa, is not generally immediately available to most physicians on a 24-hour-a-day basis. To accomplish the task of localization, in addition to the assessment of the level of consciousness, the initial neurological examination should briefly evaluate orientation, language, the cranial nerves, motor function, sensation, and coordination. This is not to suggest that a complete neurological examination is unnecessary, but only that the basics be covered first, especially when time is of the essence.

Cognition and Neglect

A brief initial assessment of cognitive status is appropriate. This should include questions related to orientation and memory. Abnormal cognition suggests bilateral or diffuse hemispheric disease. Hemispatial neglect may indicate a lesion affecting the contralateral hemisphere (particularly the parietal lobe). Neglect may be difficult to test in patients with a cognitive or language disorder. Neglect may be suspected in patients who ignore stimuli presented from one side, including those who deny an obvious deficit affecting one side of the body.

Speech and Language

In assessing speech, the distinction between an aphasia and a dysarthria can be important. Aphasia implies a lesion affecting the dominant hemisphere. Dysarthria can be caused by lesions affecting either cerebral hemisphere, the brainstem, cerebellum, lower cranial nerves, the neuromuscular junction, or structures in the oropharynx (for example, a patient may become dysarthric when dentures are removed). In contrast, patients with aphasia have a language deficit, not just a speech deficit. Different types of aphasias may affect different aspects of language. The patient with a motor aphasia may have completely intact comprehension and be able to follow written and verbal commands without difficulty. A patient with a transcortical or subcortical type of aphasia may be able to repeat verbal phrases with little difficulty (some of these individuals may be echolalic, repeating every phrase they hear). The presence of dysnomia is the *sine qua non* of the aphasic and is the single most important aspect of language to assess when differentiating aphasia from dysarthria. Patients may have particular difficulty naming parts of objects. In literate patients with unintelligible speech, dysnomia can be tested by asking them to respond in writing.

Cranial Nerves

In a cooperative patient, the assessment of visual fields can be particularly helpful. Each eye should be tested separately. A homonymous (same in each eye) visual field defect implies a lesion affecting the optic radiations as they course to the occipital lobe in the contralateral cerebral hemisphere. In noncooperative patients, visual fields can often be assessed with visual threat. The funduscopic examination may be quite helpful in certain patients. A Hollenhorst plaque detected in the fundus ipsilateral to a hemispheric stroke suggests that the stroke was embolic (from either a cardiogenic or other vascular source).[31,32]

Pupil size and pupillary light responses are assessed next. Anisocoria of more than 1 mm may be significant. If there is a ptosis on the side of the small pupil, the patient may have an ipsilateral Horner's syndrome due to a lesion affecting the sympathetic fibers innervating the eyelid and pupil. If there is a ptosis on the side of the larger pupil, or if the eye is laterally deviated, the patient may have an ipsilateral third-nerve palsy. When there are other signs suggesting a hemispheric stroke, this finding may indicate raised intracranial pressure and herniation. Nasal deviation of the eye may suggest an ipsilateral sixth-nerve palsy. The observation of a conjugate eye deviation in combination with a hemiparesis can lead to a rapid determination of whether the patient has a lesion affecting the brainstem or cerebral hemisphere.[33] In the case of a hemispheric lesion, the patient's eyes may deviate away from the side of the hemiparesis (toward the side of the hemispheric lesion). In patients with a pontine brainstem lesion, the patient's eyes deviate toward the side of the hemiparesis (away from the side of the brainstem lesion). The presence of nystagmus in combination with ataxia, dysconjugate eye movements, face or limb weakness, sensory disturbance, or isolated vertical nystagmus suggests a lesion in the posterior fossa.

The corneal response may be depressed and facial sensation altered in the setting of either a brainstem or hemispheric lesion. A lower motor neuron type of facial paresis contralateral to a motor and or sensory deficit affecting the opposite side of the body is consistent with a midpontine lesion. As with the corneal response, a depressed gag response, abnormalities of palatal movement, or tongue weakness may occur with either hemispheric or brainstem lesions. Brainstem involvement is suggested when any of these abnormalities are contralateral to a motor or sensory deficit affecting the limbs or are found in association with nystagmus or ataxia.

Motor

The motor examination involves the assessment of tone, bulk, and strength. Subtle weakness can be sought by having the patient extend both arms with palms up and checking for a downward drift with pronation of the hand. Strength is generally quantitated with the Medical Research Council grading system (0, no contracture; 1, flicker contraction; 2, active movement with gravity eliminated; 3, active movement against gravity; 4, active movement against gravity and resistance; and 5, normal power).[34] Weakness in the limbs opposite to the side of cranial nerve deficits is consistent with a brainstem lesion. Similar weakness of the face, arm, and leg in the absence of a sensory disturbance suggests a contralateral subcortical lesion. Predominant weakness of the leg is consistent with a lesion affecting the parasagittal portion of the hemisphere, whereas weakness affecting the face and arm, but relatively sparing the leg, suggests a lesion involving the lateral portion of the hemisphere. Hyperreflexia, increased tone, and a plantar extensor response (Babinski sign) are consistent with a lesion affecting the corticospinal tracts. However, in the setting of acute stroke, deep-tendon reflexes and muscle tone may be depressed in the affected limbs.

Coordination

Difficulties with coordination may be caused by weakness or a sensory deficit affecting the same limb. In the absence of a sensorimotor deficit, difficulty with coordination involving the limbs on one side of the body suggests a lesion affecting the ipsilateral cerebellar hemisphere. Although more difficult to interpret, coordination difficulties in association with an ipsilateral sensory or motor deficit may indicate a subcortial hemisphere or brainstem lesion.

Sensation

Sensation can be difficult to assess in stroke patients, particularly in the presence of a language or cognitive impairment. In patients with intact primary sensory modalities (pin-prick, light touch, proprioception, and vibration), it may be appropriate to test secondary modalities that can be abnormal in the setting of a cortical lesion (two-point discrimination, stereognosis [identification of objects placed in the patient's hand without visual clues], and graphesthesia [identification of numbers drawn on the skin]).[35] However, detailed sensory testing can be time-consuming and may not add significantly to the data required for initial management decisions.

Gait

Gait should be tested very cautiously in patients with acute stroke. Even minor positionally related changes in blood pressure may worsen an acute ischemic lesion. Gait may need to be tested in patients complaining of a gait disturbance in the absence of other findings. Isolated gait ataxia may indicate a midline cerebellar lesion. This finding should not be missed, as expansion of a cerebellar hematoma or infarction can lead to brainstem compression or obstructive hydrocephalus.

RELIABILITY OF THE NEUROLOGICAL EXAMINATION

Some portions of the neurological examination are more reliably assessed than others (see Ref. 36 for a complete discussion). For example, level of consciousness can be assessed with nearly perfect reliability, depending on the method of measurement. The precision of motor performance ratings range from slight to almost perfect, also depending on the method of measurement. In contrast, findings on physical examination that require special care or subjective judgment, such as the assessment of sensory deficits, tend to be less reliable. It is important to note that physician performance in evaluating stroke patients can be improved with training; several studies have addressed this question.[3,22,37,38] For example, a significant effect of participation in an ongoing research program is observed with improvements in global diagnostic accuracy from 61% to 87%.[3] The use of a training system using videotapes and written materials demonstrated that physicians could improve their overall rate of agreement from 41% before to 71% after training.[38] Using these standardized training methods, generalist physicians and nurses can rapidly learn to perform a reliable basic neurological assessment.[39]

In practice, anatomic diagnosis for neurologic conditions relies on the pattern of abnormal and normal findings, rather than on a single finding. For example, a right-handed patient with unilateral right facial and limb weakness might have a lesion affecting contralateral central motor pathways at any level of the neuraxis above the midpons. However, when this finding is combined with the presence of an aphasia, the clinician recognizes that the patient's deficit is the result of a lesion affecting the dominant hemisphere. Experienced physicians consider their own views of the precision of given findings (e.g., subjective sensory abnormalities tend to be unreliable) when arriving at a specific anatomic diagnosis.

ISCHEMIC STROKE SYNDROMES[40]

Common and Internal Carotid Arteries

Because of differences in collateral blood supply to the cerebral hemisphere among individuals, the effects of occlusion of the common or internal carotid artery may be variable. Collateral supply to the cerebral hemispheres can come from the contralateral carotid circulation or vertebrobasilar system via the circle of Willis, from the ipsilateral external carotid artery via the ophthalmic artery, or through leptomeningeal anastamoses. Some individuals with an occluded carotid artery may have no symptoms.[41] Others may have only mild deficits due to ischemia affecting a localized portion of the cerebral hemisphere. Watershed infarcts may occur between middle and anterior cerebral arteries, between middle and posterior cerebral arteries, and between cortical perforators and lenticulostriate vessels.[42–44] Patients with strokes involving the entire carotid territory will have a language disturbance if the dominant hemisphere is affected (and often a hemispatial neglect if the nondominant hemisphere is affected) with an ipsilateral conjugate gaze preference and contralateral paralysis and sensory loss. Because of variations in the circle of Willis, some individuals with symptomatic carotid occlusions may have relative sparing of the anterior cerebral artery territory.[45] These patients may have a clinical presentation similar to that of patients with an MCA occlusion (see below). If the contralateral anterior cerebral artery is supplied via the occluded carotid system (because of a hypoplastic or absent ipsulateral A1 segment, which can be present in 25% of individuals[45]), in addition to the signs associated with the occluded carotid artery, the patient may have weakness of the ipsilateral leg and impaired consciousness.

Middle Cerebral Artery

The lenticulostriate vessels originate from the horizontal portion of the middle cerebral artery (MI segment) to supply subcortical structures. An upper division of the middle cerebral artery (MCA) supplies the lateral portion of the frontal lobe and the anterior portion of the parietal lobe. A lower division supplies the posterior portion of the parietal lobe and the upper portion of the temporal lobe. Occlusions of the stem, upper division, lower division, and distal branches of the MCA are most commonly embolic.

Infarctions in the distribution of the upper division of the MCA result in a contalateral hemiparesis and a multimodal sensory deficit, variably affecting the face and arm to a greater extent than the leg. This may be accompanied by aphasia in the case of strokes affecting the dominant hemisphere and by a hemineglect syndrome in the case of strokes affecting the nondominant hemisphere. Occlusions of distal branches of these vessels may produce only portions of the entire syndrome.

Infarctions in the distribution of the lower division of the MCA may variably result in a contralateral visual field defect, hemisensory deficit, hemineglect syndrome, and in cases affecting the dominant hemisphere, aphasia. As with upper division infarctions, occlusions of distal branches of these vessels may produce only portions of the entire syndrome.

The lenticulostriate vessels supplying subcortical structures arise in medial and lateral groups. A variety of so-called lacunar syndromes have been ascribed to strokes resulting from local occlusion of these vessels (e.g., pure motor stroke, pure sensory stroke, ataxic hemiparesis, clumsy hand dysarthria).[46] In general, when a contralateral motor deficit is present, it affects the face, arm, and leg to a similar extent. Signs of a cortical deficit such as aphasia are generally absent. It is important to note that these are clinical syndromes and not pathophysiologic diagnoses. The same syndromes can also result from strokes in the vertebrobasilar distribution[47,48] and can have a variety of causes including emboli,[49,50] carotid stenosis,[51] hemorrhage,[52–54] neoplasm,[55] demyelinating disease,[55] and vascular malformations.[55]

Occlusions of the stem of the MCA can also have variable manifestations depending on the collateral circulation. Unlike occlusions of the common or internal carotid arteries, the obstruction in stem MCA occlusions is distal to the anterior communicating artery. Therefore, potential collateral flow may be more limited. If the occlusion is proximal to the origins of the lenticulostriate vessels, the stroke may affect both cortical and subcortical structures. As previously described, these strokes may be indistinguishable from infarctions resulting from carotid occlusion unless vascular imaging studies are performed.

Anterior Cerebral Artery

The anterior cerebral artery (ACA) has both superficial and deep territories. The superficial territory supplies the medial portions of the frontal and parietal lobe and the anterior portion of the corpus callosum. Infarctions in the ACA territory are most commonly due to emboli. ACA distribution strokes may have variable clinical manifestations including hemiparesis, mutism, and aphasia.[56] Weakness is generally more prominent than a sensory disturbance, and the leg is generally involved to a greater extent than the arm or face. The deep territory is served by numerous penetrating vessels from the stem of the ACA and supplies the anterior portion of the internal capsule, portions of the basal ganglia, and several other deep structures.[40] Infarction in this territory may be manifest by a mild, transient hemiparesis and dysarthria, agitation or abulia, and variably aphasia or a hemineglect syndrome.[40]

Anterior Choroidal Artery

The anterior choroidal artery generally arises from the intracranial portion of the internal carotid artery and supplies portions of the posterior limb of the internal capsule, basal ganglia, lateral thalamus, optic radiations, mesial temporal lobe, and the red nucleus and substantia nigra in the midbrain.[40] Occlusion of this vessel generally results in a contralateral hemiparesis affecting the face, arm, and leg to a similar extent and can be caused by either local disease or emboli.[57] Other manifestations are variable and related to infarction involving the other structures supplied by the vessel. For example, there may be an associated visual-field defect if the optic radiations are involved, an associated sensory deficit if the thalamus is involved, and ataxia if the red nucleus is affected.

Vertebrobasilar System

A detailed description of all of the syndromes due to vertebrobasilar distribution infarctions is beyond the scope of this chapter (the interested reader is directed to Refs. 58–60). These vessels supply the brainstem, cerebellum, and, via the posterior cerebral arteries, the occipital and inferior portions of the temporal lobes. One set of classic findings associated with unilateral brainstem infarction includes ipsilateral cranial nerve deficits with contralateral motor or sensory deficits affecting the limbs. For example, unilateral strokes affecting the midbrain may produce an ipsilateral third-nerve palsy and contralateral hemiparesis with or without ataxia. Unilateral strokes affecting the pons may produce an ipsilateral lower motor neuron type of facial paresis, contralateral eye deviation, and a contralateral hemiparesis. Unilateral strokes affecting the medulla may include an ipsilateral Homer's syndrome, ipsilateral palatal and tongue weakness, nystagmus with prominent vertigo, and decreased pain and temperature sensibility in the ipsilateral face and contralateral limbs.

Occlusions of the vertebral artery may result in distal emboli affecting other portions of the vertebrobasilar system or cause infarctions in the distribution of the posterior inferior cerebellar artery (PICA). PICA supplies the dorsolateral portion of the medulla, and the inferior and vermial portions of the cerebellar hemisphere. The classic features of occlusion of this vessel include findings associated with unilateral medullary lesion in addition to ipsilateral ataxia due to involvement of the cerebellum. The anterior inferior cerebellar artery (AICA) arises from the basilar artery and wraps around the pons providing circumfrential penetrating vessels, and then supplies a portion of the cerebellar hemisphere. The superior cerebellar artery (SCA) arises from the basilar artery before it bifurcates to form the posterior cerebral arteries. The SCA can give branches to the ipsilateral midbrain, and supplies the superior portion of the cerebellar hemisphere. Manifestations of occlusion of this vessel include ipsilateral ataxia and dysarthria with variable involvement of the ipsilateral midbrain.

The basilar artery gives rise to multiple large and small penetrating vessels along its course, and supplies the entire dorsal portion of the pons and portions of the midbrain and cerebellum. Clinical manifestations will vary depending on whether the main trunk of the basilar artery is occluded or the occlusion is limited to paramedian or lateral penetrating vessels. The neurological deficit will also vary depending on where along the course of the basilar artery the occlusion is located. Occlusion of the main trunk of the basilar artery from either emboli or atherothrombosis can result in massive, bilateral infarctions of the basis pontis and pontine tegmentum. Such occlusions have a very high morbidity and mortality and can lead to the "locked-in" syndrome in which the patient remains conscious (because the reticular activating system travels in the tectum and has a different vascular supply) but is unable to move the limbs, talk, or even look from side to side.[61,62] These patients are still able to communicate with coded vertical eye movements. Occlusion of the basilar artery at its tip is most commonly due to emboli and may result in variable infarctions in the territories of both superior cerebellar and both posterior cerebral arteries. Such occlusions can result in visual loss, confusion, agitation, oculomotor palsies, and sensory disturbances ("top-of-the-basilar" syndrome).[63] Occlusion of paramedian perforators from the basilar artery affects the paramedian pontine nuclei and tracts and can result in contralateral hemiparesis or, with bilateral cerebellar ataxia, quadraparesis, bilateral sensory abnormalities, and eye movement abnormalities.[40] Occlusion of the lateral perforators can cause an ipsilateral conjugate gaze palsy, facial weakness, and loss of ipsilateral facial sensation with a contralateral hemiparesis and sensory loss, as previously described. In addition, occlusion limited to small penetrating vessels can lead to lacunar syndromes similar to those that can occur with occlusion of the lenticulostriate vessels.

Posterior Cerebral Artery

The posterior cerebral artery (PCA) generally arises from the rostral portion of the basilar artery. The distribution of this vessel to the superficial portions of the cerebral hemisphere has been previously described. In addition, perforating branches of the PCA may supply portions of the ipsilateral midbrain, thalamus, and lateral geniculate bodies. It is important to note that in about 15% to 22% of individuals, the PCA arises directly from the internal carotid artery (so-called fetal origin).[45] Recognition of this potential common variant is important because, in any individual, a stroke in the PCA distribution could have arisen via the carotid or vertebrobasilar systems. Superficial PCA distribution infarction generally results in contralateral hemianopsia. Memory disturbances may also occur with involvement of the inferior and mesial portions of the temporal lobe. Language disturbance may be present in cases of dominant hemisphere involvement. Occlusion of deep perforators from the PCA can result in thalamic infarction with a contralateral sensory deficit. Proximal PCA occlusions can affect both the superficial and deep territories of the vessel.

STROKE SUBTYPE DIAGNOSIS

The history in combination with findings on general and neurological examinations can help lead to a preliminary anatomic, pathophysiologic, and etiologic diagnosis. The distinction between intracerebral hemorrhage and ischemic stroke is critical for the acute management of the patient. Studies that provide information about the accuracy of history and physical examination in distinguishing hemorrhagic from ischemic strokes indicate that clinical judgment can be used to increase or decrease the likelihood of hemorrhage, but diagnostic errors occur.[3,8,10] A simple rule for the clinical diagnosis of intracranial hemorrhage is based on the presence of at least one of the following: coma on arrival, vomiting, complaint of severe headache, warfarin therapy, systolic blood pressure >220 mm Hg, and glucose >170 mg/dL in a nondiabetic patient.[8] The presence of any of these features more than doubles the odds of hemorrhage, and the absence of any of these features drops the odds by one-third. However, neuroimaging is the only reliable method of distinguishing intracerebral hemorrhage from infarction and is mandatory to guide further management, especially if the use of anticoagulants or thrombolytics is a consideration.

The diagnosis of ischemic stroke subtype in the acute setting has proven problematic. The distinction may be irrelevant to a decision with regard to the use of t-PA (see Chap. 16).[64] However, an accurate diagnosis may be important for subsequent management, including tertiary prevention. For example, a patient with an MCA stem occlusion and a cardioembolic source who does not have evidence of carotid artery stenosis is diagnosed with an embolic stroke and may require long-term anticoagulation to prevent recurrent emboli (see Chap. 23). A patient with a nondisabling carotid distribution stroke with ipsilateral high-grade stenosis of the carotid artery may benefit from carotid endarterectomy (see Chap. 26). A patient with threatened basilar artery occlusion may require acute anticoagulation or be a candidate for thrombolytic therapy in an attempt to prevent progression to a locked-in syndrome (see Chap. 14). Even with the use of strict diagnostic rules in addition to the results of routine neuroimaging studies, differences between the initial and final (after complete diagnostic evaluation) ischemic stroke subtype diagnosis frequently occur.[65] In one such study, the initial and final diagnoses differed in 40% of 20 pairs of diagnoses by two physicians.[65] Most of these differences were due to changes from a specific stroke type to "undetermined etiology" because subsequent laboratory studies did not show supportive findings or provide data suggesting more than one potential cause. The TOAST investigators have divided ischemic stroke based on presumed mechanism into six groups (Table 2).[65] Specific diagnostic criteria have been developed to aid the diagnosis.[65] Stroke subtype diagnosis is moderately reliable when these criteria are used by experienced investigators.[66] However, the initial subtype diagnosis based on clinical features and baseline CT scan agreed with the final diagnosis at 3 months in only 62% of patients.[67] Thus, ischemic stroke subtype is often never established with certainty, and acute and long-term therapeutic decisions must often be made with the knowledge that the ischemic stroke subtype diagnosis may be inaccurate.

INITIAL LABORATORY STUDIES

A neuroimaging study is generally employed to exclude processes that may mimic stroke and to determine whether the patient's stroke-related deficit is due to ischemia or hemorrhage. Either brain CT scan or MRI is used for this purpose. In one study, routine CT scan revealed evidence of disorders other than stroke in 4% of cases.[68] A recent randomized, controlled trial of a neuroprotective agent to be given within 6 hours of carotid distribution ischemic stroke did not require a prerandomization CT scan.[69] Seventeen percent of patients were withdrawn from the target population analysis because the CT scan demonstrated hemorrhage or vertebrobasilar-territory stroke.

Routine laboratory studies including a complete blood count, serum electrolytes, sedimentation rate, urinalysis, coagulation profile, and chest x-ray are used to exclude concomitant medical problems common in stroke patients and common in the elderly. It is important to remember that patients with metabolic abnormalities such as alterations in blood glucose[70] or systemic infections can present with symptoms suggestive of acute stroke. Electrocardiography and serum cardiac enzymes are employed to exclude ischemic cardiac disease, cardiac arrhythmia, and conduction abnormalities. Additional cardiac evaluation often includes prolonged cardiac monitoring and/or transthoracic and/or transesophageal echocardiography. Depending on the individual patient, noninvasive evaluation of the extracranial cervical vessels may be performed with ultrasonography, or more recently, magnetic resonance or CT angiography. Selected patients may undergo cerebral angiography.

SUMMARY

The initial clinical evaluation of the stroke patient is critical for acute and long-term management. Clinical findings may be suggestive of stroke type, but neuroimaging is required to accurately determine whether the patient has had an intracerebral hemorrhage or ischemic stroke and to help exclude other possible causes of an acute focal neurological deficit. The early detection of patients with progressive symptoms may result in specific interventions. As will be discussed in the chapters that follow, knowledge of the presumed stroke mechanism is an important guide for therapy.

REFERENCES

1. Fieschi C, Argentino C, Lenzi GL, Sacchetti ML, Toni D, Bozzao L. Clinical and instrumental evaluations of patients with ischemic stroke within the first six hours. J Neurol Sci 1989; 91:311–322.
2. Bozzao L, Bastianello S, Fantozzi LM, Angeloni U, Argentino C, Fieschi C. Correlation of angiographic and sequential CT finding in patients with evolving cerebral infarction. AJNR 1989; 10:1215–1212.
3. Von Arbin M, Britton M, De Faire U, Helmers C, Miah K, Murray V. Accuracy of bedside diagnosis in stroke. Stroke 1981; 12:288–293.
4. Norris JW, Hachinski VC. Misdiagnosis of stroke. Lancet 1982, 1:328–331.
5. Libman RB, Wirkowski E, Alvir J, Rao TH. Conditions that mimic stroke in the emergency department. Arch Neurol 1995; 52:1119–1122.
6. Wolf PA, Kannel WB, McGee DL. Epidemiology of strokes in North America. In: Barnett HJM, Mohr JP, Stein BM, Yatsu FM, eds. Stroke. Pathophysiology, Diagnosis and Management. New York: Churchill Livingstone, 1986:19–29.
7. Heros RC. Preoperative management of the patient with a ruptured intracranial aneurysm. Semin Neurol 1984; 4:430–438.
8. Panzer RJ, Feibel JH, Barker WH, Griner PF. Predicting the likelihood of hemorrhage in patients with stroke. Arch Intern Med 1985; 145:1800–1803.
9. Caplan LR. Diagnosis and treatment of ischemic stroke. JAMA 1991; 266:2413–2418.
10. Gross CR, Shinar D, Mohr JP, et al. Interobserver agreement in the diagnosis of stroke type. Arch Neurol 1986; 43:893–898.
11. Futty DE, Conneally PM, Dyken ML, et al. Cooperative study of hospital frequency and character of transient ischemic attacks. V. Symptom analysis. JAMA 1977; 238:2386–2390.
12. Bogousslavsky J, Regli F. Cerebral infarction with transient signs (CITS): do TIAs correspond to small deep infarcts in internal carotid artery occlusion? Stroke 1984; 15:536–539.
13. Bogousslavsky J, Regli F. Cerebral infarct in apparent transient ischemic attack. Neurology 1985; 35:1501–1503.

14. Levy DE. How transient are transient ischemic attacks? Neurology 1988; 38:674–677.
15. Werdelin L, Juhler M. The course of transient ischemic attacks. Neurology 1988; 38:677–680.
16. European Carotid Surgery Trialists' Collaborative Group. MRC European Carotid Surgery Trial: interim results for symptomatic patients with severe (70–99%) or with mild (0–29%) carotid stenosis. Lancet 1991; 337:1235–1243.
17. North American Symptomatic Carotid Endarterectomy Trial Collaborators. Beneficial effect of carotid endarterectomy in symptomatic patients with high-grade carotid stenosis. N Engl J Med 1991; 325:445–453.
18. Mayberg MR, Wilson E, Yatsu F, et al. Carotid endarterectomy and prevention of cerebral ischemia in symptomatic carotid stenosis. JAMA 1991; 266:3289–3294.
19. Barnett HJM. Aspirin in stroke prevention: an overview. Stroke 1990; 21(suppl IV):40–43.
20. Gent M, Blakely JA, Easton JD, et al. The Canadian American Ticlopidine Study (CATS) in thromboembolic stroke. Lancet 1989; 1:1215–1220.
21. Hass WK, Easton JD, Adams HP Jr, et al. A randomized trial comparing ticlopidine hydrochloride with aspirin for the prevention of stroke in high-risk patients. N Engl J Med 1989; 321:501–507.
21a. CAPRIE Steering Committee. A randomized, blinded, trial of clopidogrel versus aspirin in patients at risk of ischemic events. Lancet 1996; 348:1329–1339.
21b. Diener H, Cunha L, Forbes C, Sivenius J, Smets P, Lowenthal A. European Stroke Prevention Study 2. J. Neurol. Sci 1996; 143:1–13.
22. Tomasello F, Mariani F, Fieschi C, et al. Assessment of inter-observer differences in the Italian Multicenter Study on Reversible Cerebral Ischemia. Stroke 1982; 13:32–35.
23. Kraaijeveld CL, Van Gijn J, Schouten HJA, Staal A. Interobserver agreement for the diagnosis of transient ischemic attacks. Stroke 1984; 15:723–725.
24. Calanchini PR, Swanson PD, Gotshall RA, et al. Cooperation study of hospital frequency and character of transient ischemic attacks. IV. Reliability of diagnosis. JAMA 1977; 238:2029–2033.
25. Busto R, Dietrich WD, Globus MY-T, Ginsberg MD. The importance of brain temperature in cerebral ischemic injury. Stroke 1989; 20:1113–1114.
26. Maher J, Hachinski V. Hypothermia as a potential treatment for cerebral ischemia. Cerebrovasc Brain Metab Rev 1993; 5:277–300.
27. Azzimondi G, Bassein L, Nonino F, et al. Fever in acute stroke worsens prognosis—a prospective study. Stroke 1995; 26:2040–2043.
28. Oxbury JM, Greenhall RCD, Grainger KMR. Predicting the outcome of stroke: acute stage after cerebral infarction. BMJ 1975; 3:125–127.
29. Jones HR, Millikan CH. Temporal profile (clinical course) of acute carotid system cerebral infarction. Stroke 1976; 7:64–71.
30. Jones HR Jr, Millikan CH, Sandok BA. Temporal profile (clinical course) of acute vertebrobasilar system cerebral infarction. Stoke 1980; 11:173–177.
31. Caltrider ND, Irvine AR, Kline HJ, Rosenblatt A. Retinal emboli in patients with mitral valve prolapse. Am J Ophthalmol 1980; 90:534–538.

32. Woldoff HS, Gerber M, Desser KB, Benchimol A. Retinal vascular lesions in two patients with prolapsed mitral valve leaflets. Am J Ophthalmol 1975; 79:382–385.
33. Pedersen RA, Troost BT. Abnormalities of gaze in cerebrovascular disease. Stroke 1981; 12:251–254.
34. Medical Research Council. Aids to the Examination of the Peripheral Nervous System. London: Her Majesty's Stationery Office, 1976:1.
35. Bassetti C, Bogousslavsky J, Regli F. Sensory syndromes in parietal stroke. Neurology 1993; 43:1942–1949.
36. Goldstein LB, Matchar DB. Clinical assessment of stroke. JAMA 1994; 271:1114–1120.
37. Wasson JH, Sox HC, Neff RK, Goldman L. Clinical prediction rules: applications and methodological standards. N Engl J Med 1985; 313:793–799.
38. Garraway WM, Whisnant JP, Drury I. The changing pattern of survival following stroke. Stroke 1983; 14:699–703.
39. Goldstein LB, Samsa GP. Reliability of the National Institutes of Health Stroke Scale: extension to non-neurologists in the context of a clinical trial. Stroke 1997; 28. In press.
40. Gavrilescu T, Kase CS. Clinical stroke syndromes: clinical-anatomical correlations. Cerebrovasc Brain Metab Rev 1995; 7:218–239.
41. Roederer GO, Langois YE, Jager KA, et al. The natural history of carotid arterial disease in asymptomatic patients with cervical bruits. Stroke 1984; 15:605–613.
42. Hupperts RMM, Lodder J, Heust–Van Raak EPM, Wilmink JT, Kessels AGH. Borderzone brain infarcts on CT taking into account the variability in vascular supply areas. Cerebrovasc Dis 1996; 6:294–300.
43. Bladin CF, Chambers BR. Clinical features, pathogenesis, and computed tomographic characteristics of internal watershed infarction. Stroke 1993; 24:1925–1932.
44. Mounier-Vehier F, Leys D, Godefroy O, Rondepierre P, Marchau M Jr, Pruvo JP. Borderzone infarct subyptes: preliminary study of the presumed mechanism. Eur Neurol 1994; 34:11–15.
45. Osborn AG. The circle of Willis. In: Introduction to Cerebral Angiography. Hagerstown: Harper & Row, 1980:143–165.
46. Fisher CM. Lacunar strokes and infarcts: a review. Neurology 1982; 32:871–876.
47. Chamorro A, Sacco RL, Mohr JP, et al. Clinical-computed tomographic correlations of lacunar infarction in the Stroke Data Bank. Stroke 1991; 22:175–181.
48. Nighoghossian N, Ryvlin P, Trouillas P, Laharotte JC, Froment JC. Pontine versus capsular pure motor hemiparesis. Neurology 1993; 43:2197–2201.
49. Ghika J, Bogousslavsky J, Regli F. Infarcts in the territory of the deep perforators from the carotid system. Neurology 1989; 39:507–512.
50. Cacciatore A, Russo LS Jr. Lacunar infarction as an embolic complication of cardiac and arch angiography. Stroke 1991; 22:1603–1605.
51. Tegeler CH, Fenglin S, Morgan T. Carotid stenosis in lacunar stroke. Stroke 1991; 22:1124–1128.
52. Azouvi P, Tougeron A, Hussonois C, Schouman-Claeys E, Bussel B, Held JP. Pure sensory stroke due to midbrain haemorrhage limited to the spinothalamic pathway. J Neurol Neurosurg Psychiatry 1989; 52:1427–1428.

53. Deleu D, De Waele J, Buisseret T. Dorsolateral pontine hemorrhage producing pure sensory stroke. Eur Neurol 1992; 32:222–224.
54. Groothuis DR, Duncan GW, Fisher CM. The human thalamocortical sensory path in the internal capsule: evidence from a small capsular hemorrhage causing a pure sensory stroke. Ann Neurol 1977; 2:328–331.
55. Arboix A, Martí-Vilalta JL. Lacunar syndromes not due to lacunar infarcts. Cerebrovasc Dis 1992; 2:287–292.
56. Bogousslavsky J, Regli F. Anterior cerebral artery territory infarction in the Lausanne Stroke Registry: clinical and etiologic patterns. Arch Neurol 1990; 47:144–150.
57. Leys D, Mounier-Vehier F, Lavenu I, Rondepierre P, Pruvo JP. Anterior choroidal artery territory infarcts: study of presumed mechanisms. Stroke 1994; 25:837–842.
58. Gillilan LA. The correlation of the blood supply to the human brain stem with clinical brain stem lesions. J Neuropathol Exp Neurol 1964; 23:78–108.
59. Caplan LR. Vertebrobasilar occlusive disease. In: Barnett HJM, Mohr JP, Stein BM, Yatsu FM, eds. Stroke: Pathophysiology, Diagnosis, and Management. New York: Churchill Livingstone, 1986:549–619.
60. Tatu L, Moulin T, Bogousslavsky J, Duvernoy H. Arterial territories of human brain: brainstem and cerebellum. Neurology 1996; 47:1125–1135.
61. Hawkes CH. Locked-in syndrome: report of seven cases. BMJ 1974; 4:379–382.
62. Nordgren RE, Markesbery WR, Fukuda K, Reeves AG. Seven cases of cerebromedullospinal disconnection: the "locked-in" syndrome. Neurology 1971; 21:1140–1148.
63. Caplan LR. "Top of the basilar" syndrome. Neurology 1980; 30:72–79.
64. Marler JR, Brott T, Broderick J, et al. Tissue plasminogen activator for acute ischemic stroke. N Engl J Med 1995; 333:1581–1587.
65. Adams HP Jr, Bendixen BH, Kappelle LJ, et al. Classification of subtype of acute ischemic stroke: definitions for use in a multicenter clinical trial. Stroke 1993; 24:35–41.
66. Gordon DL, Bendixen BH, Adams HP Jr, et al. Interphysician agreement in the diagnosis of subtypes of acute ischemic stroke: implications for clinical trials. Neurology 1993; 43:1021–1027.
67. Madden KP, Karanjia PN, Adams HP Jr, Clarke WR. Accuracy of initial stroke subtype diagnosis in the TOAST study. Neurology 1995; 45:1975–1979.
68. Britton M, Hindmarsh T, Murray V, Tyden SA. Diagnostic errors discovered by CT in patients with suspected stroke. Neurology 1984; 34:1504–1507.
69. Diener HC, Hacke W, Hennerici M, Rådberg J, Hantson L, De Keyser J. Lubeluzole in acute ischemic stroke—a double-blind, placebo-controlled phase II trial. Stroke 1996; 27:76–81.
70. Foster JW, Hart RG. Hypoglycemic hemiplegia: two cases and a clinical review. Stroke 1987; 18:944–946.

5

Laboratory Investigations in Acute Stroke

Ashfaq Shuaib
University of Alberta Hospital, Edmonton, Alberta, Canada

Anil Narang
George Washington University Medical Center, Washington, DC

INTRODUCTION

A number of recent advances have tremendously improved our ability to diagnose acute stroke. The introduction of cranial computed tomography (CT) scans in the early 1970s,[1,2] magnetic resonance imaging (MRI) in1980s,[3] and improvements in Doppler technology[4] have greatly enhanced our ability to confirm localization, rule out a primary hemorrhage, and define a possible etiology with very little discomfort or danger to the patient.

Acute cerebral infarction is a dynamic process. In the initial hours after an ischemic stroke the patient's condition is very unstable. Ischemia research has shown that neuronal damage is not complete at the onset of symptoms as had been previously suspected.[5] The final functional outcome may be determined by a variety of factors including fluctuations in arterial pressure, development of aspiration pneumonia, changes in serum glucose and electrolytes, body and cerebral temperature, and time to reestablishment of blood flow.[6,7] The central region (most distant territory from the occluded artery) shows irreversible necrosis early after the onset of symptoms. There is convincing experimental PET evidence that the damage in the tissue surrounding the "core of the infarction" may continue for several hours and is not complete even 24 hours after occlusion of a major artery.[8] This provides a prolonged potential treatment window. With the availability of potent experimental medications that may limit the size of an ischemic infarction and improve outcome, it has become essential to confirm the diagnosis early, rule out other etiologies that may cause confusion, and determine whether neuronal tissue is irreversibly damaged after onset of symptoms.[9]

This chapter begins with an outline of the standard nonneurological investigations that requires consideration in most patients. This is followed by a suggested plan for neurological investigations. Essential tests are discussed at the start and optional procedures that may be required in patients when diagnosis is not clear are discussed towards the end of the chapter.

DIAGNOSTIC APPROACH IN THE EMERGENCY DEPARTMENT

Despite being a common condition, investigations during an acute stroke have not been standardized and are often very haphazard. The urgency for proceeding with the investigation depends on several factors. When the time of onset of symptoms is available and the patient presents within hours of the ictus, several tests require completion and interpretation within an hour or less of presentation to the hospital. The concept of a "brain attack team" needs to be considered in hospitals that evaluate and manage a large number of patients with acute stroke. This will ensure that most major investigations are completed rapidly. The team should consist of physicians from the emergency department, radiology, neurology, and neurosurgery. Ideally a nurse-manager should supervise the program.

Essential Investigations

Nonneurological Investigations

As with all emergencies, a standard approach for every patient is essential and should include the ABCs. All patients require an electrocardiogram, chest x-ray, blood pressure measurement, and routine blood chemistry and hematology studies (including electrolytes, glucose, complete blood count, prothrombin time (PT), and partial thromboplastin time (PTT). The electrocardiogram (EKG) may provide information on the presence of arrhythmias, recent cardiac ischemia, hypertension, or left atrial enlargement. The yield on electrocardiography depends on the presence or absence of underlying heart disease. Abnormalities may be detected in 90% of patients with known heart disease, versus 17% of patients with no history of heart disease.[10] If the EKG is abnormal, continuous monitoring of cardiac rhythm is essential. Cardiac monitoring may also be important to help exclude intermittent arrhythmias, especially atrial fibrillation. Echocardiography should be considered urgently only if cardioembolism is strongly suspected and immediate confirmation may result in change of therapy.[11] Otherwise the test may be done at a later stage when the patient is stable.

There is no evidence that routine use of supplemental oxygen is of any benefit acutely after an acute stroke. There is experimental evidence that it may in fact be harmful to the brain by enhancing the generation of oxygen free radicals.[12] If hypoxia is suspected, blood gases should be ordered immediately and treatment initiated if hypoxia is detected. Hypoxemia may accelerate neuronal injury in the penumbra region. If the blood pressure is high or EKG reveals abnormalities, the patient requires continuous monitoring of blood pressure.[13,14] It is our practice to monitor blood pressure and cardiac rhythm in all patients admitted with a diagnosis of an ischemic stroke for the initial 48 hours. This may be especially important in patients with labile blood pressure.

Temperature measurements have received limited attention in the literature. It has been suggested that elderly patients with acute infections may have an increased risk of stroke.[15] Fever may also adversely affect outcome after a stroke. In a recent study, there was a significantly better outcome in patients with lower temperature on admission to hospital.[16] Although firm recommendation on the use of hypothermia may be premature, aggressive management of fever is advisable. Routine hematological studies may reveal anemia, platelet dysfunction, or a prolonged partial prothrombin time. Such abnormalities may account for the rare cause of stroke.

Other nonneurological investigations that should be considered in acute stroke include erythrocyte sedimentation rate (ESR) and urinalysis. In patients with a possible hypercoagulable state, antiphospholipid antibodies, protein C, protein S, and antithrombin III may be useful.[17] Such tests should also be considered in the young stroke patient, especially if no other etiology is apparent. Patients with sickle cell disease may need special tests. For other possible hypercoagulable states, please refer to Table 1.

Aspiration pneumonia is a common complication of acute stroke and may be seen in at least 20 to 30% of patients with an acute hemispheric stroke.[18,19] The risk is higher in patients with brain-stem stroke, bilateral strokes, and large hemispheric stroke. The presence of cranial nerve palsies, abnormal cough, and gag reflex increases the risk of aspiration. As the aspiration may frequently be silent, patients at risk must be identified early. Patients with large strokes (especially if there is a history of a previous contralateral infarction) should generally be offered nothing by mouth for the initial 24 hours after the stroke. Whenever possible a barium swallow study should be done. Patients with an abnormal study should be fed thickened fluids and soft solids for the initial several days after swallowing improves. Some patients may require gastrostomy tube feeding if the airway protection remains defective.

It is not necessary to investigate for venous thrombosis in all patients with acute stroke.[20] The use of low-dose heparin is strongly encouraged to reduce the risk of venous thrombosis. Most patients with thrombosis in the leg vein may not have the classic signs (swelling, pain, and redness) and therefore may go undetected. In patients with severe leg weakness, especially if they are not on heparin, any suggestion of venous thrombosis should be investigated with Dopplers or venography.[20]

Table 1 Hypercoagulable states which increase the risk of stroke

A. Conditions that may be seen in the young patient
   1. Anti-thrombin III deficiency
   2. Protein C deficiency
   3. Protein S deficiency
   4. Sickle cell disease
B. Conditions that can occur at any age
   1. Antiphospholipid antibodies
   2. Polycythemia vera
   3. Thrombocytosis
   4. Hypercoagulable state seen with malignancy
C. Conditions that may increase the risk of stroke (uncertain link)
   1. Plasminogen deficiency
   2. Plasminogen activator deficiency
   3. Factor XII deficiency
   4. Prekallikrein deficiency
   5. Paroxysmal nocturnal hemoglobinuria
   6. Acquired hypercoagulable platelets
D. Other hypercoagulable states.
   1. Pregnancy and oral contraceptives
   2. Thrombotic thrombocytopenic purpura
   3. Hemolytic uremic syndrome
   4. Disseminated intravascular coagulation
   5. Macroglobinemia
   6. Cryoglobinemia

The combination of Venereal Disease Research Laboratory (VDRL) and *Treponema pallidum* hemagglutination (TPHA) are the best means of detecting active syphilis. CNS syphilis, however is, a very rare cause of stroke and we do not recommend that the test be done in every patient. Urinalysis may detect bladder/kidney infection, diabetes, or other renal problems.

Essential Neurological Investigations

One important investigation that needs to be completed early after onset of symptoms is a cranial CT scan. Carotid Doppler study would help in separating patients who require further investigations for assessment of carotid stenosis. In some patients MRI/MR angiography, CT angiography, arterial angiography, echocardiography, and transcranial Doppler (TCD) blood flow studies may be helpful. These latter tests are not routine and are ordered if the diagnosis is unclear.

Cranial CT Scanning. Cranial CT has been the most significant advance in stroke diagnosis in the last 50 years. It permits the rapid distinction between an ischemic infarction and a hemorrhage. This differentiation is crucial before anticoagulants or thrombolytics can be offered to the patient. In this regard CT is superior to MRI.

CT scan is most often normal in the initial hours after the infarction. Newer CT machines have greatly improved detection, but the technology does not match the MRI ability for both early and late detection of an acute stroke. CT scans very rarely show an infarction in the initial 3 hours after an acute stroke. After 6 hours CT may show the lesion in less than a third of patients, and at 12 hours almost 50% of patients show evidence of an infarction. The location and size of the infarction are important. Over 90% of moderate to large supratentorial infarctions can be detected within 24 hours.[21] Smaller lacunar or brainstem/cerebellar infarction may escape detection in most patients.[22]

A subtle loss of gray-white matter differentiation is the earliest indicator of a cortical infarction. This and a mild hypodensity are important markers that may become evident in the initial 8 hours and offer first clues of a cortical infarction on CT scan.[23] A loss of density in the lentiform nucleus,[24] loss of density contrast in the insular cortex,[25] and hemispheric sulcal effacement[23] are other early markers seen in some patients. Over the subsequent 2 to 3 days, the infarction becomes more distinct and defines its sharp borders and characteristic wedge shape configuration in cortical infarction. The development of early hypodensity on CT scan (<4 hours) is predictive of hemorrhagic transformation.[26] While it is possible to detect hypodensity on CT scan, it is very difficult to estimate the ultimate size of the infarction with the early study within hours of the event. If, however, the CT scan shows a completed infarction in the MCA territory early after onset of symptoms, the findings may be very useful in deciding against thrombolytic therapy (see below).

A hyperdense middle cerebral artery (MCA) may sometimes be evident in the initial hours and is often helpful in diagnosis. It is highly specific but not a very sensitive sign of an acute ischemic stroke. This sign may be seen in up to 50% of patients with a proximal MCA occlusion and is very helpful with diagnosis (Fig. 1).[27,28] This is most frequently seen in the proximal segment of the MCA, is usually secondary to an acute thrombus or embolus in this region, and usually resolves within days. When seen in association with attenuation of the lentiform nucleus and loss of the insular ribbon, the hyperdense sign indicates a large MCA infarction, generally with a poor prognosis.[23]

Cerebral edema is generally not evident in the initial 24 hours. Its extent and severity are variable but are more severe in larger infarctions and with embolic disease. Edema may be more severe in patients with hyperglycemia.[29,30] Early signs for cerebral edema include effacement of sulci and the sylvian fis-

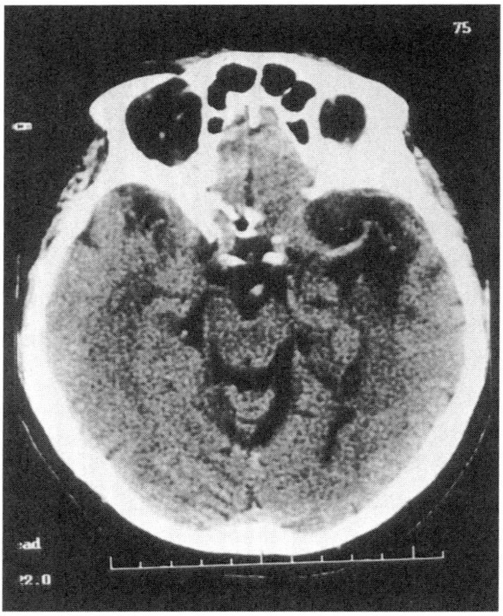

Figure 1 Axial cuts through the brain at the level of the middle cerebral artery. The middle cerebral artery on the left side shows an approximately 1-cm lesion which is hyperdense. This most frequently indicates a thrombus occluding the proximal MCS. For more details see text.

sure and a decrease in size of the ipsilateral ventricle. Edema involves both the gray and white matter and is restricted to the zone of the infarction. The edema pattern may be helpful in differentiation from brain tumor, which rarely involves the gray matter. It is important to recognize cerebral edema in patients with infarction in the cerebellum. The swelling can result in compression of the fourth ventricle and sudden increase in intracranial pressure. In the latter situation, obstruction to the CSF flow may produce acute hydrocephalus and brainstem compression or upward brain herniation. Brain edema usually subsides in 2 to 3 weeks. Sequential scans may be required in patients with acute stroke and decreasing level of consciousness to track the changes in cerebral edema.

The prognostic value of brain swelling has not been well studied. In a single study from Germany, there was a fatal outcome in 70% of patients with early focal brain swelling in the MCA distribution.[31]

Contrast infusion may sometimes be helpful in determining the age of a recent cerebral infarction. For the initial 3 to 6 days there is no enhancement with contrast infusion. Over the next 2 to 3 weeks, a characteristic enhancement is evident in most infarctions (Fig. 2). The enhancement pattern is variable from patient to patient. A curvilinear band that follows the gyri is suggestive of a subacute infarction. Contrast agents are seldom required in the early hours after an acute infarction. There are reports that the use of contrast may adversely affect

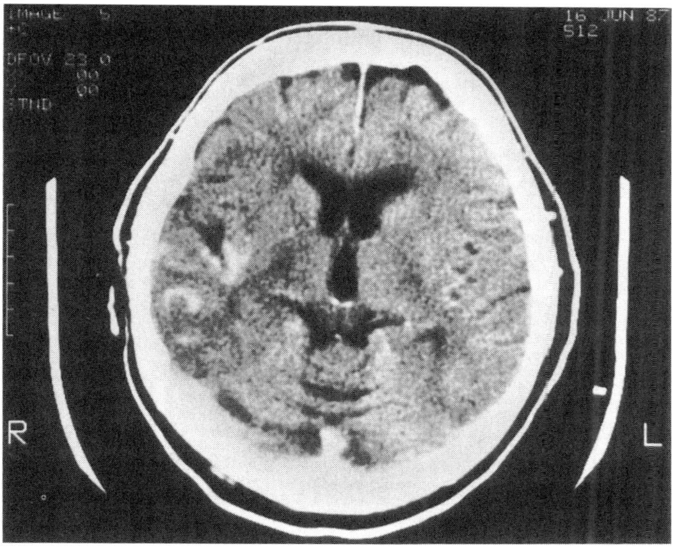

Figure 2 A typical enhancement of the borders of an infarct 1 week after the clinical event. The findings need to be differentiated from hemorrhagic transformation. In the latter instance the increased density is seen in both contrast and noncontrast.

prognosis[32] or increase edema.[33] The use of contrast agents may be necessary when the diagnosis is unclear or a neoplasm is suspected.

The location, size, and shape of a lesion identified on CT can help localize the infarction to the anterior cerebral artery (ACA), MCA, posterior cerebral artery (PCA), and other locations in the basal ganglion, thalamus, brainstem, or cerebellum. For smaller lesions, especially lacunar disease in the internal capsule or thalamus or brainstem lesions, MRI is superior to CT scans. MRI scans are, however, not widely or readily available. In most patients with lacunar disease, the history and examination are typical and therefore the MRI is seldom required. CT may show infarction within a watershed area between two major arteries. Such lesions are suggestive of hemodynamic infarction that may occur with a variety of conditions including cardiac arrhythmias, severe postural hypotension (especially in patients with cranial arterial occlusive disease), severe anemia, or thrombocytosis.

Differentiation between a primary brain hemorrhage and hemorrhage infarction is very important. In most patients with cerebral infarction, especially when secondary to an embolus, the conversion to a hemorrhagic lesion takes place over several hours to days. The underlying infarction is evident and the hemorrhage is within the vascular distribution of the stroke (Fig. 3).[34] The hemorrhage primarily involves the gray matter, with some secondary involvement of the white matter. It frequently follows the wavy contours of the cortical gyri. In contrast,

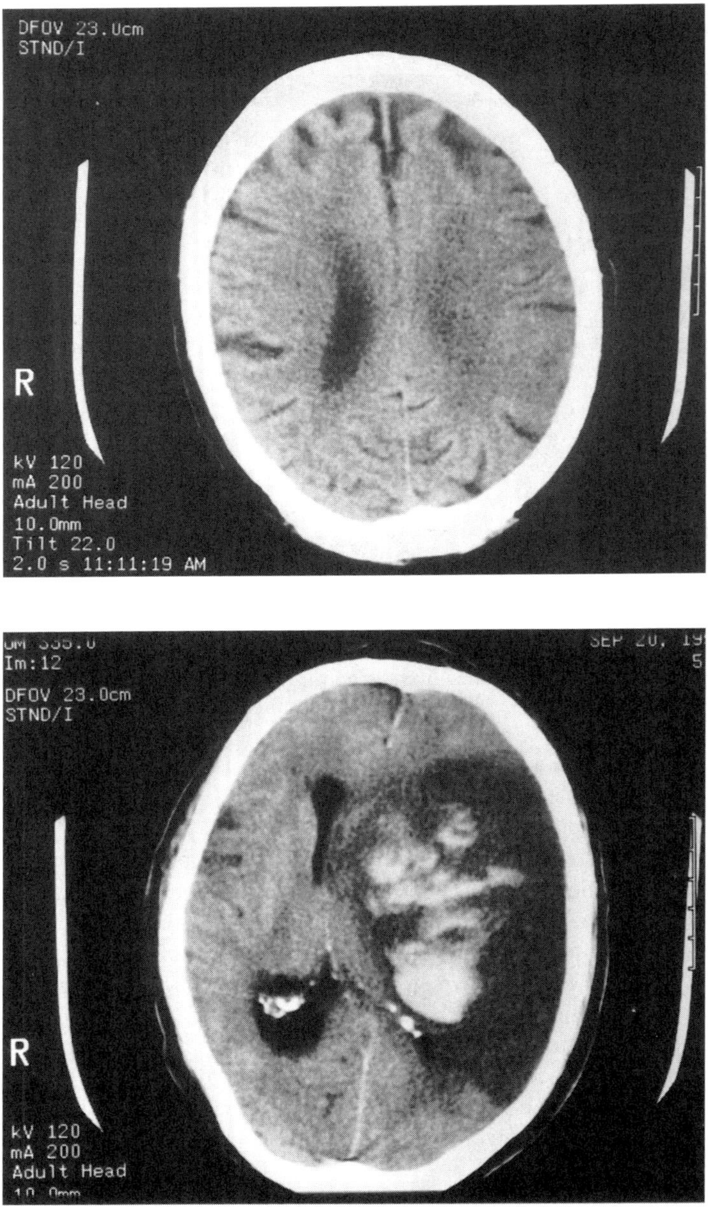

(a)

(b)

Figure 3 (a) CT scan with changes suggestive of a large infarct in the territory of the middle cerebral artery. The hypodensity affects both the gray matter and the white matter as sharply delineated from the surrounding normal tissue. (b) Three days later, the patient became drowsy and a repeat CT scan showed a large hematoma in the infarcted tissue.

a primary hematoma is a sharply demarcated, deep-sited abnormality evident from the onset of the ictus on the imaging study. However, hemorrhagic conversion may occur very early after an ischemic stroke.[35] This possibility needs to be recognized, as the underlying etiology is frequently a cardiac source and anticoagulant therapy may be required to prevent recurrences.

Computed tomography is essential in patients with acute stroke who may require treatment with tissue plasminogen activator (tPA). In addition to ruling out a hemorrhage, CT may be helpful in identifying patients at a higher risk for hemorrhage. If an infarction is clearly visible and is at least one-half the size of the MCA territory, then the age of the infarction is likely to be >3 hours or severe damage has already occurred. In such patients the risk of hemorrhage is high and the patients should not be treated with tPA. Trials are under way to determine possible benefits if treatment is initiated under 5 hours.

CT scan may at times show unexpected findings resulting in a change of diagnosis. The early hemorrhage conversion of a embolic infarction, the typical pattern of a venous infarction,[36] "direct sign" or the "delta sign" representing a clot in the sagittal sinus can be readily detected with CT scans. CT scan exposes the patient to minimal radiation and can be repeated if the clinical situation changes. Thus progression of edema or a new infarction and a hemorrhagic conversion (especially in patients on anticoagulant therapy) can easily be detected on the study.

Carotid Doppler. Patients with an acute hemispheric stroke or TIA may have severe carotid artery stenosis. Although the presence of a carotid bruit may be suggestive of an underlying stenosis, the absence of a bruit does not rule out carotid disease. In fact, many patients with severe carotid stenosis do not have bruits. Early recognition of patients with >70% stenosis is important and endarterectomy may prevent recurrences.

While there are several noninvasive methods to evaluate for carotid artery stenosis, the use of ultrasound technology has gained widespread acceptance in recent years.[37] If the test shows significant arterial narrowing, it is essential to confirm the diagnosis with cerebral angiography in surgical candidates.[38] Contrast arterial studies still remain the gold-standard for determination of the exact size and site(s) of carotid atherosclerosis (see below).[39]

There are limitations to the use of Doppler in screening for carotid atherosclerosis.[40] The Doppler imaging technique can only visualize disease in the cervical carotids and will miss more distal carotid narrowing. While the use of MR angiography and transcranial Doppler studies may improve diagnosis of intracranial disease, these tests are generally not sufficiently accurate to substitute for traditional four-vessel cerebral angiography. Doppler interpretation is dependent on the expertise of the technician who performs the test. For proper interpretation, it is essential that there be constant validation of the results of the individual Doppler laboratory.

Cerebral atherosclerosis typically affects the carotid bifurcation and the initial 2 cm of the internal carotid artery in the majority of Caucasians. Since this region is easily accessible to the Doppler probe, despite the limitations mentioned above, the procedure remains a very useful initial screening test in the evaluation of a patient presenting with an acute stroke or a TIA.

There are several different types of Doppler machines available. Ultrasound provides two types of useful information.[37] Doppler flow studies are used to detect the presence of blood flow. Flow velocity and spectral analysis are assessed to detect the presence of carotid narrowing. The B-mode imaging reveals "online" information on the contour of the blood vessel. The addition of color studies to Doppler has increased the ability to differentiate between a tight stenosis and a complete occlusion.

COLOR-DUPLEX IMAGING

The normal flow of blood in the carotid artery is laminar, resulting in a narrow-velocity spectrum. Velocity measurement, especially peak systolic velocity, is the most widely used method to gauge the severity of carotid stenosis. The velocity increases with progressive arterial narrowing until the lumen falls below 1 to 1.5 mm. Beyond this degree of narrowing, because of flow resistance, the velocity begins to fall. With milder stenosis, only the systolic velocity rises. With >50% stenosis, because of the presence of a pressure gradient, the diastolic velocity also begins to rise. The velocity readings can reliably differentiate between minor disease (<30% stenosis), moderate disease (30% to 70% stenosis), and severe disease (>70% stenosis). The B-mode study can help determine plaque composition, presence of an ulcer on the surface, intraluminal thrombus, and arterial dissection.[37,41] A fresh thrombus is not very echogenic and can therefore easily be missed. As the thrombus retracts and is invaded the fibroblasts, its echogenicity increases and becomes easier to recognize. In carotid dissections, color imaging can be very helpful in diagnosis and follow-up assessments. In most patients the diagnosis of an intraluminal thrombus or an arterial dissection requires confirmation with an arterial angiogram. The confirmation should be done rapidly as anticoagulation may be necessary for prevention of further complication in both situations. With newer color Doppler technology, it is possible to separate a very "tight" stenosis from a complete carotid occlusion by experienced technicians. The need for regular accreditation of the Doppler laboratory is important, as the procedure is very technician dependent.

Further Investigations

Additional Neurological Investigations

Cerebral Angiography. A key question that requires an early answer in patients with abnormalities on Doppler flow studies of the carotid artery is the degree of carotid stenosis. Whereas Doppler ultrasound and MRA may give an approximation of the blockage, the exact percent of stenosis can be best calculated with conventional angiography. However, angiography is an invasive procedure and should only be reserved for patients in whom a change in diagnosis would lead to a change in therapy. Besides assessing the degree of stenosis, angiography may be needed when there is clinical suspicion for an arterial dissection, aneurysm, malformation, dysplasia, or vasculitis.[42]

The most common indication for an angiogram in a patient who suffers a TIA or acute stroke is the accurate measurement of carotid stenosis. Patients with moderate and severe stenosis of the proximal internal carotid artery on Doppler flow studies should proceed to angiography. Angiography should be done as soon as possible in patients where carotid endarterectomy (CEA) is being considered, as the risk for recurrence is high in patients with severe (>70%) stenosis. Until 1991 the role of CEA was not very clear in stroke prevention. The results of the North American Symptomatic Carotid Endarterctomy Trial (NASCET) clearly indicate that in patients with recent symptoms in the distribution of the carotid artery and >70% carotid stenosis, CEA significantly reduces the risk of recurrence.[43,44] The precise measurement of the stenosis is important. The NASCET measurement calculates the percentage difference between the poststenotic normal diameter of the internal carotid minus the diameter at the stenosis multiplied by 100 to get the percentage stenosis (Fig. 4). In addition, angiography also shows the anatomy of the distal circulation. Information on the distal circulation is important, as the presence of more distal carotid stenosis or narrowing in the MCA would be a contraindication for CEA.

In addition to estimating the degree of carotid stenosis, angiography is also the best method of evaluating morphology of the diseased vessel. The presence of a thrombus can increase the risk of complications with CEA. Such thrombi can readily be diagnosed by angiography.[45] Cerebral angiography can also be very useful in the diagnosis of an arterial dissection (Fig. 5). Dissections are a common cause of stroke in the young. Often more than one lesion may be present and the dissection can involve any of the extracranial or intracranial arteries. For follow-up, MR angiography may be an alternative to contrast angiography. In the young, strokelike symptoms may develop secondary to cerebral vasculitis (Fig. 6) and can be identified on angiography.

In acute stroke the most common mechanism for the injury is an artery-to-artery or heart-to-artery embolus. If the study is being done to assess occlu-

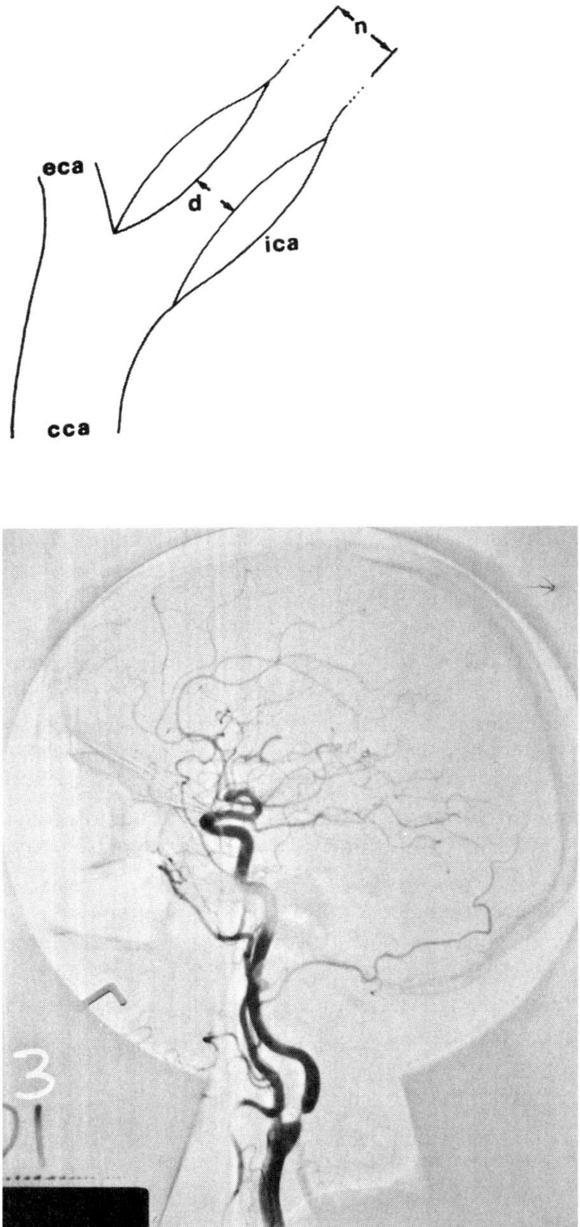

Figure 4 NASCET formula for calculating the size of carotid artery stenosis. The site of maximum stenosis is: a-[a/n] × 100%. Abbreviations: ica, internal carotid artery; cca, common carotid artery; eca, external carotid artery.

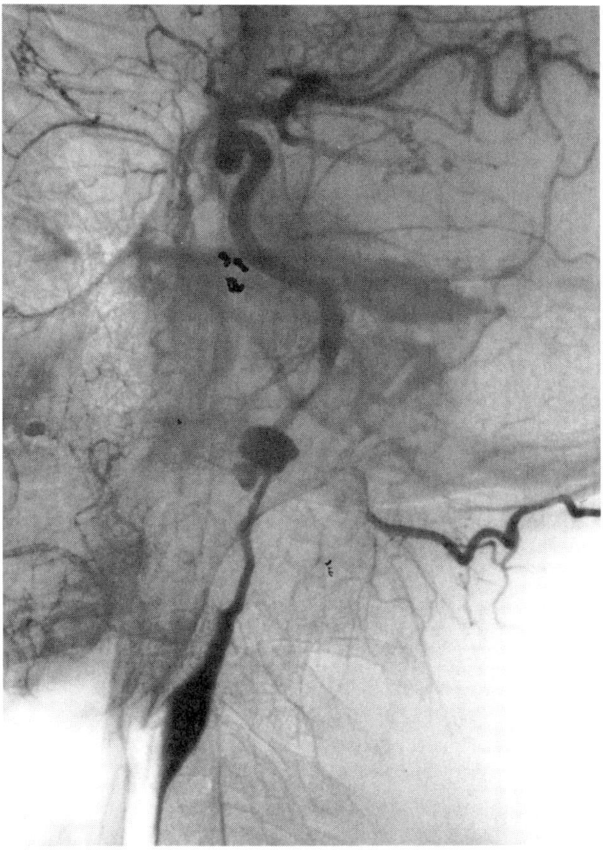

Figure 5 Carotid artery dissection distal to the carotid bifurcation. There is a narrowing of the arterial lumen "pseudo" aneurysm at the region of maximum narrowing. Distally, the vessel is of normal caliber.

sion, the timing of angiography is very important. The abrupt occlusion in an intracranial vessel can be evident on the study in >80% of patients if the study is done within 4 to 6 hours of the stroke.[46] However if the study is delayed to >24 to 48 hours, 25% of patients would have a cutoff suggestive of the embolic occlusion.[47] Presumably, spontaneous thrombolysis reopens the vessel during this time.

Cerebral angiography is an invasive procedure and may produce local or systemic complications. Focal neurological symptoms may result from dislodgment of a thrombus. There are no data indicating that the risk of complications may be higher if the procedure is done early after a stroke. The complications may be higher in elderly patients with advanced atherosclerosis. Many patients

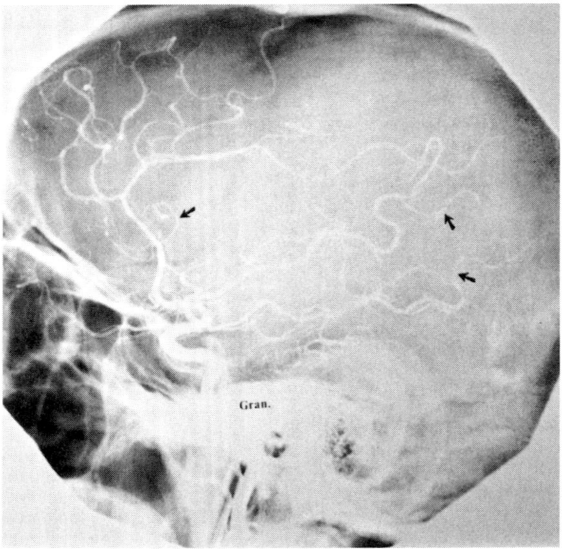

(a)

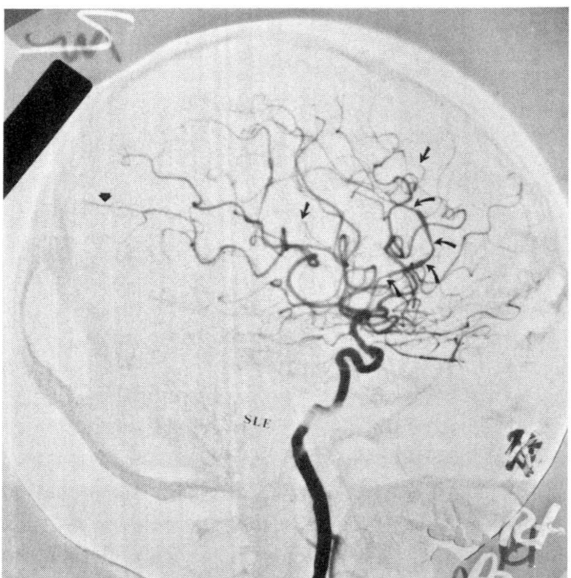

(b)

Figure 6 (a) Cerebral angiogram in a patient with narrowing and "glass-beading" of multiple vessels in the distribution of the middle cerebral artery. The black arrows highlight these sections of "narrowing and dilatation" that are seen very characteristically in CNS vasculitis. The findings are, however, by no means specific for vasculitis but may also be seen in a number of other conditions including multiple emboli, radiation-induced

may be on anticoagulants or antiplatelet agents. This may lead to local complications, which may be as high as 6%.[48] More importantly, transient (4%) and permanent (1%) complications or death (0.1%) can also develop as a direct result of the test. The test should therefore be considered only if definite indications exist and the complications have been well explained to the patient.

Magnetic Resonance Imaging. MRI has better resolution than CT and is particularly useful if small infarction or posterior fossa lesion is suspected. MRI also permits evaluation of the major intracranial blood vessels. MRI is seldom needed acutely after an acute stroke. The technology is rapidly improving, however, and its ability to define an acute infarction within a few hours of the event may prove very useful for diagnosis when treatment with newer, expensive, potentially dangerous medications are being considered.

In patients with an acute stroke, spin density-weighted (SDW), T2-weighted, and T1-weighted sequences should be completed. Within 24 hours after an infarction, 80% of ischemic strokes are visible on MRI (compared to 60% on CCT).[49] Lesions are best seen on SDW- and T2-weighted images. The increased signal is particularly evident in the gray matter and in deeper structures. The earliest lesion is usually a swelling of the gray matter with no changes in the white matter. Parenchymal enhancement is seen early and may be extensive by the second or third day after the stroke.[50] Intravascular enhancement may be seen in at least 75% of patients and may be more striking than enhancement on CCT.[50] The mechanism for parenchymal enhancement is not clear but may be related to abnormalities in the blood-brain barrier. During the follow-up the edema reabsorbs and the enhancement pattern returns toward normal. This usually occurs 4 to 6 weeks after onset. The changes in the SDW- and T2-weighted images are a result of neuronal cell death and are permanent.

An important indication for imaging after an acute stroke is to differentiate an ischemic from a hemorrhagic infarction. The presence of a hemorrhage may caution against the use of anticoagulant or thrombolytic therapy. A decreased signal on T2-weighted image is a typical finding. For diagnosis of acute hematoma, CCT is very sensitive and should remain the investigation of choice.

By its ability to detect small lesions, MRI may also be useful in the diagnosis of the underlying etiology (Fig. 7). When multiple ischemic lesions, especially of different ages, are found on MRI, one should consider the possibility of emboli from the heart. This may be particularly important if the remainder of

---

Continued damage, infections, and vasospasm. (b) Angiogram with narrowing and poststenotic dilatation in multiple branches of the middle cerebral artery in a patient with systemic lupus erythematosus. Again, similar to findings in Figure 6(a), these findings are not specific and may be seen in a variety of other conditions. Clinical examination and associated laboratory findings are therefore important in making a diagnosis.

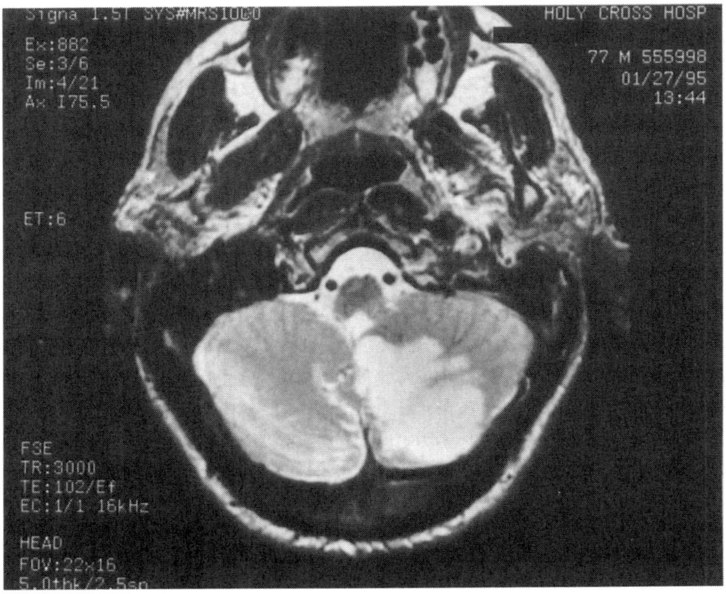

Figure 7 MRI with T2-weighted image through the posterior fossa at the level of the cerebellum. There is a clearly demarcated area of increased signal in the cerebellum, indicating an infarct. The image was obtained 8 hours after the clinical event. MRI is superior to CT scan in imaging the posterior fossa.

investigations is either normal or shows nondiagnostic changes. In one study, the presence of multiple infarctions on MRI was highly suggestive of cardioembolism, and therapy was changed to anticoagulation based on the results of the MRI.[51]

An exciting development in MRI in recent years is the ability to diagnose an acute ischemic stroke very soon after onset of symptoms with the technique of diffusion-weighted imaging. Diffusion imaging utilizes pulse sequences that are sensitive to small changes in the movement of water molecules. Experimental evidence indicates that changes secondary to ischemia can be differentiated from the normal background as early as 1 hour after the insult.[52] Clinically, the most important indication for the use of diffusion-MRI technology would be the separation of acute stroke from nonischemic mimickers. This becomes very important when thrombolytic therapy is being considered hyperacutely after a stroke.

Similar to diffusion-MRI, perfusion-MRI is a new technique that assesses cerebral blood flow and may also prove useful in defining the pathophysiology of an acute ischemic stroke. The perfusion image is performed after injection of the contrast medium (for example, gadolinium). Gadolinium causes inhomogeneity of the magnetic field, and the changes thus detected provide information on cerebral blood flow. With the development of echoplanar imaging several images can be obtained,[53] and it would become possible to improve perfusion-MRI technology to be clinically applicable.

Magnetic Resonance Angiography. Doppler is a very useful method to screen for proximal carotid stenosis. MRA technology provides a characteristic flow void over blood vessels. This is secondary to the motion of blood cells which would miss the second radiofrequency pulse, and registers as a "flowvoid" on the image.[54] There are several techniques to evaluate disease in the blood vessels. For most studies, the time-of-flight technique (TOF) is used.[55,56] The two-dimensional TOF MRA is most useful in the neck, where a wide range of velocity changes can be measured with the study. A major problem is in that the degree of stenosis may be overestimated. A number of conditions, including vessel wall motion, partial volume averaging, and shortcomings of image reconstruction may lead to such an error.[57,58] With improvements in imaging, the correlation with conventional angiography continues to improve. Recent studies indicate that up to 95% of stenosis of over 70% can be diagnosed with MRA and that the problems of overestimation of narrowing can be overcome with three-dimensional TOF methods.[58] MRA is noninvasive, has a relatively short time to complete the study (<15 minutes), and can image both the extracranial and intracranial circulation. It is increasingly being used as an alternative to Doppler flow studies. However, both technologies are expensive and not widely available. At present, we believe that the combination of a cranial CT and carotid Doppler ultrasound is sufficient for most patients. If, however, intracranial atherosclerosis is suspected, one may consider using MRA. This may be particularly important as diagnosis may result in alteration in therapy.

Transcranial Doppler. Transcranial Doppler (TCD) was initially tested in early 1980s for the diagnosis of intracranial disease. The cranial blood vessels can be insonated from several "windows," including the temporal (for MCA, ACA, PCA, and internal carotid), ocular (ophthalmic and internal carotid), and the foramen magnum (vertebral and basilar arteries). The procedure is noninvasive and provides "real-time" information for a variety of neurological conditions. TCD is used routinely in assessment of vasculature after SAH. The increase in velocities over time can alert the physicians to the development of impending vasospasm. The effects of medical and surgical therapy can be monitored repeatedly with TCD in such patients. The presence of stenosis in an intracranial blood vessel (especially internal carotid and MCA) can be detected and monitored. It is very useful in the detection of a PFO and can monitor for the presence of particulate emboli arising from the neck vessels or the heart. As better contrast agents become available, TCD will undoubtedly be used more frequently.

As the vast majority of occlusions in the MCA are embolic, a sudden loss of the blood flow signal is a characteristic TCD finding if the study is done early after the stroke. An absence of signal may also be caused by an artifact, poor insonation window, or poor technique. For diagnosis it is important that blood flow is detected in the ACA or the PCA. If increased blood flow is detected in the latter two arteries, this may indicate the recruitment of collateral blood flow to compensate for the occlusion. An increase of >20 cm/sec compared to the contra-lateral artery is suggestive of significantly increased flow. With long term monitoring, the artery recanalizes over the next 48 to 72 hours. TCD could also be used to track thrombolytic therapy with tPA in similar situations.[59]

In patients with a recent ischemic stroke, it is important to localize the source of the embolus. Perhaps the most important indication for the use of TCD in the acute stroke patient would be in the detection of cerebral emboli. With long-term monitoring, it is possible to detect asymptomatic particulate emboli in most patients with a cardiac source (for example, atrial fibrillation, prosthetic valves, mitral stenosis). The presence of asymptomatic emboli over each MCA with bilateral monitoring is very suggestive of a cardiac source.[60] Patients with symptomatic carotid stenosis may have ipsilateral emboli after an ischemic stroke. These often disappear with appropriate therapy.[61] Dissection of the cranial vessels is increasingly being diagnosed as a cause of stroke. TCD can be used to monitor for silent emboli in such patients. It could also be used to judge for efficacy of therapy when patients are anticoagulated.[62]

Air in the vascular system displays a typical signal on TCD. The air emboli signal can be detected best when the MCA is being monitored over time. Agitated saline (9.5 cc saline and 0.5 cc air) when introduced into the venous system can be tracked through the heart and is used to detect for the presence of a patent foremen ovale or other types of cardiac shunts.[63] In the past, the transthoracic flow of the air has been documented with a TEE or TTE. TCD can also be used to detect the shunts with little inconvenience to the patient. TCD may be used at the bedside and may be as sensitive as the cardiac test to rule out a cardiac source. A similar signal may be seen with cerebral and coronary artery angiography.[64] Such findings are unlikely to be of any major significance.

Blood Flow Studies. A variety of tests have been designed over the years to study the cerebral blood flow in the hours after a stroke. The major reason why the tests are ordered include confirmation of the diagnosis and to predict prognosis. With the need to treat stroke early, the use of such techniques may become important to separate ischemic stroke from conditions that may mimic it and cause confusion. The technology is rapidly improving and may prove very useful in emergency assessment of stroke patients.

Single-photon emission computed tomography (SPECT) uses the gamma-emitting properties of radioligands to monitor changes in blood flow. The images are computer generated and are displayed to highlight specific anatomical regions of the brain. The abnormalities evident on a SPECT scan are seen very early after an acute stroke and may help in separation of an acute stroke from a nonstructural lesion.[65,66] SPECT may, however, not differentiate between ischemic stroke and a primary brain hemorrhage. It is also possible that the risk of hemorrhage into an infarction in patients treated with tPA can also be predicted with SPECT study.[66]

Positron emission tomography (PET) was developed as a technique to study cerebral blood flow and metabolism in a variety of neurological disorders. Unfortunately, because of the extremely short half-lives of the radiolabeled compounds, cost, and time, PET has not gained widespread use in the diagnosis of acute ischemic stroke. There are important research studies in primates on the usefulness of PET studies acutely after an acute MCA occlusion. The progression of damage has been documented with serial studies and reveals very interesting findings. The extent of damage increases over time and may not be complete for 24 hours or longer after the insult.[8] Similar work in humans is lacking but is urgently needed. Unless better methods of producing compounds that can be used without the need of a cyclotron are developed, PET remains a research tool in the study of acute stroke.

Cerebrospinal Fluid Examination. Examination of the CSF is not required in most patients who present with an acute stroke. If SAH or bacterial meningitis is suspected, early CSF examination is essential. In patients with a focal neurological deficit and fever, especially if the patient has speech difficulty and drowsiness, the possibility of herpes encephalitis needs to be excluded. Together with abnormalities on CT (or MRI) and EEG, CSF may show characteristic findings that are helpful in making the diagnosis. Abnormalities include a bloody CSF with an increase in protein and lymphocytes. CSF examination may provide helpful information in patients who present with strokelike symptoms secondary to vasculitis, systemic lupus erythematosus, granulomatous angiitis, sarcoidosis, temporal arteritis, and other types of inflammatory conditions.[67] In most such conditions, there is an increase in proteins and lymphocyte count. Some chronic infections such as tertiary syphilis and meningeal tuberculosis may also cause small-vessel occlusion and cerebral infarction. Primary and secondary brain tumors may occasionally present with strokelike symptoms.[68] Some patients with meningeal carcinamatosis may present with strokelike symptoms and may require CSF examination.

Electroencephalography. EEG is not essential in most patients with an acute ischemic stroke. If done early after a stroke, EEG shows slowing over the site of the infarction or hemorrhage. The slowing does not differentiate between the two conditions and may remain abnormal for a long time. EEG abnormalities are present immediately after stroke onset, and the test may be of occasional value if the CT is normal and a stroke is suspected.[69,70] In a small percentage of patients, seizures are the presenting feature of the acute stroke. Many patients do not require an EEG as seizures seldom pose a chronic problem. If the seizures are persistent, an EEG may be helpful in defining a focus.

Evaluation for a Cardiac Source of Embolism

A potential cardiac source of embolism may be seen in at least 15% to 20%t of patients with acute ischemic stroke. Patients may also have symptomatic or asymptomatic ischemic heart disease that may require identification. Additional investigations are therefore necessary whenever a cardiac etiology is suspected. Because of the large number of possible tests, an organized approach is required. In patients where a valvular lesion or left ventricular pathology is suspected, transthoracic echocardiography (TTE) is usually sufficient. For assessment of the left atrium, left atrial appendage, and the ascending aorta, TTE may not provide sufficient detail. In such patients transesophageal echocardiography (TEE) may provide extremely useful information that may lead to a change in management. Cardiac arrhythmias are also a common cause of stroke. In the elderly, atrial fibrillation may present with a stroke. As the arrhythmia is sometimes intermittent, it may be missed on routine EKG. Common causes of cardiac embolism are presented in Table 2.

Echocardiography

In patients with an acute ischemic stroke, TTE readily identifies abnormalities associated with the mitral valve and left ventricular wall motion abnormalities.[71] The technique is noninvasive, can easily be performed, and can be repeated if initial results are not diagnostic.[72] The M-mode procedure has largely been replaced by two-dimensional TTE. The addition of Doppler and color has greatly improved the diagnostic powers of TTE. The technique has limitations. It is unable to access the left atrium or auricle. Both are common sources of emboli in patients with atrial fibrillation. TTE is unable to provide good images in patients with emphysema, obesity, pectus excavatum, or prosthetic valves, and in patients on assisted ventilation. Furthermore, the aorta cannot be adequately imaged. In

Table 2 The common causes of cardioembolic stroke

Conditions where TTE is sufficient:
Mitral valve stenosis and regurgitation
Aortic valve stenosis, regurgitation and calcification
Aortic valve vegetations
Left ventricular aneurysm or thrombus
Conditions where TEE is superior to TTE:
Atrial lesions (thrombus or tumor)
Atrial septal aneurysm
Patent foremen ovale
Aortic arch disease
Mitral valve vegetations

such patients TEE, despite its invasiveness, is very useful. Transesophegeal echocardiogaphy is also useful in assessment of the left atrium. Atrial and appendicular thrombi and septal defects can easily be missed even on good-quality TTE but can be diagnosed with TEE.

The most common echocardiographic findings in patients with an acute stroke is nonspecific anterior wall abnormalities of the left ventricle. These are not diagnostic of embolism and may be seen with recent or remote myocardial injury. The presence of a left ventricular thrombus, especially of recent onset, is a dramatic finding. Such a finding is common in patients with a recent anterior wall myocardial infarction and requires urgent anticoagulation. The thrombus can get dislodged (and produce symptoms) before the TTE study is completed. The absence of finding a thrombus on a TEE study does rule out the possibility of cardioembolic disease. If the initial study is normal, repeating the test may sometimes show a thrombus.[72]

A more frequent source of emboli from the heart is from thrombi in the left atrial appendage or the left atrium. These are particularly common in patients with mitral stenosis and an enlarged left atrium. Atrial fibrillation may be seen in many such patients. Atrial fibrillation is, however, more common in the absence of mitral valve disease. Such nonvalvular atrial fibrillation is becoming recognized as the commonest cause of embolic stroke.[73–76] The presence of spontaneous echo contrast on TEE increases the risk of embolism in patients with atrial fibrillation. TEE can identify small atrial or appendicular thrombi and has proved a very useful test in patients with stroke where other investigations are normal. Atrial septal aneurysms, atrial septal defects, and patent foramen ovale are easily diagnosed with TEE.[71] The aorta may contain severe atherosclerosis that may not be visible on other types of imaging. An increased thickness of the aortic wall is increasingly seen with ischemic stroke. Increased aortic atherosclerosis also increases the risk of recurrent stroke. Such lesions can be seen on TEE.

Echocardiography should not be routinely done all patients. In patients with no history of cardiac disease and normal chest x-ray and EKG, echocardiography would rarely provide useful information. It should also be considered in the young, in patients with multiple infarctions, and in patients where other investigations are nondiagnostic and a cardiac source cannot be ruled out. It is not very useful or cost-effective in patients with no clinical, radiological, or EKG evidence of a cardiac source of embolism.

Holter Monitoring. Cardiac monitoring is not recommended for all patients. In patients with no history of heart disease and a normal EKG, the yield on prolonged monitoring is usually very low. In unselected patients with stroke or TIAs, significant abnormalities are rarely found.[10] Holter monitoring may be useful in patients where a cardiac arrhythmia (especially intermittent atrial fibrillation or sick sinus syndrome) is suspected but routine investigations are normal.

It may also be useful when the patient has a history of palpitations or when the stroke is accompanied by loss of consciousness.

Other cardiac investigations that are being developed to evaluate for a cardiac source of embolism or for ischemic heart disease include indium-111-labeled platelet scintigraphy (to look for small thrombi), cardiac CT, and MRI scanning. These tests are not widely available and their role in the investigation of ischemic stroke is not clear. It is, however, important to remember that, despite a strong clinical suspicion, the diagnosis of embolic stroke cannot be confirmed in many patients. It is not uncommon to find no etiology for the infarction even when all investigations have been exhausted.

A DIAGNOSTIC APPROACH

Focal neurological deficit of sudden onset in the elderly is most likely to be secondary to an ischemic stroke. It is essential that an ischemic stroke be differentiated from a hemorrhage, brain tumor or other condition that may mimic the condition. Please refer to Table 3 for frequently used tests. A cranial noncontrast CT scan or MRI is the best test to rule out a hemorrhage and exclude other common conditions that may mimic an acute ischemic stroke. The next step is to look for a possible etiology of the infarction. Over 80% of ischemic strokes are embolic from the neck arteries or from the heart. Doppler studies are a useful screening tool to determine if carotid stenosis is present. In patients with moderate to severe stenosis, confirmation with cerebral angiography is frequently necessary. Angiography is also essential prior to surgery, as it provides information on the carotid bifurcation and may also detect additional, more distal arterial abnormalities. If Doppler studies show minimal disease in the neck, angiography is not necessary unless intracranial disease is suspected. In patients where intracranial disease is suspected, MRA may be a useful alternative test. It can detect abnormalities in the extracranial and intracranial vessels. MRA is also useful when a carotid or vertebral dissection is suspected. Cardiac investigations should be considered if EKG is abnormal or if CT scan shows multiple infarction in several vascular territories. It may also be required in young patients and where preliminary investigations fail to reveal an etiology. Such investigations have a low yield in patients with lacunar infarction. It is important to remember that etiology of the infarction may not be apparent in patients despite extensive investigations. Thus, the lack of an arterial stenosis or a cardiac source may often be seen and the problem is especially common in the young. Hematological investigations for a hypercoagulable state should only be done in the young or when other investigations are normal. These may also be necessary if the patient shows signs of systemic thrombosis.

Table 3 Frequently used tests in investigations of an acute ischemic stroke:

Diagnosis and differential diagnosis
1. Cranial CT scan: Most useful and widely available. Diagnostic test of choice to rule out a brain hemorrhage
2. MRI: More sensitive for detecting smaller lesions.

Investigating the etiology of the stroke
1. Carotid Doppler: Initial screening test for determination of carotid disease.
2. Cerebral Angiography: For accurate measurement of carotid stenosis or determination of intracranial disease.
3. Echocardiography: useful if CXR or EKG abnormal TTE reveals left ventricular abnormalities, TEE useful to image the left atrium, left auricle and the mitral valves.
4. Holter Monitor: useful if an intermittent cardiac arrhythmia suspected.
5. MRA: Non-invasive method to evaluate the cerebral vasculature. Useful for detecting dissections and intracranial arterial atherosclerotic disease.
6. Hematological evaluations usually of limited value. Tests for hypercoagulable state may be of value in young patients with no etiology or patients with signs of systemic thrombosis.

If initial investigations are normal, reevaluation at a later stage may be helpful. Although not usually indicated, a repeat CT scan may show the infarction not evident on the initial study. A change in clinical status may also require repeat CT to look for a possible hemorrhagic transformation or reinfarction. Cardiac investigations may also show a potential source that was not evident on the initial evaluation.

REFERENCES

1. Villafana T. Physics and instrumentation: computed tomography. In: Lee SH, Rao KC, Zimmerman RA. eds. Cranial MRI and CT. 3rd ed. New York: McGraw-Hill, 1992:1–39.
2. Ambrose J. Computerized transverse axial scanning tomography: clinical applications. Br J Radiol 1973; 46:1023–1047.
3. Crooks LE, Orendahl D, Kaufman L. Clinical efficiency of nuclear magnetic resonance imaging. Radiology 1983; 146:123
4. Zwiebel WJ. Duplex examination of the carotid arteries. Semin Ultrasound CT MR 1990; 11:97–135.
5. Obrenovitch TP. The ischemic penumbra: twenty years on. Cerebrovasc Brain Metab Rev 1996; 7:297–323.
6. Siesjö BK. Pathophysiology and treatment of focal cerebral ischemia. Part I. Pathophysiology. J Neurosurg 1992; 77:169–184.

7. Siesjö BK. Pathophysiology and treatment of focal cerebral ischemia. Part II. Mechanisms of damage and treatment. J Neurosurg 1992; 77:337–354.
8 Touzani O, Young AR, Derlon J, et al. Sequential studies of the severity of hypometabolic tissue volumes after permanent middle cerebral artery occlusion. Stroke 1995; 26:2112–2119.
9. NINDS rt-PA Stroke Study Group. Tissue plasminogen activator for acute ischemic stroke. N Engl J Med 1995; 333:1581–1587.
10. Bogousslavsky J, Hachinski V, Boughner DR, Fox AJ, Vinuela F, Barnett HJ. Cardiac and arterial lesions in carotid transient ischemic attacks. Arch Neurol 1986; 43:223–228.
11. Cujec B, Polasek P, Voll CL, Shuaib A. Transesophageal echocardiography in the detection of cardiac source of embolism in stroke patients. Stroke 1991; 22:727–733.
12. Balentine JD. Pathogenesis of central nervous system lesions induced by exposure to hyberbaric oxygen. Am J Pathol 1968; 53:1097–1109.
13. Shuaib A. Alteration of blood pressure regulation and cerebrovascular disease in the elderly. Cerebrovasc Brain Metab Rev 1992; 4:329–345.
14. Jorgensen HS, Nakayama H, Otto H, Olsen TS. Lancet 1994; 344:156–159.
15. Hindfelt B. The prognostic significance of subfebrility and fever in ischemic cerebral infarction. Acta Neurol Scand 1976; 53:72–79.
16. Reith J, Jogensen HS, Pedersen PM, et al. Body temperature in acute stroke: relation to stroke severity, infarct size, mortality and outcome. Lancet 1996; 347:422–425.
17. Tatlisumak T, Fisher M. Hematologic disorders associated with ischemic stroke. J Neurol Sci 1996; 1–11.
18. Horner J, Massey EW, Riski JE, Lathrop DL, Chase KN. Aspiration following stroke: clinical correlates and outcome. Neurology 1988; 38:1359–1362.
19. Alberts MJ, Horner J, Gwynn M, Hatcher N, Lynn K, Simpson S. Prevention of aspiration pneumonia following stroke. Neurology 1991; 41(suppl 1).
20. Hamilton MG, Hull RD. Pineo GF. Venous thromboembolism in neurosurgery and neurology patients: a review. Neurosurgery 1994; 34:280–296.
21. Inoue Y, Takemota K, Miyamoto T, et al. Sequential computed tomography scans in acute cerebral infarction. Radiology 1980; 135:655–662.
22. Levy LM, Killian JM, Mawad M. Acute cerebral infarction. Early diagnosis with MR. AJNR 1989; 10:872.
23. Moulin T, Cartin F, Crepin-Leblond T, et al. Early CT signs in acute middle cerebral artery infarction. Neurology 1996; 47:366–375.
24. Tomura N, Uemura K, Inugami A, Fujita H, Higano S, Sishido F. Early CT findings in cerebral infarction. Radiology 1988; 168:463–467.
25. Truwit CL, Barkovich AJ, Gean-Marton A, Hibri N, Norman D. Loss of insular ribbon: another early sign of acute middle cerebral artery infarction. Radiology 1990; 176:801–806.
26. Bozzao L, Angeloni U, Bastialleno S, Fantozzi LM, Pierallini A, Fieschi C. Early angiographic and CT findings in patients with hemorrhagic infarctions in the distribution of the MCA. AJNR 1991; 12:1115–1121.

27. Bastianello JE, Pierallini A, Colonese C. Hyperdense middle cerebral artery CT sign: comparison with angiography in acute phase of cerebral infarction. Neuroradiology 1991; 33:207–212.
28. Tomsick TA, Brott TG, Chambers AA. Hyperdense middle cerebral artery sign: efficacy in detecting middle cerebral artery thrombus. AJNR 1990; 11:473–476.
29. Berger L, Hakim AM. The association of hyperglycemia with edema in cerebral infarction. Stroke 1986; 17:865–871.
30. Candelise L, Landi G, Orazio EN, Boccardi E. Prognostic significance of hyperglycemia in acute stroke. Arch Neurol 1996; 42:661–667.
31. Von Kummer R, Buzzao L, Meyding-Lamade U, Forsting M. Sensitivity and prognostic value of computed tomography in MCA trunk occlusion AJNR 1994; 15:9–15.
32. Davis KR, Taveras JM, New PF. Cerebral infarction diagnosis by computed tomography: analysis and evaluation of findings. AJR 1975; 124:643–657.
33. Kandell BE, Pullicino P. Intravascular contrast infusion in acute stroke. II. Effect on prognosis. Neuroradiology 1980; 19:241–246.
34. Vonofakos D, Artmann H. CT findings in hemorrhagic cerebral infarction. Comput Radiol 1983; 7:75–88.
35. Bogousslavsky J, Regli F, Uske A, Maeder P. Early spontaneous hemorrhagic transformation in ischemic infarction. Is primary hemorrhage overdiagnosed? Neurology 1991; 41:837–844.
36. Jacobs K, Moulin T, Bogousslavsky J, et al. The stroke syndrome of cortical vein thrombosis. Neurology 1996; 47:376–382.
37. Zwiebel WJ. Color-duplex features of normal and abnormal arteries. In: Zwiebel WJ, ed. Introduction to Vascular Ultrasonography. Philadelphia: WB Saunders, 1992:105–122.
38. Griewing B, Morgenstern C, Drisner F, Kallwellis G, Walker ML, Kessler C. Cerebrovascular disease assessed by color-flow and power Doppler ultrasonography. Stroke 1996; 27:95–100.
39. Erdoes L, Marek JM, Mills JM, et al. The relative contribution of carotid duplex scanning, magnetic resonance angiography and cerebral angiography to clinical decision making: a prospective study in patients with carotid occlusive disease. J Vasc Surg 1996; 23:950–956.
40. Jacobs NM, Grand EG, Schellinger D, Byrd MC, Richardson JD, Cohan SL. Duplex carotid sonography: criteria for stenosis, accuracy and pitfalls. Radiology 1985; 154:385–391.
41. Bakke SJ, Smith SJ, Kerty E, Dahl A. Cervicocranial artery dissection. Detection by Doppler and MR angiography. Acta Radiol 1996; 37:528–534.
42. Lownie SP, Lee DH, Fox AJ, Pelz D. Cerebral angiography. In: Barnett HJ, Stein BM, Mohr JP, Yatsu F. eds. Stroke: Pathophysiology, Diagnosis and Management. New York: Churchill, Livingstone, 1992:215–239.
43. North American Symptomatic Carotid Endarterectomy Trial Collaborators. Beneficial effects of carotid endarterectomy in symptomatic patients with high-grade stenosis. N Engl J Med 1991; 325:445–453.
44. Streifler JY, Eliasziw M, Hachinski, V, Ferguson GG, Barnett HJ. Symptomatic high

grade carotid stenosis in the elderly—poor prognosis, high response to surgery: observations from NASCET. Stroke Cerebrovasc Dis 1992; (Suppl).
45. Buchan AM, Gates PC., Pelz D, Barnett H. Intraluminal thrombus in the cerebral circulation. Stroke 1988; 19:681–687.
46. Fieschi C, Argentino C, Lenzi GL, Sacchetti ML, Toni D, Bozzao L. Clinical and instrumental evaluation of patients with ischemic stroke within the first six hours. J Neurol Sci 1989; 91:311–322.
47. Delal PM, Shah PM, Aiyar RR. Angiographic study of cerebral embolism. Lancet 1965; II:258–261.
48. Hankey GJ, Warlow CP, Sellar RJ. Cerebral angiographic risk in mild cerebrovascular disease. Stroke 1990; 21:209–222.
49. Ida M, Mizunuma K, Hata Y, Tada S. Sub-cortical low intensity in early cerebral ischemia. AJNR 1994; 15:1387–1393.
50. Elster AD, Moody DM. Early cerebral infarction: gadopentetate dimeglumine enhancement. Radiology 1990; 177:627–632.
51. Shuaib A, Lee D, Pelz D, Fox A, Hachinski, V. The impact of magnetic resonance imaging on the management of acute ischemic stroke. Neurology 1992; 42:816–818.
52. Moseley ME, Kucharczyk J, Mintorovitch J. Diffusion-weighted MRI of acute stroke: correlation with T2-weighted and magnetic susceptibility-enhanced MRI in cats. AJNR 1990; 11:423–429.
53. Belliveau JW, Rosen BR, Kantor HL. Functional cerebral imaging by susceptibility-contrast NMR. Magn Reson Med 1990; 14:546
54. Mathews, V, Whitlow WD, Bryan RN. Cerebral ischemia and infarction. In: Atlas SC, ed. MRI of the Brain and Spine. 2d ed. New York: Lippincott-Raven, 1996:557–609.
55. Litt AW, Eidelman EM, Pinto RS. Diagnosis of carotid artery stenosis: Comparison of 2DFT, TOF MRA with contrast angiography in 50 patients. AJNR 1991; 12:149–154.
56. Riles TS, Edelman EM. Litt AW. Comparison of MRA, conventional angiography and duplex scanning. Stroke 1992; 23:341–346.
57. Lin W, Haache EM, Smith AS. Lumen definition of MRA. Magn Reson Med 1991; 1:327–336.
58. Mittl R, Broderick M, Carpenter J. Blinded reader comparison of MRA and duplex ultrasonography for carotid bifurcation stenosis. Stroke 1994; 25:4–10.
59. Karnik R, Stelzer P, Slany J. Transcranial Doppler monitoring of local intra-arterial thrombolysis in acute occlusion of the middle cerebral artery. Stroke 1992; 23:284–287.
60. Markus HS. Doppler embolus detection: stroke treatment and prevention. In: Tegeler CH, Babikian V, Gomez CR, eds. Neurosonography. New York: Mosby, 1996:239–249.
61. Sieber M, Sitzer M, Rose G. Silent cerebral emboli caused by symptomatic high grade carotid stenosis: event rates before and after carotid endarterectomy. Brain 1993; 116:1005–1015.
62. Srinivasan J, Newell DW, Sturzenegger M, Mayberg MR. Transcranial Doppler in the evaluation of internal carotid artery dissection. Stroke 1996; 27:1226–1230.

63. Yeung M, Khan KA, Shuaib A. Transcranial Doppler ultrasonography in the detection of venous to arterial shunts in acute stroke and TIAs. JNNP 1996; 61:445–449.
64. Khan KA, Yeung M, Shuaib A. Transcranial Doppler signals during cererbal angiography and cardiac catheterization. J Stroke Cerebrovasc Dis 1995; 5:187–191.
65. Giubilei F, Lenzi GL, Di Piero V, Pozzati E, Pantano P, Bastianello JE. Predictive value of brain perfusion single-photon emission computed tomography in acute ischemic stroke. Stroke 1990; 21:895–900.
66. Ueda T, Hatakeyama T, Kumon Y, Sakaki S, Uraoka T. Evaluation of risk of hemorrhagic transformation in local intra-arterial thrombolysis in acute ischemic stroke by initial SPECT. Stroke 1994; 25:298–303.
67. Fishman RA. CSF findings in diseases of the nervous system. In: Fishman RA. ed. Cerebrospinal Fluid in Diseases of the Nervous System. 2d ed. Philadelphia: Saunders, 1992:253–343.
68. Al-Twerigeri T, Shuaib A, Denath F, Amg L, Khan M. Glioblastoma multiforme presenting with recurrent neurological deficits: transient ischemic attacks or tumor attacks. J Stroke Cerebrovasc Dis 1994; 4:42–45.
69. Caplan LR. EEG findings in certain lacunar stroke syndromes. Neurology 1972; 22:403–409.
70. Yanagihara T, Houser OW, Klass DW. Computed tomography and EEG in cerebrovascular disease. Arch Neurol 1981; 38:597–600.
71. Shuaib A, Cujec B, Polasek P, Voll CL. Identification of cardiac source of embolism: Does transesophageal echo improve diagnosis? Stroke 1991; 22:147.
72. Shuaib A, Leszezynski J, Cujec B. Ataxia-hemiparesis and cardio-embolic disease. J Stroke and Cerebrovasc Dis 1991; 1:77–80.
73. Petersen P, Boysen G, Godtfredsen J, Andersen ED, Andersen B. Placebo-controlled randomized trial of warfarin and aspirin for prevention of thromboembolic complications in atrial fibrillation. Lancet 1989; 1:175–179.
74. Anonymous Preliminary report of the stroke prevention in atrial fibrillation study. N Engl J Med 1990; 322:863–868.
75. Wolf PA, Abott RD, Kannel WB. Atrial fibrillation: a major contributor to stroke in the elderly. Arch Intern Med 1987; 147:1561–1564.
76. Boston Area Anticoagulation Trial for Atrial Fibrillation Investigations. The effect of low-dose warfarin on the risk of stroke in patients with nonrheumatic atrial fibrillation. N Engl J Med 1990; 323:1505–1511.

6

Evaluation and Management of Acute Stroke: A Summary with Emphasis on Development of Critical Care Pathway

Muzaffar Mustafa Siddiqui and Ashfaq Shuaib
University of Alberta Hospital, Edmonton, Alberta, Canada

Mark Johnson
George Washington University Medical Center, Washington, D.C.

INTRODUCTION

Every year approximately 450,000 people suffer an acute ischemic stroke in the United States.[1] In the subsequent year, 150,000 are dead. Many more have lasting disability, requiring long-term care (see Chap. 1 for more details). In 1993, the cost of stroke was estimated to be over $30 billion.[2] This cost can be divided into direct cost (hospitalization, rehabilitation, medications, etc.), which accounts for approximately 57% of the cost ($17 billion), and indirect costs of 43% (lost productivity, early retirement, etc.). Early admission to hospital, efficient utilization of resources for diagnosis, and prevention of complications or recurrences may improve prognosis and result in a decrease in the cost of caring for such patients. Community and professional education, and development of the stroke care unit are strategies that have been pursued in order to meet these two goals.

Several studies have shown that patients who are admitted to a stroke unit have a decreased length of hospital stay, fewer complications, and better prognosis than individuals admitted to a general medical or neurology unit.[3,4] The presence of a highly trained group of nurses and other staff comprising an active brain attack team are important factors ensuring that stroke patients are rapidly evaluated and investigated. The team members should include members from the departments of Emergency Medicine, Neurology, Neuroradiology, and Rehabilitation. Attention to prevention of complications and early initiation of therapy promote early discharge or transfer to rehabilitation services. Hospitals with frequent admissions for stroke would benefit from the development of such units.

Utilizing the facility of the stroke care unit and team and the application of critical care pathways have proven useful in fulfilling the objectives of timely, systematic, consistent, and efficient patient care. Critical care pathways for managing stroke patients are thus becoming very popular in hospitals with a large stroke service. The use of a stroke critical care map ensures that appropriate evaluation, investigations, and consultations are completed promptly in all patients. At the end of the chapter a sample stroke critical care pathway is provided for information that may be modified according to local hospital needs (see Appendix 1).

RATIONALE FOR THE USE OF CRITICAL CARE PATHWAY

From the time the patient suffers an acute stroke to discharge from hospital, crucial assessments and diagnostic tests are carried out to help determine the underlying etiology of the stroke. A standardized approach to investigating the patient with acute stroke has been shown to be very helpful in establishing early diagnosis and in prompt initiation of therapy. Such an approach ensures both a decreased length of stay as well as improved outcome.[5–7]. This is a consequence of the timely institution of treatment as well as the prevention and treatment of complications. The data pertaining to length of stay, before and after institution of "critical care pathway," from a recent study conducted by Wentworth et al. are presented in Figure 1.

Patients who present very early after an acute ischemic stroke are potential candidates for intravenous or intra-arterial thrombolysis. These patients may be expeditiously identified and treated if the pathway includes allowance for the brain attack team. This information is more extensively detailed in Appendix 2. In addition, patients with an acute stroke are at high risk of complications, including aspiration, infections, and venous thrombosis (see Chaps. 3 and 7 for more details). Early attention to prevention would in many instances result in the avoidance of such complications. For example, in the initial days after an acute ischemic stroke, patients are at an increased risk for aspiration pneumonia. This is mostly secondary to a defective airway protection mechanism as a result of the stroke. If the critical pathway suggests that oral intake be limited until the patient has been assessed for the risk of aspiration, such a complication may be prevented in most patients.

A series of orders developed according to the needs of the local hospital would therefore be very useful and serve as a stroke critical care pathway. An organized program, if implemented for all patients, will ensure that investigations are completed on time and treatment initiated early.

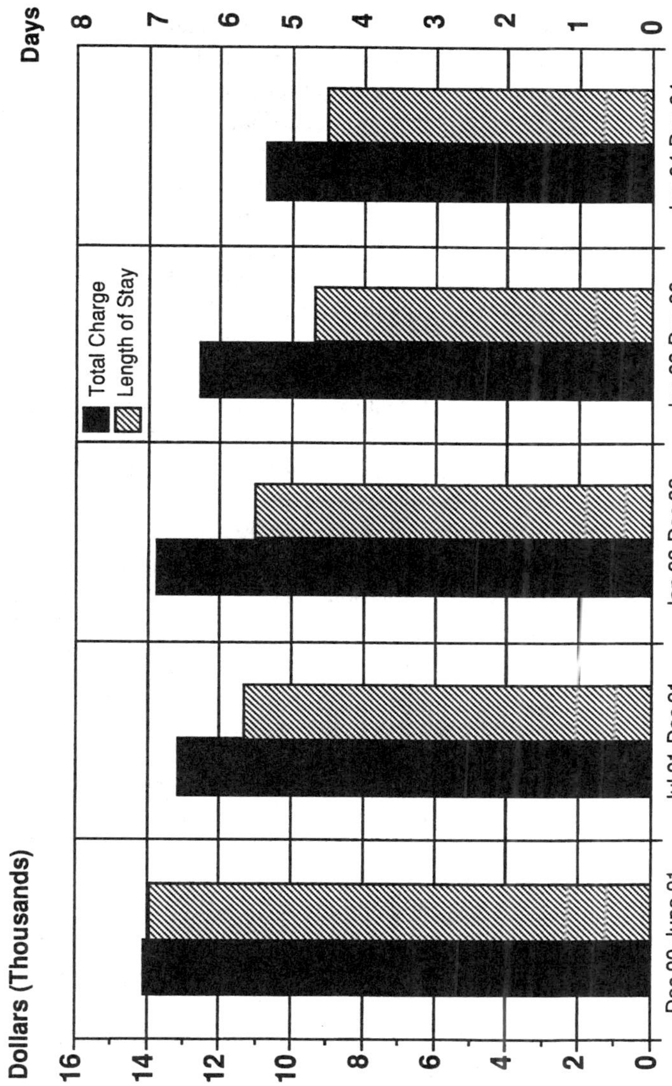

Figure 1 Comparative analysis of charges and length of stay for patients with stroke. (From Deirdre Wentworth, RN, MSN, Mercy General Hospital, 4001 J St., Sacramento, CA 95819.)

Equally important to the thorough monitoring of patients and timely intervention in the treatment of complications is the issue of prompt admission to hospital. Early admission increases the potential for effective thrombolytic treatment. Treatment with thrombolysis within hours of an ischemic stroke may improve outcome. It is therefore important to determine the percentage of patients who may benefit from thrombolytic therapy or may be candidates for neuroprotection (currently experimental therapy; see Chaps. 16 and 17). An estimate of the number of patients who may benefit from such interventions may provide useful information on the extent of the problem and allow for the development of incentives for critical pathways in a particular hospital. We recently reviewed the hospital charts of >2,002 patients from five large university hospitals across Canada.[8] The study was completed prior to the introduction of tissue plasminogen activator (tPA) as a treatment of acute stroke in Canada. The time of onset of symptoms was documented in only 889 of the 2,022 patients admitted with an acute stroke to the five university hospitals. Of these 889 patients, 307 (35%) presented to the hospital within 2 hours of onset of symptoms. Contraindications to the use of thrombolytic treatment were documented in 122 of those 307 patients. Rapid recovery of symptoms and prior use of anticoagulants were the commonest contraindications against the potential use of tPA. A further 23 patients had a hemorrhagic stroke on CT and therefore could not be candidates for tPA therapy. Excluding all such patients, 162 patients (8%) of the 2,022 patients could have been potentially treated with tPA. This number is similar to data from studies in the United States suggesting that thrombolysis is possible in <10% of patients with acute ischemic stroke.[9–11] Implementation of programs that improve awareness of stroke symptoms in the community and development of close collaboration with the paramedics and ER physicians may improve the percentage of patients arriving early to hospital after an acute stroke.[12] The assessment of patients who may benefit from thrombolysis should be a priority and requires a well-coordinated approach. The urgency of this concerted approach remains paramount regardless of whether thrombolytic therapy is instituted. Timely intervention is important in dealing with the varied complications associated with acute stroke.

This chapter summarizes the essentials of patient care from the time the patient has a stroke to admission to hospital. It highlights some points on how to improve early admission to hospital and the advantages of having a stroke unit and a stroke critical care pathway.

At the end of the chapter a protocol for the use of tPA is attached with details of how a brain attack team could function. Details of the prehospital care, emergency evaluation, examination of the patients, and the use of appropriate investigations are reviewed in greater details elsewhere (see Chaps. 2 through 5).

AWARENESS OF STROKE IN THE COMMUNITY

In order to increase the number of patients who may benefit from acute stroke therapy it is important to develop community-based stroke awareness programs that improve the perception within the local public that acute stroke is a treatable disease. Programs directed at enhancing the public's knowledge of symptoms of an impending stroke, and an explanation of how early assessment may improve outcome, may prove very helpful in the early admission of patients to hospital. The purpose of the program should include an aim to help improve the public knowledge of early acute stroke symptoms. Recent studies reveal that only a small number of the elderly subjects (who are at the greatest risk for stroke) can recognize the symptoms of an acute stroke.[13,14] With recognition, a second important factor relates to the way the patient (or family) responds to the emergency. Patients either do nothing, lie down and rest, go to sleep, or try to reach their family physicians. This nihilistic attitude of not reacting to the emergency is the commonest factor in delayed hospital admission. Strikingly, studies have shown that patients who do in fact activate the emergency 911 ambulance service arrive at the hospital significantly earlier than patients who do not.[15] We strongly advise that community programs include some education on how the local ambulance service can be approached in an expeditious manner.

It is also important to keep the local ambulance service aware of the treatment options that could be offered if the patient were seen within the initial 2 to 3 hours after an acute stroke. Various studies have been done addressing both the problems of patient education and behavior.[12–14] The awareness program should be broad based, with support from the news media (newspapers, radio, and television), community education centers, and local physicians and other health care workers. Such community programs have been very successful in improving the time to hospital in a number of communities.[12] In a recent study conducted by Alberts et al., the percentage of all patients with cerebral infarction presenting early to hospital increased from <40% to >80% after coordinated educational efforts.[12] The data from this study are presented in Table 1.

Table 1 Time of Poststroke Presentation for Patients With Cerebral Infarcts, Before and After Implementation of Community Education Program

Study	=24 hr	24-48 hr	3-7 days	8-14 days	> 14 days	Total
Initial	98 (70)	66 (48)	71 (56)	5 (5)	10 (8)	250 (187)
Follow-up[a]	136	6	14	3	0	159

Numbers in parentheses are for cerebral infarction patients excluding those with stroke in evolution.

[a]Significance probability from ridit analysis, $p = .0001$. Significance was the same whether stroke in evolution was included or excluded from cerebral infarction data.

Source: Ref. 12.

In summary, acute stroke should be perceived and managed as an emergency, similar to the way individuals with acute myocardial infarction are managed. This may improve the number of patients who could benefit from acute stroke therapy. It is also important to remember that the reason for early admission to hospital is not only to consider thrombolysis but also to provide an environment where early complications can be prevented (this may be possible through immediate admission to a stroke unit).

PREHOSPITAL CARE

The treatment of patients with an acute stroke should be initiated in the ambulance. The paramedics are the first contact with the patient and as such require to be retrained extensively on the availability of new treatment options for the patient who is evaluated within the initial minutes to hours of the insult. Advance Life Support Service (ACLS) has recently included a chapter on the management of acute stroke. This should prove to be a valuable source for retraining personnel in the management of acute stroke for paramedics and physicians. As new and safe stroke treatments become available, responsibilities of the paramedics are also likely going to increase. There are a number of steps that can be initiated early and may have positive outcome on surviving patients.

Animal research indicates that the extent of neuronal damage and the final outcome after an acute stroke depends on a number of potentially treatable factors. Hypoxemia, hyperthermia, hyperglycemia, and hypotension may all accelerate neuronal damage and require treatment as soon as possible.[16] The paramedic can initiate simple measures to ensure that the patient is not hypoxic or hypotensive. Most patients at the onset of an acute stroke would have high blood pressure. The temptation to treat hypertension should be avoided as sudden fluctuations in blood pressure may lead to an increase in the extent of neuronal injury.[17–19] As patients with acute stroke are at an increased risk for aspiration pneumonia, precautions should include not allowing for oral intake until the patient is assessed in hospital.

As discussed in greater detail in Chapters 15 and 16, unfortunately at present, only a limited number of patients with an acute stroke can be treated with thrombolytic therapy. The early identification of such individuals is of paramount importance as treatment may lead to a dramatically favorable outcome. A simple protocol is attached at the end of the chapter that may help with identification of such patients. Identification of the candidates starts with recognition by paramedics and continues through to the Emergency Department physician's assessment upon arrival to hospital, followed by rapid CT evaluation and potential thrombolysis in appropriate patients. Patients who were previously healthy and who have a defined onset of symptoms (usually <2 hours) should be triaged quickly to hospital with facilities to manage the emergency. As the ambulance nears the hospital, the Emergency Department should be notified to allow time to get the personnel and equipment ready for rapid assessment and CT scanning. We have found that early warning by paramedics is an important factor in planning treatment protocols in our emergency stroke service. All other patients who may not be candidates for rapid assessment should be evaluated in a manner explained in detail elsewhere (Chap. 5). It is important to involve ambulance services and paramedics early in the implementation of acute stroke programs. Their active involvement is the key to success.

EMERGENCY ASSESSMENT

Hospitals with a large stroke service should have a predefined set of orders that should be implemented in all stroke patients who come through the emergency doors. In hospitals where >500 patients are seen by the stroke service, a stroke observation unit in the Emergency Department can prove very useful. The unit's space could be shared with cardiology in hospitals where the volume of stroke patients is not very large.

There are numerous advantages of setting an observation room in the Emergency Department. The unit, with highly trained nursing staff, can serve as an ideal location for rapid assessment of the stroke patient and offer an excellent place where steps can be implemented to prevent complications. The stroke critical care map can be initiated in the unit. Appropriate monitoring of blood pressure, tissue oxygenation, temperature, cardiac rhythm, and serum glucose levels may improve the final outcome and could lead to shortened hospital stay. As well, the team could offer thrombolytic therapy, blood pressure management, or other treatments as required in the acute setting.

In patients who are potential candidates for thrombolysis, the time from when the patient first enters the hospital to the initiation of treatment (door-to-needle time) should ideally be <45 minutes. During this time the initial nursing assessment is completed, physician evaluation is done, and blood workup and imaging studies are carried out to rule out any contraindications to therapy. It is also important to remember that the stroke service should be available during the day and night hours and backup facilities for neurosurgical complications should be close at hand. The role of the Emergency Department in all other patients is mainly to confirm diagnosis and admit the patient to the medical or neurological service. As a cranial CT scan is essential prior to the use of thrombolytic agents, the Emergency Service should be in close contact with Radiology and with 24-hour facilities for interpretation of images. The first nurse assessment

Table 2 NINDS-Recommended Stroke Evaluation Targets for Potential Thrombolytic Candidates[a]

	Time target
Door to doctor	10 minutes
Door to CT completion	25 minutes
Door to CT read	45 minutes
Door to treatment	60 minutes
Access to neurological expertise[b]	15 minutes
Access to neurosurgical expertise[b]	2 hours
Admit to monitored bed	3 hours

[a]Target times will not be achieved in all cases, but they represent a reasonable goal.
[b]By phone or in person.

should be within <10 minutes of arrival followed within minutes by the ER physician evaluation. The CT head should be complete by 25 minutes and by this time the neurologist should either have seen the patient or be on phone contact. After the CT scan has been reviewed to rule out hemorrhage and exclude a large infarction, the patient may be a candidate for thrombolytic therapy if the time from onset to needle is <3 hours. These targets have been well delineated in a guideline recommended by the NINDS facility (see Table2)[20] and Chapter 3.

ADMISSION TO MEDICAL AND NEUROLOGICAL SERVICE

Hospitals with a large stroke service would benefit from the establishment of a designated stroke unit. We have >10 years of experience with stroke units and have found them to be very cost-effective in maintaining comprehensive patient care. The success of the unit depends on the quality and dedication of the nursing staff that runs the unit. A specified number of nurses who are designated to the unit would guarantee that patient care is effective and comprehensive. A critical care pathway of routine investigations, evaluations, and consultations is very important for the successful operation of such a unit. Such a plan in the hands of experienced nurses can limit complications and therefore promote early discharge from hospital. The essential components of any critical care pathway should include attention to the following parameters.

Patient assessment
Investigations
Treatment
Consultations
Outcome analysis

It is important to specify the time course of the various orders that are suggested in the critical pathway. Every attempt should be made to complete the investigations in the initial 24 to 36 hours after admission and to initiate treatment during this time. If the patient has a moderate-size cerebral infarction and has potential for moderate to good recovery, physiotherapy, speech therapy, and rehabilitation consultations should be initiated within the initial 2 to 3 days so that transfer to the rehabilitation service can be started early. Patients with a devastating stroke usually require compassionate care and should in most cases not be exposed to the type of investigations detailed in Chapter 5. Attention should be given to prevention of complications (especially aspiration pneumonia, venous thrombosis, infections, and bed sores, etc.). If no meaningful recovery is evident in the initial few days of admission, arrangements for transfer to a long-term facility should be planned early.

Stroke units were initially conceived three decades ago to observe patients with an acute stroke by methods that were designed for monitoring myocardial infarction victims. It became evident very early that the monitoring of cardiac rhythm did not add much to the care of the stroke patient, and therefore such units lost their popularity. In recent years stroke units are making a comeback for a variety of reasons. It has been shown in a number of studies that patients who are admitted to a unit are less likely to have medical complications, more likely to be discharged early from hospital, and have a better prognosis.[3,4,21] A number of reasons have been offered to explain this difference when compared to patients admitted to a medical (or neurological) service. Our experience shows that the presence of a group of highly trained nurses and rehabilitation personnel is a key to the better prognosis.

If the service uses a critical care stroke pathway, it makes it easy for the investigations and consultations to be completed on time while being systematically performed and documented in each patient. This allows not only an early discharge from hospital but careful analysis of patient outcome as well (see Table 3).

CASE REPORTS USING THE BRAIN ATTACK TEAM PROTOCOL

We would like to share management of two patients that were assessed by the stroke team and treated with intra-arterial thrombolysis. Whereas the outcome was striking in both patients, we have also treated patients where recovery was not as spectacular. The two examples are reported to create awareness of newer therapies that in some patients can lead to excellent outcome We would also like to use these examples to bring home the point that the development of comprehensive stroke programs is important in institutions with a large stroke service.

Table 3 Summary of the Prehospital, Emergency Care, and Admission of Patients Presenting with an Acute Ischemic Stroke

Prehospital	Emergency department	Stroke unit or neurology-medical service
Develop community programs for stoke	Identify patients who may require tPA therapy - aim for 45-min door-needle time	Continue with investigations to make etiological diagnosis
Provide ambulance supports for rapid transit to stroke-designated hospitals	Stabilize patient and prevent complications. Begin early investigations	Initiate rehabilitation consultations and therapy
		Continue treatment for prevention of recurrences
		Start risk factor management programs

Case 1

A 40-year-old female presented to the hospital with a 30-minute history of severe nausea, repeated bouts of vomiting, vertigo, and unsteadiness. Over the subsequent hour, symptoms progressed and the patient became drowsy and developed right-sided weakness. Besides being on birth control pills for 30 days prior to presentation, there were no risk factors for stroke. The stroke team was consulted by the Emergency Department. On initial examination the patient was noted to be drowsy and severely dysarthric but could obey simple commands. She had gaze-evoked nystagmus and right facial weakness. Motor examination revealed complete left-sided hemiplegia. The arm, however, was held in a dystonic posture. Examination of the left upper extremity revealed mild coordination deficits. A cranial CT scan was reported as normal. A presumptive diagnosis of basilar artery thrombosis was made and the patient was evaluated with immediate cerebral angiography. Angiography showed a left vertebral artery dissection and complete occlusion of the basilar artery (Fig. 2a). As the angiography studies were being completed, the patient became comatose and developed intermittent decerebrate posturing. The patient was intubated and paralyzed, so the procedure could continue. The angiogram catheter was used for direct intra-arterial treatment with tissue plasminogen activator (tPA). Treatment was started with 20 mg tPA intra-arterial injection over 2 minutes and the angiogram repeated to assess patency. Angiography showed mild improvement in basilar artery filling. Repeated doses of tPA followed by angiography were done over the next 1 hour. A total of 70 mg tPA was used for successful opening of the artery (Fig. 2b,c). As the artery opened up, the patient awoke and the vital signs stabilized. Despite the high dose of tPA, a small clot remained in the basilar artery . The patient was started on heparin and transferred to the neurointensive care unit. The

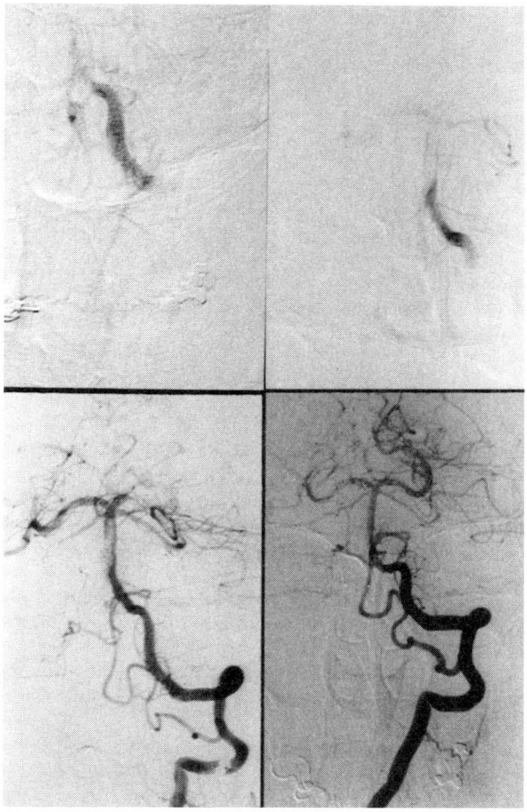

Figure 2 Cerebral angiography, Case 1: a. Vertebral artery dissection, basilar occlusion; b,c. Treatment with repeated doses of tPA; d. Follow-up angiogram (24 h post-treatment).

next day the patient was fully awake, with minimal neurological deficits. A repeat angiogram (Fig. 2d) showed no evidence of the intraluminal thrombus and resolution of the left vertebral occlusion. The whole procedure from onset of symptoms to completion of angiography and treatment with tPA lasted 5 hours. Follow-up at 2 months showed very trivial deficits in fine motor movements of the right arm and mild difficulty with tandem gait. An MRI showed three small infarctions in the cerebellum but was otherwise normal (Fig 3).

Comment

Acute occlusion and thrombosis of the basilar artery carries a grave prognosis with >80% of patients dead or severely disabled within days of the event. Open-

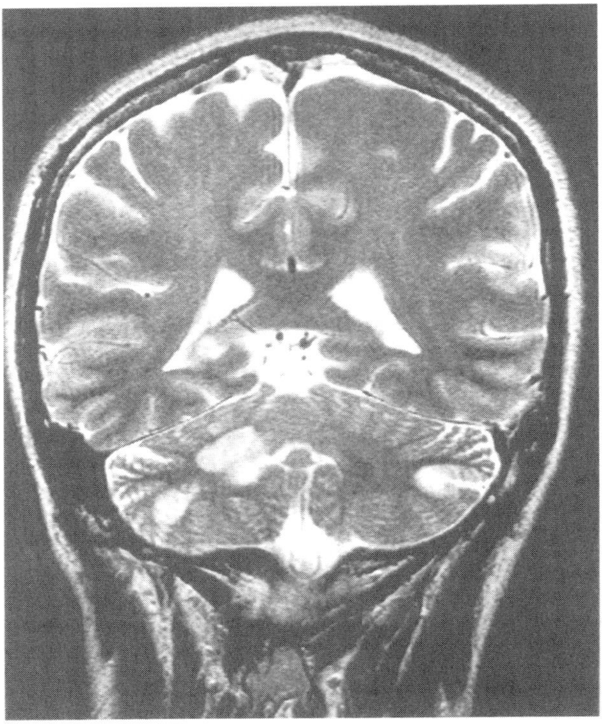

Figure 3 Case 1: Follow-up MRI (3 months post-treatment).

ing of the artery has been shown to significantly improve prognosis.[22] Quick assessment and intervention by the team from the Emergency Department and collaboration between Neurology and Neuroradiology were instrumental in getting the patient treated with the intra-arterial therapy.

Case 2

This 62-year-old patient with a previous history of a mild stroke a few years earlier developed a sudden onset of speech difficulty and right-sided weakness while undergoing coronary angiography. Examination revealed drowsiness, left-gaze preference, and a complete left-sided hemiplegia. The stroke team assessed the patient within 20 minutes of the event, and cerebral angiography showed a complete occlusion of the proximal middle cerebral artery (MCA) on the left side (Fig. 4a). Cranial CT scan was normal. Selective catheter was inserted into the MCA and thrombolysis was initiated with intra-arterial urokinase. After approximately 120 minutes and a 500,000-unit infusion of urokinase, there was recanali-

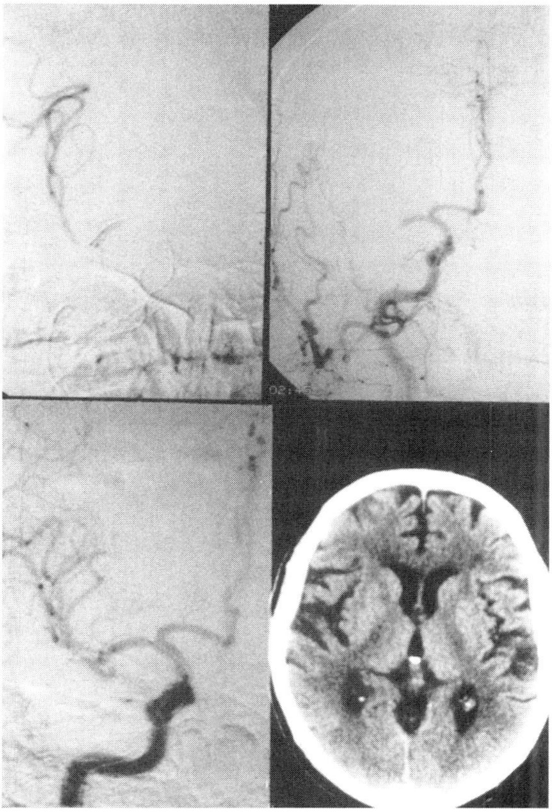

(a) (b) (c) (d)

Figure 4 Cerebral angiography, Case 2: a. Complete occlusion proximal MCA; b,c. Treatment with intra-arterial urokinase; d. Follow-up CT.

zation of the MCA (Fig. 4b,c) and the patient recovered speech and motor strength. Examination revealed minimal right-sided weakness that may have been residual from the previous stroke. Repeat cranial CT (Fig. 4d) showed no new infarction. (We are grateful to Drs. Mary Lou Myles and Derrick Emery for the second patient case study.)

Comment

While in-hospital strokes are rare, early interventional therapy in selective patients may have dramatic effects. The second patient was discharged from hospital with very small neurological deficits.

(*continued on page 114*)

Appendix 1 A Sample Stroke Critical Care Pathway That Could Be Adapted for Local Use

Patient demographics:
Name:____________________
Age:____________________
Sex: M/F
Patient Identifier:____________________
Initiated by M.D.__________ Date:__________ Time:__________
Expected LOS:____________
Reviewed by Case Manager:__________ Date:__________
Actual LOS:__________

Patient Information	Discharge Outcomes	Date Achieved/Signature
Complications	*Neurological*	Date:_______________
	No increasing deficits (past 24 hours)	Sign:_______________
	Cardiopulmonary	
	Systolic BP within	Date:_______________
	mm Hg from baseline	Sign:_______________
	Heart rate controlled	
	(__ beats/min)	
	Lungs clear	
	GI/Nutrition	Date:_______________
	Tolerating prescribed diet	Sign:_______________
	Renal/GU/fluid and	Date:_______________
	Electrolyte balance	Sign:_______________
	Foley catheter-free	
	Means of voiding pattern established	
	Complication prevention	Date:_______________
	Afebrile	Sign:_______________
	No evidence of venous thrombosis	
	Stroke prophylaxis Established	
	Integument	Date:_______________
	No evidence of hospital acquired pressure sores	Sign:_______________
Mobility	Home environment assessment	Date:_______________
	complete and safety issues resolved	Sign:_______________
Learning Needs	Pt./family/significant other	Date:_______________
	verbalized understanding of:	Sign:_______________
	Medication	
	Life-style changes	
	Smoking program	
	Signs and symptoms of depression	

Appendix 1 Continued

	Local chapter of heart and stroke association Follow-up care Safety Diet		
Multidisciplinary Action Plan	Emergency Department (0-6 hrs) Date/time of symptoms onset: __/__/__-__________ ED arrival time: Primary care MD:	Day 1 Date:__________ Primary care MD:__________	Day 2 Date:__________ Primary care MD:__________
Consults	Neurology Consider: Cardiology Subspecialty Interventional Neuroradiology	Speech pathology Social work PT OT Rehabilitation	Dietary
Tests	PT/PTT, CBC with diff. Electrolyes, Na^+, Ca^{2+}, Mg^{2+}, liver/ renal function, urinalysis EKG, CXR Head CT—Consider ECHO/Holter monitor Consider angiogram	Guiaic all stools Consider MRI/MRA, carotid/ TCD Doppler	Guiaic all stools PTT (if on heparin)
Assessments	Preliminary Diagnosis made VS q 15 min. to q 2 h if stable Temp q 4 Neurocheck q 2	VS q 2, Temp q 4 Neurocheck q 2 I & O q 4 (check post void residuals) Pulse oximetry Consider: cardiac monitoring, TCD monitoring Speech: swallowing and speech assessment	VS, Neurocheck q 4, Temp q Shift, I & O q 4 (Keep void volume <500 cc) OT: ADL evaluation ADL support (home needs) Splint supports PT: Mobility evaluation

(*continued*)

Appendix 1 Continued

Multidisciplinary Action Plan	Emergency Dept. (0–6 Hours) Date:__________	Day 1 Date:__________	Day 2 Date:__________
		Maintain pulse ox>92%	Speech language pathology if needed Postvoid residual urine vol < 500 cc
Treatment	IV access, consider IV fluids	Consider IV fluids Teds/SCD while in bed Chest PT as indicated	D/C IV fluids if tolerating liquids Teds/SCD while in bed Bowel program init Chest PT as indicated No clinical evidence of venous thrombosis
Medications	Refer to brain attack team Type of stroke Hemorrhagic Ischemic Thrombotic Embolic Lacunar Venous occlusive Uncertain Other (specify): Consider tPA (if <3 h from sympt onset) Consider therapy with neuroprotect agents	Medicate according to diagnosis: Consider: ASA Ticlopidine Hep/warfarin Medicate for nausea prn Continue with prescribed medical regimen	Continue with prescribed medical regimen
Nutrition	NPO	NPO if swallowing impaired; progress according to swallowing evaluation *Swallowing not impaired*	Progress according to swallowing evaluation
Activity/safety	Bed rest Falls prevention	Activity as tolerated Falls prevention	OOB activity Falls prevention

Appendix 1 Continued

Multidisciplinary Action Plan	Emergency Dept. (0–6 Hours) Date:__________	Day 1 Date:__________	Day 2 Date:__________
	Program	Program	Program
	Aspiration	Aspiration	Aspiration
	Precautions	Precautions	Precautions
	HOB 30°	HOB 30°	HOB 30°
	Seizure precautions	Seizure precautions	Seizure precautions
Teaching	Provide patients family with stroke educational materials	T/L	T/L
		Speech:	Speech:
		Aphasic/dysphasic	Asphasic/dysphasic
		Teaching	Teaching
		PT:	PT:
		Give info to pt. fam. on:	Give info to pt. fam. on:
		Mobility	Mobility
		Aides	Aides
		Falls	Falls
		Prevent.	Prevent.
		Home	Home
		Safety	Safety
		OT:	OT:
		Give info. to pt. fam. on:	Give info. to pt. fam. on:
		Functional	Functional
		Transfer	Transfer
		Training	Training
		Assist	Assist
		devices	devices
		Positioning	Positioning
		needs	needs
		RN:	RN:
		Give info. to pt. fam. on:	Give info. to pt. fam. on:
		Unit intro.	Unit intro.
		Medication	Medication
		Smoking	Smoking
		program	program
		Safety	Safety
		Diet	Diet
		Aspiration	Aspiration

(continued)

Appendix 1 Continued

Multidisciplinary Action Plan	Emergency Dept. (0–6 Hours) Date:__________	Day 1 Date:__________	Day 2 Date:__________
		precautions Falls Prevention Seizure precautions	Precautions Falls Prevention Seizure Precautions
Psychosocial	Determine whether the patient has the capacity to make his own health care decisions. Identify surrogate: (specify): Determine status of advance directive	Emotional support	Encourage family involvement with patient's care.
Discharge Plan	Pt./family verbalizes understanding of plan of care Plan of care mutually set with pt. family	SW: discharge needs assessment Identify supports	SW: discharge needs assessment cont. Identify home equipment, needs/supports MD: determine disposition of patient

Multidisciplinary action plan	Day 3 Date:__________ Primary care MD:__________	Day 4 Date:__________ Primary care MD:__________
Consults		
Tests	PT/PTT if on heparin Guiaic all stools	
Assessments	VS. temp, neuro check q shift I & O q shift	VS, temp, neuro check q shift I & O q shift
Treatment	Teds/SCD while in bed Chest PT as indicated SLP: Tx bedside/dept OT: Tx bedside/dept PT: Tx bedside/dept	D/C IV access
Medications	Continue with prescribed medications	Continue with prescribed medications
Nutrition	Advance as tolerated	Advance as tolerated

Appendix 1 Continued

Multidisciplinary action plan	Day 3 Date:__________ Primary care MD:__________	Day 4 Date:__________ Primary care MD:__________
Activity/Safety	Increase as tolerated Falls prevention program Aspiration precautions HOB 30° Seizure precautions	Increase as tolerated Falls prevention program Aspiration precautions HOB 30° Seizure precautions
Teaching	T/L SLP: Aphasic/ dysphasic Teaching RN: Pt/fam view stroke video D/C medication training Support groups Signs and symptoms of depression OT: Safety ADL training Positioning *Pt/Family verbalizes* *Understanding of:* *available support groups* *Signs and symptoms of* *depression* *Discharge medications* *Safety*	T/L SLP: Aphasic/ dysphasic Teaching RN: D/C instructions Medications Emerg. tel. numb. Follow-up care PT: Mobility Falls prevention Positioning
Psychosocial	Provide emotional support Encourage family involvement in care	
Discharge plan	SW: confirms D/C plan with pt. family MD: determines disposition of the patient *Verbalizes understanding of* *and agrees with discharge* *plan* *Disposition determined*	Discharge

Appendix 2 Brain Attack Team Protocol

Purpose: Definition of a uniform rapid response team comprising members from the Emergency Department, Neurology, Neuroradiology, and Neurosurgery in clinical assessment, investigation, and management of patients with a suspected acute stroke

Plan of Action:

Prehospital:

911 called for possible stroke. Paramedics make 'first contact' and inform 'stroke hotline' of suspected stroke and informs of category (see below). Training of the paramedics for early recognition of signs of acute stroke. If patient candidate for tPA or neuroprotection therapy, the paramedics would call the Emergency Department (ED) in advance. Only patients that are possible candidates for the brain attack team intervention would be urgently transported to the ED. All other patients would go to hospitals closest to pickup.

The following essential information would be required at the initial paramedic contact with the ED:

1. Time of onset of process
   Reliability of information?
2. Presence of a headache
3. Level of consciousness:
   Awake
   Drowsy
   Comatose
4. Arm/leg weakness:
   No weakness
   Partial weakness
   No movements
5. Speech
6. Blood pressure and pulse

Hospital:

All patients with suspected stroke would be admitted to the stroke observation unit in the Emergency Department. After admission the following steps would be undertaken so that rapid assessment can be assured.

Step 1. Primary Assessment (time 0–10 minutes)

ED physician to confirm judgment of the paramedic/nurse, perform history and physical exam, and categorize the patient to one of the following five categories (Modified Rankin Scale; see below). Please note that the Rankin scale is to be used in defining the prestroke clinical status.

Category 1

Definite acute stroke
Onset <3 hrs
Rankin score 0, 1, 2, 3

Appendix 2 Continued

Category 2
Definite stroke
Onset <12 hours
Rankin score 0, 1, 2, 3

Category 3
Definite acute stroke
Onset >12 hours
Rankin score 4–6

Category 4
Patient with neurological deficits of uncertain origin (metabolic, toxic problems)

Category 5
Patients with suspected subarachnoid hemorrhage

Step 2: Detailed Evaluation

Category 1, 2, 5:

a. Emergency evaluation of vital signs
b. Neurological central brain attack team (BAT) notification
c. Clinical monitoring:
   IV access (normal saline to keep vein open)
   Blood sent for CBC, Chemistry, INR and PTT
   Dextrostick and temperature monitoring
   Oxygenation only if pulsox <90%
   EKG/BP/cardiac monitor
d. CT examination (25–40 minutes) (scan reviewed by radiologist and BAT)

Category 3, 4 would be evaluated in routine manner until better treatment options become available.

Step 3: Treatment

Category 1, 2:
Treatment options including the use of tPA and experimental therapies to be discussed with patient and family.
tPA to be delivered per protocol by BAT.
Experimental treatment offered if patient eligible and gives informed consent. Stroke team to administer medications per protocol.

Category 5:
To be transferred to neurosurgery if preliminary investigation reveals SAH.

(continued)

Appendix 2 Continued

Modified Rankin Scale

Grade	Description
0	No symptoms
1	No significant disability despite symptoms. Able to carry out all usual duties and activities.
2	Slight disability: Unable to carry out all previous activities but able to look after own affairs without assistance.
3	Moderate disability: Requires some help but able to walk and able to attend to own body needs.
4	Moderately severe disability: Unable to walk with assistance and to attend to own body needs.
5	Severe disability: Bedridden, incontinent, and requiring constant nursing care and attention.

Appendix 3 Protocol for tPA Administration in Stroke

(*Note*: This protocol is a summary of the sequence and procedure of patient evaluation; treatment with tPA, detailed instructions on preparation/administration, and equipment have not been included.)

Goal of Therapy

The goal of therapy is to attempt to limit irreversible ischemic damage during an acute ischemic stroke caused by an arterial occlusion. Thrombolysis will promote reperfusion of viable tissue. Time is Brain!

The Emergency Department nurse and physician have the prime responsibility to rapidly identify suspected acute ischemic stroke. Time delay means greater viable tissue loss.

Prior to Infusion of tPA

History and physical exam consistent with an acute ischemic stroke

Compatibility with the inclusion/exclusion criteria

Baseline laboratory investigations: e.g., CBC, electrolytes, ECG, pregnancy test for females of childbearing age

CT scan of head with contrast on 3rd or 4th generation scanner

IV access

Consent

No IV heparin or ASA for the first 24 hours

Patient/Family Education and Consent

It is essential that the patient and his family be advised *from the beginning* that the patient is having an acute ischemic stroke. Thrombolytic therapy is *not* experimental and

(*continued*)

Appendix 3 Continued

does not require written consent, but consent will be required in order to indicate understanding of treatment.

Patients must be advised that bleeding/bruising is anticipated (although not usually life-threatening) and that they should report any new bruising.

Damage sustained *prior to* the administration of the drug will remain; successful therapy prevents further damage from occurring at the time of administration.

Inclusion Criteria (must have both)

Patient presenting with symptoms and signs of acute cerebral hemispheric, brainstem, or cerebellar ischemic stroke.

Onset known to be within 3 hours

Symptoms not rapidly improving

CT Inclusion Criteria

No intracranial hemorrhage

No "early infarct signs" or edema involving >1/3 middle cerebral artery territory or cerebellar hemisphere

No mass effect (midline shift)

No hypodensity which may represent evolving infarction (e.g., hemorrhagic transformation)

No evidence of tumor, aneurysm, or arteriovenous malformation (AVM)

Exclusion Criteria

Active bleeding

Severe hypertension (systolic >185, diastolic >105) persisting despite therapy as per protocol

Intracranial bleeding risk (history of subarachnoid hemorrhage not definitively treated; head trauma or surgery within the preceding 3 months)

Known bleeding diathesis (including the presence of petechiae, advanced liver or renal disease)

Anticoagulation therapy with PT/PTT above normal

GI or GU hemorrhage in the preceding 3 weeks

Surgery, biopsies, trauma, or subclavian punctures within the previous 3 weeks

History suggestive of aortic dissection

History suggestive of subarachnoid hemorrhage

Seizures at stroke onset

Glucose <2.7 or 22.2 mmol/L

Relative Contraindications

Pregnancy, postpartum >6 weeks

Infective endocarditis or acute pericarditis

Diabetic proliferative retinopathy; history of laser photocoagulation

Tissue Plasminogen Activator (tPA)

0.9 mg/kg intravenous (to maximum of 90 mg)

(*continued*)

Appendix 3 Continued

Give 10% of total dose as *bolus*
Infuse remaining 90% of total dose over 60 minutes

Physicians/Nursing Orders
Blood pressure q 15 minutes × 3 then q 30 min × 12 then q 1 h × 16 then q 2 h
Report systolic BP >185 or diastolic BP >105 on two readings 5 to 10 minutes apart
Neuro vital signs q 1 h × 4 then q 4 h × 6 if stable
Observe for bruising and bleeding
Avoid unnecessary venous and arterial puncture, and IM injections
Saline lock unused IV sites—use for blood work (no unnecessary punctures)

DO NOT GIVE HEPARIN, COUMADIN, OR ANTIPLATELET DRUGS IN FIRST 24 HOURS

Follow-up
Daily neurological assessment after first 24 hours by stroke neurologist

CT Scan: Repeat CT scan after 24 h (POSTINITIAL CT SCAN TIME)

Treatment of Complications
Bleeding (most common complication)

Any bleeding that can be controlled by pressure or that does not put the patient at risk should be observed and noted in the patient's chart.

If the patient develops a bleeding complication that cannot be controlled, i.e., frank GI or GU bleeding, intracranial bleeding, retroperitoneal or periaccess hemorrhage, the tPA and heparin infusions must be immediately discontinued. Due to the short half-life of the drug, most will be out of the circulation in 30 to 40 minutes.

Hct and/or Hgb values should be followed on a thrombolytic patient and transfusions given if indicated.

The attending physician must be notified STAT and approriate measures taken to control the bleeding. Transfusion of blood products, PRBCs, FFP, or cryoprecipitate will help to return the coagulation system to normal.

Nausea/Vomiting

Approximately 25% of the patients experience nausea and/or vomiting which may be related to tPA, the underlying illness, reperfusion, or analgesics. IV Gravol is recommended.

REFERENCES

1. Sacco RL, Lipset CH, Stroke Risk Factors: Identification and modification, M. Fisher (ed), Stroke Therapy, 1995 Butterworth-Heinemann, Washington, USA, pp. 1–28.
2. Anonymous. National Stroke Association. Cost of stroke. Stroke Clin Updates 1994; 5:9–12.

3. Indredavik B, Bakke F, Slordahl SA, Rokseth R, Haheim LL. Stroke unit treatment improves long-term quality of life: a randomized controlled trial. Stroke 1998; 29:895–899.
4. Langhorne P, Williams BO, Gilchrist W, Howie K. Do stroke units save lives? Lancet 1993; 342:395–398.
5. Bowen J, Yaste C. Effect of a stroke protocol on hospital costs of stroke patients. Neurology 1994; 44(10):1961–1964.
6. Wentworth DA, Atkinson RP. Implementation of an acute stroke program decreases hospitalization costs and length of stay. Stroke 1996; 27(6):1040–1043.
7. Brickman R, Axelrod R, Roberson D, Flanagan C. Clinical process improvement as a means of facilitating health care system integration. Joint Commun J Qual Improv 1998; 24(3):143–153.
8. Hakim AM, Lebrun L, Phillips S, Shuaib A. Factors influencing time from onset of stroke to hospital arrival for five Canadian cities. Can J Neurol Sci 1998; 25:s14–s15.
9. Hachinski V. Thrombolysis in stroke between the promise and the peril. JAMA 1996; 276:995–996.
10. NINDS TPA Stroke Study Group. Generalized efficacy of t-PA for acute stroke; subgroup analysis of the NINDS t-PA stroke trial. Stroke 1997; 28:2119–2125.
11. Zoppo GJ. Mechanism of thrombolysis. In: Ginsberg M, Bogousslavsky J, eds. Cerebrovascular Disease: Pathophysiology, Diagnosis, and Management. Vol. 1. Malden, MA: Blackwell Science, 1998; 665–681.
12. Alberts MJ, Perry A, Dawson DV, Bertels C. Effect of public and professional education on reducing the delay in presentation and referral of stroke patients. Stroke 1992; 23(3):353–356.
13. Pancioli AM, Broderick J, Kothari R, Brott T, Tuchfarber A, Miller R, Khoury J, Jauch E. Public perception of stroke warning signs and knowledge of potential risk factors. JAMA 1998; 279(16):1307–1309.
14. Feldman E, Gordon N, Brooks JM, Brass LM, Fayad PB, Kara LS, Nazareno F, Levine SR. Factors associated with early presentation of acute stroke. Stroke 1993; 24(12):1805–1810.
15. Williams LS, Bruno A, Rouch D, Marriot DJ. Stroke patient's knowledge of stroke: influence on time to presentation. Stroke 1997; 28:912–915.
16. Adams JP, Brott TG, Crowell RM, Furlan AJ, Gomez CR, Woolson RF, et al. Guidelines for the management of patients with acute ischemic stroke. Stroke 1994; 25:1901–1914.
17. Slivka AP. Hypertension and hyperglycemia in experimental stroke. Brain Res 1991; 562:66–70.
18. Phillips SJ. Pathophysiology and management of hypertension in acute ischemic stroke. Hypertension 1994; 23:131–136.
19. Carlberg B, Asplund K, Hägg E. Course of blood pressure in different subsets of patients after acute stroke. Cerebrovasc Dis 1991; 1:281–287.
20. Recommendations: Acute Hospital Care Panel, in: Proceedings of the National Symposium on Rapid Identification and Treatment of Acute Stroke, Dec. 12-13 1996, The National Institute of Neurological Disorders and Stroke-NIH, Bethesda, MD. 1998.

21. Kalra L. The influence of stroke unit rehabilitation on functional recovery from stroke. Stroke 1994; 25:821–825.
22. Brandt T, von Kummer R, Muller-Kuppers M, Hacke W. Thrombolyic therapy of acute basilar artery occlusion. Variables affecting recanalization and outcome. Stroke 1996; 27(5):875–881.

7

Medical Complications of Acute Stroke

Ahmar Aziz Butt
Brooklyn Hospital Center, New York University School of Medicine, Brooklyn, New York

Acute stroke can be devastating because it usually occurs in a relatively elderly population who often have several comorbid conditions. A significant amount of mortality and morbidity can result from secondary complications. Medical complications are important because many are preventable. Detection of predisposing factors may help identify the patients at risk .

Risk factors for poststroke complications include: increasing age, atrial fibrillation, urinary incontinence, prestroke disability and type of stroke (total anterior circulation syndrome and hemorrhagic strokes).[1] Fever,[2,3] preexisting diabetes and strokes associated with hyperglycemia have been associated with a higher poststroke mortality.[3,4] Increased complications were also reported to occur if the length of stay at the hospital was >30 days, if the Glasgow coma scale was < 4 (eye) or < 6 (motor) and the Oxford Handicap Score was >2.[1]

Secondary complications of acute stroke include: cardiac complications (acute myocardial infarction and arrhythmias), respiratory complications (dysphagia, aspiration pneumonia), vascular complications (deep-vein thrombosis and pulmonary embolism), urinary complications (incontinence and infections), gastrointestinal complications(ulcers and hemorrhage), endocrine abnormalities (hyperglycemia and SIADH), and depression. Miscellaneous complications such as poststroke seizures, pain syndromes, falls, skin breaks, and pyrexial illness have been reported to occur with varying frequencies and may impact adversely on clinical outcomes.

CARDIAC COMPLICATIONS

Coronary artery disease and cerebrovascular disease often coexist. Cardiac complications usually occur within the first 72 hours poststroke and account for 17% of deaths in acute stroke.[5] Coincident myocardial infarction and stroke occurs in 12.7% of patients admitted for stroke as evidenced by serial electrocardiograms and cardiac enzyme measurements, with a 64% 1-year mortality for combined myocardial infarction and stroke as compared to 42% for stroke alone.[6,19] Conversely there is a 2.4% (with a range of 1% to 8.6%) incidence of stroke in patients hospitalized for an acute MI,[5,7] most probably due to embolic events from anterior wall mural thrombi. Creatinine kinase has been reported to be elevated in 44% of patients with stroke, and CK-MB elevation was noted in 11%.[8]

Electrocardiographic abnormalities are common in acute stroke and most commonly constitute repolarization disorders such as inverted T-waves, peaked T-waves, U-waves, and prolonged QT intervals.[9,10] Ventricular arrhythymias such as ventricular ectopy, ventricular tachycardia, and ventricular asystole have also been described. These occur most commonly in intracranial hemorrhages, particularly subarachnoid hemorrhage,[10,11] but may occur in ischemic strokes involving anterior circulation.[11] With the exception of prolonged QT intervals and persistent U-waves, most of these changes usually revert to normal within 48 to 72 hours. QT interval prolongation occurs particularly in sub-arachnoid hemorrhages and can lead to torsades de pointes and ventricular fibrillation.[10] Poststroke atrial fibrillation occurs infrequently, is usually transient but may predispose to deep-vein thrombosis and pulmonary thromboembolism[12,13] in addition to causing cardioembolic strokes. Supraventricular tachycardia is probably more common in right hemisphere strokes while left-hemisphere strokes tend to cause ventricular arrhythmias.[14] Most of these cardiac abnormalities are transient and may resolve spontaneously but require monitoring because of the risk of sudden death.[9]

Sudden death usually occurs within the first 7 to 10 days with the peak at the second or third day. The insular cortex is thought to play a central role in the pathogenesis of cardiac complications . The parietoinsula plays an important part in autonomic equilibrium. Stimulation of the left insular cortex results in bradycardia and depressor responses while right insular stimulation produces tachycardia.[15,17] Conversely, heart rate increases after left-hemisphere inactivation by amobarbital and decreases following right-hemisphere inactivation.[16,17] Hemispheric strokes involving the insular cortex can alter parasympathetic vs. sympathetic homeostasis, resulting in arrhythmias and, conceivably, cardiac damage.

Acute stroke is associated with increased plasma norepinephrine levels.[18] Sympathetic overactivity has been known to cause structural myocardial damage. There is subendocardial myofibrillar degeneration or necrosis that may cause elevation of cardiac enzymes or myocardial infarction, or lead to the disruption of the Purkinje system, leading to repolarization abnormalities, ventricular ectopy, ventricular tachycardia, and heart blocks.[5,19] The ventricular arrhythmias do not respond well to conventional antiarrhythmic drugs but respond to beta blockers.This further suggests a role for sympathetic overactivity in their pathogenesis.[5] Admission to a cardiac monitoring unit with serial electrocardiograms and cardiac enzyme measurements for the first 72 hours following an acute stroke is recommended for all patients.[6,8,9,11,19]

PULMONARY COMPLICATIONS

Pneumonia from all causes occurs in 12% and is recurrent in 11% of stroke patients.[1] It accounts for 29% of stroke deaths.[5] Dysphagia occurs in 25% to 50% of stroke patients.[26,28] Aspiration probably occurs in 20% to 38% of patients and is frequently silent.[26,27] Indeed, one study reported that those who aspirated had actually a lower prevalence of subjective complaints of swallowing difficulty then the ones who did complain of swallowing problems.[28] The incidence is understandably higher (50% to 54%) in those referred for speech and swallowing evaluation.[27,29] Unrecognized aspiration may lead to aspiration pneumonia in about 12% to 15% of these patients.[26,27] A high index of suspicion, a careful clinical and neurological evaluation, and liberal use of fluoroscopic swallowing studies are probably appropriate.[26] Aspiration precaution thus forms an important part of management of strokes. The patient should take nothing by mouth for 24 hours following an acute stroke. This is followed by a clinical speech and swallowing evaluation. Those with gross swallowing abnormalities and those with normal swallowing do not require fluoroscopic swallowing studies.[26] Patients with a poor cough reflex, dysarthria, and dysphonia are at a much higher risk for aspiration than those with these reflexes intact.

However an impaired gag reflex has not been associated with an increased risk for aspiration.[28,29] Dysphagia and aspiration occur with equal frequency in unilateral right- and left-hemispheric infarcts but are more frequent in bilateral strokes and lower brainstem strokes with multiple cranial nerve paralyses. The exact lesions and pathways have been much debated but remain undefined.[26–29]

All patients with mild to moderate dysphagia or multiple risk factors for aspiration require swallowing studies. For those deemed to have significant aspiration risk by clinical and/or radiological evaluation, a soft nasogastric feeding tube can be placed for 10 to 14 days , then swallowing reevaluated.[26] Most patients recover normal swallowing within 2 weeks.[27] If swallowing does not improve, a permanent gastrostomy tube is recommended. For patients undergoing rehabilitation and judged to have mild to moderate risk of aspiration, limited patient and family training regarding use of diet modification and compensatory swallowing techniques are as effective as therapist controlled techniques.[30] Using a multidisciplinary approach (biofeedback; laryngeal adduction exercise; Valsalva maneuver; Mendelson's maneuver; postural modifications, etc.), the incidence of aspiration pneumonia has reportedly been reduced by several investigators,[26] but the efficacy of each of these has not been firmly established. A more detailed discussion in presented in Chapter 12.

URINARY COMPLICATIONS

Urinary incontinence occurs in 44% to 66% of patients with acute strokes and 37% of patients admitted for stroke rehabilitation. The incidence then drops to 42% and 29%, respectively, at 4 and 12 weeks.[31–33] Incontinence is prevalent in patients with large infarcts, cognitive impairment, dysphasia, and functional disability. Neither age, sex, or side of stroke is associated with an increased risk.[33] Bladder hyperreflexia is probably the cause of urinary incontinence in 37% of patients, detrusor-sphincter dyssynergy in 5%, and bladder hyporeflexia in 21%. Diabetes mellitus and anticholinergic medications are reported to be the most common cause of bladder hyporeflexia.[32] Simple discontinuation of these medications results in improvement of symptoms.

Preexisting urinary incontinence may exist and should be investigated because it is frequently treatable.[33] Anticholinergic drugs such as oxybutyrin chloride are only effective if bladder symptoms occur due to involuntary bladder contraction and reflex relaxation of the external sphincter. Unfortunately, urinary incontinence is commonly treated by the insertion of a Foley's catheter. The indwelling catheter than predisposes to urinary tract infections and septicemia. Urinary tract infections occur in 16% to 77% of patients with strokes and are among the most frequent of all post-stroke complications.[1,5] Subsequent septicema accounts for 5% of deaths in stroke patients.[5] Scheduled voiding can be used as a first-line treatment in most incontinent patients.[32] Intermittent bladder catheterization is safer than an indwelling foley catheter and most patients can be taught this technique.[5] Biofeedback-assisted bladder retraining may be useful in selected patients.[35] For further details, please refer to Chapter 12.

DEPRESSION

The prevalence of depressive illness after stroke is 23% to 32%.[36–38] Major depression occurs in 13% to 15% of patients and minor depression in 5% to 11%.[36] Poststroke depression as evaluated by using the Hamilton Depression Rating Scale occurs in 41% of all stroke patients and 33% of first-stroke patients.[38] Vast majority (79% to 80%) of depressions occur in the first few weeks to months after stroke,[39] show a decline at 1 to 2 years and then rise again at 3 years.[33] Depression that occurs early tends to resolve, while late depressions tend to be more chronic.[36,38,39]

Significant risk factors for developing a depressive illness include impairment of daily activities, social activities, impaired intellect,[39] history of previous stroke, history of previous depression, female gender, living alone, and prestroke social distress.[40] Predictors of immediate poststroke depression are left anterior circulation infarcts and dysphasia,[38] but this correlation has not been found with major depression.[37,40] Later depression is more related to right-hemisphere infarcts, dependence in activities of daily living, and fewer social contacts.[37,38] Most stroke patients do not tolerate daytime somnolence or urinary incontinence caused by traditional tricyclic antidepressants, and these agents should be used judicously.[37,40] Alternative agents such as trazodone[41] or serotonin reuptake inhibitors such as citalopram[42] show more promise. The latter is also effective in post-stroke pathological crying, which is thought to occur due to serotonin depletion.[40,42]

GASTROINTESTINAL COMPLICATIONS

The incidence of serious gastrointestinal hemorrhage is probably low (0.1% to 3%) and does not seem to pose as an independent risk factor for increased mortality.[43,44] However, 10 of 18 patients who did bleed in a large study died, with hemorrhage contributing directly to death in three.[44] Hemorrhage occurred due to gastric, duodenal, or esophageal ulceration. Risk factors for gastrointestinal hemorrhage include increasing age, urinary incontinence, large infarcts or total anterior circulation syndrome, hemorrhagic stroke, and a prestroke Oxford handicap score of >2.[43,44] The use of anticoagulant agents has not been reported to increase the risk of this complication. The routine use of H_2 antagonist as prophylaxis for gastrointestinal hemorrhage is not indicated for stroke patients unless they have a coagulopathy and/or are on mechanical ventilation.[43–45]

PAIN SYNDROMES

Central poststroke pain is relatively common, occurring in 8% of patients with stroke.[46] The lesion is most often in the spinothalamic pathways. The patients can be divided into three groups: those with somatosensory deficits and central pain (classic thalamic pain syndrome); those with central pain but normal sense perception (analgetic thalamic syndrome); and those with somatosensory impairment alone(pure algetic thalamic syndrome). The location of the lesion is important. A paramedian or anterolateral thalamic lesion might be an indicator for the development of central pain especially when somatosensory evoked potential are intact. A patient with a posterolateral thalamic lesion and a loss of cortical somatosensory evoked potentials is probably at low risk for developing central pain.[47] Other authors believe that allodynia or dysesthesia combined with partial sensory loss is a prerequisite for the diagnosis of the thalamic syndrome. A spinothalamic tract deficit does not appear to be as important as was previously considered. Whatever the symptom complex or location of lesion, the pain is related to hyperalgesia or dysesthesia, suggesting a deafferentation phenomenon. Subsequent secondary central sensitization of third- or higher-order neurons that have lost part of their afferent input then leads to dysesthesias.[46] Central pain is also reported to occur in brainstem or sensory cortical infarctions.[48] The pain may appear 1 week to 6 months (mean 69 days) after the stroke.[47] Treatment with carbemezepine or phenytoin is variably successful .[48] Tricyclic antidepressants or the newer serotonin uptake inhibitors may be more effective.[46,48]

Shoulder pain occurs in 12% to 72% of patients with hemiparesis. It occurs more often in patients having spasticity (88%) than in those with flaccidity (22%). Anteroinferior subluxation, rotator cuff tear, and shoulder-hand syndrome/ reflex sympathetic dystrophy syndrome (RSD) also predispose to shoulder pain.[49] RSD is present in only 20% of cases with shoulder pain; stroke accounts for 27% cases of RSD. Trauma, inadvertent or otherwise, to the shoulder or the paretic limb is thought to be important in the pathogenesis of the shoulder-hand syndrome.[50] Roentgenographic evaluation should be done on all patients with shoulder pain, and every effort made to treat spasticity and subluxation as early as possible. Physical and occupational therapy, antispastic drugs (such as tizanidine, benzodiazopines), and shoulder girdle injections of lidocaine or alcohol can be tried.[49] Avoiding shoulder trauma is preventive. Established RSD responds to 7 to 10 days of steroid therapy if initiated early.[50] In later stages skin atrophy and contractions of joints may occur.

FALLS

Falls are common after stroke, occuring in 22% to 46% of hospitalized patients[1,51]. Six months after discharge to home this incidence rises to 73%.[51] In patients admitted for rehabilitation 39% suffer falls.[52] Fortunately, only 1% to 4% of the falls result in fracture or serious injury.[51,52] However, multiple falls are frequent (48% to 66%), and the risk of injury, both minor and serious, in these "fallers" is higher (44% and 8%, respectively). Fallers are defined as those that fall two or more times in an index year.

History of fall during hospitalization is the most significant predictor of subsequent falls.[51] Depressed mood and degree of motor disability (Barthel index score of 16 or less) are also closely related to falls.[51] Right-hemisphere strokes are frequently cited as predisposing to falls because of their left hemispatial neglect syndromes but regardless of site of lesion impulsivity and rightward orienting bias seem to be important predisposing conditions.[53,54]

Comorbidity such as heart disease, diabetes, chronic obstructive lung disease, previous stroke, prestroke history of fall, hypertension, or poor eyesight does not increase the risk of falls.[51]

The risk of fall-related mortality and bleeding complications in anticoagulated patients undergoing stroke rehabilitation is reportedly low,[55] but long-term prevalence is not known. Fall prevention requires a multidisciplinary approach with physician, physical therapist, home care, family support and awareness.

ENDOCRINE COMPLICATIONS

Diabetes is a risk factor for stroke and is known to increase stroke mortality . It occurs in 35% of patients with cerebrovascular accidents.[5] What is less known is that impaired glucose tolerance as evidenced by a raised HbA_1C concentration and without a prior history of diabetes occurs in 42% patients with stroke.[56] It may also be a major risk factor for stroke and stroke mortality. Transitory reactive hyperglycemia has been reported to occur in as many as 28% of patients and may be linked with severity, location, and type of stroke.[5,57] Other investigators have reported a prevalence of 6% undiagnosed diabetes in stroke and 14% cases of hyperglycemia overall. Diabetes was responsible for a surprising 39% early mortality in this study population.[3] Hyperglycemia, whether chronic or transitory, is associated with increased cerebral edema, reduced cerebral blood flow, and larger infarct size.[4] Blood sugars should be carefully monitored and kept under fairly tight control in the setting of acute stroke. However, hypoglycemia also causes cerebral damage and should be avoided.

Inappropriate antidiaretic hormone secretion (SIADH) occurs in 10% of cerebral infarctions and 14% of cerebral hemorrhages. This may lead to reduced sodium concentration and clinical deterioration or seizures. Treatment is with fluid restriction. However, most cases of hyponatremia are incidental and asymptomatic and require no treatment.[4] Fluid restrictions or hydration must be done judiciously, as dehydration exacerbates neurological deficit and overhydration worsens cerebral edema, which may itself cause SIADH.[5]

MORTALITY AND MISCELLANEOUS DISORDERS

High fever is a poor prognostic feature in stroke, and the longer the fever lasts, the worse the prognosis. About 43% of fevers occurs within the first 7 days of stroke, and of these 64% occur in the first 2 days.[2] Presence of fever in stroke may be an isolated finding or an indication of underlying infection or inflammation and warrants a search for pneumonia, urinary tract infection, or deep-vein thrombosis. Pyrexial illness, defined as a temperature elevation > 37.5°C for >24 hours without an underlying cause, occurs in 4% of patients.[1] High fever (>37.9°) is an independent risk factor for a worse prognosis, as is degree of conscious impairment.[2] Whether the poorer prognosis occurs due to direct neurological damage from the increase in temperature remains unclear.[2]

There is a 20% mortality following acute stroke. It follows a bimodal pattern. Deaths in the first week are usually due to the transtentorial herniation. The second peak occurs at the end of the second week and is most often due to pneumonia, sepsis, and pulmonary embolism. Cardiac death peaks in the first week[5] but continues to occur throughout the first month.[58]

Thus, recognition is important as complications result in prolongation of hospital stay, slower recovery, and increased morbidity and mortality despite many of these conditions being potentially preventable.

REFERENCES

1. Davenport RJ, Dennis MS, Wellwood I, Warlow CP. Complications after acute stroke. Stroke 1996; 27:415–420.
2. Azzimondi G, Bassein L, Nonino F, Fiorani L, Vignatelli L, Re G, D'Alessandro R. Fever in acute stroke worsen prognosis. A prospective study. Stroke 1995; 26(11): 2040–2043.
3. Oppenheimer SM, Hachinski V. Complications of acute stroke. Lancet 1992; 339:721–724.
4. Oppenheimer SM, Hoffbrand BI, Oswald GA, Yudkin JS. Diabetes mellitus and early morbidity from stroke. Lancet 1984; 291.
5. Weinberger J. Management of the complications of stroke. In: Batjet HH et al eds. Cerebrovascular disorders. Lippincott Raven. 1997; 655–673.
6. Chin PL, Kaminski J, Rout M. Myocardial infarction coincident with cerebrovascular accidents in the elderly. Age Ageing 1977; 6(1):29–37.
7. Komad MS, Coffey CE, Coffey KS, McKinnis R, Massey EW, Califf RM. Myocardial infarction and stroke. Neurology 1984; 34:1403–1409 .
8. Norris JW, Hachinski VC, Myers MG, Callow J, Wong T, Moore RW. Serum cardiac enzymes in stroke . Stroke 1979; 10(5):548–553.
9. Oppenheimer SM, Cechetto DF, Hachinski VC. Cerebrogenic cardiac arrhythmias. Arch Neurol 1990; 47:513–519.

10. Roth E. Heart disease in patients with stroke: incidence, impact, and implications for rehabilitation. Part 1. Classification and prevalence. Arch Phys Med Rehabil 1993; 74:752–760.
11. Mikolich JR, Jacobs C, Fletcher GF. Cardiac arrhythmias in patient with acute cerebrovascular accidents. JAMA 1981; 246(12):1314–1317.
12. Vingerhoets F, Bogousslavsky J, Reglis F, Van Melle G. Atrial fibrillation after acute stroke. Stroke 1993; 24:26–30.
13. Noel P, Gregoire F, Capon A, Lehert P. Atrial fibrillation as a risk factor for deep venous thrombosis and pulmonary emboli in stroke patients. Stroke 1991; 22(6):760–762 .
14. Lane RD, Wallach JD, Petrosky PP, Schwartz GE, Gradman AH. Supraventricular tachycardia in patients with right hemisphere strokes. Stroke 1992; 23(3):362–368.
15. Oppenheimer SM, Gelb A, Girvin JP, Hachinski V. Cardiovascular effects of human insular cortex stimulation. Neurology 1992; 42:1727–1732 .
16. Zamrini EY, Meador KJ, Loring DW, Nichols FT, Lee GP, Figueroa RE, Thompson WO. Unilateral cerebral inactivation produces differential left/right heart rate responses. Neurology 1990; 40:1408–1411.
17. Hachinski VC. The clinical problem of brain and heart. Stroke 1993; 24(12)(suppl 1):1–12.
18. Myers MG, Norris JW, Hachniski VC, Sole MJ. Plasma norepinephrine in stroke. Stroke1981; 12(2):200–204.
19. Dimant J, Grob D. Electrocardiographic changes and myocardial damages in patients with acute cerebrovascular accidents. Stroke 1977; 8:448–455.
20. Warlow C, Ogston D, Douglas AS. Venous thrombosis following strokes. Lancet 1972; i:1305–1306.
21. McCarthy ST, Robertson D, Turner JJ, Hawkey CJ. Low-dose heparin as a prophylaxis against deep-vein thrombosis after acute stroke. Lancet 1977; 2(8042): 800–801.
22. Sioson ER, Crowe WE, Dawson NV. Occult proximal deep vein thrombosis: its prevalence among patients admitted to a rehabilitation hospital. Arch Phys Med Rehabil 1988; 69:183–185.
23. Wieslaw J, Oczkowski WJ, Ginsberg JS, Shin A, Panju A. Venous thromboembolism in patients undergoing rehabilitation for stroke. Arch Phys Med Rehabil 1992; 73:712–716.
24. Miyamoto AT, Miller LS. Pulmonary embolism in stroke:prevention by early heparinization of venous thrombosis detected by iodine-125 fibrinogen leg scans. Arch Phys Med Rehabil 1980; 61(12):584–587.
25. Turpie A, Hirsh J, Jay R, Andrew M, Hull R, Levine M, Carter C, Powers PJ, Magnani HN, Gent M. Double-blind randomised trail of ORG 10172 low-molecular-weight heparinoid in prevention of deep-vein thrombosis in thrombotic stroke. Lancet 1987; 8532: 523–526.
26. Alberts MJ, Horner J. Dysphagia and aspiration syndrome. In: Bogousslavsky J, Caplan L, eds. Stroke syndromes. Cambridge Press, 1995; 213–222.
27. Gordon C, Hewer RL, Wade DT. Dysphagia in acute stroke. BMJ 1987; 295:411–413.

28. Horner J, Massey EW. Silent aspiration following stroke. Neurology 1988; 38:317–319
29. Horner J, Massey EW, Riski JE, Lathrop DL, Chase KN. Aspirations following stroke: clinical correlates and outcome. Neurology 1988; 38:1359–1362.
30. DePippo KL, Holas MA, Reding MJ, Mandel FS, Lesser ML. Dysphagia therapy following stroke: a controlled trial. Neurology 1994; 44(9):1655–1660.
31. Henriksen T. Urinary incontinence after apoplexy. Ugeskrift Laegar 1993; 155(15):1107–1109.
32. Gelber DA, Good DC, Laven LJ, Verhulst SJ. Causes of urinary incontinence after acute hemispheric stroke. Stroke 1993; 24(3):378–382.
33. Borrie MJ, Campbell AJ, Caradoc-Davies TH, Spears GF. Urinary incontinence after stroke: a prospective study. Age Ageing. 1986; 15(3):77–81.
34. Dromerick A, Reding M. Medical and neurological complications during inpatient stroke rehabilitation. Stroke 1994; 25(2):358–361.
35. Middaugh SJ, Whitehead WE, Burgio KL, Engel BT. Biofeedback in treatment of urinary incontinence in stroke patients. Biofeedback Self Regul 1989; 14(1):3–19.
36. Burvill PW, Johnson GA, Jamrozik KD, Anderson CS, Stewart-Wynne EG, Chakera MH. Prevalence of depression after stroke: the Perth Community Stroke Study. Br J Psychiatry 1995; 166:320–327.
37. House A. Depression after stroke. BMJ 1987; 294:76–78.
38. Astrom M, Adolfsson R, Asplund K. Major depression in stroke patients: a 3-year longitudinal study. Stroke 1993; 124 (7):976–982.
39. Anderson G, Vestergaard K, Riis JO, Lauritzen L. Incidence of post-stroke depression during the first year in a large unselected stroke population determined by using a valid standardized rating scale. Acta Psychiatr Scand 1994; 90:190–195.
40. Anderson G, Vestergaard K, Ingermann-Nielsen M, Lauritzen L. Risk factors for post-stroke depression. Acta Psychiatr Scand 1995; 92:193–198.
41. Reding MJ, Orto LA, Winter SW, Fortuna IM, Di Ponte P, McDowell FH. Antidepressant therapy after stroke. Arch Neurol 1986; 43:763–765.
42. Anderson G, Vestergaard K, Lauritzen L. Effective treatment of poststroke depression with the selective serotonin reuptake inhibitor citalopram. Stroke 1994; 125(6):1099–1104.
43. Wijdicks EFM, Fulgham JR, Batts KP. Gastrointestinal bleeding in stroke. Stroke 1994; 25(11):2146–2148.
44. Davenport RL, Dennis MS, Warlow CP. Gastrointestinal hemorrhage after acute stroke. Stroke 1996; 27:421–424.
45. Cook DJ, Fuller HD, Gordon GH, Marshall JC, Leasa D, Hall R, Winton TL, Rutledge F, Todd JRT, Roy P, Lacroix J, Griffith L, Willan A. Risk factors for gastrointestinal bleeding in critically ill patients. N Engl J Med 1994; 330:377–381.
46. Jensen TS, Lenz FA. Central post-stroke pain: a challenge for the scientist and the clinician. Pain 1995; 61:161–164.
47. Wessel K, Vieregge P, Kessler CH, Kompf D. Thalamic stroke: correlation of clinical symptoms, somatosensory evoked potentials, and CT findings. Acta Neurol Scand 1994; 90:167–173.
48. Leijon G, Boivie J. Central post-stroke pain—a controlled trial of amitriptyline and carbamazepine. Pain 1989; 36(1):27–36.

49. Ouwenalller VC, Laplace PM, Chantriaine A. Painful shoulder in hemiplegia. Arch Phys Med Rehabil 1986; 67(1):23–36.
50. Braus DF, Krauss JK, Strobel J. The Shoulder-Hand Syndrome after stroke: a prospective clinical trial. Ann Neurol 1994; 5:728–733.
51. Forster A, Young J. Incidence of consequences of falls due to stroke: a systematic inquiry. BMJ 1995; 311:83–86.
52. Nyberg L, Gustafson Y. Patient falls in stroke rehabilitation . A challenge to rehabilitation strategies. Stroke 1995; 26(5):838–842.
53. Rapport LJ, Webster JS, Kirstin L, Flemming KL, Lindberg JW, Godlewski MC, et al. Predictors of falls among right-hemisphere stroke patients in the rehabilitation setting. Arch Phys Med Rehabil 1993; 74(6):621–626.
54. Webster JS, Roades LA, Morrill B, Rapport LJ, Abadee PS, Sowa MV, Dutra R, Godlawski MC. Rightward orienting bias, wheelchair maneuvering, and fall risk. Arch Phys Med Rehabil 1995; 76(10):924–928.
55. Stein J,Viramontes BE, Kerrigan DC. Fall-related injuries in anticoagulated stroke patients during inpatient rehabilitation. Arch Phys Med Rehabil 1995; 76(9):840–843.
56. Riddle MC, Hart JH. Hyperglycaemia, recognised and unrecognised, as a risk factor for stroke and transient ischaemic attacks. Stroke 1982; 13(3):356–359.
57. Melamed E. Reactive hyperglycaemia in patients with acute stroke. J Neurosci 1976; 29(2–4):267–275.
58. Silver, FL, Norris JW, Lewis AJ, Hachinski VC. Early mortality following stroke: a prospective review. Stroke 1984; 15(3):492–496.

8
Progressing Stroke

Carmelo Graffagnino
Duke University Medical Center, Durham, North Carolina

INTRODUCTION

Physicians who care for stroke patients have long recognized that a proportion of such patients may worsen clinically over the first few days. This phenomenon has been referred to as deteriorating, or progressing, stroke. Since Millikan first introduced the concept of progressing stroke over 30 years ago, controversy has surrounded this clinical phenomenon.[1]

The reported frequency of stroke progression varies from 26% to 43%.[2–7] Some of the variability may relate to a lack of uniformity in the methods used to quantify neurological deficits; this is particularly true of earlier reports. The development of standardized measurement scales has now allowed a more precise definition of clinically significant worsening.[8] A second factor contributing to the variability in reported rates of progressing stroke relates to the timing of the observed events. Patients whose symptoms progress at 6 hours may do so for reasons other than those deteriorating at 48 or 96 hours. Finally, stroke is a heterogeneous condition. Progression of symptoms among patients with cerebral infarction may result from processes different from those associated with intracerebral hemorrhage. Studies carried out prior to the development of CT scanning may have included patients with a variety of stroke types.

DIFFERENTIAL DIAGNOSIS

Deteriorating neurological function may result from primary neurological processes, systemic causes (medical conditions that impact brain function), or ia-

Table 1 Differential Diagnosis of Deteriorating Stroke

Iatrogenic	Neurological	Systemic medical factors
Drugs	Ischemic Infarctions	Respiratory
Sedative/hypnotic agents	Early events (0–72 hours)	Airway obstruction
Benzodiazepines	Progression of infarction at the cellular level	Hypercarbia
Opiates	Progression of thombosis	Hypoxia
Barbiturates	Seizure (postictal state)	Pulmonary
Analgesic drugs	Cerebral edema	Pneumonia
Opiates	Hemorrhagic transformation	Pulmonary embolism
Anesthetics	Hydrocephalus	Atelectasis
Propofol	Late events (>72 hours)	Neurogenic pulmonary edema
Other drugs	Seizure (postictal state)	Cardiovascular
Anticonvulsants	Hemorrhagic transformation	Dysrhythmias with hypotension (tachy and brady)
Intravenous phenytoin may cause transient sedation	Recurrent infarction	Endocrinological
Misdiagnosis	Cerebral Hemorrhage	Hypoglycemia
Infections	Early events (0–72 hours)	Hyperglycemia
Encephalitis	Rehemorrhaging	Hyponatremia (SIADH and neurogenic salt wasting)
Meningitis	Hydrocephalus (obstructive)	Infections
Other vascular conditions	Cerebral edema	Pneumonia
Subarrhachnoid hemorrhage	Seizure (postictal state)	Urinary tract infection
Subdural hematoma	Secondary cerebral infarction from compression of intracerebral blood vessels	Septicemia
Seizures	Late events (>72 hours)	Fever
Nonconvulsive status epilepticus	Same as above	Regardless of etiology results in poor neurological function

trogenic interventions such as the administration of sedating medications (Table 1). All patients with progressing neurological symptoms should be evaluated for the presence of one or more of these factors to correctly select the appropriate therapeutic intervention.

MECHANISMS OF PROGRESSING STROKE

Neurological Mechanisms

Ischemic Strokes

The neurological processes that result in progressing stroke may be regarded as being either *directly* due to ischemia or *indirectly* due to the effects of the infarcted tissue on the adjacent healthy brain. Direct mechanisms may include worsening ischemia secondary to thrombus propagation or progression of ischemia due to secondary or delayed cell death. Indirect neurological mechanisms include cerebral edema, hemorrhagic transformation, and seizures.

Direct Mechanisms

Clot Propagation Propagation of a thrombus which then leads to more profound ischemia and eventually to a larger volume of infarction is commonly considered as a cause of progressing stroke.[9] Although this is an attractive theory, there is little evidence to support it. Angiographic studies of patients with progressing stroke have not shown evidence of thrombus propagation.[10] However, because of the belief that a propagating thrombus is responsible for the deterioration, anticoagulation with heparin has long been recommended as a treatment of progressing stroke. Early case reports suggested that patients who were treated with heparin in this setting had good outcomes.[11] However, there are no controlled clinical trials that have proven the efficacy of such therapy. Most of the studies utilizing heparin were either not randomized,[12] too small, or lacked clearly defined endpoints.[13–15] The one double-blind, placebo-controlled trial of heparin therapy in patients with acute stable stroke failed to show any benefit for heparin in halting or preventing the progression of stroke symptoms.[16]

Delayed Cell Death Cerebral ischemia and infarction is a dynamic process in which a sequence of molecular events eventually leads to cell death. Reversal of the process is possible if intervention occurs prior to a pivotal point. The degree of ischemic injury to a neuron (and thus the reversibility of the deficit) depends directly on the severity and duration of cerebral blood flow (CBF) impairment. In regions where the CBF is <10 mL/100/g/min, the tissue becomes damaged irreversibly resulting in an area which is referred to as the ischemic core.[17] Surrounding this area of irreversibly damaged tissue is a region that has come to be referred to as the ischemic pneumbra, and ultimately into infarcted tissue.[18,19] The neurons in this region display impaired functional activity resulting from failure of membrane pumps and loss of electrical activity.[20–22] Failure to reestablish blood flow eventually results in cell death. It has been proposed that the clinical phenomenon of "progressing stroke" corresponds, at the cellular level, to the conversion of functioning brain tissue into the ischemic pneumbra and ultimately into infarcted tissue. It is at this level that clinical interventions need to be targeted to reverse the process of cell death and stop the accompanying clinical deterioration.

Cerebral Edema The development of cerebral edema is another potential cause of clinical worsening. The earliest event is the failure of membrane pumps resulting in cellular swelling (cytotoxic edema). With continued ischemia, injury occurs to the microcirculation, resulting in damage to the blood-brain barrier and vasogenic edema. Cytotoxic edema may develop as early as 90 minutes from the onset of ischemia whereas vasogenic edema typically peaks at 48 to 72 hours.[23–25] Compression of the adjacent tissue due to progressing edema may then result in worsening clinical function (Fig. 1). It is this shift in brain tissue and not increased intracranial pressure that results in clinical deterioration, often manifesting by impairment in consciousness.[25,26] Edema may also cause worsening through compression of intracranial vessels, resulting in secondary ischemic injury. Finally, cerebral edema may result in compression of the ventricular outflow system, resulting in clinical deterioration due to the development of hydrocephalus.

Hemorrhagic Infarction Ischemic injury to the microvascular circulation produces necrotic vessels that may lead to petechial hemorrhage or less commonly large hematomas (Fig. 2). The latter may be associated with clinical worsening. Although petechial hemorrhages are common, clinical deterioration is seen in only 10% of patients.[27,28] The incidence of symptomatic hematoma among patients with acute ischemic stroke ranges from 0.6% to 2.4%.[29,30] This can increase to 6% among patients treated with tPA within 3 hours of their stroke[30] and up to 24% in patients treated up to 6 hours after stroke onset.[29]

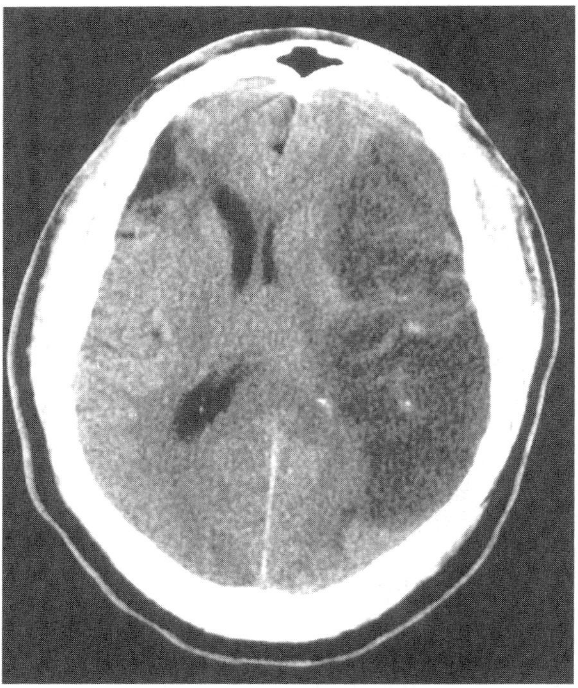

Figure 1 Malignant cerebral edema 72 hours following the onset of ischemic stroke.

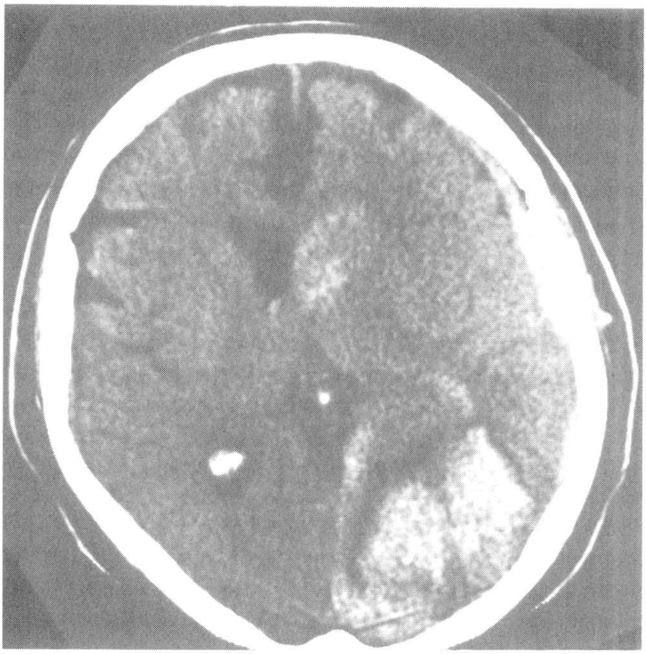

Figure 2 Hemorrhagic transformation of an ischemic cerebral infarction.

Indirect Mechanisms

Seizures Up to 6% of patients with an ischemic stroke will have a seizure within the first week.[31] Most of these seizures are of the simple partial type, and status epilepticus is quite rare.[32,33] Although it is often believed that seizures are more common with cardioembolic strokes, the evidence supporting this contention is inclusive.[32–34] Patients with focal motor seizures and postictal Todd's paralysis may appear to be clinically worsening. This is particularly confusing when the seizure is not witnessed. Most often patients have only a single seizure and thus anticonvulsants are not indicated. Patients who experience multiple seizures should be considered for chronic antiepileptic drug treatment.[31,32,35]

Reinfarction Stroke recurrence is most likely within the first 30 days following a cerebral infarction.[36] The risk varies from 2.2% to 7.9% depending on the type of stroke. Atherothrombotic strokes have the highest risk while lacunar infarctions are least likely to recur in the early period. Cardioembolic strokes recur at a rate of 1% per day up to a cumulative maximum of 10% to 12% after 2 weeks.[37,38]

Hemorrhagic Strokes

Rebleeding Although intracerebral hemorrhage is less prevalent than ischemic infarction, it is associated with a higher mortality rate. As is the case with cerebral infarction, these patients may also worsen after the acute presentation. Rebleeding is often seen during the first 24 hours.[39–41] Poorly controlled hypertension is associated with a higher rate of rebleeding; thus it is critical to control hypertension early in order to reduce the likelihood of subsequent bleeding and preventing clinical worsening.[42,43]

Hydrocephalus Intracerebral hemorrhage with ventricular extension may result in the development of communicating hydrocephalus and secondarily elevated intracranial pressure. Obstruction of the ventricular system, particularly the third ventricle in the case of basal ganglion or thalamic hemorrhages and the fourth ventricle in the case of cerebellar hemorrhages, may result in obstructive hydrocephalus.

Brainstem Compression The ascending reticular activating system, located in the brainstem from the midpontine level to the midbrain, is vulnerable to direct compression from an enlarging cerebellar mass such as a parenchymal hemorrhage or edematous infarcted cerebellar tissue. In such cases clinical deterioration may occur quite quickly, often resulting in irreversible brainstem damage and in some cases death. Supratentorial edema or large parenchymal hemorrhages may also result in herniation of the uncus with compression of the midbrain and secondary impairment of consciousness.

Systemic Mechanisms

Systemic medical complications associated with stroke (ischemic and hemorrhagic) may cause a change in clinical status mimicking progressing stroke (Table 1). Respiratory and airways problems present the most acute and life-threatening situations. Patients with impaired level of consciousness (Glasgow coma scale <11) often experience significant respiratory difficulties, which may lead to development of hypercarbia and/or hypoxia. Both of these states may cause further damage to the already ischemic brain. Hypercarbia results either from airway obstruction or reduced ventilatory drive. Hypoxia is less common in the acute stroke period. Some patients may develop hypoxia in the setting of neurogenic pulmonary edema.[44] This is seen more often in patients with subarrachnoid and intracerebral hemorrhage than in those with ischemic strokes.[44] Pneumonia occurs in nearly one-third of all patients with stroke and is often associated with clinical deterioration.[45] Pulmonary embolism is another respiratory complication that may result in clinical deterioration and secondarily impaired neurological function. This is most often seen within the first week following onset of stroke symptoms, although it remains a risk as long as the patient remains immobile.

Cardiovascular complications of acute stroke include tachy- and brady-dysrrhythmias as well as acute coronary syndromes.[46,47] The associated hypotension may increase the extent of cerebral ischemia and result in worsening neurological function.

Metabolic abnormalities that may result in impaired neurological function include hypoglycemia, hyperglycemia, and hyponatremia. The latter may result from neurogenic salt wasting or SIADH (syndrome of inappropriate antiduretic hormone).

Iatrogenic Mechanisms

Not all patients who present with focal neurological deficits have a stroke (Table 1). The differential diagnosis for stroke includes seizures, migraines, infections, and metabolic abnormalities (hypoglycemia). Failure to make the proper diagnosis may result in clinical worsening, thus mimicking progressing stroke.

Drugs that impair the patient's level of consciousness should not be used in the acute or subacute phases of a stroke. The sedating effects of the drugs may be misdiagnosed as progression of stroke symptoms and lead to unnecessary diagnostic tests and clinical interventions. The most commonly used medications with such effects include benzodiazepines, opioid analgesics, and major tranquilizers such as phenothiazines.

CLINICAL DIAGNOSIS

As progression of stroke symptoms may result from mechanisms that vary depending on the stroke type and duration from onset of symptoms, an accurate clinical history and evaluation of the extent of neurological impairment at the time of presentation are critical. Close clinical monitoring by trained personnel is essential to detect any clinical changes. When a patient experiences a decline in neurological status, a search for the cause should immediately take place. It must then be determined whether the change is due to neurological, systemic, or iatrogenic causes (Table 1).

All medications should be reviewed, and if possible, those with centrally acting effects should be discontinued (i.e., benzodiazepines, opiates, phenothiazines, barbiturates, and dopamine agonists such as metoclopramide). A comprehensive physical examination with particular attention to the fundamental ABCs of resuscitation is essential. Ensuring that the patient has a patent airway and is ventilating adequately is the first and most important component of the initial evaluation. Pulse oxymetry provides a rapid method of assessing oxygenation until the results of arterial blood gas evaluation are available. A stable cardiac rhythm and adequate systemic blood pressure must be maintained. As ventricular arrhythmias are seen in up to 35% of patients with acute stroke, all such patients should have continuous cardiac monitoring during the first 72 to 96 hours.[46] Tachydysrhythmias such as atrial fibrillation, paroxysmal atrial tachycardia, supraventricullar tachycardia, and ventricular tachycardia may result in hypotension and worsening cerebral ischemia.[47] Ventricular tachycardia may deteriorate into ventricular fibrillation and result in death. Although less common, bradyarrhythmias may also result in hypotension with the same consequences as the tachyarrhythmias.

As listed in Table 1, there are many metabolic abnormalities that may be associated with clinical worsening. Of these, hypoglycemia may manifest as worsening focal deficits as well as global impairment of function. Early evaluation for metabolic abnormalities such as hypoglycemia and hyponatremia should routinely be performed in cases of clinical worsening.

All patients with clinical worsening following a stroke should have a comparison neuroimaging study. CT scanning has the advantage of being widely available and requiring a relatively short time to conduct. The vast majority of structural neurological causes for progressing stroke can be diagnosed using a CT scan.

Most often, patients who deteriorate following a seizure will recover once the period of postictal neuronal dysfunction (Todd's paralysis) has passed. There are, however, some patients who may either continue to have subclinical seizures and thus fail to improve. An EEG may aid with the diagnosis of nonconvulsive status epilepticus.

TREATMENT

Identified hypoxemia, hypercarbia and metabolic abnormalities should be treated immediately. Maintaining an adequate cerebral perfusion pressure by not overtreating hypertension is also critical. In ischemic stroke patients, it is generally recommended that the systolic blood pressure be allowed to fluctuate as high as 200 mm Hg and the diastolic blood pressure to be as high as 100 mm Hg. In patients with intracerebral hemorrhage, hypertension should be treated if the systolic pressure is >180 mm Hg. These values represent commonly used practice guidelines by a number of neurocritical care physicians. After completing the respiratory and circulatory evaluation and treating any abnormalities noted, the focus of attention should be directed at the neurological evaluation. The results of neuroimaging may be critical.

The optimal way to treat raised intracranial hypertension remains controversial. Venous return from the brain may be improved by raising the head of the bed (up to 20°) and keeping the head pointed forward to prevent jugular obstruction. Hyperventilation may rapidly reduce ICP by 25% to 30%. The beneficial effects may last for hours, but as the pH of the cerebral spinal fluid reaches equilibrium, the vascoconstrictive effects of hyperventilation become less evident. It is generally recommended to keep the pCO_2 between 30 and 35 mm Hg until the ICP improves. A slow correction is recommended to prevent rebound intracranial hypertension.

Hyperosmolar therapy is the next form of therapy utilized in controlling raised ICP. Hyperosmolar therapy only works in the setting of an intact blood-brain barrier so that the free water is extracted from the healthy brain. In North America, the osmolar agent of choice remains mannitol. It is given as a bolus of 0.5 to 1.0 g/kg and then continued at 0.25 to 0.5 g/kg every 3 hours. Serum osmolarities should be checked every 3 hours. If the serum osmolarity is >310 m.osmol then the mannitol therapy is held.

Serum electrolytes should also be closely monitored as hyponatremia may also be associated with mannitol therapy. Steroid therapy has never been demonstrated to be of help in treating edema related to cerebral infarction.[48–50] Complications such as pneumonia[49,50] and sepsis have been associated with corticosteroid use in the setting of stroke. Barbiturate therapy, although effective in reducing intracranial hypertension, is associated with numerous complications including hypotension, infections, and decubital ulcers.[51] Insertion of an intraventricular catheter may be both diagnostic and therapeutic. Cerebrospinal fluid can be drained continuously to maintain ICP below a predetermined level. ICP monitoring via ventriculostomy is associated with several potential complications including parenchymal hemorrhage at the time of insertion and ventriculitis. In cases of severe cerebral edema, the ventricles may be fully drained and therefore collapsed. CSF no longer flows and ICP recordings may be inaccurate.

Experimental approaches for managing malignantly raised intracranial hypertension include hemicraniectomy and induced moderate hypothermia. A pilot study of hemicraniectomy for patients with massive hemispheric infarcts demonstrated a reduction in mortality from a predicted 80% to 35%.[52] A more recent report of hemicraniectomy within the first 24 hours (early hemicraniectomy) of a completed middle cerebral artery infarction showed a survival rate of 73. These results are promising and warrant further study. Hypothermia has long been recognized to be neuroprotective in experimental studies; however, it is now known whether such therapy improves outcome after massive cerebral infarction.

CONCLUSION

Progressing stroke is not the result of a single pathophysiological process. Worsening cerebral ischemia, cerebral edema, hemorrhagic transformation, and seizures are among the most common neurological causes, while hypoxia, hypercarbia, hypotension, fever, and infections are frequent systemic medical causes. Appropriately directed therapy depends on identifying the underlying cause(s).

REFERENCES

1. Millikan C, Siekert R. Studies in cerebral vascular disease. IV. The syndrome of intermittent insufficiency of the carotid arterial system. Proc Staff Mayo Clin 1955; 30:186–191.
2. Gilman S. Ingravescent cerebral infarction. Q J Med 1960; 29:611.
3. Jones H, Millikan C. Temporal profile (clinical course) of acute carotid system cerebral infarction. Stroke 1976; 7:64–71.
4. Hachinski V, Norris JW. The deteriorating stroke. In: Anonymous. The Acute Stroke. Philadelphia: F.A. Davis, 1985:123–140.
5. Britton M, Reden A. Progression of stroke after arrival at hospital. Stroke 1985; 16:629–632.
6. Davalos A, Cendra E, Turuel J, Martinez M, Genis D. Deteriorating ischemic stroke: risk factors and prognosis. Neurology 1990; 40:1865–1869.
7. Toni D, Fiorelli M, Gentile M, et al. Progressing neurological deficit secondary to acute ischemic stroke. Arch Neurol 1998; 52:670–675.
8. Lyden P, Lau G. A critical appriasal of stroke evaluation and scoring scales. Stroke 1991; 22:1345–1352.
9. Millikan C, McDowell F. Treatment of progressing strokes. Stroke 1981; 12:397.
10. Irino T, Watanabe M, Nishide M, Gotoh M, Tsuchiya T. Angiographical analysis of acute cerebral infarction followed by "cascade"-like deterioration of minor neurological deficits. What is progressing stroke? Stroke 1983; 14:363–368.
11. Millikan C, Siekert R, Shick R. Studies in cerebrovascular disease. III. The use of anticoagulant drugs in the treatment of insufficiency or thrombosis within the basilar arterial system. Proc Staff Mayo Clin 1955; 30:116–126.
12. Haley E, Kassell N, Torner J. Failure of heparin to prevent progression in progressing ischemic infarction. Stroke 1988; 19:10–14.
13. Carter A. Anticoagulant treatment in progressing stroke. Br Med J 1961; 2:70–73.
14. Baker R, Broward J, Fang H, et al. Anticoagulan therapy in cerebral infarction: report on cooperative study. Neurology 1962; 12:823–835.
15. Dobkin B. Heparin for lacunar stroke in progression. Stroke 1983; 14:421–423.
16. Duke R, Bloch R, Turpie A, Trebilcock R, Bayer N. Intravenous heparin for the prevention of stroke progression in acute partial stable stroke: a randomized controlled trial. Ann Intern Med 1986; 105:825–828.
17. Fisher M, Takano K. The penumbra, therapeutic time window and acute ischemic stroke. In: Hachinski V, ed. Balliere's Clinical Neurology, Cerebrovascular disease. London: Balliere Tindall, 1995:279–296.
18. Astrup J, Symon L, Siesjo B. Thresholds in cerebral ischemia: the ischemic penumbra. Stroke 1981; 12:723–725.

19. Symon L, Branston N, Strong A, et al. The concepts of thresholds of ischemia in relation to brain structure and function. J Clin Pathol 1977; 30(suppl 11):149–154.
20. Hakin A. The cerebral ischemic penumbra. Can J Neurol Sci 1987; 14:557–559.
21. Hossmann K. Viability thresholds and the penumbra of focal ischemia. Ann Neurol 1994; 362:557–559.
22. Ginsberg M, Pulsinelli W. The ischemic penumbra, injury thresholds and the therapeutic window for acute stroke. Ann Neurol 1994; 36:553–554.
23. Shaw C-M, Alvord EJ, Berry R. Swelling of the brain following ischemic infarction with arterial occlusion. Arch Neurol 1959; 1:161–177.
24. Ropper A, Shafran B. Brain edema after stroke; clinical syndrome and intracranial pressure. Arch Neurol 1984; 41:26–29.
25. Frank J. Large hemispheric infarction, deterioration, and intracranial pressure. Neurology 1995; 45:1286–1290.
26. Schwab S, Aschoff A, Spranger M, Albert F, Hacke W. The value of intracranial pressure monitoring in acute hemispheric stroke. Neurology 1996; 47:393–398.
27. Hornig C, Dorndorf W, Agnoli A. Hemorrhagic infarction: a prospective study. Stroke 1998; 17:179–185.
28. Hornig C, Bauer T, Simon C, Trittmacher S, Dorndorf W. Hemorrhagic transformation in cardioembolic cerebral infarction. Stroke 1993; 24:465–468.
29. Hacke W, Kaste M, Fieschi C, et al. Intravenous thrombolysis with recombinant tissue plasminogen activator for acute hemisphere stroke. JAMA 1995; 274:1017–1025.
30. National Institute of Neurological Disorders and Stroke rt-PA Stroke Study Group. Tissue plasminogen activator for acute ischemic stroke. N Engl J Med 1995; 333:1581–1587.
31. So E, Aegers J, Hauser W, O'Brien P, Whisnant J. Population-based study of seizure disorders after cerebral infarction. Neurology 1996; 46:350–355.
32. Gupta S, Naheedy M, Elias D, Rubino F. Postinfarction seizures: a clinical study. Stroke 1988; 19:350–355.
33. Kilpatrick C, Davis S, Tress B, Rossiter S, Hopper J, Vandendriesen M. Epileptic seizures in acute stroke. Arch Neurol 1990; 47:157–160.
34. Giroud M, Gras P, Fayolle H, Andre N, Soichot P, Dumas R. Early seizures after acute stroke: a study of 1640 cases. Epilepsia 1994; 35:959–964.
35. Adams H Jr, Brott T, Crowell R, et al. Guidelines for the management of patients with acute ischemic stroke: a statement for healthcare professionals from a special writing group of the Stroke Council, American Heart Association. Stroke 1994; 25:1901–1914.
36. Gasecki A, Ferguson G, Eliasziw M, et al. Early endarterectomy for severe carotid artery stenosis after a nondisabling stroke: results from the North American Symptomatic Carotid Endarterectomy Trial. J Vasc Surg 1994; 20:288.
37. Sherman D, Dyken M, Fisher M, et al. Antithrombotic therapy for cerebrovascular disorders. Chest 1989; 95:104S.
38. Yatsu F, Hart R, Mohr J, Grotta J. Anticoagulation of embolic strokes of cardiac origin: an update. Neurology 1988; 38:314.
39. Broderick J, Brott T, Tomsick T. Ultraearly evaluation of intracerebral hemorrhage. J Neurosurg 1990; 72:195.

40. Brott T, Broderick J, Kothari R, et al. Early hemorrhage growth in patients with intracerebral hemorrhage. Stroke 1997; 28:1.
41. Fujii Y, Tanaka R, Ueguchi T, et al. Hematoma enlargement in spontaneous intracerebral hemorrhage. J Neurosurg 1994; 80:51.
42. Arakawa S, Saku Y, Ibayashi S, Nagao T, Fujushima M. Blood pressure control and recurrence of hypertensive brain hemorrhage. Stroke 1998; 29:1806–1809.
43. Gonzalez-Duarte A, Cantu C, Ruiz-Sandoval J, Barinagarrementeria F. Recurrent primary cerebral hemorrhage; frequency, mechanisms, and prognosis. Stroke 1998; 29:1802–1805.
44. Drislane F, Samuels M. How cardiorespiratory problems are caused by neurologic disease. J Respir Dis 1988; 9:31.
45. Horner J, Massey E, Riski J, et al. Aspiration following stroke: clinical correlates and outcome. Neurology 1988; 38:1359.
46. McDermott M, Lefevre F, Arron M, Martin G, Biller J. ST segment depression detected by continuous electrocardiography in patients with acute ischemic stroke or transient ischemic attacks. Stroke 1994; 25:1820–1824.
47. Mikolich J, Jacobs W, Fletcher G. Cardiac arrhythmias in patients with acute cerebrovascular accidents. JAMA 1981; 246:1314–1317.
48. Anderson D, Cranford R. Corticosteroids in ischemic stroke. Stroke 1979; 10:623–628.
49. Norris J. Steroid therapy in acute cerebral infarction. Arch Neurol 1976; 33:69–71.
50. Norris J, Hachinski V. Megadose steroid therapy in ischemic stroke. Stroke 1985; 16:150.
51. Neuwelt E, Kikuchi K, Hill S. Barbiturate inhibition of lymphocyte function. Differing effects of various barbiturates used to induce coma. J Neurosurg 1982; 56:254–259.
52. Rieke K, Schwab S, Krieger D, von Kummer R, Aschoff A, Hacke W. Decompressive surgery in space-occupying hemispheric infarction: results of an open prospective trial. Crit Care Med 1995; 23:1576–1587.

9

Stroke in Neonates, Infants, and Children

Jerome Y. Yager
University of Saskatchewan, Saskatoon, Saskatchewan, Canada

INTRODUCTION

Although relatively uncommon during childhood, it has become evident in recent years that cerebrovascular accidents affect the lives of individuals in all age groups.[1] When stroke occurs during childhood, the impact can have dramatic consequences, with reported mortality rates varying from 6% to 15%[2–4] and residual neurologic morbidity ranging from 60% to 90% of survivors of ischemic brain injury.[3,4] Consequently, the impact of cerebrovascular accidents in childhood is immense, exacting a heavy toll not only for the individual whose future cognitive and motor development may be impaired for the remaining 50 to 70 years of their lives, but also on today's society on which an extremely heavy emotional and economic burden is placed.

With our improved understanding of the risk factors and pathophysiologic mechanisms that cause vascular lesions, stroke in childhood is clearly emerging as unique from that which occurs in the adult. Whereas stroke in the adult is most frequently related to atherosclerosis and hypertension, in children stroke is associated with a vast array of conditions (Table 1) in which congenital heart defects, vasculopathies, infectious and autoimmune vasculitides, coagulopathies, and inherited metabolic disorders are most prominent. Recent evidence relating to the extent of substrate utilization, the ontogeny of neurotransmitter function, and the maturation of intrinsic neuroprotective mechanisms has also clearly shown the important role developmental factors play in the age-specific vulnerability of the brain to ischemic events. Even the definition of stroke in childhood is less clear and may vary with the age of onset. In the adult population, a stroke de-

Table 1 Predisposing Conditions to Stroke in Childhood and Adolescence

Cardiac disease	Vascular dysplasias
Congenital	Moyamoya syndrome
Cyanotic disease with right-to-left shunt	Fibromuscular dysplasia
Aortic & mitral valve stenosis	Neurofibromatosis
Patent ductus arteriosus	Marfan syndrome
Ventricular septal defects	Ehrlos Danlos syndrome
Valvular disease (mitral valve prolapse)	Sturge Weber syndrome
Acquired	Tuberous sclerosis
Endocarditis	Metabolic/genetic
Cardiomyopathy	Homocystinuria
Arrhythmia	Fabry's disease
Atrial myxoma	Sulfite oxidase deficiency
Surgical correction	MELAS syndrome
(hypothermia: Catheterization	
Rheumatic heart disease	Hematologic causes
Infectious/inflammatory	Hemoglobinopathy
Meningitis	(Sickle cell disease)
Bacterial	Antithrombin III deficiency
Viral	Protein C & S deficiency
Sepsis (with dehydration)	Lupus anticoagulant
Immunologic disorders	Anticardiolipin antibody
Systemic lupus erythematosus	Oral contraceptives
Takayasu arteritis	Iron deficiency
Mixed connective tissue disease	Hyperlipidemia
Henoch-Schonlein purpura	Trauma
Kawasaki disease	
Hemolytic uremic syndrome	
Polyarteritis nodosa	
Rheumatoid arthritis	
Vasospasm	
Migraine	
Drugs	
Cocaine	
Wasp sting	

notes the sudden onset of a *focal* neurologic deficit, as a result of the interruption of blood flow to a specific part of the brain. In childhood and particularly as regards the newborn infant, stroke is often referred to as a hypoxic-ischemic insult; the consequence of a *global* reduction in blood flow to the brain, usually in association with an impairment in gas exchange (asphyxia). Moreover, sinovenous thrombosis is a frequent cause of venous infarcts in childhood, accounting for up to 25% of reported cases compared to adults, in whom it is a rare occurrence.[3,5,6]

For purposes of the present chapter, the working definition of stroke will include global cerebral ischemia of either venous or arterial origin, along with ischemia confined to a single arterial distribution. With the exception of a brief mention, primary hemorrhagic events will not be included. Cerebrovascular disease in the newborn (up to 1 month of age) will be differentiated from that which occurs in infants and children up to ~15 years of age. It is the intent of this review to leave the reader with an outline of the major causes of stroke in children, a more complete understanding of age-related differences in stroke pathogenesis, and finally, a comprehensive approach to the child with stroke.

EPIDEMIOLOGY

The overall incidence of cerebrovascular disease in infants and children appears to have remained remarkably constant over the past quarter-century. Schoenberg et al.[4] were the first to document the incidence of childhood stroke in a well-defined population of children. Of their 15,834 children, 69 (2.52/100,000/year) between the ages of 0 and 14 years suffered a stroke. Of these. 63/100,000/year were ischemic, while the remaining 1.89/100,000/year were hemorrhagic. Broderick et al.[2] found an overall yearly incidence of 2.7 strokes per 100,000 children. Incidence rates for hemorrhagic and ischemic strokes were 1.5 and 1.2 per 100,000/year, respectively. In the latter study, the overall incidence was similar both for males and females and for blacks and whites. Neither of these studies included newborn or premature infants, nor did they include venous occlusive disease.

Though not frequently acknowledged in stroke statistics, cerebrovascular accidents in term and preterm infants is a common occurrence. Of infants born at <35 weeks' gestation, cerebrovascular accidents occur in 20% to 30%—a most unfortunate figure when compared to an incidence of 1.2% in the >65-year-old age group.[7] Indeed, the incidence in premature infants appears to be increasing as vigilant care of the very sick premature newborn has improved survival, but not morbidity over the last decade.[8] Recently, the Canadian Pediatric Stroke Registry[3] identified 156 children <18 years of age with nonhemorrhagic stroke due to arterial occlusion (75%) or sinovenous thrombosis (25%). This represents an annual incidence of 1.0/100,000 children, and remains constant with previously published data. Interestingly, 24% of their cohort were neonates.[3] In all likelihood, the clinical incidence of stroke in children underestimates its true occurrence, given the finding by Banker[9] that up to 8.7% of pediatric autopsies displayed significant cerebrovascular disease.

ETIOLOGY

Much of our knowledge regarding the etiology of cerebrovascular accidents in children has been clarified only recently, with the advent of improved techniques of neuroradiologic imaging together with a recognition of the important role genetic, metabolic, and systemic factors play in the pathogenesis of stroke in this age group. Even so, 25% to 30% of children experiencing a cerebrovascular accident continue to have no known cause for their insult.[3,10,11]

Stroke In the Newborn

Global ischemia (hypoxic-ischemic encephalopathy) consequent to asphyxia, hypoxia, or ischemia is the most common cause of neurologic morbidity in the newborn. Conditions that predispose the infant to the insult arise from complications of either pregnancy, labor and delivery, or the early postpartum period (first month of life). By and large, these events (Table 2) quite clearly differ significantly from those that might occur after the first month, and certainly from those that occur later in life.

Just prior to and during labor and delivery, any condition of the mother or the birth process that interrupts uterine or placental blood flow will predispose the infant to a global ischemic insult. As described later in this chapter, in the preterm infant (24 to 32 weeks' gestation) this results in ischemia to the watershed areas of the periventricular regions, and in "periventricular leukomalacia" (PVL) or damage to subcortical white matter structures (Fig. 1). Clinically, this entity is responsible for the onset of spastic diplegia or quadriplegia in later life, and these neonates are diagnosed with cerebral palsy. Radiographically one sees the development of a porencephalic cyst, as a result of destruction of tissue in the periventricular zone and communication with the underlying lateral ventricle, often extending to the cortex (Fig. 2). In the term infant, compromise of the more mature cerebrovascular system results in ischemia to watershed or parasagittal regions which correspond to border zones of circulation between the anterior, middle, and posterior cerebral arteries. Clinically, these insults result in the more "classic" forms of focal cerebral infarction, or stroke, with sudden-onset hemiparesis, seizures, and/or aphasia.

Of those newborn infants who have not been subjected to an overt asphyxial insult, only 25% will have a definite cause identified. Among these causes is an embolic phenomenon arising from the placenta. Because the fetal circulation sends blood directly to the brain without being filtered through the lungs, placental emboli may have direct access to the cerebral circulation.[11,12] Indirect trauma to the pregnant woman may also be an underrecognized cause of fetal stroke. And certainly, exposure of the fetus to vasoconstrictive agents (cocaine) crossing the placenta may result in cerebral infarction. Ascending prenatal in-

Table 2 Predisposing Conditions to Stroke in the Fetus and Newborn Infant

	Prepartum	Intrapartum (labor & delivery)	Neonatal (1st month of life)
Maternal		Obstetric	
Toxemia	Placenta previa	Precipitous delivery	Prematurity
Diabetes mellitus	Abruptio placenta	Difficult delivery (Forceps, vacuum extraction)	Respiratory disease
Drugs (cocaine)	Multiple pregnancy	Intrauterine growth retardation	Congenital heart disease (right-to-left shunt)
Cardiovascular disease	Prolapsed umbilical cord		Sepsis/shock
Infection (amnionitis)	Premature rupture of Membranes (chorioamnionitis)		
Isoimmunization			

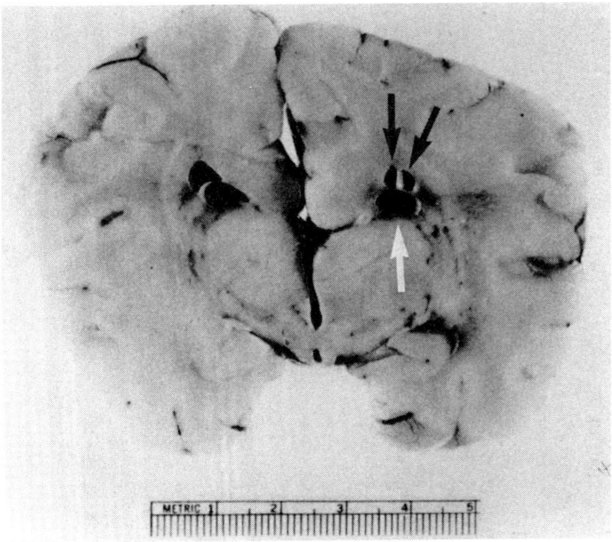

Figure 1 Coronal section of newborn infant brain. White arrow indicates lateral ventricle dilated as a result of atrophy. Black arrows indicate cystic formation due to white-matter necrosis in a region of periventricular leukomalacia (PVL).

fections (chorioamnionitis) can cause a vasculitis or coagulopathy that leads to a cerebral infarction.

Thrombosis of the deep cortical veins accounts for a large percentage (25%) of ischemic infarctions in the neonate[3] (Fig. 3). Presenting most commonly within the first 2 weeks of life, 40% are of undetermined etiology; the remainder are usually due to sepsis, dehydration, and shock.[5]

Stroke in the Infant and Child

A comprehensive list of disorders predisposing the young infant and child to cerebral infarction is contained in Table 1. While impressively long, 25% of cases remain classified as idiopathic. Many of the conditions in this list are readily eliminated in the majority of children, with the appropriate history and physical examination. Nonetheless, the underlying etiologies do differ significantly from those that occur in adults.

Cardiac Disease

Both congenital and acquired forms of heart disease account for between 20% and 30% of arterial strokes in childhood.[3,4] The underlying mechanisms by which

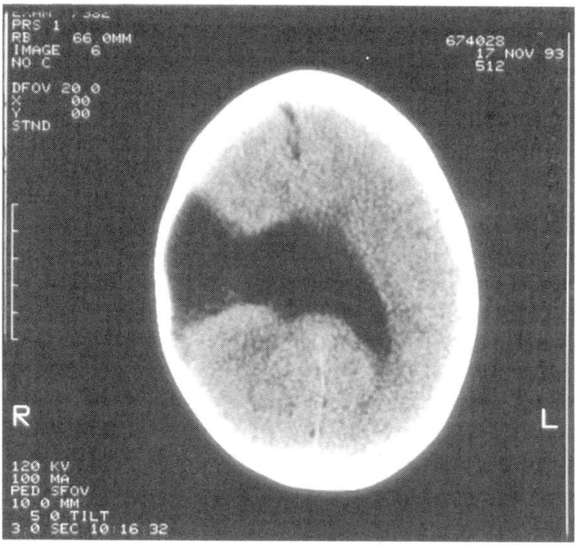

Figure 2 CT scan of brain revealing the development of a porencephalic cyst as a result of early periventricular leukomalacia. Note the communication of cyst with the lateral ventricle.

children with cardiac disease suffer cerebral injury are predominantly related to structural anomalies, the hematological response to chronically low oxygen tensions, and the surgical intervention, per se. Cardiac anomalies in which there are large right-to-left intracardiac shunts lead to hypoxemia, manifest by microcytosis and anemia in children under 4 years of age, and polycythemia in older children. Both can lead to thrombotic or embolic phenomena and are reasons to advocate iron supplementation in young children with congenital cardiac anomalies[13] and to pursue early surgical intervention in cyanotic heart disease. Major admixture lesions also can result in direct access of returning venous blood to the cerebral circulation and, as it does in the fetus, bypasses the filtering system of the lungs, leading to embolic stroke.

Surgical procedures, including primary repair under deep hypothermia, lead to a state of hypercoagulability and clearly place the child at risk for stroke.[14] In addition, children with congenital heart disease are susceptible to emboli from sources such as arrhythmias and infective endocarditis.

Infectious Inflammatory

Infectious etiologies are the second most common cause of stroke in childhood, responsible for 15% of the series by deVeber and colleagues.[3] Direct infection

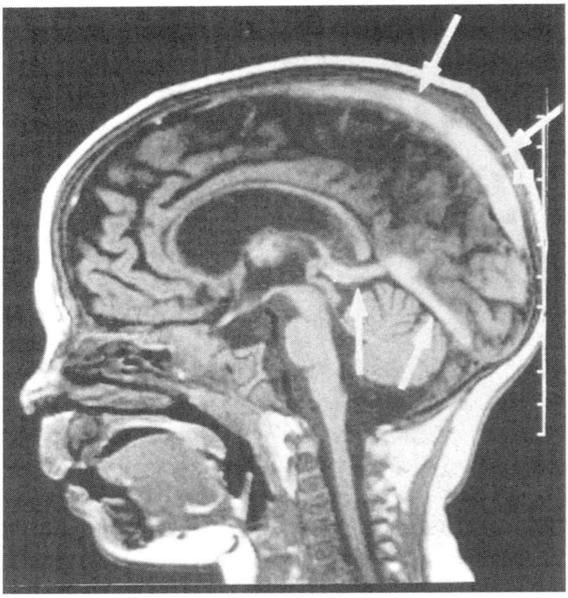

Figure 3 Magnetic resonance image, sagittal section. Eighteen-month-old child with superior sagittal sinus thrombosis (top arrows), together with involvement of the straight sinus (lower left and right arrows). Thrombosis was the result of severe iron deficiency.

of the central nervous system by bacteria or viruses can lead to perivascular inflammation of arteries with narrowing and occlusion, or to venous thrombosis. Deep, cavernous vein thrombosis can also arise as a result of infections of the head and neck, and has been described with otitis media, mastoiditis, and cat-scratch disease with progressive regional lymphadenopathy.

A host of systemic viral infections have been associated with childhood stroke. Most often these have been the common childhood exanthems, including chickenpox, rubella, mumps, influenza, Coxsackie virus, and Epstein-Barr virus.[15,16] Indeed, the vast majority of children who develop sagittal sinus thrombosis do so in the context of an acute viral illness with dehydration.[5]

Autoimmune disorders in children make a small but significant contribution to the incidence of stroke. Cerebrovascular disease in systemic lupus erythematosis is probably the most frequently recognized cause. Previously thought to be the result of a central nervous system vasculitis, infarction is now believed to more likely be the result of lupus anticoagulants and anticardiolipin antibodies. Although first noted in patients with SLE, these antibodies have since been described in patients with and without autoimmune disorders—even in children as young as 9 months.[17] Stroke may also occur with a variety of other immune disorders including Takayasu disease[18] and mixed connective tissue disease.[19]

Neurologic sequelae of cerebral infarction have been associated with a number of other, relatively common infectious/inflammatory diseases in childhood. Among them, necrotizing arteritis has been found in the cerebral vessels of children with Henoch-Schonlein purpura, Kawasaki's disease, and hemolytic uremic syndrome, in which up to 5% of children may have focal infarctions.

Hematologic Causes

While hematologic disorders leading to emboli or thrombosis have been described in all age groups, they occur most frequently in childhood and adolescence. Sickle cell disease is the most common hemoglobinopathy associated with cerebrovascular disease in childhood, which occurs with an annual incidence of 700/100,000 children, which is 500 to 700 times more common than in the general population.[20]

The absence of specific serum proteins which act as inhibitors of coagulation may also lead to stroke in children. Deficiencies of antithrombin III, or protein C or S are autosomal dominant and have been associated with childhood arterial and venous occlusive disease.[11,21] Antithrombin III is an alpha$_2$-globulin which binds irreversibly to thrombin and stabilizes the clot. Acquired deficiencies can occur with protein-losing gastrointestinal or renal disorders, and with the use of L-aspariginase in the treatment of acute leukemias. Protein C and its cofactor protein S inhibit the activated forms of Factors V and VIII. Deficiency of either of the two leads to a hypercoagulable state.

Iron deficiency was recently identified as a relatively common cause of stroke in childhood. In their series of 53 children between 0 and 17 years of age, Hartfield et al.[22] described six infants who developed a stroke (either venous thrombosis or arterial occlusion). All six were between 6 and 18 months of age, were iron deficient (though not necessarily anemic), and had an associated mild viral illness with no CNS involvement. This group accounted for 11% of the total number of strokes seen and, interestingly, accounted for almost 40% of those children in whom a cause of stroke had not been found.

Vascular Dysplasias

Congenital or inherited abnormalities of the vessel wall comprise between 1% and 2% of strokes in children. Of these moyamoya syndrome is the best known. From the Japanese meaning "something hazy like a puff of smoke," moyamoya disease is most commonly seen in children under 15 years old, and is six times more common in females than males. Pathologically, the disorder is characterized by progressive narrowing of the supraclinoid internal carotid arteries, usually in a bilateral, symmetrical fashion. Proliferation of collateral vessels, which appear as a fine vascular network from the external carotid artery, give the appearance of rising smoke on angiography. Clinically the disorder is progressive, with frequent TIAs, mental deterioration, and seizures occurring.

Fibromuscular dysplasia can occur in cerebral vessels and often involves multiple sites. Pathologically it appears as focal zones of fibrous and muscular hyperplasia of the media, and gives a "string-of-beads" appearance on angiography. Dysplastic vessels with dissection or aneurysmal formation has also been described with neurofibromatosis, Marfan syndrome, and Ehrlos-Danlos syndrome.

Metabolic/Genetic

Homocystinuria is an autosomal-recessive disorder caused by one of three possible enzyme deficiencies of homocysteine metabolism. The disorder is characterized by a marfanoid appearance (tall, thin habitus), developmental delay, ocular lens dislocation, and thromboembolic disease. Biochemically, serum levels of homocysteine and methionine are elevated, the former of which can injure vascular endothelium which subsequently becomes a nidus for thrombus formation. Ischemia can occur as a result of either the thrombus formation or embolization to a distant focus. Heterozygosity for the disorder has also been shown to predispose to premature arteriosclerotic disease.[23] Treatment is by dietary restriction aimed at lowering serum homocysteine levels, and by pyridoxine (B_6) administration.

Fabry's disease, or angiokeratoma corporis diffusum, is an X-linked disorder resulting from a deficiency of alpha-galactosidase. Deposition of the sphingolipid trihexoside, in the kidney, vascular endothelium, and cornea causes distinctive rash, burning pain in the extremities, renal failure, and stroke. Symptoms usually begin in late childhood or early adolescence.

Sulfite oxidase deficiency, a disorder of sulfur amino acid metabolism, is an autosomal-recessive disease which results in the accumulation of serum sulfites. Children with this disorder also suffer from mental retardation, seizures, lens displacement, and stroke. The cause of the cerebrovascular involvement in these children is unknown. Treatment with dietary restriction to reduce sulfite accumulation has not been successful.

A newly recognized group of metabolic diseases, the mitochondrial encephalomyelopathies, have also been associated with recurrent stroke in childhood. In particular, MELAS syndrome (mitochondrial myopathy, lactic acidosis, and stroke) presents in the second decade of life and is due to a mutation of mitochondrial DNA, inherited solely through maternal transmission. Additional neurologic manifestations include proximal muscle weakness, recurrent vomiting, seizures, and mental deterioration. Neuropathologic findings have shown cystic cavities and necrosis of the cortex, especially the posterior cerebrum, with sparing of white matter. The disorder is most commonly associated with a deficiency of complex I of the electron transport chain (for review see Ref. 24).

Other Causes

Unsuspected trauma, particularly of the neck, may be an important, overlooked cause of stroke in childhood and adolescence. Kalapurackal et al.[25] found that 20% of the children in their series of ischemic strokes (excluding meningitis and leukemia) had a history of trauma within the 24 hours prior to presentation. In other series, brainstem and cerebellar strokes in children have been attributed to vertebral artery trauma secondary to traction injuries of the neck at the C-1 and C-2 levels.[26]

Although not frequently associated with stroke in the young, Glueck et al.[27] brought attention to the prevalence of hyperlipidemia among children. Of 11 pediatric victims of unexplained nonhemorrhagic stroke, only one child had normal lipid and lipoprotein profiles. Seven of the children had low serum HDL levels, four had high triglycerides, and two had high LDL levels. In addition, their study showed a familial clustering of vascular disease at a young age, including myocardial infarctions, stroke, and migraine.

PATHOGENESIS

The pathophysiologic mechanisms underlying stroke have been extensively reviewed elsewhere in this text (see Beneviste) and pertain to children as well as they do to adults.[28] In the next few paragraphs I will briefly review the pathogenesis of ischemic brain damage. It is important to recognize, however, that the effects these mechanisms have on cerebral injury are extremely age dependent. As a result, this section will be followed by a review of those mechanisms which are now recognized as being exquisitely sensitive to age and how they may affect stroke outcome.

The basis of those alterations which culminate in neuronal and glial cell death is a reduction of regional or global cerebral blood flow (CBF) below a critical level, causing a curtailment of oxygen and substrate supply to the brain. In the absence of these substrates, normal energy reserves can no longer be maintained and the metabolic demands of the cell must depend entirely on its endogenous energy reserves, phosphocreatine and ATP, and on the energy derived from anaerobic glycolysis. Under these circumstances, a rapid depletion of high-energy phosphate stores occurs concurrent with the accumulation of lactic acid, leading to a progressive tissue acidosis. This resultant energy failure[28] is associated with a shift in transmembrane potential, cell depolarization, inactivation of the Na-K^+ ATPase pump, and the development of cytotoxic edema.

Concurrent with these alterations, glutamate, the predominant excitatory amino acid in the brain, accumulates within the synaptic cleft to concentrations toxic to the surrounding brain cells. The effect of glutamate, under these pathologic circumstances, is to perpetuate neuronal swelling by enhancing the influx of sodium and chloride through voltage-oated channels, and to stimulate receptor-mediated calcium (Ca^{2+}) channels causing a rapid elevation of intracellular Ca^{2+}.[29,30] The accumulation of intracellular Ca^{2+}, occurring in concert with a continued energy debt, promotes a cascade of catabolic processes which eventually culminate in cell disintegration.

Even under circumstances in which oxygen and substrate supply to the brain are replenished, lingering alterations in cellular homeostasis may contribute to and exacerbate the extent of brain damage. Convincing evidence points to a role for the formation of oxygen free radicals in the pathogenesis of postischemic injury. (A free radical is a molecule that contains an uneven number of electrons and is therefore unstable.) The major site of free-radical production is the mitochondria, where reactive intermediates including the superoxide radical (O_2^-) and hydrogen peroxide (H_2O_2) arise from the oxygen used in the electron transport chain due oxidation of substrates to form ATP and water. These intermediates then interact with transition metals such as iron to result in the formation of the highly reactive hydroxyl radical (OH^-). Oxygen free radicals perpetuate brain injury by causing the disruption of cell membranes through lipid peroxidation, DNA damage, reduced glutamate reuptake, inhibition of sodium-potassium ATPase, and the elevation of intracellular Ca^{2+}. Under physiologic conditions, the brain contains a number of endogenous mechanisms by which scavenging of free radicals takes place. These include enzymes such as superoxide dismutase and glutathione peroxidase, and endogenous free radical scavengers such as glutathione and vitamin E. During ischemia and following resuscitation, these endogenous mechanisms are rendered ineffective, and the generation of oxygen free radicals occurs unabated. The propagation of these events following H-I result in the phenomenon of delayed neuronal death.[31,32]

Recent evidence suggests that delayed cell death may occur via two separate pathways. The first, characterized by the loss of membrane integrity, signs of organelle damage, and loss of lysosomal contents, is consistent with "necrosis." The second, characterized by the preservation of membrane integrity, organelle structure, and lysosomal contents, but with diminution of cell volume, chromatin condensation, and nuclear fragmentation, has been termed 64 "apoptosis."

This latter type of cell death appears to be a form of "programmed cell death" and occurs at thresholds of injury less than that required for cell necrosis. Moreover, apoptosis is induced or inhibited as an active process of the cell, occurring via a number of newly recognized gene products (i.e., C-fos, Bcl-2, Bax, C-jun).[33,35]

Aging and Stroke Outcome

While the basic mechanisms underlying ischemic injury may be similar in different age groups, the extent to which a reduction in cerebral blood flow (ischemia) to the brain affects neuropathologic outcome at different ages is controversial. Data from early studies[36,37] has led to the long-held belief that the developing animal was far more resistant to the damaging effects of cerebral hypoxia-ischemia than was its adult counterpart. Recent experimental evidence, however, has questioned these earlier conclusions. To elucidate the role of aging on ischemic brain damage in vivo, Yager et al.[38] developed a model whereby the neuropathologic effects of an identical ischemic insult to the brain could be examined at different ages. Wistar rats ranging in age from 10 days (equivalent to human newborn) to 6 months (adult) were exposed to a global hemispheric hypoxic-ischemic insult. Measurement of systemic blood pressure and cerebral blood flow indicated that all animals, regardless of age, received the same degree of ischemia to the brain. Surprisingly, the results indicated that brain damage did not increase linearly with age, as had been previously suggested. Rather, cerebral injury was most pronounced in the youngest age groups (1 and 3 weeks old), least in those rats that were "middle aged" (6 and 9 weeks old), and then increased again in the oldest animals (6 months old) (Fig. 4). In addition, the distribution of injury also differed with age. The neocortex revealed more extensive injury in the two younger age groups (1 and 3 weeks old) compared to the others. In the age groups most sensitive to ischemic injury, the neocortex and hippocampus were equally damaged in the 1-week-old rats. In the 3-week- and 6-month-old animals, however, the hippocampus was more sensitive to injury than was the neocortex, particularly in the 6-month-old animals.

Support for the above findings arise also from work in the neurobehavioral field during which the effects of brain plasticity were investigated in different age groups of rats. In numerous studies, during which specific regions of the rat brain were surgically removed, Kolb and Whishaw[39,40] have shown that recovery of function is greatest in animals 7 to 10 days of age, compared to those in which surgery was performed at 1 day of age. Thus, not only might damage from a specific insult be age related, but so too might recovery of function, and younger animals may do less well than previously anticipated.

Ontogeny of Excitatory Amino Acids

Several recent studies have outlined a number of cerebrovascular and metabolic changes that occur with age,[41–45] many of which may play an important role in

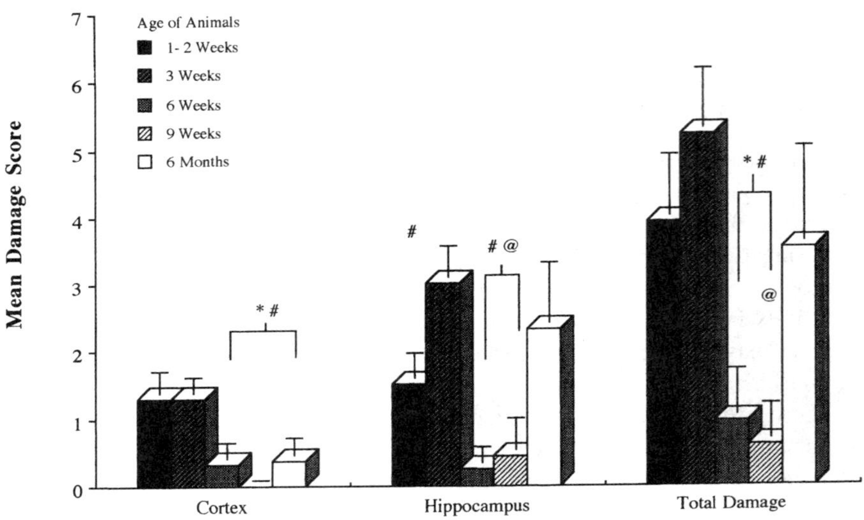

Figure 4 Graph depicting the mean and SEM damage score for the cortex and hippocampus of all animals, together with the total damage score. The neocortex was significantly more damaged in the 1- and 3-week animals. Hippocampal damage was greatest in the 3-week animal followed by the 6-month and 1-week groups. Within age groups, the hippocampus was injured to a greater extent than the neocortex in the 3-week and 6-month animals, whereas the neocortex and hippocampus were equally damaged in the 1-week animals. *P < .05 vs. 1 week; $^{\#}$P < .05 vs. 3 weeks; $^{@}$P < .05 vs. 6 months.

the complex nature of hypoxic-ischemic brain damage. Ontogenic factors regarding the excitatory neurotransmitters may have a profound effect on the age-related susceptibility to hypoxic-ischemic damage. Evidence suggests that the younger brain is more susceptible to damage due to enhanced postsynaptic development of the NMDA receptor.[46–48] Tremblay et al.[48] demonstrated a significantly increased binding to glutamate receptors in the hippocampus at 8 days of age, continuing through to 22 days of age, in comparison to the adult. This was further substantiated in experiments in which direct injections of the excitatory amino acid analog NMDA into the corpus striatum of 7-day- and 3-month-old rats produced damage in the younger animals that was 21 times greater than that seen in the adults.[46] Ikonomidou et al.[49] also demonstrated that vulnerability to either hypoxia-ischemia or injections of NMDA into the brain peaked at 6 days of age and diminished thereafter. In addition, glutamate concentrations in the brain of the immature rat have been shown to be elevated to 150% to 200% of adult values during the first month of life.[43] Taken together, the evidence supports in vivo findings that the infant brain may indeed be more sensitive to injury than previously recognized, and that the lack of tolerance may be due, at least in part, to an enhancement of the toxic effects of the excitatory amino acids.

Development, Substrate Utilization, and Stroke

The brain is one of the major energy-consuming organs of the body. During the neonatal period, infancy, and childhood, specific substrate requirements vary in accordance with the developing brain's stage of myelinogenesis, synaptogenesis, and dendritic arborization. Whereas the adult brain normally derives almost all of its energy from the aerobic oxidation of glucose, the newborn and infant brain additionally utilize alternate substrates (ketone bodies, lactate, and acids) in order to meet the specific requirements of growth and development.[50,51]

Insight into the age-specific differences in substrate utilization as it pertains to hypoxic-ischemic brain damage arises from work related to glucose supplementation. Investigations in *adult animals* have convincingly shown that glucose supplementation (*hyperglycemia*) prior to or during focal and/or global ischemia profoundly *accentuates brain damage*.[52,53] The pathophysiologic mechanism by which increased blood glucose concentrations worsen brain damage in adult animals has been related to the excess production of tissue lactic acid[54] due to an acceleration of anaerobic glycolytic flux during hyperglycemic cerebral ischemia.

Data available in *newborn animals* has shown that *in contrast to the adult, hyperglycemia* both prolongs survival and *has a beneficial effect* on neuropathologic outcome. A series of experiments by Vannucci's group of collaborators[55,56] points out the contrasting nature of the perinatal brain with respect to glucose supplementation and ischemic brain injury. Preliminary studies showed that glucose supplementation prolonged hypoxic survival of developing 7-day-old rats from 3.5 to 8 hours. In follow-up studies blood glucose concentrations were elevated five to sixfold during the hypoxic-ischemic episode. In contrast to adult animals, the hyperglycemia resulted in a significant reduction in brain damage. Similar results were obtained by Hattori and Wasterlain,[57] who induced profound hyperglycemia following severe forebrain ischemia in the immature rat, and found a 63% reduction in infarct volume of the cerebral cortex and virtually complete attenuation of injury to the striatum and hippocampus. Pathophysiologically, glucose supplementation in immature animals has been shown to reduce ATP utilization during ischemia[58] and to enhance the $CMRO_2$ postasphyxia.[59]

Biochemical support for the notion that glucose supplementation may actually be beneficial rather than deleterious to the perinatal brain exposed to hypoxia-ischemia stems from recent investigations in our laboratory exploring the oxidation-reduction state of mitochondria as a reflection of substrate availability.[60,61] As anticipated, the cytoplasmic redox state ($NAD^+/NADH$) was reduced compared to controls, as a reflection of an accumulation of reducing substances in this compartment of the cell. The mitochondria, however, were found be oxidized. Concurrent measurements of brain glucose, pyruvate, and α-ketoglutarate indicated that the upward shift in mitochondrial $NAD^+/NADH$ (oxidation) was the result of a depletion of substrate supply to the mitochondria. An analogous situation occurs in adult brain during severe hypoglycemia, in which cellular oxidation is observed.[62] The alterations in the mitochondrial redox state of the immature brain during hypoxia-ischemia appear to mimic state II respiration, as described by Chance and Williams,[63] in which substrate, rather than oxygen supply, is deficient in the perinatal brain. This is further substantiated by both human and animal studies indicating the comparatively low metabolic requirements for oxygen of the fetus and young infant compared to the adult.[36,64]

During recent years, a large body of information has come forward regarding the ability of the developing nervous system to utilize alternative substrates. It is now well documented, for example, that glucose transport across the blood-brain barrier in suckling rats is only 1/5 that of the adult, and glucose utilization is even lower (1/10).[50,65] In contrast, the transport capacity of beta-hydroxybutyrate in suckling rats is at least four times the value obtained in adults and, according to data by Nehlig et al.,[66] contributes between 40% and 60% of total energy metabolism of the immature brain, compared to only 10% to 15% at weaning (21 days). Several studies have also shown lactate to be an important contributor to the metabolic demands of the neonatal brain.[51,67] In fact, lactate utilization by neonatal rat brain is much higher than that of either glucose or beta-hydroxybutyrate.[66]

Under pathologic conditions, the immature brain is clearly capable of utilizing alternative substrates. In the newborn rat, lactate can enter the brain during anoxia or hypoxia and is able to substitute for glucose as an energy substrate during recovery.[67] Ketone bodies supplemented either exogenously or via fasting have a marked protective effect on the newborn brain.[56,68,69]

White-Matter Injury in the Premature Infant

Given the tremendously high incidence of cerebrovascular accidents in the premature infant (see above), mention should be made of the differences in topographic localization of strokes in this group compared to their more mature counterparts. The most common cerebrovascular lesion affecting the premature asphyxiated infant is damage to the subcortical white matter, and is pathologically referred to as periventricular leukomalacia (PVL). Overall, it has been reported to occur in up to 75% of premature infants weighing <1,500 g. Pathologically, PVL appears as both focal or diffuse areas of white-matter necrosis. Focally, PVL occurs in a classic distribution around the anterior horns and trigone of the lateral ventricle,[70,71] sites which in the developing brain are border zones between penetrating branches of the middle, posterior, and anterior cerebral arteries. Within 1 to 3 weeks of the hypoxic-ischemic insult, small, often multiple cavities can be visualized pathologically or by cranial ultrasound in surviving infants (Fig. 1). Subsequently, subcortical white-matter loss and areas of focal ventricular dilation can be seen. Microscopically, in the human, oligodendroglial deficiency is the dominant cellular finding, along with loss of myelin and astrogliosis.

Clinically, the long-term sequelae resulting from PVL are the spastic cerebral palsies, particularly spastic diplegia. This clinicopathologic correlation is evident when one considers the distribution of the lesion, which "interrupts" descending fibers from the motor cortex, known to function in the control of the upper and lower extremities. More diffuse lesions follow the anatomic representation of the homunculous on the motor cortex, increasing involvement to the upper extremities and resulting in spastic quadraplegia, and eventually involving the muscles controlling the face, speech, and glutition (pseudo-bulbar palsies).

Although PVL is restricted almost entirely to the immature CNS of the 26- to 36-week'-gestation infant, the underlying predisposition for this selective vulnerability remains unknown. Ontogenically, as the brain matures, the gray-matter regions of the cerebral hemispheres become the primary target of ischemic insults resulting in laminar necrosis of layers 3, 5, and 6, as well as hippocampal and striatal selective neuronal necrosis or infarction. This evolution in the distribution of lesions of the developing brain suggests not only that regional susceptibility to hypoxic-ischemic damage of the brain varies with age, but also that in certain situations, oligodendrocytes (those cells responsible for the production of myelin in the CNS) or their precursors can be preferentially affected over neurons following perinatal or prenatal insults.

Pathogenetically, several factors likely contribute to the production of PVL in the premature infant. As previously indicated, vascular factors play a major contributory role in the selective distribution of PVL. Thus, DeReuck and colleagues[72] have clearly demonstrated the presence of arterial "border zones" between the centripedal and centrifugal arteries within the periventricular regions of the white matter. Moreover, as a result of the developmental pattern of the arterial microvascular network,[73] these "watershed regions" are most prominent in the least mature infants, accounting for the prevalence of this disease almost exclusively in the 26- to 36-weeks'-gestation neonate. As maturation of the fetus occurs, extensive anastomosis between the penetrating vessels of the cerebral cortex occurs, augmenting blood flow to the white matter and enhancing its tolerance to ischemia. In contrast, border zones arise between the major cerebral arteries (anterior, middle, and posterior), leaving the interface between these vessels as watershed zones and, in later gestation (>36 weeks), predisposing the parasagittal regions of the cerebral cortex to ischemic insults.

In combination with the above information, which suggests an inherent predisposition to damage in the border zone regions of the periventricular white matter, the cerebral circulation of the immature infant and in particular that of the sick newborn, is pressure passive. In animal studies investigators[74] have shown a direct correlation between systemic blood pressure and cerebral blood flow during hypoxia-ischemia. In addition, subcortical white matter has consistently demonstrated a more profound selective hypoperfusion than other cortical gray-matter and brainstem structures. Similar alterations in cerebral blood flow have been documented in the distressed human neonate. In that regard, Lou et al.[75] utilizing the ^{133}Xe clearance technique, were the first to show a pressure-passive cerebral circulation in asphyxiated newborn infants at birth. Hence, reductions in systemic blood pressure due to asphyxia, sepsis, myocardial failure, or apnea with bradycardia, will be reflected in a reduction in cerebral blood flow, and inevitably to ischemic injury in vulnerable regions of the brain such as the periventricular white matter.

While vascular factors and ischemia are the predominant influence in determining the topography of tissue injury (i.e., periventricular white matter), recent evidence suggests that the intrinsic vulnerability of the oligodendrocyte per se significantly contributes to the pathogenesis of PVL. Oka et al.[76] exposed differentiating oligodendroglia to 2-mM concentrations of L-glutamate, and observed a dramatic loss of cells (>90%) compared to controls. Interestingly, the authors also showed that cell death was not due to a receptor-mediated mechanism but rather to a depletion of intracellular cystine, and subsequent reduction in concentrations of gluthathione, an important free-radical scavenger. Protection from injury was afforded this cell line by culturing the cells in medium enriched with vitamin E, or idebenone. More recently, Back et al.,[77] in the same laboratory, observed that this form of oligodendroglial cell death likely occurs as a result of apoptosis, rather than necrosis. That glutamate-induced injury may occur in vivo is suggested by the fact that the earliest neuropathologic change seen with PVL is, in fact, axonal disruption. Such axonal death could result in the release of high concentrations of glutamate into the extracellular space of the periventricular region, causing free-radical-induced oligodendroglial apoptosis.

Further evidence demonstrating the susceptibility of the oligodendrocyte to oxidative stress has been suggested during experiements in which the oligodendrocyte has been shown to be exquisitely sensitive to hyperthermia and hypoxia.[78,79] This appears to be due to more reactive oxygen species (ROS) being generated in oligodendroglial cells in part because of the high iron content of the cells (23 times higher in oligodendrocytes than astrocytes) and, in part, because of the low reduced-glutathione (GSH) content of these cells.[80] As previously stated, GSH plays an important role in the glutathione peroxidase (GPx) reaction whereby peroxides are reduced to water and molecular oxygen. Oligodendrocytes have further been demonstrated to have <10% the activity of glutathione peroxidase compared to astrocytes.[81]

CLINICAL PRESENTATION AND DIAGNOSTIC EVALUATION

Newborn

Evidence of a hypoxic-ischemic injury to the newborn as a result of asphyxia generally manifests as a global encephalopathy. In moderately to severely affected infants, diffuse hypotonia is the most common motor deficit, usually accompanied by decreased reflexes, in a baby who appears lethargic and difficult to arouse. In premature infants, features of periventricular leukomalacia may arise shortly thereafter. This results in weakness evolving to hypertonia, predominantly involving the lower extremities as a result of damage to fibers descending from the motor strip, which subserve the legs. In term infants, parasagittal watershed infarct is often manifest as late-onset hemiparesis with weakness of the proximal upper extremities predominating.

While injury in the newborn is often bilateral, focal seizure is a frequently identified clinical feature indicating the presence of a stroke.[32] This is particularly true of the term infant, who may have few if any other neurological signs in the first days of life. Infants who do not present until later in the first year do so with pathologic early hand preference, often with no other symptoms. Once fully manifest, children frequently develop signs of hemi- or quadriparesis, which seldom improves.[83]

Given the association of intrauterine events with alobal cerebral ischemia in the newborn with stroke, investigations are often of limited value. Cranial ultrasound and/or CT scan confirm the diagnosis, and differentiate a hemorrhagic from a nonhemorrhagic event. Computed tomographic scanning with contrast or MRI may be utilized in infants in whom a sagittal sinus thrombosis is suspected. Further studies should be directed at ruling out possible risk factors in the mother which may have led to compromising fetal blood flow and to a premature delivery. Newborns who experience stroke are seldom at risk for a recurrence later in life.

Infants and Children

Clinical presentation in the infant or child >1 month of age differs significantly from that of the newborn. Typically, onset is with an acute neurologic deficit (usually acute hemiparesis) with or without seizures.[83] The motor deficit is usually most severe at onset, but improves with time. Unlike adults, who experience transient ischemic events as a prodrome, headache is a more common feature heralding the onset of stroke in childhood.[84]

Once stroke is suspected, confirmation should be obtained utilizing computed tomography (CT) or magnetic resonance imaging (MRI). MRI, particularly with diffusion-weighted images, provides greater resolution and structural detail early in the evolution of a stroke. If, however, this technology is not available, and the stroke has occurred within a short peroid of time prior to admission (<24 hours), an electroencephalogram may be of some benefit, often giving rise to periodic laterizing epileptiform discharges (PLEDs) over the hemisphere experiencing a vascular accident. This may be particularly helpful in the early stages of a stroke, to help rule out other possibilities in the differential diagnosis of acute hemiplegia in childhood including a subdural or epidural hemorrhage, postictal Todd's paralysis, hemiplegic migraine, hypoglycemia, or alternating hemiplegia of childhood.

Laboratory investigations should be initiated to evalutate the stability of the infant or child and to determine the underlying etiology. Figure 5 outlines a step-by-step scheme for evaluating the infant or child in whom the diagnosis of stroke has been confirmed. A hematological screen will quickly rule out the possibilty of underlying infection or iron deficiency anemia, and act as a screen for coagulation disorders. Blood glucose and assessment of acid/base status will uncover hypoglycemia as a possible cause, and may direct one's attention toward an underlying metabolic disturbance. Cerebrospinal fluid can be examined, with caution, in children whose symptoms support a suspicion of CNS infection. A toxicology screen should be done in all children in whom drugs are suspected.

If these initial investigations are not helpful in determining a diagnosis, a more in-depth search should be undertaken. Echocardiograms provide important information regarding the structure of the heart, its function, and the presence or absence of any vegetations from which an embolus may be thrown. Systemic inflammatory or metabolic causes should be sought, as many of them are not only treatable but run a high risk of recurrence if not adequately treated. CSF and serum lactate are particularly helpful as a screen for the mitochondrial disease; however, if clinically suspected, one should pursue a muscle biopsy in search of abnormal respiratory chain complexes and ragged-red fibers to rule out the possibility of MELAS. Similarly, a metabolic screen and white blood cell enzymes can be obtained if signs or symptoms suggest an underlying inborn error of metabolism or lysosomal storage disease.

Finally, angiography should be performed to evaluate central nervous system vasculature. This will be particularly helpful in those suspected of moyamoya disease, fibromuscular dysplasia, or a dissection. MR angiography has been particularly helpful, and less invasive in its assessment of blood flow and structure of the larger cervical and intracranial vessels.[86]

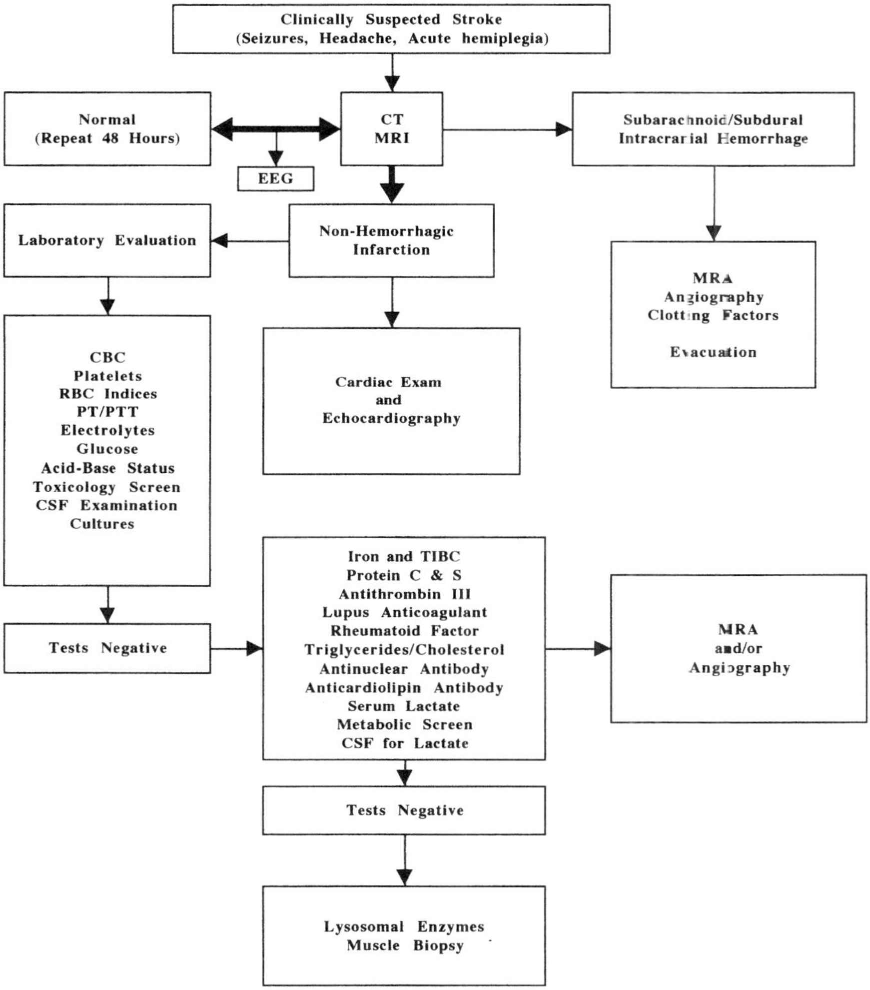

Figure 5 Diagnostic evaluation flow chart for the investigation of stroke in a child.

THERAPEUTIC APPROACHES

The literature abounds with experimental evidence regarding the management of stroke. While this topic has been discussed thoroughly in subsequent chapters of the text (see Section B), the following paragraphs focus on potential new modalities in the newborn and young child (see Refs. 87–89 for reviews).

Newborn

Despite the tremendous gains in our understanding of the pathogenesis of hypoxic-ischemic encephalopathy in the newborn infant, a rational approach to its management does not exist. A number of factors have stood in the way of pursuing therapeutic avenues, not the least of which is the relative inaccessibility of the at-risk infant in the late stages of labor and delivery, and the ethical dilemma posed by administering unproven agents to both the mother and fetus. Of further hindrance is our lack of understanding of how many of these agents might affect the "developing" nervous system, particularly during the initial periods of synaptogenesis and myelination. Nonetheless, a number of animal studies have been undertaken which at least begin to investigate the potential role of several therapeutic agents.

Whether cerebral edema per se contributes to the brain injury following an ischemic event remains controversial. In the newborn, Lupton et al.[90] showed that maximal brain swelling occurs 24 to 72 hours after the insult. This was also shown to be true in studies in the newborn rat.[91] Treatment of cerebral edema, however, with hyperosmolar agents has had no effect on outcome.[92]

The mechanism by which glucocorticoids influence the extent of brain damage is unknown. Early studies in both adults and newborns suggested that the glucocorticoids may have a deleterious effect on the brain. More recently, studies in the immature animal have shown that dexamethasone administered up to 24 hours prior to an hypoxic-ischemic insult virtually prevented brain injury from occurring. Further investigations showed that its administration >24 hours prior to or following the ischemic event was ineffective in ameliorating brain damage. Of particular interest was the fact that this neuroprotective effect was also age dependent. In their ongoing series of investigations, Tuor et al.[93] delivered dexamethasone to 2- and 4-week-old rats, 24 and 5 hours prior to hypoxia-ischemia. While the glucocorticoids lessened cerebral infarction by 90% in the 2-week-old animals compared to controls, no effect was seen in the 4-week-old group. The reason for this difference in response in the two age groups is unknown.

Reducing the metabolic rate of the brain, or enhancing its ability to meet its energy demands, has also been viewed as a potential method of reducing neuronal injury to the newborn brain. Indeed, animal studies have shown that barbiturates do favorably influence the outcome of perinatal asphyxia, but only when delivered prior to an ischemic insult.[94] In human newborns, a controlled clinical trial was undertaken by Goldberg et al.,[95] who administered thiopental at 2-hour-old to term infants who had experienced an asphyxial event at birth. Despite the barbiturate therapy, no improvement in mortality or neurologic morbidity was noted compared to controls at 1 year of recovery.

Hypothermia as a mechanism of reducing the metabolic demands of the brain has been shown to be effective neuroprotection in both the adult and newborn. In the newborn animal, reductions of 3 to 6°C has been shown to be highly neuroprotective when applied systemically[96] or focally to the brain[97] during an ischemic insult. Postischemically, hypothermia appears effective only in those instances when the insult is of mild to moderate severity (unpublished data).

Enhancing the brain's ability to meet its energy requirements, particularly following an ischemic event, when energy reserves are depleted, is an important potential avenue of therapeutic manipulation. This is particularly true of the newborn brain, which is ideally suited to the utilization of alternate substrates. As pointed out earlier in this chapter, while hyperglycemia is profoundly detrimental to the adult brain, it may be beneficial to the newborn.[56] A number of authors have also pointed out the potential role of ketone bodies as an alternative substrate during or following hypoxic-ischemic brain injury. Indeed, the newborn brain is well adapted to benefit from the effects of ketone bodies. Not only is the capacity of the immature blood-brain barrier to transport ketone bodies from blood into brain threefold greater than its capacity for glucose transport,[98] but those enzymes linked to ketone body metabolism in brain display a rapid increase after birth to levels far exceeding those seen later in life.[90] Yager et al.[68] also showed that fasting of newborn animals was neuroprotective. Subsequent studies in their laboratoy suggested that this protective effect may well be due to the induction and utilization of ketone bodies by the brain under conditions of hypoxia-ischemia.[69]

The excitatory amino acid antagonists have received a great deal of attention due to the clear role glutamate plays as a neurotoxic agent in stroke. As in adults, investigations in immature rats have demonstrated that glutamate receptor antagonists are beneficial. When administered systemically, MK-801 prevents the tissue necrosis seen following the direct injection of the glutamate agonist NMDA.[46] This appears to be true even if the drug is administered for up to 1 hour postischemia.[100] Interestingly, this effect of MK-801 was found to be exquisitely age dependent, having a far greater neuroprotective effect in the very immature animal than in its mature counterpart; the difference was likely related to the age-specific enhancement of glutamate binding and receptors in this age group.[43] Others have shown beneficial effects from a host of excitatory amino acid antagonists including L-kynurenine, probenecid, and the AMPA antagonist NBQX.[89]

Studies in recent years have focused on protecting the brain from the secondary effects of oxygen free radical production and delayed neuronal death. In the newborn rat, allopurinol, a free-radical scavenger, was shown to be effective when administered both prior to and following a hypoxic-ischemic insult.[101,102] This same group of investigators reported a beneficial effect of deferoxamine, an iron chelator, following hypoxia-ischemia.[103] In the newborn pig lamb, therapeutic efficacy has been shown utilizing superoxide dismutase as an antioxidant.[104,105] Enhancing the brain's ability to scavenge oxygen free radicals may also be important to the premature infant, who is primarily at risk for white-matter damage in the form of periventricular leukomalacia (see above).

New groups of compounds appear frequently, and at least in animal studies, many provide evidence of a neuroprotective effect. Among these are the anti-inflammatories. Current evidence indicates that the inflammatory response plays a role in determining the extent of brain damage following an ischemic insult in the newborn[106] and that, as part of this response, there is a marked stimulation of interleukin-1B release.[107] To block this reaction, Martin et al.[108] administered a competitive interleukin antagonist before and after hypoxia-ischemia in the neonatal rat, and showed marked neuroprotection. Similarly, Palmer et al.[109] inhibited the inflammatory response by the injection of antineutrophil serum 4 hours prior to an ischemic insult in the neonatal rat, and again found a reduction in brain damage.

Growth factors that have trophic actions on the brain are an exciting area of promise, particularly in the newborn, whose brain is still undergoing extensive maturation. Nozaki et al.[110] displayed a dose-dependent neuroprotective effect of basic fibroblast growth factor in neonatal rats prior to hypoxia-ischemia. And the exogenous administration of GM_1 gangliosides, which probably have a host of effects, including the stimulation of neural growth, to fetal sheep before ischemia reduced neuronal damage.[111]

Infants and Children

Given the vast array of stroke etiologies in infants and children >1 month of age, the therapeutic approach must involve resolution of the underlying disorder. In children with congenital heart disease, prevention of recurrent cerebrovascular accidents should involve correction of the defect. Anticoagulants should be utilized in individuals with chronic valvular abnormalities, though the efficacy of long-term warfarin in children, due to the increased risk of trauma, particularly in toddlers, has yet to be evaluated.

Similarly, treatment of cerebral venous thromboses causing stroke has not been determined. To date, most children with large-vein thrombosis are treated conservatively[5] with good outcome.

In general, stroke as a result of metabolic disease has no specific therapy. Children with homocystinuria should be provided with a diet low in homocysteine. Individuals with abnormalities of coagulation factors are treated best with anticoagulants of daily aspirin therapy, though again, no specific clinical trials evaluating their efficacy have been undertaken to determine outcome as a result of long-term therapy.

OUTCOME

Most of the information compiled to date regarding outcome of stroke or hypoxia-ischemia comes from the neonatal literature. Perhaps one of the most extensive follow-up studies comes from work done by Robertson and colleagues,[112,113] who examined 226 full-term infants experiencing a hypoxic-ischemic event. Each infants had been categorized with either a mild, moderate, or severe encephalopathy.[114] According to their follow-up data at 3.5 and 8 years of age, none of the infants in the mild category experienced any neurologic sequelae (cerebral palsy, mental retardation, seizures, deafness, blindness). Of those in the moderate and severe groups, mortality rates were 6% and 80%, respectively. A neurologic handicap occurred in 20% of those who were moderately affected, and in 100% of those with a severe encephalopathy.

Outside the newborn age group, outcome data are sparse. DeVeber et al.[3] reported a 6% mortality rate in their group of children, which included neonates. Of the survivors, 57% displayed neurolologic sequelae and 36% were normal. Multiple or recurrent strokes occurred in 11%. In a study of 42 children aged 3 months to 13 years, Lanska et al.[83] reported a normal outcome in 24%. Seventy-five percent had a residual hemiparesis, and 19% developed late-onset seizures.

CONCLUSIONS

Stroke in the newborn, infant, and child is not as uncommon a problem as was once considered. The wide range of underlying etiologies reflects the dynamics of a developing and maturing cerebral vascular system and its neuroglial network. The ongoing changes within this system make it uniquely different from the adult, and provide the challenge for future development of agents that can provide benefit to the stroke victim without compromising the normal physiologic maturation of the brain.

REFERENCES

1. Bogousslavsky J, Pierre P. Ischemic stroke in patients under age 45. Neurol Clin 1992; 10:113–124.
2. Broderick J, Talbot GT, Prenger E, Leach A, Brott T. Stroke in children within a major metropolitan area: The surprising importance of intracerebral hemorrhage. J Child Neurol 1993; 8:250–255.
3. DeVeber G. Canadian Pediatric Stroke Registry: An updated analysis. Can J Neurol Sci 1995; 22:S24.
4. Schoenberg BS, Mellinger JF, Schoenberg DG. Cerebrovascular disease in infants

and children: A study of incidence, clinical features and survival. Neurology 1978; 28:763–768.
5. Barron TF, Gusnard DA, Zimmerman RA, Clancy RR. Cerebral venous thrombosis in neonates and children. Pediatr Neurol 1992; 8:112–116.
6. Jaillard AS, Hommel M, Mallaret M. Venous sinus thrombosis associated with androgens in a healthy young man. Stroke 1994; 25:212–213.
7. U.S. Department of Health, Education and Welfare. National Survey of Stroke. NIH publication No. 80-2069, 1980.
8. Volpe JJ Brain injury in the premature infant: is it preventable? Pediatr Res 1990; 27:528–533.
9. Banker BQ. Cerebral vascular disease in infancy and childhood. I. Occlusive vascular disease. J Neuropathol Exp Neurol 1961; 20:127.
10. Kerr LM, Anderson DM, Thompson JA, Lyver SM, Call GK. Ischemic stroke in the young: evaluation and age comparison of patients six months to thirty-nine years. J Child Neurol 1993; 8:266–270.
11. Riela AR, Roach S. Etiology of stroke in children. J Child Neurol 1993; 8:201–220.
12. Nelson KB. Prenatal origin of hemiparetic cerebral palsy: how often and why? Pediatrics 1991; 88:1059–1061.
13. West DW, Scheel JN, Stover R, et al. Iron deficiency in children with cyanotic congenital heart disease. J Pediatr 1990; 117:266–268.
14. Reed RL, Bracey AW, Hudson JD, Miller TA, Fischer RP. Hypothermia and blood coagulation: dissociation between enzyme activity and clotting factor levels. Circ Shock 1990; 32:141–152.
15. Baker FJ, Kotchmar GS, Foshee WS, Sumaya CV. Acute hemiplegia of childhood associated with Epstein-Barr virus infection. Pediatr Infect Dis 1983; 2:136–138.
16. Gold AP, Carter S. Acute hemiplegia of infancy and childhood. Pediatr Clin North Am 1976; 23:413–433.
17. Roddy SM, Giang DW. Antiphospholipid antibodies and stroke in an infant. Pediatrics 1991; 87:933–935.
18. Kohrman MH, Huttenlocher PR. Takayasu arteritis: a treatable cause of stroke in infancy. Pediatr Neurol 1985; 2:154.
19. Graf WD, Milstein JM, Sherry DD. Stroke and mixed connective tissue disease. J Child Neurol 1993; 8:256–259.
20. Ohene-Frempong K. Stroke in sickle cell disease: demographic, clinical, and therapeutic considerations. Semin Hematol 1991; 28:319.
21. Isreals SJ, Seshia SS. Childhood stroke associated with protein C or S deficiency. J Pediatr 1987; 111:562–564.
22. Hartfield DS, Lowry NJ, Keene D, Yager JY. Iron deficiency: a cause of stroke in infants and children. Pediatr Neurol 1997; 1:50–53.
23. Boers GHJ, Smals AGH, Trijbels FJM, et al. Heterozygosity for homocystinuria in premature peripheral and cerebral occlusive arterial disease. N Engl J Med 1985; 313:709–715.
24. Natowicz M, Kelley RI. Mendelian etiologies of stroke. Ann Neurol 1987; 22:175–192.

25. Kalapurackal M, Shuaib A, Lowry NJ. Ischemic stroke in children: relationships to unsuscepted trauma. J Stroke Cerebrovasc Dis 1994; 4:57–62.
26. Hart RG, Easton JD. Dissections of cervical and cerebral arteries. Neurol Clin 1983; 1:155–182.
27. Glueck CJ, Daniels SR, Bates S, Benton C, Tracy T, Third JLHC. Pediatric victims of unexplained stroke and their families: familial lipid and lipoprotein abnormalities. Pediatrics 1982; 69:308–316.
28. Vannucci RC. Experimental biology of cerebral hypoxia-ischemia: relation to perinatal brain damage. Pediatr Res 1990; 27:317–326.
29. Rothman SM, Olney JW. Glutamate and the pathophysiology of hypoxic-ischemic brain damage. Ann Neurol 1986; 19:105–111.
30. Silverstein FS, Naik B, Simpson J. Hypoxia-ischemia stimulates hippocampal glutamate efflux in perinatal rat brain: an in vivo microdialysis study. Pediatr Res 1991; 30:587–590.
31. Chan PH. Role of oxidants in ischemic brain damage. Stroke 1996; 27:1124–1129.
32. Ginsberg MD, Watson BD, Busto R, et al. Peroxidative damage to cell membranes following cerebral ischemia: a cause of ischemic brain injury? Neurochem Pathol 1988; 9:171–194.
33. Bredesen DE. Neural apoptosis. Ann Neurol 1995; 38:839–851.
34. Charriaut-Marlangue C, Pollard H, Ben-Ari Y. Is ischemic cell death of the apoptotic type? Adv Neurol 1996; 71:425–431.
35. Chen S, Soares HD, Morgan JI. Novel molecular correlates of neuronal death and regeneration. Adv Neurol 1966; 71:433–450.
36. Duffy TE, Kohle SJ, Vannucci RC. Carbohydrate and energy metabolism is perinatal rat brain: relation to survival in anoxia. J Neurochem 1975; 24:271–276.
37. Jilek L, Fischer J, Virulich L, Trojan S. The reaction of the brain to stagnant hypoxia and anoxia during ontogeny. Prog Brain Res 1964; 9:113–131.
38. Yager JY, Shuaib A, Thornhill J. The effect of age on susceptibility to brain damage in a model of global hemispheric hypoxic-ischemia. Dev Brain Res 1996; 93:143–154.
39. Kolb B, Whishaw IQ. Earlier is not always better: Behavioral dysfunction and abnormal cerebral morphogenesis following neonatal cortical lesions in the rat. Behav Brain Res 1985; 17:25–43.
40. Kolb B, Holmes C, Whishaw IQ. Recovery from early cortical lesions in rats. III. Neonatal removal of posterior parietal cortex has greater behavioral and anatomical effects than similar removals in adulthood. Behav Brain Res 1987; 26:119–137.
41. Bickler PE, Gallego SM, Hansen BM. Developmental changes in intracellular calcium regulation in rat cerebral cortex during hypoxia. J Cereb Blood Flow Metab 1993; 13:811–819.
42. Chugani HT, Hovda DA, Villablanca JR, Phelps ME, Xu W-F. Metabolic maturation of the brain: a study of local cerebral glucose utilization in the developing cat. J Cereb Blood Flow Metab 1991; 11:35–47.
43. Hattori H, Wasterlain CG. Excitatory amino acids in the developing brain: ontogeny, plasticity, and excitotoxicity. Pediatr Neurol 1990; 6:219–228.

44. Stolk JA. Olsen JI, Reeves PM, et al. In vivo [^{31}P]NMR studies on the influence of age on rat brain hypoxia. Brain Res 1989; 482:1–11.
45. Zhang J-R, Andrus PK, Hall ED. Age-related regional changes in hydroxyl radical stress and antioxidants in gerbil brain. J Neurochem 1993; 61:1640–1647.
46. McDonald JW, Johnston MV. Physiological and pathophysiological roles of excitatory amino acids during central nervous system development. Brain Res Rev 1990; 15 41–70.
47. Represa A., Tremblay E, Ben-Ari Y. Transient increase of NMDA binding sites in human hippocampal during development. Neurosci Lett 1989; 99:61–66.
48. Tremblay E, Roisin MP, Represa A, Charriaut-Marlangue C, Ben-Ari Y. Transient increased density of NMDA binding sites in the developing rat hippocampus. Brain Res 1988; 461:393–396.
49. Ikonmidou C, Mosinger JL, Salles SK. Sensitivity of the developing rat brain to hypobaric/ischemic damage parallels sensitivity to N-methyl-D-aspartate neurotoxicity. J Neurosci 1989; 9:2809–2818.
50. Cremer JE. Substrate utilization and brain development. J Cereb Blood Flow Metab 1982; 2:394–407.
51. Young RSK, Petroff OAC, Chen B, Aquila WJ, Gore JC. Preferential utilization of lactate in neonatal dog brain: in vivo and in vitro proton NMR study. Biol Neonate 1991; 59:46–53.
52. Pulsinelli WA, Waldman S, Rawlinson D, Plum F. Hyperglycemia converts neuronal damage into brain infarction. Neurology 1982; 32:1239–1246.
53. Yip PK, He YY, Hsu Cy, Garg N, Marangos P, Hogan EL. Effect of plasma glucose on infarct size in focal cerebral ischemia-reperfusion. Neurology 1991; 41:899–905.
54. Rehncrona S, Rossen I, Siesjo BK. Excessive cellular acidosis: an important mechanism of neuronal damage in the brain? Acta Physiol Scand 1989; 110:435437.
55. Vannucci RC, Mujsce DJ. Effect of glucose on perinatal hypoxic-ischemic brain damage. Biol Neonate 1992; 62:215–224.
56. Vannucci RC, Yager YJ. Glucose, lactic acid, and perinatal hypoxic-ischemic brain damage. Pediatr Neurol 1992; 8:3–12.
57. Hattori H. Wasterlain CG. Post-hypoxic glucose supplement reduces hypoxic-ischemic brain damage in the neonatal rat. Ann Neurol 1990; 28:122–128.
58. Laptook AR, Corbett RJT, Arencibia-Mireles O, Ruley J. Glucose-associated alterations in ischemic brain metabolism of neonatal piglets. Stroke 1992; 23:1504–1511.
59. Rosenberg AA, Murdaugh E. The effect of blood glucose concentration on postasphyxia cerebral hemodynamics in newborn lambs. Pediatr Res 1990; 27:454–459.
60. Yager JY. Brucklacher RM, Vannucci RC. Cerebral oxidative metabolism and redox state during hypoxia-ischemia and early recovery in the immature rat. Am J Physiol 1991; 262:H1102–H1108.
61. Yager JY, Brucklacher RM, Vannucci RC. Paradoxical mitochondrial oxidation in perinatal hypoxic-ischemic brain damage. Brain Res 1996; 712:230–238.

62. Bryan RM, Jobsis FF. Insufficient supply of reducing equivalents to the respiratory chain in cerebral cortex during severe insulin-induced hypoglycemia in cats. J Cereb Blood Flow Metab 1986; 6:286–291.
63. Chance B, Williams GR. Respiratory enzymes in oxidative phosphorylation I-III. J Biol Chem 1955; 217:383–427.
64. Altman DI, Perlman JM, Volpe JJ, Powers WJ. Cerebral oxygen metabolism in newborn infants measured with positron emission tomography. J Cereb Blood Flow Metab 1989; 9:S25.
65. Fuglsang A, Lomholt M, Gjedde A. Blood-brain transfer of glucose and glucose analogs in newborn rats. J Neurochem 1986; 46:1417–1428.
66. Nehlig A, Vasconcelos AP. Glucose and ketone body utilization by the brain of neonatal rats. Prog Neurobiol 1993; 40:163–221.
67. Hellmann J, Vannucci RC, Nardis EE. Blood-brain barrier permeability to lactic acid in the newborn dog: lactate as a cerebral metabolic fuel. Pediatr Res 1982; 16:40–44.
68. Yager JY, Heitjan DF, Towfighi J, Vannucci RC. Effect of insulin induced and fasting hypoglycemia on perinatal hypoxic-ischemic brain damage. Pediatr Res 1992; 31:138–142.
69. Yager JY. Protective effects of fasting and ketone body supplementation on hypoxic-ischemic brain damage in the immature rat. Ann Neurol 1994; 36:540
70. Volpe JJ. Neurology of the Newborn III. Philadelphia: W.B. Saunders, 1995.
71. Rorke LB. Pathology of Perinatal Brain Injury. New York: Raven Press, 1982.
72. DeReuck J. The human periventricular arterial blood supply and the anatomy of cerebral infarctions. Eur Neurol 1971; 5:321–334.
73. Takashima S, Taraka K. Development of cerebrovascular architecture and its relationship to periventricular leukomalacia. Arch Neurol 1978; 35:11–16.
74. Young RSK, Hernandez MJ, Yagel SK. Selective reduction of blood flow to white matter during hypotension in newborn dogs: a possible mechanism of periventricular leukomalacia. Ann Neurol 1982; 12:445–448.
75. Lou HC, Lassen NA, Friis-Hanson B. Impaired autoregulation of cerebral blood flow in the distressed newborn infant. J Pediatr 1979; 94:170–173.
76. Oka A, Belliveau MJ, Rosenberg PA, Volpe JJ. Vulnerability of oligodendroglia to glutamate—pharmacology, mechanisms, and prevention. J Neurosci 1993; 13:1441–1453.
77. Back SA, Yonezawa M, Gan XD, Rosenberg PA, Volpe JJ. Oligodencrocyte death induced by cystine deprivation occurs via apoptosis. Ann Neurol 1995; 38:502A.
78. Husain J, Juurlink BHJ. Oligodendroglial precursor cell susceptibility to hypoxia is related to poor ability to cope with reactive oxygen species. Brain Res 1995; 698:86–95.
79. Juurlink BHJ, Husain J. Hyperthermic injury of oligodendrocyte precursor cells—implications for dysmyelination disorders. Brain Res 1994; 641:353–356.
80. Thorburne SK, Juurlink BHJ. Low glutathione and high iron govern the susceptibility of oligodendroglial precursors to oxidative stress. J Neurochem 1996; 67:1014.

81. Juurlink BHJ, Schultke E, Hertz L. Glutathione release and catabolism during energy substrate restriction in astrocytes. Brain Res 1996; 710:229–233.
82. Levy SR, Abroms IF, Marshall PC, Rosquete EE. Seizures and cerebral infarction in the full-term newborn. Ann Neurol 1985; 17:366–370.
83. Lanska MJ, Lanska DJ, Horwitz SJ, Aram DM. Presentation, clinical course, and outcome of childhood stroke. Pediatr Neurol 1991; 7:333–341.
84. Eeg-Olofsson O, Ringheim Y. Stroke in children. Clinical characteristics and prognosis. Acta Pediatr Scand 1983; 72:391–395.
86. Wiznitzer M, Masaryk TJ. Cerebrovascular abnormalities in pediatric stroke: assessment using parenchymal and angiographic magnetic resonance imaging. Ann Neurol 1991; 29:585–589.
87. Palmer C, Vannucci RC. Potential new therapies for perinatal cerebral hypoxia-ischemia. Clin Perinatol 1993; 20:411–432.
88. Vannucci RC. Current and potentially new management strategies for perinatal hypoxic-ischemic encephalopathy. Pediatrics 1990; 85:961–968.
89. Tuor UI, Del Bigio MR, Chumas PD. Brain damage due to cerebral hypoxia/ischemia in the neonate: pathology and pharmacological modification. Cerebrovasc Brain Metab Rev 1996; 8:159–193.
90. Lupton BA, Hill A, Roland EH, Whitfield MF, Flodmark O. Brain swelling in the asphyxiated term newborn: pathogenesis and outcome. Pediatrics 1988; 82:139–146.
91. Vannucci RC, Christensen MA, Yager JY. Nature, time-course and extent of cerebral edema in perinatal hypoxic-ischemia brain damage. Pediatr Neurol 1993; 9:29–35.
92. Mujsce DJ, Towfighi J, Stern D, Vannucci RC: Mannitol therapy in perinatal hypoxic-ischemic brain damage. Stroke 1990; 21:1210–1214.
93. Tuor UI, Chumas PD, Del Bigio MR. Prevention of hypoxic-ischemic damage with dexamethasone is dependent on age and not influenced by fasting. Exp Neurol 1995; 132:116–122.
94. Cockburn F, Daniel SS, Dawes GS. The effect of pentobarbital anesethesia on resuscitation and brain damage in feral rhesus monkeys asphyxiated on delivery. J Pediatr 1969; 75:281–291.
95. Goldberg RN, Moscoso P, Bauer CR. Use of barbiturate therapy in severe perinatal asphyxia; a randomized controlled trial. J Pediatr 1986; 109:851–856.
96. Yager JY, Towfighi J, Vannucci RC. Influence of mild hypothermia on hypoxic-ischemic brain damage in the immature rat. Pediatr Res 1993; 34:525–529.
97. Towfighi J, Housman C, Heitjan DF, Vannucci RC, Yager JY. The effect of focal cerebral cooling on perinatal hypoxic-ischemic brain damage. Acta Neuropathol 1994; 87:598–604.
98. DeVivo DC, Leckie MP, Agrawal HC. The differential incorporation of beta-hydroxybutyrate and glucose into brain glutamate in the newborn rat. Brain Res 1973; 55:485–490.
99. Page MA, Krebs HA, Williamson DH. Activities of enzymes of ketone-body utilization in brain and other tissues of suckling rats. Biochem J 1971; 121:49–53.
100. Hattori H, Morin AM, Schwartz PH, Fujikawa DG, Wasterlain CG. Post-hypoxic

treatment with MK-801 reduces hypoxic-ischemic damage in the neonatal rat. Neurology 1989; 39:713–718.
101. Palmer C, Towfighi J, Roberts RL, Heitjan DF. Allopurinol administered after inducing hypoxia/ischemia reduces brain injury in 7-day old rats. Pediatr Res 1993; 33:405–411.
102. Palmer C, Vannucci RC, Towfighi J. Reduction of perinatal hypoxic-ischemic brain damage with allopurinol. Pediatr Res 1990; 27:332–336.
103. Palmer C, Roberts R, Bero C. Deferoxamine posttreatment reduces ischemic brain injury in neonatal rats. Stroke 1994; 25:1039–1045.
104. Armstead WM, Mirro R, Thelin OP, et al. Polyethyleneglycol superoxide dismutase and catalase attenuate increased blood-brain barrier permeability after ischemia in piglets. Stroke 1992; 23:755–762.
105. Rosenberg AA, Murdaugh E White CW. The role of oxygen free radicals in postasphyxia cerebral hypoperfusion in newborn lambs. Pediatr Res 1989; 26:215–219.
106. Towfighi J, Zec N, Yager J, Housman C, Vannucci RC. Temporal evolution of neuropathological changes in an immature rat model of cerebral hypoxia-ischemia (HI): a light microscopic study. Acta Neuropathol 1995; 90:375–386.
107. Szaflarski J, Burtrum D, Silverstein FS. Cerebral hypoxia-ischemia stimulates cytokine gene expression in perinatal rats. Stroke 1995; 26:1093–1100.
108. Martin D, Chinookoswong N, Miller G. The interleukin-1 receptor antagonist (rhIL-1ra) protects against cerebral infarction in a rat model of hypoxia-ischemia. Exp Neurol 1994; 130:362–367.
109. Palmer C, Roberts RL, Young PI. Neutropenia before but not after hypoxia-ischemia reduces brain injury in neonatal rats. J Cereb Blood Flow Metab 1995; 15:S291.
110. Nozaki K, Finklestein SP, Beal MF. Basic fibroblast growth factor protects against hypoxia/ischemia and NMDA neurotoxicity in neonatal rats J Cereb Blood Flow Metab 1993; 13:221–228.
111. Tan WKM, Williams CE, Gunn AJ, Mallard CE, Gluckman PD. Pretreatment with monosialoganglioside GM_1 protects the brain of fetal sheep against hypoxic/ischemic injury without causing systemic compromise. Pediatr Res 1993; 34:18–22.
112. Robertson CMT, Finer NN. Term infants with hypoxic-ischemic encephalopathy: outcome at 3.5 years. Dev Med Child Neurol 1985; 27:473–484.
113. Robertson CMT, Finer NN, Grace MGA. School performance of survivors of neonatal encephalopathy associated with birth asphyxia at term. J Pediatr 1989; 114:753–760.
114. Sarnat HB, Sarnat MS. Neonatal encephalopathy following fetal distress—a clinical and electroencephalographic study. Arch Neurol 1976; 33:695–706.

10
Stroke in Young Adults

Enrique C. Leira and Harold P. Adams, Jr.
University of Iowa, College of Medicine, Iowa City, Iowa

Betsy B. Love
Indiana University, College of Medicine, Indianapolis, Indiana

INTRODUCTION

While ischemic stroke is often considered a disorder of the middle-aged or elderly, it is also an important neurological disease in young adults. The frequency of stroke in young adults may be increasing due to factors such as better recognition and an increased prevalence of risk factors such as drug abuse. Among young women, stroke appears to be more common than myocardial infarction. Stroke in young adults is especially expensive in terms of health care costs and lost productivity. The young person who has stroke is often otherwise healthy without other disability or chronic illness; thus, the economic consequences of stroke in this group are high due to lost productivity since these individuals are often vital contributors to the work force. Finally, the personal losses and costs are great among young adults. Stroke affects not only the individual, but also the family. The definitions used when studying young adults vary. Usually, this young-adult population is defined as those between 15 and 45 years of age. However, some have further divided this group into those <30 years and those ≥ 30 years.[1]

EPIDEMIOLOGY

The incidence of stroke in the young population in the United States varies from 5 to 10 per 100,000.[2] The age-specific cerebral infarction rate in persons <45 years of age is <11/100,000.[3] Stroke mortality rates have declined since 1968 for both whites and nonwhites in the United States.[4] However, it is clear that nonwhites have a significantly higher mortality rate than whites in the 25-to-44-year age group. In 1988, the mortality rates were three to five times higher among nonwhites than whites.[4]

One study of young adults with acute ischemic stroke showed a 30-day mortality of 6.6%, which is substantially less than the mortality reported with older adults. In this series, patients with a cardiac source of stroke had the greatest mortality.[5] In another series, the prognosis was slightly better among patients 16 to 30 years than among patients who were 31 to 45 years of age.[1] Among the young group, 60% of patients had either no or minor disability, compared to 51% of the older group.[1]

The risk of stroke recurrence in the young has not been studied extensively. The Stroke Data Bank estimated that the 2-year cumulative recurrence of stroke in patients < age 44 years was 6.9%.[6]. When only patients with no prior history of stroke were studied, the 2-year cumulative risk was 5.2%.

Studies that address the quality of life after stroke in the young are relatively few. One study showed that after rehabilitation, approximately 80% of young adults resume their previous jobs within 6 months afer discharge.[7] However, other series report that while 75% to 80% of young stroke survivors have minimal or no disability, less than half of these patients return to work, due to their neurologic impairments.[8,9] In addition, a majority of survivors in one series reported emotional, social, or physical residuals that lessened the quality of life.[8]

ETIOLOGY

The list of etiologies for cerebral infarction in young adults is diverse and complex (Table 1). Unusual causes for cerebral ischemia are found more frequently in patients <45 years of age than in older patients, in whom atherosclerosis plays an overwhelming role in pathogenesis. The mechanisms for stroke in young adults (with approximate frequency in parenthesis) are:

1. Atherosclerosis (20–30%)
2. Cardioembolism (20%)
3. Nonatherosclerotic arteriopathies (20–30%)
4. Secondary to vasospasm (<5%)
5. Hematological (<5%)
6. Hypoperfusional states (<5%)
7. Metabolic abnormalities (inherited or acquired) (<5%)
8. Cryptogenic (10–40%)

Atherosclerotic lesions account for 20% to 30% of the infarcts, depending on the series and criteria utilized.[10,11] Since the prevalence of atherosclerosis in-

Table 1 Etiological Classification of Strokes in the Young Based on Physiopathology

- Atherosclerosis
  - Extracranial/intracranial[10]
  - Thromboembolism/artery-artery embolism[10]
- Embolism
  - Cardiac origin
    - Valvular lesions:prosthetic valve, mitral stenosis, infective endocarditis, Libman-Sacks endocarditis, calcified aortic stenosis, mitral annual calcification, mitral valve prolapse[17]
    - Atrial fibrillation[19]
    - Sick-sinus syndrome[18]
    - Hypokinetic segment/myocardial infarction[19]
    - Mural thrombus[29]
    - Left atrial myxoma[19]
    - Cardiomyopathy: idiopathic, Friedreich's, peripartum, viral, cocaine-induced, hereditary[20,21]
    - Rhabdomyoma (tuberous sclerosis)[22]
    - Rhabdomyosarcoma[68]
    - Papillary fibroelastoma[23]
    - Wolff-Parkinson-White syndrome[24]
  - Paradoxical
    - Cardiac anomalies capable of producing a right-to-left shunt
      - Atrial septal defect[18]
      - Ventricular septal defect[18]
      - Patent foramen ovale[17]
      - Fallot's tetralogy[30]
    - Sources of paradoxical embolism
      - Air embolism (venous lines, surgery)[18]
      - Talc embolism (IV drug abuse of heroin and methylphenidate)[25]
      - Decompression sickness (Caisson's disease)[69]
      - Pulmonary AVM (including Rendu-Osler-Weber syndrome)[26]
      - Pulmonary vein thrombosis[31]
      - Pulmonary and mediastinal tumors[31]
      - Fat embolism[27]
      - Venous thrombosis[28]
      - Extracorporeal circulation[70]

(continued)

Table 1 Continued

C. Artery-artery embolism (nonatherosclerotic)
- Transient embologenic aortitis[71]
- Embolism distal to unruptured aneurysm[31]

Nonatherosclerotic arteriopathies
- Inflammatory
  - Noninfectious
    - Takayasu disease[31]
    - Primary angiitis of the nervous system (PANS)[32]
    - Drug-induced (cocaine, amphetamine)[32]
    - Giant cell arteritis[33]
    - Associated with systemic disease (systemic lupus erythematosus, Wegener disease, panareteritis nodosa, rheumatoid arthritis, Sjogren syndrome, scleroderma, Dego disease, Bechet syndrome, acute rheumatic fever, inflammatory bowel disease)[7,27]
    - Susac microangiopathy of brain and retina[12]
    - Eale disease[72]
    - Acute posterior multifocal placoid pigment epitheliopathy (APMPPE)[73]
    - Neurosarcoidosis[74]
  - Infectious:
    - Syphilis, HIV, Lyme, herpes zoster, herpes simplex, tuberculosis, malaria, mucomycosis, cysticercosis, associated to amygdalitis[31,32,34,75–78]
- Noninflammatory
  - Spontaneous arterial dissection[79]
  - Fibromuscular dysplasia[79]
  - Moyamoya syndrome[36]
  - Fabry disease[37]
  - CADASIL (cerebral autosomal-dominant arteriopathy with subcortical infarcts and leukoencephalopathy)[35]
  - Homocystinuria[38]
  - Spontaneous aneurysms[16]
  - Marfan syndrome[29]
  - Enchondromatosis (Ollier disease)[10]
  - Ehlers-Danlos syndrome type IV[80]
  - Neurofibromatosis[22]
  - Postirradiation vasculopathy[81]
  - Thromboangiitis obliterans (Buerger disease)[82]
  - Neoplastic angioendotheliosis[83]
  - Osteopetrosis[84]
  - Amyloid angiopathy[31]
- Traumatic
  - Traumatic dissection (trauma, neck surgery)[10]
- Extraluminal compression
  - External neck pressure[10]
  - Neck malignancy[10]

Table 1 Continued

Secondary to vasospasm
- Subarachnoid hemorrhage[85]
- Drugs (e.g., cocaine, ergots, amphetamines, ephedrine, methylphenidate, lysergic acid diethylamide, marijuana)[31,54]
- Iatrogenic (secondary to cerebral arteriogram)[55]
- Hypertensive encephalopathy[27]
- Migraine[56]
- Skull base surgery[57]
- Vasospasm secondary to trauma[85]

Hematological
- Hyperviscosity states
  - Corpuscular proliferation (polycytemia, myeloproliferative)[19]
  - Dysproteinemias (multiple myeloma, Waldestrom macroglobulinemia, cryoglobulinemia)[39]
  - Sickle cell disease[40]
- Procoagulant States
  - Primary
    - Lupus anticoagulant, Sneddon syndrome, anticardiolipin antibodies[10,41,42]
    - Protein C deficiency[10,48]
    - Protein S deficiency[10,48]
    - Antithrombin III deficiency[43]
    - Hyperfibrinogenemia[10]
    - Factor VIII deficiency[31]
    - Familial C2 deficiency[31]
    - Thrombotic thrombocytopenic purpura[44]
  - Secondary
    - Alcohol intoxication[46]
    - Nephrotic syndrome[10]
    - Oral contraceptives[31]
    - Postpartum[10]
    - Hyperfibrinogenemia[10]
    - Paroxysmal nocturnal hemoglobinuria[47]
    - Crohn's disease[48]
    - Ulcerative colitis[49]
    - Snake bite[50]
    - Chronic diffuse intravascular coagulation[51]
    - Platelet hyperaggregability[52]
    - Exogenous testosterone[86]
    - Chemotherapeutic agents[76]

Hypoperfusional states
- Secondary to cardiac arrest/arrhythmias[58]
- Shock[59]

(*continued*)

Table 1 Continued

Iatrogenic (antihypertensive drugs, carotid surgery, extracorporeal pump devices)[87–89]
Illicit drugs (e.g., opioids)[25]
Severe anemia,[16] thalassemia[24]
Traumatic brain injury[30]
Secondary to venous occlusion
Cortical sinus or vein thrombosis[60]
Inherited metabolic abnormalities
MELAS[61]
Kearns-Sayre syndrome[10]
Leigh disease[22]
Acquired metabolic abnormalities
Primary hypoglycemia[90]
Hypoglycemia secondary to insulinoma[62]

Source: Ref. 31.

creases with age, the probability of finding relevant atherosclerosis lessens as age decreases.[12,13] An accelerated picture of atherosclerosis in the young can be seen in cases of familial hyperlipidemia, diabetes mellitus, heavy tobacco use, homocystinuria, or following organ transplantation.[14] Atherosclerotic lesions can result in infarction by mechanisms of thrombosis, artery-to-artery embolism, or hypoperfusion.

Embolism of cardiac origin is another important source of strokes in the young, with a prevalence comparable to atherosclerosis in most series. Although several different lesions have been related to stroke, their acceptance as sources of cardioembolism varies with the abnormality. Some valvular lesions like mitral stenosis or a hypokinetic ventricular segment are widely considered "high-risk" lesions. Others, such as a patent foramen ovale or mitral valve prolapse, are found frequently in normal subjects and therefore have an uncertain role in the pathogenesis of stroke. The increased use of transesophageal echocardiography for evaluating young adults with stroke has generated new abnormalities (e.g., fibrin strands) of uncertain significance. Since the evaluation for the cause of stroke is often inconclusive in young adults, it is easy to fall in the temptation to ascribe the stroke to these "soft," probably controversial, echocardiographic findings. More data are needed to better delineate the relationship between some of these potential emboligenic lesions and stroke.[15–18]

Cardiac embolism can also result from dysrhythmias such as atrial fibrillation, sick-sinus syndrome, or Wolff-Parkinson-White syndrome. Cardiomyopathies of several etiologies and intracardiac tumors are potential sources of embolism. In the presence of a right-to-left shunt (atrial septal defect, ventricular septal defect, tetralogy of Fallot, patent foramen ovale, or pulmonary arteriovenous malformation), paradoxical embolism can be attributed to embolus from fat, air, or thrombosed peripheral veins.[16–33]

Nonatherosclerotic arteriopathies are also encountered frequently in young patients, and are divided in inflammatory and noninflammatory causes. They account for approximately 20% to 30% of strokes. Inflammatory vasculopathies (vasculitis) are subdivided into several categories; they can be infectious, autoimmune, drug-related, or idiopathic. Topographically, the several types of vasculitis have a predilection for large/medium vessels (Takayasu), small vessels (primary angiitis of the nervous system), or capillaries (Susac's syndrome). They can present either as a primary central nervous system process or as a multisystem process with secondary brain involvement.[7,12,27,31–34]

Noninflammatory, nonatherosclerotic arteriopathies can be hereditary or sporadic. The most common sporadic nonatherosclerotic vasculopathy is an arterial dissection, which can be spontaneous or secondary to trauma. A genetic cause includes the recently mapped condition of cerebral autosomal-dominant arteriopathy with subcortical infarcts and leukoencephalopathy (CADASIL).[35] The arteriopathic process can be also secondary to systemic connective-tissue abnormalities, such as Marfan syndrome or fibromuscular dysplasia. Neoplastic processes can affect the vessels by direct infiltration (e.g., neoplastic angiodotheliosis) or by producing external compression over the vessels (e.g., neurofibromas in Von Recklinghausen syndrome). Radiation over the cervical area can also induce postradiation arteriopathy.[10,29,35–38]

Hematological causes for stroke are more common in young patients than older persons, but are still relatively infrequent. Hematological predisposition to stroke can occur by means of hyperviscosity of the blood itself, or through the development of a procoagulant state. For instance, hyperviscosity can be the result of corpuscular proliferation (e.g., polycythemia) and/or dysproteinemias (e.g., multiple myeloma). Structural deficiencies in the red blood cell itself (sickle cell anemia) also result in an impaired flow.[19,39,40] Procoagulant states can be either primary or secondary. Primary procoagulant states are produced by the presence of antiphospholipid antibodies, which include the lupus anticoagulant and anticardiolipin antibodies. Procoagulant states can also be the result of protein deficiencies, such as protein C, protein S, antithrombin III, C2 or Factor VIII. Although protein C and S deficiencies are correlated with venous thrombotic events, the extent of their relationship with arterial strokes remains unclear. Whether directly promoting arterial thrombosis, or through paradoxical embolization from venous clots, each protein deficiency has been linked to strokes in the young. Hyperfibrinogenemia and thrombotic thrombocytopenic purpura can result in cerebral infractions.[10,31,41–45] Secondary procoagulant states can be transiently seen with acute alcohol intoxication, the postpartum state, snake bites, disseminated intravascular coagulation, and paroxysmal nocturnal hemoglobinuria. Chronic secondary procoagulant states can be seen with nephrotic syndrome, oral contraceptive use, exogenous testosterone intake, Crohn's disease, or ulcerative colitis.[10,31,46–53]

Vasospasm is a potential but infrequent pathophysiological mechanism of cerebral ischemia in the young. Vasospasm can be triggered by different stimuli, such as subarachnoid hemorrhage, cerebral angiography, hypertensive encephalopathy, or surgery at the base of the skull. Although strokes occurring during migraine attacks were traditionally believed to occur through a vasospastic mechanism, this association remains controversial.[27,31,54,55–57]

Hypoperfusional states can account for brain ischemia, which will have a border zone distribution in normal subjects, or a lateralizing focality if an underlying structural abnormality is present. Pump failure can be produced by an arrhythmia, cardiac arrest, septic shock, or drugs. Severe anemia can result in cerebral ischemia, especially in an hypoxic environment.[16,24,25,30,58,59]

Venous infarctions can result from occlusion of the major venous drainage pathways of the brain. Venous infarctions can be idiopathic. Hypercoagulable states, dehydration, or infiltration of the venous sinuses can predispose to venous obstruction. The obstruction of the venous drainage can result in secondary infarction by means of flow stagnation and retrograde transmission of hydrostatic pressure.[60]

Acquired metabolic derangements can lead to cerebral ischemia. Hypoglycemia, either primary or secondary to tumors (e.g., insulinoma), can result in focal neurological ischemia. Inherited mitochondrial disorders, such as mitochondrial encephalopathy lactic acidosis and strokelike episodes (MELAS), Kearns-Sayre syndrome, or Leigh's disease, may also present with acute strokes[10,22,61]

A substantial number of strokes (10% to 40%) cannot be attributed to any particular etiology despite a thorough evaluation.[10,11] This wide range may be explained by differences in the approach to diagnostic workup, and also be personal preferences of the physician in establishing a cause-and-effect relationship between certain findings and the clinical picture. Future research may provide more unified criteria and hopefully minimize the frequency of cryptogenic stroke.[10,11,15]

DIAGNOSIS

The success in finding the cause for stroke in the young adult relies on the combination of a careful history, a thorough neurological exam, and a judiciously selected battery of ancillary diagnostic tests. A random approach that includes all tests available is likely to be excessively expensive, to generate a considerable amount of data of uncertain significance, and to create additional questions rather than provide answers.

The history gives important clues. Questions regarding family history should focus specifically on strokes, myocardial infarction, and migraine, with special emphasis on the age of presentation. A family history of spontaneous miscarriages, deep venous thrombosis, or pulmonary embolism should prompt a specific search for a primary procoagulant state. A family history of children or adolescents suffering from encephalopathy, myopathy, seizures, and/or strokes following a pattern of maternal inheritance should raise the possibility of a mutation in the mitochondrial DNA, such in MELAS or Kearns-Sayre syndrome[10,16] A hereditary, dominant pattern of migraines (often "complicated"), progressive dementia, and strokes occurring in young adults can lead to the probably underdiagnosed condition of cerebral autosomal dominant arteriopathy with subcortical infarcts and leukoencephalopathy (CADASIL).[35] The ethnic background may be also relevant in certain cases, such as Crohn's disease (Ashkenazi Jews), thalassemia (Mediterranean descent), or sickle cell disease (African-Americans).

The social history can delineate any present or past use of illicit drugs, tobacco, exogenous hormones, and alcohol. Alcohol intake in the hours before the stroke is an important piece of information.[46] A sexual history, including risk factors for HIV, should be obtained. Exposure to tick bites can be relevant in areas where Lyme disease is common. A travel history should be explored, as it can suggest exposure to foreign pathogens (e.g., malaria). Contact sports, such as martial arts, can result in traumatic arterial dissection. An unexplained carotid dissection in a young woman should raise the suspicion of nonreported physical abuse.

The review of systems aims at detection of systemic factors that might relate to stroke. For example, a history of recent fluctuating fevers can be the clue leading to the diagnosis of infectious endocarditis. Constitutional symptoms can lead to the diagnosis of an infectious, neoplastic, or connective-tissue disease process. Episodic chest pain in a young patient with a stroke should be considered ischemic until proven otherwise. A cardiological evaluation may identify a potential source of embolism. Palpitations can suggest transient dysrhythmias, as with thyrotoxicosis or Wolff-Parkinson-White syndrome.[19,24] Neck and ear pain can indicate a carotid dissection. Headaches and cognitive symptoms often are complaints in nervous system vasculitis. Lower gastrointestinal symptoms suggest Crohn's disease or ulcerative colitis. Dry eyes, dry mouth, and sensory dysesthesias can be elicited in Sjogren's syndrome. Edema can be the manifestation of nephrotic syndrome or a dilated cardiomyopathy. New onset of headaches with decreased level of consciousness is a hallmark of a cerebral sinus vein occlusion. Recurrent episodes of symptoms attributed to hypoglycemia could point to an insulinoma as a cause of the stroke.[62]

Certain physical findings on the general examination point toward a specific etiological condition. For example, an elongated body habitus and joint hypermobility suggests an underlying connective-tissue abnormality (Marfan syndrome, homocystinuria).[63] Skin examination may detect the presence of livedo reticularis, which is a hallmark of Sneddon's syndrome. Other relevant skin lesions are those rashes suggestive of herpes zoster, syphilis, or Lyme disease. Osler's nodes (maculopapular hemorrhagic or erythematous lesions) can be seen with infective endocarditis.[63] Petechiae can be seen in cases of disseminated intravascular coagulation. The presence of lesions suggestive of repetitive venous puncture ("railroad tracks") can uncover drug use habits. Tattoos can sometimes be strategically placed to disguise such lesions. Also, certain tattoos are markers of membership to particular subculture groups, and can be indirect evidence of drug abuse.[63]

The blood pressure should be measured in both arms, as an asymmetry may indicate subclavian steal syndrome. An elevated blood pressure, if accompanied by signs of chronic hypertension such as vascular retinal changes and other end-organ damage, suggests atherosclerotic damage. Ocular examination should also look for lens dislocation, which can point to Marfan's syndrome or homocystinuria. Changes in the lens can provide clues for diseases such as Fabry's disease that can cause stroke. Fundoscopic exam should concentrate on detecting microemboli (cholesterol, talc) or retinal lesions (mitochondrial disorders). An abnormal pulse can uncer a rhythm abnormality. An absent temporal artery pulse or an inflamed tender artery can occur in the context of an arteritis. Careful cardiac auscultation may uncer bruits from valvular disease, or right-to-left shunting abnormalities. Auscultation of the extracranial and intracranial arteries may also detect bruits. Chest auscultation (outside the cardiac dull area) may reveal bruits suggestive of pulmonary arteriovenous malformation. Renal bruits may lead to the discovery of fibromuscular dysplasia. The elicitation of calf pain after passive dorsiflexion of the foot (Homan's sign) may suggest the presence of deep venous thrombosis as a possible source of paradoxical embolization.[63] Besides finding signs that correlate with the severity and location of the stroke, the neurological examination can give clues to the causes of stroke. For example, a painful polyneuropathy may be found in patients with Fabry's disease.

Every young patient presenting with an acute stroke should have a basic array of diagnostic tests that includes a noncontrast computerized tomography (CT) of the brain, an electrocardiogram, chest x-ray, complete blood count with differential, electrolytes, and PT and PTT (Table 2). A quick determination of glucose by finger stick should be considered if the results of the blood glucose are likely to be delayed. If a hypercoagulable state is suspected, hematological

Table 2 Initial Tests in Evaluation of Acute Ischemic Stroke in the Young

CBC
Electrolytes/glucose finger-stick
Prothrombin time, partial thromboplastin time, bleeding time
Chest x-ray
Electrocardiogram
Telemetry cardiac monitoring
Sedimentation rate
Drug screen
Syphilis test
Pregnancy test
Lipid profile
Noncontrast CT scan
Transthoracic echocardiography, transesophageal echocardiography
Magnetic resonance imaging/angiogram/venogram
Cerebral angiogram

tests should be drawn before any anticoagulant medication is started, as the administration of medications may preclude a reliable determination. In addition, the stroke itself may influence some of the results of special hematological studies. A sedimentation rate, blood lipid determination, VDRL, drug screen, and pregnancy test for females should probably be included.

Echocardiographic evaluation should be considered if there is history of cardiac disease. Although transthoracic echocardiogram is noninvasive, it is unlikely to show abnormalities in a young patient without history of cardiac disease.[64] Conversely, transesophageal echocardiogram is a very sensitive test that efficiently visualizes the left atrium and ascending aorta, and is therefore more likely to show abnormalities. The two forms of echocardiography are complementary, as they study the heart from different perspectives. The decision of performing either form of echocardiography should be based on the clinical characteristics of the case. For example, in a patient who had a stroke following a myocardial infarction, a transthoracic echocardiogram usually is sufficient to visualize a left ventricular thrombus. On the other hand, an acute stroke stroke occurring concomitantly with embolization to the fingers and toes may warrant a transesophageal echocardiogram to rule out the possibility of a mobile aortic plaque. More data are needed before establishing an algorithm for echocardiographic evaluation that would wisely combine health cost issues with the effective detection and management of treatable cardiac sources of embolism.

Brain magnetic resonance imaging (MRI) should be considered in patients in whom the localization of the stroke is uncertain by either clinical or CT findings. MRI is able to visualize ischemic lesions earlier than CT, and it may also be useful if a nonischemic pathology is suspected. However, the test should be performed only if management is likely to be changed based on potential results. MRI may also provide the highest yield in diagnosing carotid artery dissections.[65] Magnetic resonance angiogram (MRA) can visualize both the arterial and venous vessels for screening purposes.

Cerebral angiography should be considered strongly in the young adult in whom the etiology of the stroke is not apparent after the proposed initial evaluation. The probability of finding an abnormality by arteriography is approximately 70% in young patients.[55,66] The importance of performing early angiography has been stressed, because the yield diminishes the later the test is performed.[66]

If no etiology can be found after the initial evaluation, the use of more specific diagnostic tests should be considered based on the historical, exploratory, and laboratory findings listed above. A list of the available diagnostic tests is outlined in Table 3. The conditions that can be mistaken with stroke in the young adult are listed in Table 4.

TREATMENT

Young adults are more likely than older patients to have a cause for the stroke that warrants specific treatment; for example, conditions such as central nervous system vasculitis can be treated with immunosuppressant drugs. Infective diseases such as Lyme disease or syphilis are treated with antibiotics. Moyamoya syndrome can be treated with several surgical revascularization and bypass procedures.

The acute treatment of the ischemic stroke in young adults is not substantially different from that of the elderly. Since younger patients tend to have fewer underlying medical problems, they are more likely to meet the inclusion criteria for treatment with intravenous r-tPA, and they might have a lower rate of complications.[67]

Younger patients can benefit from carotid endarterectomy for stroke prophylaxis due to a lower surgical risk than older patients. The pharmacological prevention of stroke is not substantially different in the young. Aspirin should be the first-line agent for stroke prophylaxis in patients with no cardiac source of embolism. Ticlopidine is generally considered to be a second-line agent, although women and diabetic patients may benefit from it more than they do from aspirin. Warfarin should be used whenever a cardiac source of embolism is suspected. The usefulness of warfarin in patients with intracranial stenosis or certain procoagulant states needs further investigation. Warfarin is a teratogenic drug, particularly in the first trimester. Pregnant woman that require anticoagulation

Table 3 Possible Tests in the Evaluation of Acute Ischemic Stroke in the Young

Test	Indications
Blood cultures	infective endocarditis
Sickle cell testing/hemoglobin electrophoresis	sickle cell anemia
Serum protein electrophoresis	dysproteinemia
Complement levels	familial C2 deficiency
Cerebrospinal fluid examination	inflammatory arteriopathies
Human immunodeficiency virus, Lyme, tuberculosis testing	infective arteriopathies
Platelet aggregation tests	platelet hyperaggregability
Antinuclear antibodies	systemic lupus erythematosus
Cardiac stress testing/catheterization	ischemic heart disease
Holter monitoring	cardiac arrhythmias
Urine protein determinations	nephrotic syndrome
Factor VIII assay	Factor VIII deficiency
Antithrombin III	antithrombin III deficiency
Antiphospholipid antibodies	Sneddon syndrome
Proteins C and S	protein C and S deficiency
Fibrinogen determinations	Hyperfibrinogenemia
Homocysteine	Homocystinuria
Cystathione B-synthetase in tissue	Homocystinuria
Connective tissue biopsy	noninflammatory vasculopathies
Brain biopsy	vasculitis
Venous duplex lower extremities	paradoxical embolization
Chromosomal/mitochondrial deoxyribonucleic acid	mitochondrial diseases, CADASIL
Colonoscopy/biopsy	Crohn's disease, ulcerative colitis
Neck computed tomogram/magnetic resonance imaging	extraluminal compression/dissection
Chest computed tomogram with contrast	pulmonary arteriovenous malformation
Temporal artery biopsy	giant cell arteritis
SS-A, SS-B antibodies	Sjogren syndrome
Schirmer's test/gland biopsy	Sjogren syndrome
Ophthalmological examination (iritis)	Bechet syndrome

Table 4 Conditions Simulating Acute Ischemic Stroke in the Young

Brain hemorrhage
Todd paralysis (epilepsy)
Migraine
Multiple sclerosis
Trauma
Brain tumor/metastasis
Abscess
Subdural/epidural hematoma
Encephalitis/meningitis
Hypoglycemia
Conversion disorder/malingering

should probably be switched to subcutaneous heparin, at least for the first 3 months of pregnancy.

REFERENCES

1. Bogousslavsky J, Pierre P. Ischemic stroke in patients under age 45. Cerebral ischemia: treatment and prevention. Neurol Clin 1992; 10:113–124.
2. Broderick JP, Phillips SJ, Whisnant JP, et al. Incidence rates of stroke in the eighties: the end of the decline of stroke? Stroke 1989; 20:577–582.
3. Love BB, Orencia AJ, Biller J. Stroke in children and young adults: overview, risk factors and prognosis. In: Biller J, Mathews KD, Love BB, eds. Stroke in Children and Young Adults. Boston: Butterworth-Heinemann, 1994:1–13.
4. Modan B, Wagener DK. Some epidemiological aspects of stroke: mortality/morbidity trends, age, sex, race, socioeconomic status. Stroke 1992; 23:1230–1236.
5. Biller J, Adams HP Jr, Bruno A, et al. Mortality in acute cerebral infarction in young adults—a ten year experience. Angiology 1991; 42:224–230.
6. Hier DB, Foulkes MA, Swinontoniowski M, et al. Stroke recurrence within 2 years after ischemic infarction. Stroke 1991; 22:155–161.
7. Adunsky A, Hershkowitz M, Rabbi R, et al. Functional recovery in young stroke patients. Arch Phys Med Rehabil 1992; 73:859–862.
8. Kappelle LJ, Adams HP, Heffner ML, et al. Prognosis of young adults with ischemic stroke. Stroke 1994; 25:1360–1365.
9. Chancellor AM, Glasgow GL, Ockelford PA, et al. Etiology, prognosis and hemostatic function after cerebral infarction in young adults. Stroke 1989; 20:477–482.
10. Adams HP, Kappelle LJ, Biller J, Gordon DL, Love BB, Gomez F, Heffner M. Ischemic stroke in young adults. Arch Neurol 1995; 52:491–495.
11. Alvarez J, Matias-Guiu J, Sumalia J, Molins M, Insa R, Molto JM, Martin R, Codina

A, Martinez-Vazquez JM. Ischemic stroke in young adults: analysis of the etiological subgroups. Acta Neurol Scand 1989; 80:28–34.
12. Bogousslavsky J, Pierre P. Ischemic stroke in patients under age 45. Neurol Clin 1992; 10(1):113–124.
13. Barinagarrementeria F, Figueroa T, Huebe J, Cantu C. Cerebral infarction in people under 40 years. Cerebrovasc Dis 1996; 6:75–79.
14. Bruno A, Adams HP. Neurological problems in transplant recipients. Neurol Clin 1988; 6(2):305–325.
15. Adams HP, Love BB. Transesophageal echocardiography in the evaluation of young adults with ischemic stroke: promises and concerns. Cerebrovasc Dis 1995; 5:323–327.
16. Adams HP, Butler MJ, Biller J, Toffol GJ. Nonhemorrhagic cerebral infarction in young adults. Arch Neurol 1986; 43:793–796.
17. Besson G, Bogousslavsky J, Hommel M, Stauffer JC, Siche JP. Patent foramen ovale in young stroke patients with mitral valve prolapse. Acta Neurol Scand 1994; 89:23–26.
18. Love BB, Biller J. Stroke in the young: cardiac causes. Stroke Clin Updates 1990; 1:4.
19. Leno C, Berciano J, Combarros O, Sedano C, Alvarez C, Merino J, Quintana F, Martin-Duran R, Rebollo M, Pascual J, Polo JM. Etiologic study of stroke in 95 young adults. Neurologia 1995; 10:283–287.
20. Lisovoski F, Rousseaux P. Cerebral infarction in young people. A study of 148 patients with early cerebral angiography. JNNP 1990; 54:576–579.
21. Petty GW, Brust JCM, Tatemichi TK, Barr ML. Embolic stroke after smoking “crack” cocaine. Stroke 1990; 21:1632–1635.
22. Natowicz M, Kelley RI. Mendelian etiologies of stroke. Ann Neurol 1987; 22:175–192.
23. Topol EJ, Biern RO, Reitz B. Cardiac papillary fibroelastoma and stroke: echocardiographic diagnosis and guide to excision. Am J Med 1988; 80:129–132.
24. Carolei A, Marini C, Ferranti E, Frontoni M, Prencipe M, Fieschi C. A prospective study of cerebral ischemia in the young. Stroke 1993; 24:362–367.
25. Kokkinos J, Levine SR. Neurological complications of drug and alcohol abuse: stroke. Neurol Clin 1993; 11:577–590.
26. Jessurum GA, Nossent JC. CVA at a young age in Rendu-Osler-Weber S.: a survey in the Netherlands Antilles. Nederlands Tidschrift Voor Geneeskunde. 1992; 136:428–431.
27. Zavadenko. Causes of ischemic strokes in young patients. Zhurnal Nevropatologii I Psikhiatrii Imeni S-S-Korsakova 1986; 86:931–937.
28. Chariof EL, Campbell BE, Smith RB III. Paradoxical embolism and acute arterial occlusion: rare or unexpected. J Vasc Surg 1984; 20:372–384
29. Bevan H, Sharma, Bradley DM. Stroke in young adults. Stroke 1990; 21:382–386.
30. Hindfelt B, Nilsson O. Brain infarctions in young adults. Acta Neurol Scand 1977; 55:145–157.
31. Hart RG, Miller VT. Cerebral infarction in young adults: a practical approach. Stroke 1983; 14:110–114.

32. Calabrese LH, Furlan AJ, Gragg LA, Ropos TJ. Primary angiitis of the central nervous system: diagnostic criteria and clinical approach. Cleve Clin J Med 1992; 59:293–306.
33. Warlow C. The young stroke. Br J Hosp Med 1979; 22:252–259.
34. Kitagawa Y, Gotoh F, Koto A, Okayasu H. Stroke in systemic lupus erythematosus. Stroke 1990; 21:1533–1539.
35. Tournier-Lasserve E, Joutel A, Melki J, et al. Cerebral autosomal dominant arteriopathy with subcortical infarcts and leucoencephalopathy maps to chromosome 19q12. Nat Genet 1993; 3:256–259.
36. Lloyd AR Gatenby PA, Lamond TS, Dorsch NWC, Basten A. Moyamoya disease causing recurrent cerebrovascular episodes in a young adult. Med J Aust 1987; 146:379–381.
37. Grewal RP. Stroke in Fabry disease. J Neurol 1994; 241:153–156.
38. Visi JM, Le Coz P, Chadefaux B, Fressinaud C, Woimant F, Marquet J, Zittoun J, Visy J, Vallat JM, Haguenau M. Homocystinuria due to 5,10-methyllenetetrahydrofolate reductase deficiency revealed by stroke in adult siblings. Neurology 1991; 41:1313–1315.
39. Rossner S, Kjellin KG, Mettinger KL, Siden A, Sodestrom CE. Dyslipoproteinemia in patients with ischemic cerebrovascular disease: a study of stroke before 55. Atherosclerosis 1978; 30:199–209.
40. Childs JW. Sickle cell disease: the clinical manifestations. J Am Osteopath Assoc 1995; 95:593–598.
41. Lee MK, Cheng HM, Ng SC, Menaka N, Tan CT, Wang F. Antiphopholipid antibodies and stroke in the young: a study of three cases. Med J Malaysia 1993; 48:3.
42. Barbut D, Boret JS, Wallerson D, Ameisen O, Lockshin M. Anticardiolipin antibody and stroke: possible relation of valvular heart disease and embolic events. Cardiology 1991; 79:99–109.
43. Graham JA, Daly HM, Carson PJ. Antithrombin III deficiency and cerebrovascular accidents in young adults. J Clin Pathol 1992; 45:921–922.
44. Wijdicks EM. Silent brain infarct in the thrombocytopenic purpura. (Letter.) Stroke 1994; 25:1297–1298.
45. Barinagarrementeria F, Cantu-Brito C, De la Pena A, Izaguirre R. Prothrombotic states in young people with idiopathic stroke: a prospective study. Stroke 1994; 25:287–290.
46. Bevan H, Sharma K, Bradley W. Stroke in young adults. Stroke 1990; 21:382–385.
47. Al Hakim M, Katirji B, Osorio I, Weisman R. Cerebral venous thrombosis in paroxysmal nocturnal hemoglobinuria: report of two cases. Neurology 1993; 43:742–746.
48. Mevorach D, Goldberg Y, Gomori JM, Rachmilewitz D. Antiphospholipid syndrome manifested by isquemic stroke in a patient with Crohn's disease. J Clin Gastroenterol 1996; 22:141–143.
49. Mayeux R Fahn S. Strokes and ulcerative colitis. Neurology 1978; 28:571–574.
50. Bashir R, Jinkins J. Clinical infarction in a young stroke following a snake bite. Stroke 1985; 16:328–331.
51. Mulder LJMM, Spierings ELH. Stroke in a young adult with *Mycoplasma*

pneumoniae infection complicated by intravascular coagulation. Neurology 1987; 37:1430–1431.
52. Lou HC, Nielsen JD, Bomholt A, Gormsen J. Platelet hyperaggregability in young patients with completed stroke. Acta Neurol Scand 1977; 56:326–334.
53. De Marini S, Arnett EN. Cerebrovascular occlusion in a transsexual man taking mestranol. Arch Intern Med 1978; 138:1732–1733.
54. Zachariah SB. Stroke after heavy marijuana smoking. Stroke 1991; 22:3.
55. Mani RL, Eisenberg RL, McDonald EF, Pollock JA, Mani JR. Complications of cerebral arteriography: analysis of 5000 procedures. I. Criteria and incidence. AJR 1978; 131:861–865.
56. Bogousslavsky J, Regli F, Van Melle G, Payot M, Uske A. Migraine stroke. Neurol 1988; 38:223–226.
57. Smith PG, Killeen TE. Carotid artery vasospasm complicating extensive skull base surgery: cause prevention and management. Otolaryngology. 1987; 97:1–7.
58. Zapson DS, Riviello JJ, Bagwell S. Supraventricular tachycardia leading to stroke in childhood. J Child Neurol 1995; 10:239–241.
59. Kerr LM, Anderson DM, Thompson JA, Lyver SM, Call GK. Ischemic stroke in the young: evaluation and age comparison of patients six months to thirty nine years. J Child Neurol 1993; 8:266–270.
60. Bogousslavsky J, Regli F. Ischemic stroke in adults younger than 30 years of age: cause and prognosis. Arch Neurol 1987; 44:479–482.
61. Danks RA, Dorevitch M, Cummins JT, Byrne E. Mitochondrial myopathy, encephalopathy, lactic acidosis and stroke-like episodes (M.E.L.A.S.): adolescent onset with severe cerebral edema. Aust NZ J Med 1988; 18:69–72.
62. Lazarov G, Manolov D, Iankov I, Lichkov V. Malignant insulinoma with a cerebral stroke at young age. Vutreshni Bolesti 1979; 18:124–127.
63. Sapira JD. The Art and Science of Bedside Diagnosis. Baltimore: Williams & Williams, 1990.
64. Leira EC, Davis PH, Romont AA, Adams HP. Age and cardiac disease as predictors of the yield of echocardiography in patients with ischemic stroke or transient ischemic attacks. 22d Joint International Conference on Stroke and Cerebral Circulation (poster). American Heart Association, Feb 1997.
65. Bakke SJ, Smith HJ, Kerty E, Dahl A. Cervicocranial artery dissection: detection by Doppler ultrasound and MR angiography. Acta Radiol 1996; 37:529–534.
66. Smoker WRK, Biller J, Hingtgen WL, Adams HP, Toffol GT. Angiography of nonhemorrhagic cerebral infarction in young adults. Stroke 1987; 18:708–711.
67. Adams HP, Brott TG, Furlan AJ, Gomez CR, Grotta J, Helgason CM, Kwiatkowski T, Lyden PD, Marler JR, Torner J. Guidelines for thrombolytic therapy for acute stroke: a supplement to the guidelines for the management of patients with acute ischemic stroke. Stroke 1996; 27:1711–1718.
68. Awad M, Dunn B, Al Halees Z, Mercer E, Akhtar M, Hainau B, Duran C. Intracardiac rhabdomyosarcoma: transesophageal findings and diagnosis. J Am Soc Echocardiog 1992; 5:199–202.
69. Wilmshurst PT, O'Doherty MJ, Nunan TO. Cerebral perfusion deficits in divers with neurological decompression illness. Nucl Med Commun 1993; 14:117–120.

70. Furlan AJ, Brever AC. CNS complications of open heart surgery. Stroke 1984; 15:912–916.
71. Wickremasinghe HR, Peiris JB, Theibadu PN, Sheriffdeen A. Transient emboligenic aortoarteritis: noteworthy new entity in young stroke patients. Arch Neurol 1978; 35:416–422.
72. Mishra UK, Jha S, Kalita J, Sharma K. Stroke, a rare presentation of eales disease: a case report. Angiology 1996; 47:73–76.
73. Comu S, Verstraeten T, Rinkoff JS, Busis NA. Neurological manifestations of acute posterior multifocal placoid pigment epitheliopathy. Stroke 1996; 27:996–1001.
74. Zadra M, Brambilla A, Erli LC, Grandi R, Finazzi G. Neurosarcoidosis, stroke and antiphospholipid antibodies—a case report. Eur J Neurol 1996; 3:146–148.
75. Rangel-Guerra et al. Cysticercosis vasculitis. 12th International Congress of Neurology, Kyoto. Sep 1981.
76. Sancho J, Lopez-Trigo J, Martin R, Romero A, Cervello A. Accidentes cerebrovasculares isquemicos en adultos jovenes: revision de neustra casuistica. In: Yaya, Sancho, and Lainez, eds. Accidentes Cerebrovasculares Isquemicos en Adultos Jovenes. Edictorial MCR S.A., 1987:261–270.
77. Abduljabbar M, Ghozi I, Haq A, Korner H. Sudden stroke-like onset of hemiparesis due to herpetic encephalitis. Can J Neurol Sci 1995; 22:320–321.
78. Liau CT, Yang TS, Wang CH, Hsueh S. Intra-abdominal desmoplastic small cell tumors: report of two cases. Anti-Cancer Drugs 1996; 7:228–232.
79. Hart RH, Easton JD. Dissections of cervical and cerebral arteries. Neurol Clin 1983; 1:155–182.
80. North KN, Whiteman DAH, Pepin MG, Byers PH. Cerebrovascular complications in Ehlers-Danlos syndrome type IV. Ann Neurol 1995; 38:960–964.
81. Elerding SC, Fernandez RN, Grotta J, Lindberg RD, Causay LC, McMurtrey MJ. Carotid artery disease following external cervical irradiation. Ann Surg 1981; 194:609–615.
82. Kessler C, Reuther R, Berlit P, Carls C, Hofmann W. CAT scan and immunohistochemical findings in a case of cerebral thromboangiitis obliterans (Buerger's disease). Eur Neurol 1984; 23:7–11.
83. Yamamura Y, Akamizu H, Hirata T, Kito S, Hamada T. Malignant lymphoma presenting with neoplastic angioendotheliosis of the CNS. Clin Neurophatl 1983; 2:62–68.
84. Martin GJV, Loakes RK, Pelz D, Drake CG, Barnett HJM. Major cerebral arterial and venous disease in osteopetrosis. Stroke 1986; 17:1.
85. Martin NA, Doberstein C, Zane C, Caron MJ, Thomas K, Becker DP. Posttraumatic cerebral arterial spasm: transcranial doppler ultrasound, cerebral blood flow, and angiographic findings. J Neurosurg 1992; 44:575–583.
86. Nagelberg SB, Lowe L, Loriau L, Liu L, Sherin RJ. Cerebrovascular accident associated with testosterone therapy in a 21 years old hypogonadal man. NEJB 1986; 314:1649–650.
87. Shah AR, Passalacqua BR. Case report: sustained-release verapamil overdose causing stroke: an unusual complication. Am J Med Sci 1992; 304:357–359.

88. Pedrini L, Pisano E, Sacca A, Magnoni F, D'Addato M. Carotid endarterectomy in young adults. Int Angiol 1991; 10:220–223.
89. Masai T, Shimazaki Y, Kadoba K, Miyamoto Y, Sawa Y, Matsuda H, Satoh M, Kashiwabara S. Clinical experience with long term use of the Toyobo left ventricular assist system. ASAIO J 1995; 41(3):522–525.
90. Wallis WE, Scott RS, Donaldson I, Wilson J. Hypoglycemia masquerading as cerebrovascular disease. Ann Neurol 1985; 18:510–512.

11

Management of Stroke in the Elderly

Ashfaq Shuaib
University of Alberta Hospital, Edmonton, Alberta, Canada

INTRODUCTION

The risk of stroke increases with age, and the underlying etiology may vary with age. It is important therefore to specifically evaluate the elderly as a separate high-risk group for stroke. This chapter highlights some of the salient features of stroke in the elderly.

Due to an increase in living standards, there has been a progressive increase in life expectancy during the last five decades. In 1985, 12% (or 28.6 million) of the U.S. population was over 65 years old; this is expected to increase to 19.5% (or 58.7 million) by 2025.[1] The fastest-growing segment of the population is people over the age of 80 years. This group included 6.2 million people in the United States in 1985 and is expected to increase to over 14.5 million by 2025. It is believed that after reaching maturity, humans show progressive decline in all physiological processes to an extent that limits the ability to survive.[2] At age 74 to 79 only 40% of women and 16% of men are living independently, and up to 40% of people over the age of 80 years may suffer from cognitive deficits.[3]

As the elderly segment of the population increases, one can expect a rise in debilitating conditions, including cerebrovascular diseases. The incidence of stroke is approximately 30 per 100,000 population before age 44 years. This increases to 1,230 per 100,000 after age 75 years.[4] The increase in stroke is secondary to a combination of factors, including progressive carotid artery stenosis, increasing frequency of cardiac arrhythmias and other cardiac problems, decreased responsiveness to beta stimulation, and abnormal baroreceptor reflexes.[5]

We begin with an overview of the risk factors for stroke in the elderly followed by a discussion on the common underlying etiologies, investigation, and management strategies in this group of patients.

CAROTID ATHEROSCLEROSIS AND AGING

Carotid arteries show progressive narrowing of the lumen with aging. Up to 30% of the population over the age of 70 years may have Doppler evidence of stenosis of the carotid arteries [6]. In addition, autopsy studies have shown that with increasing carotid stenosis, there is progressive increase in associated complications such as ulceration, intraplaque hemorrhage and thrombus formation. With severe stenoses the majority of patients have such complications[7].

Risk Factors

The risk for stroke can be divided into correctable and noncorrectable factors. For the purpose of this chapter only selected correctable risk factors will be discussed in brief.

Numerous studies have shown that hypertension is a risk factor for stroke.[8] The risk of stroke increases with increasing severity of hypertension. The systolic blood pressure increases by an average of 5 to 10 mm Hg and the diastolic by 5 to 6 mm Hg per decade between the ages of 40 and 70. This increase is more severe in blacks and in women. The risk of stroke increases with increasing age in hypertensive individuals.[9] The incidence of isolated systolic hypertension also increases with age (systolic pressure >160 mm Hg and diastolic <90 mm Hg). Isolated systolic hypertension accounts for 70% of hypertension in individuals >65 years.[10] There is a fivefold increase in cardiovascular and cerebrovascular mortality with systolic hypertension.[11,12] Diagnosing hypertension can sometimes be difficult in the elderly. Treatment of "pseudo-hypertension" may sometimes lead to severe hypotension and symptomatic cerebral ischemia.[13]

Management of hypertension decreases cerebrovascular mortality and morbidity.[8] Several large prospective studies have shown that treating asymptomatic hypertensive individuals leads to a decrease in stroke. This decrease is seen in treating both diastolic and systolic hypertension.[14-16] The lowering of blood pressure in the elderly should, however, be a gradual process. Whenever possible it should begin with nonpharmacological methods. Because of altered cerebral autoregulation, the blood pressure should be lowered slowly to a systolic level of no lower than 140 mm Hg and a diastolic of 80 mm Hg.[17] Nocturnal hypotension may be seen in the elderly and lead to an increase risk of stroke.[18] The use of diuretics and angiotensin-converting enzyme blockers or calcium channel blockers is usually effective and presents few side effects. It is important to avoid postural hypotension.

It is becoming apparent that lack of exercise may be an important risk factor for stroke and cardiac disease.[19,20] People who exercise tend to eat well, not be obese, have an elevation in HDL cholesterol, have better control of their blood pressure, and frequently be nonsmokers. The risk of stroke in people who exercise is dependent on the intensity and regularity of exercise.[19] Increasing exercise correlates with a progressive decline in stroke rate. However, with frequent strenuous exercise, there may be an increase in cardiac morbidity, especially in individuals with underlying cardiac disease.[19] Implementation of an exercise program therefore needs to be gradually initiated and medically supervised in the elderly.

Smoking is an important risk factor for stroke and heart disease.[21-23] The risk increases with the duration and number of cigarettes smoked.[21] The risk reduction occurs rapidly with smoking cessation in both the young and the elderly [24]. The risk increases if other risk factors are also present.[25]

The incidence of carotid bruit increases with age.[26] It is a marker of generalized atherosclerosis. The risk of stroke depends on the severity of the carotid stenosis and the rate of progression of disease.[27] Aggressive management of risk factors and the use of antiplatelet agents may slow progression of this disease. The role of carotid endarterectomy in asymptomatic disease is unclear. While there is recent evidence for the support of carotid endarterectomy in asymptomatic stenosis, the benefits from the procedure may be very small in the elderly. At present carotid endarterectomy is rarely indicated in the management of asymptomatic carotid stenosis.[28]

PATHOPHYSIOLOGICAL CHANGES PROMOTING STROKE IN THE ELDERLY

Cardiovascular Changes

Cardiac Muscle

In the absence of heart disease, aging may have no effect on the heart muscle.[29] The aging normal cardiac muscle maintains its ability to develop tension. However, with increasing age, cardiac responses to beta adrenergic stimulation decrease strikingly.[29,30] This is manifest by a reduced inotropic response, arterial vasodilation, and changes in heart rate. In older individuals, noninvasive studies have shown a prolongation of the duration of contraction and a delayed relaxation phase during the cardiac cycle. Although these changes usually do not affect the resting cardiac muscle,[31] they may compromise subendothelial blood flow during tachycardia with resultant serious arrhythmias and ventricular thrombus formation. The increased sympathomimetic stimulation during an acute cerebral infarction can result in tachy- or bradyarrhythmias and other complications in the elderly.[32] The arrhythmias or syncope can lead to cerebral hypoperfusion and may be responsible for the watershed infarctions that are seen with increasing frequency in the elderly.

Arrhythmias

There is a progressive loss of conduction tissue and pacemaker function with aging,[33] predisposing to bundle branch block and atrial and ventricular arrhythmias. These changes can be present without associated ischemic heart disease. Cardiac arrhythmias, especially atrial fibrillation, are a common cause of cardioembolic stroke.[34] Also, elderly stroke patients with atrial fibrillation have been found to have a poor prognosis for recovery.[35,36]

Valvular Heart Dysfunction

Degenerative changes in the aortic valves increases with age, and in the elderly these changes may lead to calcific aortic stenosis.[37] These patients may be at increased risk of bacterial endocarditis or cardioembolism.

Carotid Sinus Hypersensitivity

Massage or compression of the carotid sinus frequently results in slowing of the heart rate and a mild decrease in blood pressure. In the elderly, "carotid hypersensitivity," with marked slowing of the heart rate or hypotension, can lead to syncope.[38] A combination of acute slowing of the heart rate and hypotension, especially after an acute stroke, can exacerbate the neurological deficit.

Baroreceptor Function

The mechanoreceptors in the aortic arch and the carotid sinus are major afferent pathways for control of circulatory dynamics. With an increase in arterial pressure, there is an increased activation of nerve fibers arising from these receptors, which results in a decrease in muscle tone of blood vessels and a slowing of the heart rate. The reverse occurs if the blood pressure suddenly decreases. With aging, the progressive loss of function of such mechanoreceptors results in hemodynamic dysfunction. The mechanism for such lowered sensitivity is not fully understood. Evidence suggests that this decrease may be due to decreased distensibility of the aortic vessel at the site of the baroreceptor.[5,39] Physicians must realize the clinical importance of this decreased receptor sensitivity when blood pressure is lowered in an elderly patient suffering an acute stroke.

Cerebral Autoregulation

Cerebral blood flow decreases gradually with aging. This decrease in blood flow may occur more rapidly in patients at risk for stroke.[40] The decreased blood flow may be secondary to a loss of neurons, or a loss of hemodynamic reserve. A failure of cerebral autoregulation may be a predisposing factor to cerebrovascular ischemic disease, especially for hypertensive patients in whom the blood pressure is reduced rapidly .

Altered Metabolism and Drug Interactions

With increasing age, there are changes in gastric emptying, intestinal absorptive surface, liver size and absorption, and elimination of most drugs.[41] A decrease in plasma albumin, as seen in the elderly, may result in increased activity of "free and unbound" fraction of drugs leading to complications.[42] The anticoagulant effect of warfarin can therefore be more severe in the elderly.

About 10% of all patient admissions to geriatric units are the result of adverse drug reactions.[43] The incidence of drug reactions increases with age. Physicians must become aware of such problems, which develop acutely in elderly patients with cerebrovascular diseases.

STROKE TYPES SEEN WITH INCREASING FREQUENCY IN THE ELDERLY

Stroke with Atrial Fibrillation

The frequency of nonvalvular atrial fibrillation increases with age.[44] In the Framingham study, atrial fibrillation's prevalence increases from 0.2 per 1,000 in individuals 30 to 39 years of age to 19 per 1,000 among those 74 to 84 years of age.[45] The proportion of stroke associated with atrial fibrillation also increases, from 6.7% among people in their sixth decade to 36.2% among those >80 years of age.[45] In most such individuals, the mechanism is cardioembolic. The risk appears to be highest amongst patients with a large left atrium, a history of hypertensive heart disease, previous embolic events , or echocardiographic abnormalities.

Until recently, most patients with nonvalvular atrial fibrillation and no neurological complications were simply observed. Four large studies have clearly shown that the risk of embolism is very high and the patients require anticoagulant or antiplatelet therapy.[44] In the elderly with no risk factors, acetylsalicylic acid (ASA) 325 mg may be adequate.

Stroke with Other Types of Heart Disease

Cardioembolic stroke may account for 15% to 25% of ischemic strokes. The incidence of cardioembolic stroke increases with age. Early recognition of cardiac source is important, as anticoagulant therapy may prevent recurrences.[5]

Hypotension and Watershed Infarction

Watershed infarction occurs between the territories of two main arteries. Although bilateral infarctions frequently develop after severe hypotension, unilateral watershed infarction may also occur in patients with severe ipsilateral carotid disease and hypoperfusion.[46] Such infarctions are common in patients with cardiac dysfunction or postural hypotension. The incidence of severe cardiac disease, hypotension, or an increased hematocrit can be as high as 75% in individuals with watershed infarctions.[46] Management of the underlying cardiac condition or hypotension may prevent recurrences.

Amyloid Disease and Stroke or Cerebral Hemorrhage

Cerebral amyloid angiopathy exists in the absence of systemic amyloidosis. The incidence of cerebral amyloid angiopathy increases with age. It may be seen in >90% of patients with advanced Alzheimer's disease.[47] Such patients may remain asymptomatic or develop recurrent cerebral hemorrhages. Amyloid angiopathy-related cerebral hemorrhage is the commonest cause of spontaneous cerebral hemorrhage in patients over the age of 65.[48] These hemorrhages tend to occur at the junction of gray and white matter and are commonly located in the parietal or occipital lobes. Patients may sometimes present with small infarctions. Unfortunately, treatment at present is symptomatic, and recurrences cannot be prevented.

Cancer-Related Stroke

The incidence of stroke in patients with cancer may be as high as 30%.[49] Following cerebral metastasis, it accounts for the most common neurological findings in patients with cancer. Nonbacterial thrombotic endocarditis and intravascular coagulation are the commonest causes in end-stage "cancer-related stroke." In such patients the presentation of cerebrovascular disease may frequently be a diffuse encephalopathy and therefore often missed. Also, patients are at an increased risk of subdural hematomas. In the elderly, cancer-related stroke should be suspected in patients presenting with progressive encephalopathy, especially when associated with other focal signs.

Multi-infarct Dementia

Patients with repeated strokes may present with progressive cognitive deficits. In many patients progression is "stepwise," and focal signs may also be evident on examination. In the elderly, multi-infarct dementia may account for up 40% of dementias in the community.[50] Early diagnosis, aggressive risk factor management, and the use of antiplatelet drugs may slow progression of the disease.[51]

MANAGEMENT OF ACUTE STROKE IN ELDERLY PATIENTS

Evaluations and Investigation

A detailed examination of the neurological and cardiac system is essential at all ages. It is important to fully document the currently used medications in all patients. Their blood pressure should be checked both lying down and standing to detect any postural hypotension. Patients may be hypertensive acutely after a stroke.[52-54] The temptation to reduce blood pressure should be avoided, as blood pressure will decrease within 4 to 6 days in most patients.[52] Elderly patients often have compromised cognition and may become further disorientated after an acute stroke. Such patients may become severely confused in the "new environment" of the hospital and may require urgent medical attention. Cardiac rhythm abnormalities need careful assessment.

Investigations in all patients (regardless of age) should include a complete blood count, measurement of serum electrolytes, kidney and liver function studies, measurement of serum glucose, a urinalysis, electrocardiography, and chest x-ray. Echocardiography and Holter monitoring may become very useful in patients with a history suggestive of cardiac disease. The increasing use of transesophageal echocardiography may increase detection of cardiac abnormalities.[55]

Neurological investigations should include CT within the initial hours to rule out an intracranial hemorrhage or a subdural hematoma. MRI scan may be more sensitive and may sometimes be helpful in detection of underlying etiology.[56] Carotid Doppler can be used to screen patients for the extent of arterial stenosis. In patients with abnormal Doppler, cerebral angiography is indicated, as carotid endarterectomy may prevent recurrences.[57]

Patients with acute stroke are at an increased risk of aspiration pneumonia. Recent evidence suggests that this may be frequently silent and result in a pneumonia in the days following a stroke.[58] It is our practice to do barium swallow studies in all patients with a large hemispheric infarction.

In large Stroke units, the diagnosis of "acute stroke" may be incorrect in up to 13% of patients.[59] Conditions frequently mistaken for an acute stroke include seizures with Todd's paralysis, brain tumors, and subdural hematomas. Functional paralysis may be especially important to rule out when thrombolytic medications are being considered in patients presenting within 3 hours of the onset of stroke.

Medical and Surgical Management

With the availability of thrombolytic therapy for acute ischemic stroke, all patients who present within 3 hours of the event and have no contraindications to therapy are potential candidates for such medications. Old age should not pose a contraindication for tissue plasminogen activator (tPA). If the patient presents within 3 hours of the event and fulfills all the entry criteria, the therapy should be offered to the patient. (Details on thrombolytic therapy are discussed in Chap. 16).

The patient should be admitted to a specialized acute stroke unit or an acute medical care facility where specially trained nurses can do regular evaluations and detect complications.[60] To decrease the risk of joint contractures and venous thrombosis, occupational and physiotherapy assessments should be done early so that the patient can be mobilized as soon as possible. There is no justification for prolonged bed rest after a stroke.

The blood pressure should not be lowered unless there is clear evidence of end-organ compromise (e.g., hypertensive encephalopathy or congestive heart failure). In two-thirds of stroke patients an elevated blood pressure will return to normal within a week without intervention.[52] In elderly patients, because of compromised cerebral autoregulation and decreased sensitivity of the baroreceptors, a sudden decrease in blood pressure can result in an increase in the cerebral infarction.[61]

Fecal impaction is frequent in patients with acute stroke. The lack of oral intake and decreased mobility contribute to this problem. The routine use of bladder catheters should be discouraged, as they increase the risk of bladder infection. In most male patients condom catheters will solve the problem. Women with urinary incontinence may require diapers.

Because of an increased risk for venous thrombosis, prophylaxis with subcutaneous heparin is recommended. Anticoagulant therapy should only be used in patients with definitive cardiac embolism.[62] In patients with ischemic stroke ASA, 1,300 mg/d will decrease the recurrence by 25% to 35%. Lower doses may not be so effective.[63] Ticlopidine is a new antiplatelet agent that has been shown to be effective in stroke prophylaxis.[64] It is indicated in patients who cannot tolerate ASA or have symptoms while on ASA.

SUMMARY

The evaluation and management of elderly stroke patients need particular attention. Age-related changes in the heart, vasculature, and cerebral autoregulation may be of pathophysiologic significance in the development of stroke in the elderly. Cardioembolism, watershed infarction, and stroke in association with cancer occur more frequently with increasing age. Amyloid angiopathy and related hemorrhage are the most common causes of cerebral hemorrhage. Careful control of hypertension and other risk factors, early and aggressive treatment of TIAs and atrial fibrillation, and prevention of complications after acute stroke will help to decrease the morbidity and mortality rates of strokes in the elderly. With the availability of thrombolytic therapy, patients with acute stroke who present to the hospital within the initial 3 hours should be treated with tPA if there are no contraindications.

BIBLIOGRAPHY

1. Torrey B, Kinsella K, Tacuber CM. Washington, DC:Bureau of Census, 1987.
2. Martin GR, Danner DB, Holbrook NJ. Aging—causes and defenses. Annu Rev Med 1993; 44:419–429.
3. Evans DA, Funkenstein HH, Albert MS. Prevalence of Alzheimer's disease in a community population of older persons. JAMA 1989; 262:2551–2556.
4. Millikan CH, McDowell F, Easton JD. Stroke. Philadelphia: Lea & Febiger, 1987:63.
5. Shuaib A, Hachinski V. Mechanisms and management of elderly stroke patients: a review. CMAJ 1991; 145:433–445.
6. Niederkorn K. Asymptomatic carotid artery disease detected by duplex scanning: incidence and correlation with risk factors, cerebral blood flow and CT findings. Eur Neurol 1990; 30:61–66.
7. Svindard A, Torvic A. Atherosclerotic carotid disease in asymptomatic individuals. Acta Neurol Scand 1988; 78:506–517.
8. Shuaib A. Alteration of blood pressure regulation and cerebrovascular disorders in the elderly. Cerebrovasc Brain Metab Rev 1992; 4:329–345.
9. Psaty BM, Koepsell TD, Monolio TA. Risk ratios and risk differences in estimating the effect of risk factors for cardiovascular disease in the elderly. J Clin Epidemiol 1990; 43:961–970.
10. Winker MA, Murphy MB. Isolated systolic hypertension in the elderly. JAMA 1991; 265:3301–3302.
11. Vokonas PS, Kannel WB, Cupples LA. Epidemiology and risk of hypertension in the elderly. Am J Public Health 1988; 6(suppl 1):s3–s9.
12. Borhani NO. Isolated systolic hypertension in the elderly. J Hypertens 1988; (suppl 4:s15–s19.

13. Spence DJ. Pseudohypertension. In: Laragh JH, Brenner BM, eds. Hypertension: Pathophysiology, Diagnosis and Management. New York: Raven Press, 1990:1407–1414.
14. Potter JF., High RA. Benefits of anti-hypertensive therapy in the elderly. Br Med Bull 1990; 46:77–93.
15. SHEP Cooperative Research Group. Prevention of stroke by antihypertensive drug treatment in older persons with systolic hypertension. JAMA 1991; 265:3255–3264.
16. Dahlof B, Lindholm L, H., Hansson L, Schersten B, Ekbom T, Wester P. Morbidity and mortality in the Swedish Trial in Old Patients with Hypertension (STOP-Hypertension). Lancet 1991; 338:1281–1285.
17. Desforges J, F. How far should blood pressure be lowered? N Engl J Med 1992; 326:251–254.
18. Watanabe N, Imai Y, Nagai K, et al. Nocturnal blood pressure and silent cerebrovascular lesions in elderly Japanese. Stroke 1996; 27:1319–1327.
19. Wannamethee G, Shaper AG. Physical activity and stroke in British middle aged men. Br Med J 1992; 304:597–601.
20. Fletcher GF, Blair SN, Blumenthal J, et al. Statement on exercise. Benefits and recommendations for the physical activity programs for all Americans. Circulation 1992; 86:340–344.
21. Wolf PA, D'Agostino R, Kannel WB, Bonita R, Belanger AJ. Cigarette smoking as a risk factor for stroke: the Framingham study. JAMA 1988; 259:1025–1029.
22. Shinton R, Beevers G. Meta-analysis of relation between cigarette smoking and stroke. BMJ 1989; 298:789–794.
23. Donnan GA, You R, Thrift A, McNeil JJ. Smoking as a risk factor for stroke. Cerebrovasc Dis 1993; 3:129–138.
24. LaCroix AZ, Lang J, Scherr P, et al. Smoking and mortality among older men and women in three communities. N Engl J Med 1991; 324:1619–1625.
25. Manson J,E, Tosteson H, Ridker PM, et al. The primary prevention of myocardial infarction. N Engl J Med 1992; 326:1406–1416.
26. Norris JW, Zhu CZ, Bornstein NM, Chambers BR. Vascular risks of asymptomatic carotid stenosis. Stroke 1991; 22:1485–1490.
27. Chambers BR, Norris JW. Outcome in patients with asymptomatic neck bruits. N Engl J Med 1986; 315:860–865.
28. Hobson RW, Weiss DG, Fields WS, et al. Efficacy of carotid endarterectomy for asymptomatic carotid stenosis. N Engl J Med 1993; 328:221–227.
29. Weisfeldt ML, Leoven WA, Shock NW. Resting and active mechanical properties of cardiac muscles from aged male rats. Am J Physiol 1977; 220:1921–1927.
30. Fleish JH. Further studies of the effect of aging on beta-receptor activity in the rat aorta. Br J Pharmacol 1971; 43:311–314.
31. Harrison T, R., Dixon K, Russell RO, et al. The relation of age to the duration of contraction, ejection, and relaxation of the normal heart. Am Heart J 1964; 67:189–194.
32. Myers MG, Norris JW, Hachinski V, Sole MJ. Plasma norepinephrine in stroke. Stroke 1981; 12:200–204.
33. Lev M. The pathology of complete arterioventricular block. Prog Cardiovasc Dis 1964; 6:317–334.

34. The Boston Area Anticoagulation Trial for Atrial Fibrillation Investigators. The effect of low-dose warfarin on the risk of stroke in patients with nonrheumatic atrial fibrillation. N Engl J Med 1990; 323:1505–1511.
35. Friedman PJ. Atrial fibrillation and stroke in the elderly. Stroke 1991; 22:209–214.
36. Candelise L, Pinardi G, Morabito A, Italian Stroke Study Group. Mortality in acute stroke with atrial fibrillation. Stroke 1991; 22:169–174.
37. Weisfeldt ML, Gerstenbith G. Cardiovascular aging and adaptation to disease. In: Hurst JD, ed. The Heart. New York: Saunders, 1990:1488–1496.
38. Eagle KA, Pruett R. Syncope. In: Eagle KA, Haber E, DeSantis RW, Austen WG. eds. The Practice of Cardiology. Boston: Little Brown and Company, 1989:45–61.
39. Johnson RH, Lambie DG, Spalding JM. Neurocardiology. New York: Saunders. 1984:1.
40. Shaw TG, Mortel KF, Meyers JS, Rojers RL, Hardenberg J, Cutaia M, M. Cerebral blood flow changes in benign aging and cerebrovascular disease. Neurology 1984; 34:855–862.
41. Tregaskis BF, Stevenson I. Pharmacokinetics in old age. Br Med Bull 1990; 46:9–21.
42. Shepherd AM, Hewick DS, Moreland TA, Stevenson, I. Age as determinant of sensitivity to warfarin. Br J Pharmacol 1982; 37:398–403.
43. Williamson J, Chopin JM. Adverse reactions to prescribed drugs in the elderly. Age Aging 1980; 9:73–80.
44. Pritchett EL. Management of atrial fibrillation. N Engl J Med 1992; 326:1264–1270.
45. Wolf PA, Abbot RD, Kannel WB. Atrial fibrillation: A major contributor to stroke in the elderly. Arch Intern Med 1991; 147:1561–1564.
46. Bogousslavsky J, Regli F. Unilateral watershed cerebral infarction. Neurology 1986; 36:373–377.
47. Cosgrove GR, Leblanc R, Meagher-Villemure K, Ethier R. Cerebral amyloid angiopathy. Neurology 1985; 35:625–631.
48. Regli F. Cerebral amyloid angiopathy. In: Vinkin PJ, Bruyn GW, Klawans HL, eds. Handbook of Clinical Neurology. Vol 10(54). Amsterdam: Elsevier Science Publishing, 1989:333–344.
49. Graus F, Rogers LR, Posner JB. Cerebrovascular complications in patients with cancer. Medicine 1985; 64:16–35.
50. Skoog I, Nilsson L, Palmertz B, Andreasson L, Svanborg A. A population-based study of dementia in 85-year-olds. N Engl J Med 1993; 328:153–158.
51. Erkinjuntti T, Hachinski VC. Rethinking vascular dementia. Cerebrovasc Dis 1993; 3:3–23.
52. Wallace JD, Levy LL. Blood pressure after stroke. JAMA 1981; 246:2177–2180.
53. Hertz L, Drejer J, Schousboe A. Energy metabolism in glutaminergic neurons, GABAergic neurons and astrocytes in primary culture. Neurochem Res 1988; 13:605–610.
54. Petito CK, Juurlink HJ, Hertz L. In vitro models differentiating between direct and indirect effects of ischemia on astrocytes. Exp Neurol 1991 Sept; 113(3)364–372
55. Cujec B, Polasek P, Voll CL, Shuaib A. Transesophageal echocardiography in the detection of cardiac source of embolism in stroke patients. Stroke 1991; 22:727–733.

56. Shuaib A, Lee D, Pelz D, Fox A, Hachinski, V. The impact of magnetic resonance imaging on the management of acute ischemic stroke. Neurology 1992; 42:816–818.
57. North American Symptomatic Carotid Endarterectomy Trial Collaborators. Beneficial effects of carotid endarterectomy in symptomatic patients with high-grade stenosis. N Engl J Med 1991; 325:445–453.
58. Horner J, Massey EW, Riski JE, Lathrop DL, Chase KN. Aspiration following stroke: clinical correlates and outcome. Neurology 1988; 38:1359–1362.
59. Norris JW, Hachinski, V. Misdiagnosis of stroke. Lancet 1982; 1:328–331.
60. Langhorne P, Williams BO, Gilchrist W, Howie K. Do stroke units save lives? Lancet 1993; 342:395–398.
61. Dempsey AJ, Combs DJ, Edwards Maley J, Cowen DE, Roy MW. Moderate hypothermia reduces post-ischemic edema development and leukotriene production. Surgery 1987; 21:177–181.
62. Yatsu FM, Hart RG, Mohr JP, Grotta JC. Anticoagulation of embolic strokes of cardiac source: An update. Neurology 1988; 38:314–316.
63. Dyken ML, Barnett H, Easton JD, et al. Low-dose aspirin and stroke: "It ain't necessarily so." Stroke 1992; 23:1395–1399.
64. Gent M, Easton JD, Hachinski V, et al. The Canadian American ticlopidine study (CATS) in thromboembolic stroke. Lancet 1989; 1:1215–1220.

12

Rehabilitation After Stroke

Gregory Scott and David C. Good
Wake Forest University School of Medicine,
Winston-Salem, North Carolina

INTRODUCTION

Prevention is the best strategy to limit the personal and social and consequences of stroke. When prevention fails, an increasing armamentarium of acute interventions is available to reverse the pathophysiologic manifestations of stroke. However, despite improvements in prevention and acute management, neurological impairment from stroke remains a major public health problem. Stroke remains the most common cause of disability among adults. While this has long been the situation in developed countries, improving health care and longer life expectancies in developing countries have made disability due to stroke a major problem in all parts of the world.[1]

In addition to the personal burden of disability born by persons who have suffered a stroke, the social and economic implications of their disease[2] are enormous. Forty-two percent of stroke-related costs are due to direct costs associated with stroke and its medical complications; the remainder is attributable to indirect costs, including such factors as loss of employment and cost of long-term care.

Rehabilitation for stroke therefore remains an important topic. Traditional approaches remain an important strategy to minimize disability and improve quality of life for stroke victims. There is convincing evidence from a number of trials that coordinated stroke care, including rehabilitation, results not only in lower mortality but also in improved functional outcomes in persons with stroke.[3–8]

The final chapter in stroke rehabilitation has not been written. Exciting discoveries have resulted in new insights into the molecular, cellular, and neuronal network reorganizations that occur in the days, weeks, and months following stroke. In addition, advances in the understanding of basic aspects of learning in normal and brain-damaged individuals have occurred. Neuroimaging techniques now permit the sequential evaluation of cerebral blood flow and metabolism following stroke. Data from these and other lines of investigation raise the possibility of rationally designed, new training approaches and pharmacological interventions to enhance functional recovery.

SCOPE OF REHABILITATION

Rehabilitation may be defined as a process through which a person with acquired impairments due to injury or disease obtains the maximum physical, functional, and psychosocial recovery possible within the limits imposed by those impairments. Thus, rehabilitation is a holistic approach concerned not only with minimizing pathophysiological processes, but also with facilitating function within the home and community, and maximizing psychological and social adaptation. Another characteristic of rehabilitation is its focus on the needs of the individual, which may vary widely from person to person. For some stroke patients, the goal may be complete restoration of independence at home, in the community, and at the workplace. For others, the goal may be to return home with modified independence, with the help of family or caretakers. Another hallmark of rehabilitation is its use of the multidisciplinary team approach.[9]

Difference health care professionals bring their expertise to bear on the problems of the individual patient. In theory, the whole is greater than the sum of the parts, with the techniques of each discipline integrating with those of the others for the betterment of the patient. Therefore, traditional rehabilitation is often very labor-intensive and expensive. The modern health care environment may result in limited access to rehabilitation care. There is increasing need to identify patients who benefit most from rehabilitation services, and to determine the intensity of services that will provide the most value to both patients and third-party payers. Outcome measurement has long been an important focus of medical rehabilitation. However, predicting outcome in individual patients is still challenging. Recent novel approaches at predicting functional outcomes following stroke may assist in the task of choosing appropriate rehabilitation candidates, and the specific rehabilitation strategies that will be most successful for individual patients.

There are many types of rehabilitation services, which may be delivered at various sites and at different intensities. The specific approach chosen may be influenced by many factors, including the interval since stroke, the severity of stroke-related impairments, and the presence of preexistent or concurrent medical conditions. Nonmedical factors including the availability of family or care givers, age, and the source of financial payment all influence the scope of rehabilitation services provided. About three-fourths of stroke survivors in the United States receive some form of rehabilitation care.[10]

Rehabilitation should begin as soon as the patient has been medically stabilized following stroke. Serious physical and functional consequences can be avoided by early interventions. These interventions include passive range of motion to prevent contractures, active range of motion against minimal resistance to prevent disuse atrophy, frequent turning and careful repositioning to prevent pressure ulcers, feeding and aspiration precautions to prevent pneumonia, and prophylaxis for deep venous thrombosis. As their condition stabilizes, the patients begin to take a more active role in participating in the recovery process. Active mobilization is critical to minimize the many medical consequences of immobility. With continued medical improvement and increased endurance, a tailored rehabilitation plan is formulated, based on the patient's individual rehabilitation goals. While early rehabilitation efforts usually occur at bedside, mobilization permits transportation to specialized rehabilitation evaluation and treatment areas. A decision must then be made regarding the appropriate site for additional rehabilitation. Is the patient a candidate for an intensive, multidisciplinary, hospital-based rehabilitation program? Or, would a home-based or outpatient clinic approach be more appropriate? If the patient exhibits poor endurance, slow recovery is anticipated, or if there is limited care giver support, rehabilitation in a skilled nursing facility may be needed. As time passes, the patient's status should be reassessed at intervals, and the rehabilitation program changed to accommodate changes in the patient's condition. Eventually, a decision will be made regarding discontinuation of professional therapy services, although patient- or family-directed exercise programs and environmental adaptations may need to continue indefinitely. Decisions regarding discontinuing therapy services are based on knowledge of natural recovery of stroke, the patient's progress, concurrent medical conditions, patient motivation, availability of social support systems, and the influence of third-party payers.

In summary, rehabilitation for stroke begins early after the stroke and continues for a variable period of time which may range from days to months depending on individual patient goals and resources. Strategies may be simple or complex, and services may be provided at a number of different locations.

Traditional rehabilitation programs seek to improve adaptation in the following areas: mobility; activities of daily living (ADLs); instrumental (community) living skills; language and cognition; vocational skills; avocational (leisure) activities; and psychosocial adjustment.

EARLY REHABILITATION FOLLOWING STROKE

Patients should be mobilized as soon as they are medically stable. Patients with reasonable alertness, stable vital signs, and adequate oxygenation can usually be out of bed with assistance by 48 hours. Immobility results in a variety of preventable problems. One of the most devastating functional consequences of immobility is disuse weakness and muscle atrophy. Disuse weakness compounds weakness caused by hemiparesis, and results in a slower rate of recovery and a longer period of rehabilitation. With complete inactivity, a muscle loses 10% to 15% of strength and bulk per week.[11] A patient immobilized for 3 to 5 weeks loses one-half of his or her muscle strength.[12] While muscle atrophy and weakness during immobilization occur at all ages, the effects are more pronounced in the elderly.[13] For an elderly person already at threshold strength for climbing stairs and getting out of bed, even a 10% of loss of strength may make the difference between dependence and independence. Disuse atrophy is prevented by short periods of daily muscle contraction of only 20% to 30% of maximal tension.[14] One disuse atrophy and weakness occur, a graduated exercise program is indicated to restore strength and bulk. The strengthening process is much slower than the loss that occurs during inactivity, usually taking about twice as long.[15] For elderly persons the recovery process is even slower,[13] but muscle strength and bulk can increase during an exercise program even in the very old.[15,16] The importance of early mobilization and avoidance of prolonged bed rest cannot be overstressed. In situations where bed rest is unavoidable, such as lengthy stays in an intensive care unit, an active range of motion program twice daily should be prescribed for all cooperative patients.

Another important complication of stroke is contracture, which is defined as lack of full active or passive range of motion due to joint, muscle, or soft-tissue limitations.[12] The most common cause is joint immobilization, which can be prevented by proper positioning in a bed or chair, and an active or passive range of motion program. Three to five full range-of-motion movements of each joint twice daily is adequate, except in patients with significant spasticity. In these cases, proper positioning is even more important, and splints may need to be applied. Nursing staff and family can be instructed in the proper techniques. The position of the paretic limb should be changed every few hours.

Contractures can result in major functional disability. Upper-extremity dressing is difficult for a person with a shoulder or elbow contracture. Hygiene of the hand may be a problem for a person with flexion contractures of the fingers. A patient with a knee flexion contracture has a biomechanical disadvantage during ambulation, with shortened stride length and compensatory hip flexion. An ankle plantar flexion contracture prevents adequate heel strike, resulting in abnormal "push-off" when walking, and impedes toe clearance during the swing phase of gait. Hip and knee contractures impair transfers. Contractures also cause weight to be distributed over bony prominences, increasing the risk of pressure ulcers.

Once contractures are established, treatment is often prolonged and painful. Terminal stretching of 30 minutes or more at least twice a day combined with vigorous active and passive range-of-motion programs is necessary. Serial casting is sometimes attempted in difficult cases.[17–19] The cast is applied after prolonged stretching. It is removed after several days, the stretching is repeated, and a new cast is applied. The process is repeated until the contracture is reduced, which may take weeks. Dynamic splints are also available for treating both upper- and lower-extremity contractures. These may be individually prefabricated and also are commercially available.[17] As a last resort, contractures may be treated surgically using a variety of techniques.[20,21]

Finally, a number of other medical conditions can result from immobility.[22,23] These include pneumonia, pressure ulcers, and DVT and will be discussed shortly.

In summary, early passive range of motion, positioning, and mobilization are critical but often overlooked features of an early rehabilitation program for stroke patients.

MEDICAL COMPLICATIONS AND OTHER SPECIAL PROBLEMS

There are several well-recognized early medical complications after stroke. The most common and those with the greatest risks of morbidity and mortality include venous thromboembolism, dysphagia and aspiration pneumonia, pressure ulcers, spasticity, bowel dysfunction, and bladder dysfunction.

Venous Thromboembolism

Epidemiology

Venous thromboembolism consists of two associated conditions. These are deep venous thrombosis (DVT) and pulmonary embolus (PE). There is a reported 59% to 73% incidence of DVT within 10 days poststroke.[24–29] While much more prevalent in the paralyzed leg alone (50%), DVT is also found in the nonparalyzed leg (7%) and bilaterally (43%). Many cases are clinically unsuspected. Pulmonary embolism is the most feared complication of DVT, and occurs in 16% to 37% of stroke patients.[30–32] Approximately 2.5% of pulmonary emboli are fatal. Sudden and unexpected death on a rehabilitation service is often due to PE.

Risk Factors

A large number of risk factors predispose to DVT formation (Table 1). In a review of 1231 patients with recognized DVT, 96% had one or more of these risk factors.[31] Prior thromboembolism carries with a risk of recurrence of 10% after the first episode and 20% after more than one episode. Another way of stating

Table 1 Risk Factors Predisposing to DVT Formation

Prior thromboembolism
Age >40 years
Paralytic stroke
Hypercoagulable state
Prolonged immobility
Obesity
Myocardial infarction
Congestive heart failure
Major surgery
Fracture of hip or leg
Varicose veins
Malignancy
Estrogens
Parturition

this is that the patient with a history of DVT is eight times more likely to develop a DVT than a similar patient without a prior history of DVT. Age >40 has been described as a risk factor, but the relationship between age and DVT is not linear. The risk after age 40 doubles with each decade, and increases by a factor of 200 between age 20 and 80.

Diagnosis

Distal thrombi in the calf are often thought to be the most frequent site of inception, but proximal thrombi are actually the most frequent source of PE. Less than a third of DVTs present with the classic syndrome of calf pain, swelling, venous distension, and a Homan's sign.[33,34] Over half with these complaints have an alternate explanation. The differential diagnosis includes musculoskeletal trauma, cellulitis, impaired venous flow, impaired lymphatic flow, heterotopic ossification, acute arthritis, and inflammatory popliteal cysts. Pulmonary embolus has a classic presentation of tachycardia (HR>90), hypoxemia (PO_2<80), dyspnea, chest pain, and rales. In the rehabilitation setting the symptoms have been stated to be different and include back pain, unusual facial skin color, anxiety, and fevers (101°F).[35] The traditional test for DVT is venography,[33,34] which can detect both proximal and distal thrombi. The major disadvantages of venography are invasiveness, cost, and difficulty in serial examinations. However, because of its high sensitivity and specificity it remains the gold standard by which other diagnostic procedures are judged.

Impedance plethysmography is performed by measuring the electrical impedance between two electrodes attached to the calf. Proximal DVTs are detected by the decreased impedance secondary to the presence of an electrical conductor, in this case blood. The sensitivity ranges from 22% for asymptomatic DVTs to 92% for symptomatic DVTs. The specificity is 95% to 98%. The major limitations are insensitivity to calf and nonocclusive proximal thrombi.[34]

Ultrasonography is more sensitive, with 59% sensitivity for asymptomatic DVTs and 97% for symptomatic DVTs. Specificity is 97% to 98%. The major limiting factor is the skill of the operator.

Magnetic resonance venography, while stated to have a high sensitivity (96%) and specificity (>99%), is expensive and has a limited availability.[34]

In patients with normal ultrasound studies, anticoagulant therapy can be withheld unless the clinical index of suspicion is high. Conversely, abnormal studies justify treatment. Screening of asymptomatic patients is not warranted.[33] If DVT remains suspected despite initially normal studies, then the studies should be repeated.

The standard for diagnosis of pulmonary embolism remains ventilation/perfusion scanning; chest x-ray is often negative. If clinical suspicion is high and the ventilation/perfusion scan is negative, pulmonary angiography is recommended.

Prevention

Of those who die from PE, two-thirds survive <30 minutes after the event. Therefore the emphasis should be on prevention of DVT, which may be accomplished by either physical or pharmacologic methods.[31,36] Pharmacologic methods include a variety of heparin and heparinoid products, warfarin, dextran, and antiplatelet agents. Physical methods are as varied as elastic compression hose, intermittent pneumatic compression, and vena cava interruption. Low-dose heparin (LDH) has been available since the 1930s and has been recommended prophylaxis since 1986 in stroke patients in whom hemorrhage has been excluded. It has been proven to reduce both DVT and PE (both fatal and nonfatal). It is typically given as 5,000 units subcutaneously twice or three times daily. For patients with a stroke it is recommended that it be given three times a day.[33] Hemorrhagic side effects are uncommon as long as there is no systemic bleeding diathesis.[37]

Low-molecular-weight heparin is obtained by either the chemical or enzymatic degradation of heparin. It is available in many commercial preparations. In comparison to unfractionated heparin, it shows greater availability, a longer and more predictable plasma half-life, and reduced platelet-associated side effects.[36] It is typically administered once to twice a day. It is as effective as unfractionated heparin,[38] but is more expensive. There have been claims of fewer bleeding complications in comparison to unfractionated heparin.

Fixed low-dose warfarin has been tested prophylactically in patients with a high risk for DVTs. These studies found that a dose of 1 mg daily was ineffective.[39–42] although it is effective in the prevention of subclavian vein thrombosis in cancer patients with indwelling subclavian catheters.[43]

Aspirin use has a small benefit when compared to other agents. Its use as the sole mode at DVT prophylaxis can not be recommended.[44]

Dextran is a glucose polymer that has been used as a prophylactic agent. In addition to decreased fibrin polymerization, it decreases plasma viscosity and platelet function. It was originally introduced as a blood volume expander. The major drawbacks to its use are that it is an intravenous preparation, is expensive, precipitates rare but serious allergic reactions, and can be renal toxic.[31]

Physical means of prevention are recommended for those with contraindications to anticoagulation. These are typically thought to be less effective. Improper application of pneumatic compression devices may be the reason for failure of this form of prophylaxis and is described in 22% of patients in intensive care units and 52% of patients on general wards.[45] Elastic compression hose are thought to be less effective than properly applied pneumatic compression hose.

Treatment

Therapy for known DVT should begin with heparin at an adequate dose to achieve anticoagulation.[46] Failure to reach the prescribed intensity in 24 hours increases the risk of embolism by 15 times.[46] Heparin therapy followed by warfarin is regarded as conventional therapy. Asymptomatic extension of thrombosis in 8%[47] and symptomatic PE in 0.5% of patients being treated with heparin is expected.[48]

Use of warfarin without use of heparin is not recommended as the risk of either symptomatic extension or recurrence is 20%.[47] It has recently been reported that there are fewer complications and nearly as rapid a response when beginning therapy with 5 mg warfarin as opposed to 10 mg/day.[49] Warfarin is given in doses to prolong the prothrombin time to International Normalized Ratio (INR) of 2.0 to 3.0. With an INR of >3.0, there is an increasing rate of bleeding complications.[33] Recommendations vary from 3 to 6 months of anticoagulation after a first episode of DVT.

When a DVT already exists, adjusted-dose heparin is often used. The dose is adjusted to obtain a high normal partial thromboplasmin time (PTT). While effective, it does require laboratory monitoring of PTTs, platelets, and dosage adjustments. As with any heparin product, instances of thrombocytopenia have been reported.

It is possible to restore venous patency by surgical thrombectomy. There is significant reocclusion and this procedure probably should be reserved for patients in whom the occlusion is limb threatening.[50]

The use of thrombolytics is more effective in the restoration of early patency of the vein.[51,52] It does not, however, provide more protection against PE than anticoagulation.[53] There is a two to four times greater risk of intracranial bleeding associated with thrombolysis.[51,52] For those with contraindications to anticoagulation, vena cava filter placement is a viable option. The risk of pulmonary embolism after placement of a filter is 2% to 3%. Complications include filter migration (3% to 69%), insertion complications (2% to 28%), IVC penetration (9% to 24%), vena cava obstruction (6% to 30%), and venous insufficiency (5% to 59%).[54]

Dysphagia and Aspiration

The prevalence of dysphagia ranges from 25% to 32% in patients with stroke. In patients with dysphagia following stroke, the frequency of aspiration ranges from 51% to 73%[55] and is clinically silent in 42% to 52%[56,57] Intermittent or persistent aspiration may cause cough, intermittent fever, tracheobronchitis, atelectasis, pneumonia, and empyema. Some studies have found little difference in the nature of the swallowing disorder according to stroke location,[58] but this is not universally accepted.[59] Aspiration occurs in patients with unilateral and bilateral, hemispheric stroke and brainstem stroke.[59–61] It is, however, twice as common in those with bilateral signs (66%).[61]

Diagnosis

Clinical evaluation is of limited use in distinguishing between groups of patients who aspirate and those who don't aspirate. Abnormal sputum, noncardiac chest pain, fever, and wet dysphonia are more prevalent in aspirators, but are not exclusive to that group.[61] A poor gag response is also of limited value[61] and has not been a universal finding.[62] Single chest roentogram is not able to clearly differentiate between the groups.[61] The gold standard for evaluation of aspiration is the videofluoroscopic modified barium swallow (MBS). It is not practical to perform as a screening exam due to expense, need for radiological support, and radiation exposure. Screening examinations have been devised that will identify >90% of patients with dysphagia and aspiration. The Burke Dysphagia Screening Test takes into account seven different factors, which are noted to be either present or absent[63]: (1) bilateral stroke; (2) brainstem stroke; (3) history of pneumonia during acute stroke phase; (4) coughing associated with feeding or during a 3-oz water swallow test; (5) failure to consume one-half of meals; (6) prolonged time required of feeding; and (7) nonoral feeding program in progress. The presence of any feature constitutes failure. After failure of the screen the patient should be referred for MBS.

Distinct categories of pneumonia associated with aspiration in rehabilitation patients are chemical pneumonitis from gastric secretions, and infections due to oropharyngeal bacteria. The most common lung segments involved in pneumonia secondary to aspiration are the posterior segments of the upper lobes and the superior segments of the lower lobes.[64] Gastric acid and enzymes are the primary agents causing pneumonia after aspiration of gastric contents.[65] In pneumonia due to oropharyngeal bacteria, anaerobes constitute 90% of the infectious agents.[66] The syndromes have somewhat different presentations. Acute dyspnea, hypoxemia, and lower-lobe infiltrates predominate with chemical pneumonia. Cough, purulent sputum, fever, and infiltrates in dependent segments are typically found with pneumonia due to oropharyngeal bacteria. Infectious pneumonia is more likely to have an indolent course.[67]

Treatment

Initial severity of the dysphagia and patient age are not predictive of improvement. The anatomic location of stroke is predictive. Improvement of dysphagia in one study was stated to occur in 65% of patients with cortical stroke, 31% with subcortical stroke, 20% with brainstem stroke, and 12.5% with multiple strokes.[68] Since a certain percentage will not improve, compensatory methods must be taught. Patients are instructed to sit upright during feeding to capitalize on the effects of gravity, and to turn their head toward the weak side while tilting toward the strong side.[69,70] This increases the anterior-posterior opening diameter resulting in a greater percentage of the food bolus being swallowed.[69,70] As widening of the vallecular space slows entry of material into the pharynx, they are also instructed to tuck their chin.[71] Postural changes have been shown to be of benefit in 77% of patients.[72,73] Not all patients have the same abnormalities of swallowing. Certain classes of patients are instructed to use one postural change in preference to another. The benefit of head rotation has been reported in studies of patients with medullary infarcts that resulted in unilateral pharyngeal paresis.[69,70] The chin tuck technique has been found to work in most patients with delayed pharyngeal triggering of swallowing demonstrated by videofluoroscopy.[74] Thermal stimulation of swallowing has been studied but has not shown long-term benefit.[75] A technique for improving a weak swallow is the Mendelsohn maneuver, a volitional prolongation of laryngeal elevation during midswallow.[76] In addition to postural changes, dietary modifications are often recommended. These modifications include thickened liquids and soft homogenous solids. Pureed foods are the easiest to swallow.[72,73] Thin liquids and dry solids are reported to be the most difficult to manage.[77,78] Exercise programs for swallowing rehabilitation are available. Many of these emphasize oral exercise to improve tongue and lip function or vocal cord adduction. The effectiveness is unknown.[76]

Treatment of pneumonia is based on general medical principles. These include appropriate antibiotics for probable agents, pulmonary toilet to aid in clearance of secretions, and, if possible, prevention of future episodes.

Pressure Ulcers

Pressure ulcers have been defined as areas of unrelieved pressure over a localized area, usually a bony prominence, resulting in ischemia, cell death, and tissue necrosis.[79] The differential diagnosis includes stasis or ischemic ulcers, vasculitis, cancer, radiation injury, and other dermatologic conditions. Lesions due to such disorders require specific interventions and should be distinguished from pressure ulcers.[80] Estimates of pressure ulcer prevalence in hospitalized patients ranges from 3% to 14%.[79,81,82] The incidence in another study was 12.9% after a median time of 9 days from admission[83]. The in-hospital mortality rate for those with pressure ulcers is between 23% and 37%.[84,85] Pressure ulcers are given a grade or stage based on several characteristics (Table 2). These include erythema and depth of ulceration.[82,86,87]

Risk Factors and Etiology

Several different risk factors have been described for the development of pressure ulcers. The most important of these is immobility.[88] Fecal incontinence, diarrhea, fractures, urinary catheter use, decreased weight, dementia, and hypoalbuminemia are also associated with the development of pressure ulcers.[82,86,87] Some of these factors are not clearly causative, but represent markers of underlying disability and nutritional state. Changes in aging skin may also contribute to skin breakdown. These include loss of elastic fibers, thinning of the epidermis, loss of dermal vessels, and flattening of the dermal-epidermal interface.[89]

Four primary mechanical factors have been identified in the production of pressure ulcers: pressure, shearing forces, friction, and moisture.[82,87] Degeneration of muscle fibers begins after 1 or 2 hours of exposure with pressures of 60

Table 2 National Pressure Ulcer Advisory Panel Classification of Pressure Ulcers

Stage	Description
Stage I	Nonblanchable erythema of intact skin.
Stage II	Partial-thickness skin loss involving epidermis and/or dermis. The ulcer is superficial and presents clinically as an abrasion, blister, or shallow crater.
Stage III	Full-thickness skin loss involving necrosis of subcutaneous tissue which may extend down to, but not through, underlying fascia. The ulcer presents clinically as a deep crater with or without undermining of adjacent tissue.
Stage IV	Full-thickness skin loss with extensive destruction, tissue necrosis, or damage to muscle, bone, or supporting structures (e.g., tendon, joint capsule, etc.)

to 70 mm Hg.[90] The areas of greatest risk are over bony prominences. In one study of 1604 pressure ulcers in 649 patients, the ischial tuberosity had the highest occurrence rate (28%), followed by the trochanter (19%), sacrum (17%), heel (9%), malleolus and pretibial region (5% each), and patella (4%). Other sites accounted for 13%.[91] Pressure under these prominences may be as high as 100 to 150 mm Hg on a typical mattress. This pressure is sufficient to cause injury with prolonged exposure due to decreased transcutaneous oxygen tension.[92,93] The time necessary for pressure to cause injury is decreased by any of the other causative factors. It has been stated that friction and moisture are the most important factors in the development of superficial skin breakdown, whereas injury due to pressure and shearing typically begins in the deeper tissues.[94]

Prevention

As damage can occur after as little time as 1 or 2 hours of exposure to pressure, prevention is clearly important. This has led to the recommendation of patient repositioning at least every 2 hours in those at highest risk.[80,90,95] This will not prevent all cases of ulceration, and more frequent repositioning may be needed. Sheepskin or "egg crate" mattresses are not sufficient by themselves to prevent ulceration. The use of foam padding, wheelchair cushions, and preventive repositioning may decrease the incidence of ulceration.[96,97]

Treatment

Clinical staging should guide the management of pressure ulcers. Stage I or II ulcers will generally heal in days to weeks if causative factors are removed and treatment is initiated. Stage III or IV ulcers may take weeks to months to heal and may not do so completely without surgical intervention.

Local wound care is aimed at debridement of necrotic tissue which results in lower bacterial counts. This can typically be accomplished by the use of wet to dry dressings two to three times per day or sharp surgical debridement in cases with considerable overlying escar. Recently, vacuum-assisted closure of chronic and difficult wounds was reported to be efficacious. This technique entails placing an open cell foam dressing into the wound cavity and applying a controlled subatmospheric pressure of 125 mm Hg below ambient pressure.[98,99] This technique is not widely available at present. Antiseptics are available which decrease the bacterial count but are also cytotoxic. Among these are povidone-iodine, acetic acid, hydrogen peroxide, and Dakin's solution (sodium hypochlorite).[94] Enzymatic agents are useful in debridement but may also damage healthy granulation tissue. Once the ulcer is clean, a moist environment facilitates healing. Surgical procedures include myocutaneous flaps, split-thickness skin grafts, and primary closure. A surgical consultation should be considered if the patient's condition and stage of ulceration are thought to warrant possible intervention. Specialized beds are an expensive treatment but in one study demonstrated a fivefold increase in the odds of improvement.[85] Either air-fluidized or low-air-loss beds may be used. Low-air-loss cushions may be fitted on a frame similar to a standard hospital bed. This enables bed positioning and transfer of patients to be more easily accomplished. Nutritional status of the patient is important. Protein intake at baseline is a good predictor of improvement in pressure ulcers.[85] Ascorbic acid supplementation (500 mg twice daily) has demonstrated a significant positive effect. In one study the reduction of ulcer size was 84% in the treatment group compared to 43% in the placebo group.[100] Zinc has been shown to be of benefit in wound healing.[101,102]

Bacterial colonization of pressure ulcers is not uncommon. Systemic antibiotics are indicated only when there is evidence of cellulitis, sepsis, or osteomyelitis. Topical antibiotics are not cytotoxic and may have a role during the time that the wound is being debrided.

Spasticity

Spasticity has been defined as a motor disorder characterized by a velocity-dependent increase in tonic stretch reflexes (muscle tone) with exaggerated tendon jerks.[103] It is caused by lesions in the cerebrum, brainstem, or spinal cord. It is thought to result at least in part from abnormal intraspinal processing of primary afferent input in combination with hyperexcitability of the Ia pathway to motor neurons. This processing abnormality is due to damage to descending suprasegmental control of interneuronal systems in the spinal cord.[104] With each patient, the degree of spasticity varies. This variation can be due to fatigue, changes in temperature, pain, noxious stimuli, and time of day. Any sudden increase in spasticity should alert the clinician to search for possible provoking factors. These include urinary tract infection, fecal impaction, pressure ulcer, and improper positioning.

Treatment

Therapy should not automatically be instituted. Spasticity may be useful, as in the hemiplegic whose extended leg may act as a crutch or brace. The relief of spasticity, however, may reduce pain and facilitate care and hygiene.

Physical treatments are considered first. Regular range of motion and stretching exercises decrease tone and the incidence of contractures. The reason for the reduction in tone is not clear. The effect lasts several hours. Other physical treatments are topical application of cold and topical anesthesia. Casting and splinting are valuable in extending joint range due to hypertonicity.[105]

Baclofen, diazepam, and dantrolene are the major pharmacologic agents for the treatment of spasticity[106]. Alternative medications include clonidine and tizanidine.[107,108] Baclofen acts as a agonist at GABA B receptors, leading to an inhibition of release of excitatory amino acid neurotransmitters. There is typically complete absorption after oral administration. Excretion is by the renal route. The half-life is approximately 3.5 hours. Seizures are considered a contraindication. Hallucinations as well as seizures may occur with abrupt withdrawal after long-term administration.[109] Side effects include hallucinations, confusion, sedation, hypotonia, and ataxia.[110] Dosage begins at 5 mg twice or three times daily by mouth. The maximal dosage range is 80 to 120 mg in four divided doses.[111] Intrathecal administration by implanted pump may be useful, especially in persons with spinal cord disorders.

Diazepam acts by modulating GABA transmission at the GABA A receptor. This results in presynaptic inhibition of excitatory neurons.[112] It is generally well tolerated except for its sedative effects. The half-life is 27 to 37 hours. It is less than optimal in treatment of spasticity of cerebral origin due to its effects on attention and memory.[113] Physiologic dependence may occur and withdrawal symptoms may appear with discontinuance. Dosage begins at 2 mg by mouth twice daily, and may be increased to 60 mg/day in divided doses.[111]

Dantrolene acts directly on muscle tissue by decreasing the release of calcium into the sarcoplasmic reticulum thereby decreasing the force of excitation-contraction coupling. It has little effect on smooth and cardiac muscle tissues. It is metabolized in the liver with a half-life of 8.7 hours.[114] It is less likely to cause cognitive changes than baclofen or diazepam and may be the preferred drug for spasticity due to cerebral causes.[115] Hepatotoxitiy may occur in approximately 1% of patients, with fatal hepatitis being reported in 0.1% to 0.2% of patients treated for >60 days.[116] It also may cause malaise, nausea and vomiting, dizziness, sedation, and diarrhea. Dosage begins at 25 mg/day increasing up to 400 mg/day.[114]

Tizanidine acts at the α2-adrenergic receptor. Its activity results in the impairment of excitatory amino acid release from spinal interneurons and concomitant inhibition of coeruleospinal pathways.[117] It principally affects polysynaptic reflexes. It may increase muscle strength, in contrast to the other medications mentioned. It has been shown to be equivalent to both baclofen and diazepam in reduction of spasticity. Treatment should begin with a low dose and be gradually titrated upward. The average dose is 12 to 24 mg/day, but it may be used up to 36 mg/day in divided doses. Common side effects include mild hypotension, sleepiness, and dry mouth.[118,119] Clonidine is also an α2-adrenergic receptor agonist. It presumably acts in a similar fashion as tizanidine. It has been shown to be effective in reduction of spasms and spasticity.[120] It may have cognitive side effects, and occasionally causes hypotension, sleepiness, and dry mouth.[111] In animal models clonidine delays recovery from stroke.

Injections of various solutions have been used to treat increased tone. Phenol injection at the motor end plate produces a chemical neurolysis.[121,122] Its effects may last up to 6 months. The problems associated with phenol are a 10% incidence of dysesthesias and causalgia in addition to possible protein coagulation and necrosis at the site of injection.[123] Intramuscular botulinum toxin injection is supplanting phenol block. The effects typically last 3 to 6 months. With either of these treatments, only selected muscles should be injected in order to lessen the cumulative dose.

Surgical options include both orthopedic and neurosurgical procedures. Tendon lengthening, tendon transfer, and selected join fusion may be useful.[124] The complexity of movement limits usefulness in the upper extremities.[125] Lower-extremity tendon transfer is the most successful orthopedic procedure in hemiplegia. The operation is usually a combination of anterior tibial transfer (to reduce supination) and Achilles tendon lengthening.[126] Neurosurgical techniques have included myelotomy and rhizotomy. The success of both of these techniques is hampered by recurrent spasticity.[124]

Peripheral neurectomy abolishes tone at the expense of any residual function and sensation.[127] Selective neurectomy has been performed preserving some voluntary muscle activity and sensation.[128]

Bladder Dysfunction

The results of a stroke on the genitourinary system can be devastating.[129] After stroke voluntary voiding is often impaired.[130] When seen in the elderly with preexisting voiding dysfunction (stress incontinence in females and prostatism in males), the resulting problem is challenging to diagnose and treat. Urinary incontinence has been shown to be the single best initial predictor of eventual disability (sensitivity of 60% and specificity of 78%)[131]. It has also been shown to be a prognosticator for poor survival, with half of the incontinent patients dying with 6 months of their stroke.[132]

Presentation

The effect of stroke on micturition depends on the degree, size, and location of the lesion. After a stroke, a period of initial detrusor areflexia or urinary retention occurs. The reasons for this are unclear,[133,134] but may be due to direct neurologic consequences, restricted mobility, or temporary detrusor failure due to overdistension.[135] In addition to these factors, prior urologic conditions and medications may play a role.[136] As time passes, bladder dysfunction develops into complaints of frequency, urgency, and urge incontinence. The symptoms are usually the result of detrusor hyperreflexia.[137,138]

The reported incidence of poststroke incontinence is between 57% and 83%.[139,140] In one study, the initial incontinence rate was 60%, falling to 29%

by 12 weeks.[135] In another study, incontinence had resolved in 80% of patients by 6 months.[141]

Supraspinal influences on the urinary tract are only partially understood. Input to the pontine micturition center is derived from the cerebral cortex, basal ganglia, cerebellum, and spinal cord.[142] The frontal cortex is the area involved in voluntary control of the external sphincter and bladder detrusor muscle in humans.[142,143] Lesions in frontal areas are characterized by a hyperactive detrusor reflex. Lesions in the basal ganglia or thalamus result in involuntary bladder contractions. In animal studies, the cerebellum plays an inhibitory role in the bladder-filling phase and a facilitatory role in the voiding phase.[144] Similar effects are postulated in humans, but remain unproven. No effect of hemispheric dominance has been seen.[145,146]

Evaluation

The approach to the patient who has suffered a stroke must be a multidisciplinary one with attention to all aspects of care including micturition.[147] Evaluation begins with a premorbid voiding history. This should include information regarding preexisting medical conditions and medications. Reversible causes of urinary retention, frequency, urgency, or urge incontinence, such as fecal impaction or urinary tract infection, need to be corrected if they are identified. Thorough physical examination of the genitourinary systems of both men and women should be performed. If available, bedside bladder ultrasound should be used to identify patients with large postvoid residual urine. Alternatively, a postvoid catherization should be performed. Given that a large number of patients will spontaneously improve, urodynamic testing is not indicated as a screening tool. It patients fail to improve, then a urodynamic evaluation including uroflow study, postvoid residual, filling and voiding cystometrogram, abdominal pressure measurement, and assessment of leak point pressure should be performed.[129,148] Treatment is based on these findings. Follow-up studies are recommended at 4 weeks, 3 months, and 1 year to evaluate change in urologic status.

Management

Diagnosis of the cause and management of voiding dysfunction before the patient leaves the acute care facility is desirable as urinary dysfunction may complicate rehabilitation.[146] In the immediate poststroke period, when retention is the primary symptom, intermittent catherization is appropriate.[149] While <50 mL of residual is normal, postvoid residuals of 100 mL are probably acceptable in deciding to terminate catheterization. In men with preexisting bladder outlet obstruction, transurethral resection of the prostate should be delayed for 6 months to 1 year after the stroke. In one study 50% of those who had suffered a stroke and underwent early prostatectomy had unsatisfactory results.[150] Detrusor hyperreflexia as evidenced by urgency, frequency, and urge incontinence (not due to urinary tract infection) is typically managed with timed voiding, fluid restriction, and anticholinergics. Among these anticholinergics are oxybutynin, dicyclomine, and imipramine. DDAVP has been used in patients with refractory nocturia. Sphincter dyssynergia occurs when the external or internal sphincter fails to relax as the bladder contracts. Medical treatment is typically with baclofen or diazepam. Spincterotomy is an option in some patients.

For those who have failed medical management and are poor surgical candidates, the options of indwelling catheter, suprapubic catheter, and external collection device exist. With indwelling catheters, recurrent urinary tract infection (UTI) and damage to the urethra (including fistula) can occur. A suprapubic catheter, in addition to risk of UTIs, has the associated complications of bladder stones and squamous cell carcinoma of the bladder. External devices are difficult to maintain, may cause skin excoriation, and are also associated with recurrent UTI. Patients with appropriate manual dexterity or an able assistant may be able to perform clean intermittent catheterization with little increase in the rate of UTI.

Bowel Dysfunction

Bowel dysfunction is the loss of voluntary control of defecation. It may result in either fecal incontinence or difficulty with evacuation. Fecal incontinence or impaction is found in 0.3% to 5% of the general population. Difficulty with evacuation is found in 10% to 50% of hospitalized or institutionalized elderly.[151,152] Fecal incontinence decreases the return-to-home rate for stroke patients.[152,153]

Evaluation

A wide range of normal bowel patterns occur, from several times per day to once a week. The majority of individuals have a frequency between three times per week and three times per day. The premorbid bowel pattern including frequency, consistency, and time should be ascertained. Medications and gastrointestinal disease history should also be obtained. Excessively large-caliber hard stool can be determined by a history of toilet plugging.[154] The patient's goals and willingness to alter prior patterns need to be established.[155] Physical examination begins with inspection of the anus. A patulous anus may indicate previous or ongoing dysfunction. Rectal examination should be performed to assess the presence or absence of impaction. External anal sphincter and puborectalis tone and control may be evaluated during this exam.

Management

The goals of management are social continence and the avoidance of complications. Social continence can be defined as scheduled adequate defecations, without incontinence at other times.[156] Colonic transit time and fecal elimination are enhanced by softer stool. Some degree of stool firmness must be tolerated to prevent incontinence.[156] Fiber softens stool more consistently than docusate. It also adds bulk, which can help stimulate defecation.[157,158] Adequate emptying is accomplished by (1) making stools easier to move by softening, (2) adding bowel stimulant medication if needed, and (3) triggering defalcation at consistent desired times.[156] The use of chronic bowel stimulant medications has been questioned, as some cathartics have been shown to damage myenteric neurons.[159,160] The bowel should be emptied if stool is present in the vault or is palpable proximal to the descending colon. This may be accomplished by the use of either enemas or oral cathartics. Enemas, digital stimulation, and rectal stimulant suppository use have all been used. An increasing enema volume needed for defecation may be a warning of chronic rectal overdistension.[154] Local rectal stimulants do not carry the same risks as oral stimulants.[156] Once an effective bowel program is established, it should be continued after hospital discharge.

REHABILITATION IN THE LATER STAGES FOLLOWING STROKE

There is general agreement that rehabilitation is useful for teaching compensatory techniques to persons following stroke, and to train family or care givers to assist with care. Whether rehabilitation is truly "restorative," in the sense of promoting beneficial reorganization of neuronal networks, is still a matter of discussion. Certainly, there is increasing evidence of "plasticity" of neuronal networks in normal individuals, as well as in persons following stroke. In primate models of brain injury, both the somatosensory and motor cortices are capable of considerable rearrangement, which is in part determined by the experience of the animal. In one recent study[161] a specific motor training program was associated with considerable reorganization of motor cortex following local injury. New neuroimaging techniques to evaluate brain function in intact humans have provided additional insights. The best studied are positron emission tomography (PET) and functional magnetic resonance imaging (fMRI). Persons exhibiting good motor recovery from subcortical strokes exhibit widespread PET and fMRI activation of bilateral primary motor and motor association areas during simple motor tasks, a phenomenon not observed in normal persons. Using transcortical magnetic stimulation to activate cortical motor neurons, it can be demonstrated that expansion of the cortical area associated with hand function correlates with good motor recovery. Whether these "plastic" changes are truly the substrate of a motor recovery, or simply an interesting epiphenomenon, is not known. Nevertheless, the mere demonstration of remarkable plastic changes in cortical motor networks has caused considerable excitement. The possibility that beneficial patterns of reorganization can be facilitated through specific training paradigms or pharmacologic intervention is exciting.

There is evidence that currently available stroke rehabilitation programs are effective in decreasing mortality and improving functional outcomes in persons following stroke.[3–8] Most reported studies have been from Europe, and have usually compared patients randomized to "stroke units" (which included both acute stroke care and multidisciplinary rehabilitation) to patients randomized to general medical wards. Patients randomized to stroke units have lower mortality and better ability to perform activities of daily living up to 1 year following stroke. The authors of these studies have been unable to demonstrate any significant difference in medical treatment between experimental and control groups, leading to the hypothesis that multidisciplinary rehabilitation was the key factor in promoting better outcomes.

Major problems in assessing the effectiveness of rehabilitation interventions are the natural clinical variability of stroke and the considerable spontaneous recovery that occurs in many patients. Several independent variables may interact to influence the final outcome. the severity of the initial neurologic deficit is clearly a major factor.[162,163] Other independent variables are age, history of prior stroke, concurrent medical illness, dementia, and the presence of incontinence.[164–167] Attempts to identify a group of variables that could collectively predict outcome using multivariant analyses have had only limited success.[168–173]

MEASURING OUTCOME

There is no single correct measurement of outcome for stroke. The ultimate goal is overall quality of life, but this is difficult to define and subject to individual variation. More specific outcomes are more appropriate for rehabilitation, especially measures of mobility and independence in activities of daily living (ADLs). Measures of mobility and ADLs generally define the degree of assistance that a person needs and predict ability to return home, an important outcome in itself. Multifaceted assessment scales are widely used as outcome measures in rehabilitation. Most commonly used are the Barthel Index (BI) and its revised and expanded version, Functional Independence Measure (FIM). Both scales have been rigorously evaluated for reliability and validity in stroke rehabilitation. The BI has been the most intensively studied. A score >90 generally ensures that a person with stroke can function at home independently.[174] A score >60 correlates with ability to return home with the assistance of a spouse or a care giver for ambulation and ADLs.[165,175] A BI score of <20 correlates with total dependence. In addition, low BI or FIM hospital admission scores correlate with low discharge scores, and patients with low scores recover more slowly than those with higher scores.[163,175,176] Other outcome measures used for stroke rehabilitation include measures of ambulation (e.g., the ability to walk unassisted for 150 feet), comprehensive measures of motor abilities (e.g., the Fugl-Meyer motor assessment scale[177]), and measures of focal disability (the Frenchay test of arm function[178,179] and the Arm Motor Activity Test.[180]) The ability to perform community activities (instrumental living skills) is also important. The Nottingham Scale samples a variety of community activities (e.g., paying bills, using transportation, community socialization, etc.).[181]

Functional scales have found widespread acceptance in stroke rehabilitation settings to track patient progress and assist therapists in setting goals. Multifaceted scales, especially the FIM, have been incorporated into large databases for rehabilitation. The best known in North America is the Uniform Data Set, which provides individual centers with regional and national "benchmark" data of inpatient outcome. As previously mentioned, the ultimate goal for stroke patients is an adequate quality of life. Several studies have demonstrated a significant decline in the perception in the quality of life in persons who have had stroke.[182–185] Improvement in ADLs, mobility, and community living skills doesn't guarantee a satisfactory quality of life. It is also important to address financial, family, and other psychosocial issues.

REHABILITATION TREATMENT STRATEGIES

Motor Function

Approximately 70% to 88% of patients with ischemic stroke have some degree of motor impairment,[164,186,187] and attempts to facilitate motor function are a major part of traditional rehabilitation programs. Spontaneous recovery shows considerable individual variation, but most patients have some residual dysfunction.

The most common way to improve motor function is through programs of physical therapy. A rather surprising number of philosophies and techniques have been developed.[188] An example of an older approach is the neurodevelopmental treatment technique (NDT) developed by Bobath.[189] This technique seeks to facilitate normal patterns of motor movements by inhibiting pathologic reflexes, synergy movements, and spasticity. More recent approaches, such as that formulated by Carr and Shepherd,[190] stress the practice of motor activities in a "task-specific" environment. While task-specific training programs are most consistent with modern theories of motor learning, there is no clear evidence that one approach to physical therapy is superior to the others.[191–195] A recently proposed treatment for hemiparesis is the "forced-use" approach whereby the unaffected extremity is restrained, forcing the individual to use the affected upper extremity.[196,197] At least a minimal degree of motor function is necessary for this approach to be attempted. An analogous approach in the lower extremities is treadmill training with body weight partially supported by an overhead pulley.[198,199] A therapist initially guides the patient's feet along a moving treadmill. The amount of body weight applied to the treadmill and the speed of the treadmill are gradually increased. This approach has been successful in small clinical trials and is being studied on a larger cohort of patients.

In addition to physical therapy, other strategies to enhance motor function are available. Assistive devices make waking safer by increasing base of support and redistributing weight from the legs to the arms.[200] A variety of canes are available, from simple "j" canes to wide-based quad canes and "hemiwalkers."

Orthoses (braces) may also improve function following stroke.[201,202] The most commonly utilized is the ankle-foot orthosis (AFO). The most common reasons to use an AFO are to improve toe clearance during the swing phase of gait (by improving dorsiflexion or inhibiting excessive plantar flexion), to correct ankle inversion, or to control force moments at the knee (thereby correcting recurvatum and other gait deviations in some patients). In order to provide these functions, most stroke patients require a custom-fabricated AFO, which can be expensive and must be carefully designed to prevent skin breakdown. Clinicians and patients should have realistic expectations regarding what the AFO will accomplish, and it should be used only to address a specific component of gait. An AFO will not improve gait in a patient whose most critical problem is neglect or balance impairment, nor will it improve ambulation when the critical deficit is weakness of hip flexion, which prohibits the patient from advancing the leg.

About 80% of patients with stroke will eventually be able to ambulate.[203] For those who cannot ambulate, wheelchair mobility is a reasonable goal. A person with hemiparesis should be prescribed a chair with a seat height 1 to 2 inches lower than the standard adult wheelchair.[200] This allows the patient to use the unaffected leg to help propel the chair. Many other wheelchair features are available to improve mobility and safety for persons with hemiparesis. These include removable leg rests, removable arm rests (to facilitate transfers in and out of the chair), brake extenders to lock the wheelchair on the hemiparetic side, and a variety of cushions.

Multichannel microprocessor-based systems of electrical stimulation have been used in a small number of paraplegic patients to improve gait, and in tetraplegic patients to improve arm function. A prototype system has been designed to assist hemiparetic patients, but is not practical for widespread use. Functional electrical stimulation systems are costly, and require an extraordinarily motivated patient.

Activities of Daily Living

The ability to perform ADLs is a major determinant of whether a person can return to community living.[175] In addition, a person's ability to perform self-care engenders pride and self-confidence. Inability to perform ADLs correlates well with lower overall life satisfaction.[183] Basic ADLs include bathing, dressing, toileting, grooming, and transferring. In the context of the rehabilitation team, all members address these issues, but training proficiency in ADLs is the major focus of occupational therapy. Each task is broken down into its components, and practiced. When independence in an ADL activity is impossible, equipment may substitute, or caregivers can be instructed to provide the remainder of the activity. Examples of simple adaptive devices include special eating utensils, denture brushes, and specially adapted clothing and shoes.[200] Simple devices such as commodes and bathtub benches make simple ADL activities easier for many persons with stroke. The patient's home may need special adaptations including ramps, wider doorways, rearrangement of furniture, and adaptation of the kitchen. A visit by a trained therapist to a patient's home is often useful to identify specific needs.

SPEECH AND LANGUAGE DISORDERS

A variety of speech and language disorders may follow stroke. Aphasia is the most common problem and may affect as many as 23% of stroke patients.[203] A bedside or clinic examination may reveal a great deal about a person's language ability. However, because social skills and automatic responses are often preserved, a rigorous evaluation should include tests of comprehension, repetition, naming, reading, and writing. Speech and language pathologists utilize a variety of comprehensive batteries to better quantify aphasia, and thereby assist in directing treatment.

As with many aspects of stroke, aphasia improves with time in many patients, even without specific treatment.[204] As a general rule, recovery correlates with the severity of initial aphasia, but there are individual exceptions.

The most important goal in treating persons with aphasia is establishing communication. This does not necessarily involve language function, and the temptation to focus solely on "speaking" should be avoided. Formal speech therapy for aphasia remains controversial.[205–207] Studies of the effectiveness of speech therapy are difficult to interpret, but many have failed to provide clear evidence of benefit. Specific techniques are sometimes useful for individual patients, including using melodies or rhythm to facilitate verbal output.

The other large class of speech disorders following stroke is disorders of articulation and phonation. A number of compensatory techniques are available including instruction in controlling the rate of speech, and "overpronouncing" words. Practicing breath support may also be helpful for some persons.

For some patients with expressive aphasia or severe dysarthria, augmentative communication devices are available.[205] These range considerably in sophistication, from simple communication boards to complex, computer-based systems which generate synthesized speech. Careful assessment by speech and language pathologists experienced in use of these devices is necessary before one is recommended. Success depends on overall cognitive status and motivation to use the device.

SETTINGS FOR REHABILITATION

Rehabilitation services can be provided in many locations, including the acute care hospital, special rehabilitation hospitals and units, outpatients facilities, skilled nursing facilities, and the patient's own home. Depending on location, programs different considerably in focus and intensity. During the acute hospital stay early after stroke, rehabilitation programs concentrate on range of motion, positioning, mobilization, and prevention of the many medical complications that can occur early after stroke. After the patient improves, an intensive rehabilitation inpatient hospital program may be recommended. Multidisciplinary patient-focused rehabilitation in this setting may extend over several weeks. According to the Uniform Data System (UDS), the average length of stay for stroke patients in this setting across the United States was 23 days in 1995.[208] The major purpose of these programs is to facilitate independence in ADLs and mobility, with the goal of returning home. Patients in rehabilitation hospitals or units generally receive 3 to 5 hours of therapy per day, and there are close medical supervision and intensive rehabilitation nursing. Many stroke patients are elderly, have concurrent medical illnesses, and cannot tolerate intensive programs. For those persons, a rehabilitation program located in a skilled nursing facility (SNF) is often more appropriate. Skilled nursing facilities may be either hospital-based or located in a nursing home. Rehabilitation in such facilities is often termed "subacute." While there is no precise definition of subacute, services provided are generally intermediate in scope and intensity between those provided in rehabilitation hospitals and units, and those provided at traditional "nursing homes." Patients receive 1 to 3 hours of therapy a day in most subacute programs.

Outpatient rehabilitation services are available in a wide variety of settings, including hospital-based programs, small outpatient clinics, and comprehensive multidisciplinary outpatient programs. Outpatient service is sometimes confined to a single discipline, for example, an aphasic patient requiring only speech and language therapy. On the other extreme, programs may be intensive and multidisciplinary, approaching the services provided by inpatient rehabilitation hospitals. This concept of a "day hospital" allows patients to be dropped off in the morning and picked up at night, retaining much of the benefit of inpatient programs, at less cost.

Rehabilitation services provided by home health agencies is a popular option, especially for elderly patients with decreased mobility. In the United States, Medicare and third-party payers require that persons receiving these services be "home-bound," meaning that they are able to leave their home only periodically and with the assistance of another person. The focus of home health rehabilitation is function within the home environment, usually concentrating on activities of daily living. The training of a spouse or care giver to assist with the patient's needs often receives a high priority.

The most appropriate setting for rehabilitation for an individual patient depends on a number of factors. Most important is the setting in which the rehabilitation goals can best be met. For example, a younger patient with a stroke may hope to regain complete independence in mobility and activities of daily living, and hope to eventually return to work or school. For such an individual, an intensive rehabilitation hospital setting followed by a prolonged outpatient program focusing on community mobility and vocational issues would be most appropriate. On the other hand, an elderly stroke patient with multiple medical problems and limited mobility from other causes (osteoarthritis, etc.) whose goal is to return home with the care of a spouse might best receive home health rehabilitation with an emphasis on education and training of the spouse. The same patient without an available care giver might receive rehabilitation services in an SNF. Therefore, the neurological status of the patient, age, concurrent medical illnesses, personal rehabilitation goals, and presence or absence of a caregiver all determine the appropriateness of a particular level of care. Most rehabilitation programs have written admission criteria based on their specific focus and the type of patients that they can most appropriately treat.

For many years, third-party payers, especially Medicare in the United States, have had a profound influence on the setting in which patients receive rehabilitation services. The current environment of providing health care in the least costly environment is forcing reexamination of costs. There has been considerable pressure to provide rehabilitation services in SNFs, outpatient programs, and the home, rather than in costly inpatient programs.

Since stroke is largely a disease of the elderly, the most important third-party payer in determining payment for rehabilitation services in the United States is Medicare. The Tax Equity and Fiscal Responsibility Act (TEFRA) of 1982 excluded rehabilitation services from Medicare's prospective payment system. This resulted in rapid expansion of all rehabilitative services in the United States. For example, between 1986 and 1994, the number of rehabilitation hospitals grew 149%, and the number of rehabilitation units in general acute care hospitals generally grew 71%.[209] Skilled nursing facility and home health rehabilitation services have grown even faster. For example, total Medicare expenditures for home health care increased from $2 billion in 1988 to $12.7 billion in 1994, accounting for 8% of the total Medicare budget.[210] This growth led to payment reform including in the Balanced Budget Act of 1997. This legislation specified that all postacute services will be reimbursed through prospective payment systems. This will result in changes in location of service delivery for older patients, and will have major financial ramifications for rehabilitation providers.

In order for Medicare patients to receive rehabilitation services in hospitals or units, patients must be medically stable, have had an illness or injury resulting in a decline from prior functional abilities, have reasonable rehabilitation goals (often this means returning to community living), and be able to tolerate 3 hours of therapy daily for a minimum of 5 days per week. For home health services, Medicare requires "skilled" services (defined as physical therapy, registered nursing, or speech and language pathology). If one of these services is required, then payment may also be available for occupational therapy or social service, if required. Medicare requires that care be needed only intermittently, that it be approved by a physician and renewed every 2 months, that the services "reasonable," and that the person be home-bound.

In the past, other third-party payers have generally followed Medicare guidelines for payment of services. Given the current emphasis on health care cost containment, the shift toward less expensive levels of care will likely continue for the foreseeable future. In response to present and future market conditions, rehabilitation providers are increasingly part of integrated delivery systems which provide rehabilitation services in all the settings previously described. Theoretically, patients can then receive services in the most cost-effective setting within a single delivery system.

Studies comparing outcomes between traditional hospital-based rehabilitation and other settings are few. In an nonrandomized comparison of stroke patients receiving rehabilitation in a traditional rehabilitation hospital and in a free-standing skilled nursing facility, one study showed substantially greater gains in functional abilities in patients treated in the rehabilitation hospital, but the cost for successful discharge to the community was twice as high as for the subacute facility.[211] In a carefully performed prospective study, Medicare patients admitted to a rehabilitation hospital or a skilled nursing facility were studied prospectively for 6 months.[212] Return to community living and proficiency in ADLs were evaluated. When outcomes were adjusted for premorbid residence and function, care giver availability and comorbid illness, stroke patients admitted to rehabilitation hospitals were more likely to have favorable outcomes than those treated in SNFs. However, improved outcomes were again achieved at higher costs. The relative inability of subacute facilities to closely monitor medically unstable patients, and the relative lack of medical ancillary services, has raised the issue of whether the patients in such facilities have higher morbidity and mortality rates.[213] Overall, available evidence suggests that outcomes in subacute facilities are less favorable than those in rehabilitation hospitals, but the cost is 50% to 65% lower in subacute facilities.[211,212] Studies comparing outcomes of patients treated at home to those treated in other settings are lacking, partially because of differences in patient populations. Home health rehabilitation services usually occur longer after the onset of stroke, and are often used "in sequence" with hospital SNF services.[214] Studies comparing rehabilitation outcomes of those treated in outpatient programs with those treated in other settings are also limited. One study showed similar performance in household and community activities in stroke patients treated at home and those treated in outpatient facilities.[215]

In summary, the "ideal" setting for the provision of rehabilitation services for persons with stroke remains uncertain. While there is mounting evidence that a coordinated team approach to patients with stroke is effective and that outcomes from stroke patients treated in intensive rehabilitation programs are better than those treated in SNFs, detailed information regarding outcomes among other rehabilitation settings is limited. In lieu of careful studies, these decisions will often continue to be made on a financial basis.

SUMMARY

Rehabilitation for stroke remains an important component for the care of persons with stroke. The major goals of rehabilitation are to maximize recovery in mobility, activities of daily living, community activities, language and cognition, and psychosocial adjustment. These goals are accomplished by teaching compensatory techniques, utilizing adaptive equipment, specific training paradigms to "restore" function, and training care givers to assist with care when needed. Rehabilitation is individually focused, is goal directed, and represents a multidisciplinary effort. The rehabilitation process should begin early after stroke, when the focus is on maintaining range of motion, mobilization, and preventing the medical complications of inactivity. At this stage, it is almost impossible to distinguish between "rehabilitative" and "general medical" aspects of care. Issues that must be addressed include preventing complications of immobility, dysphagia and aspiration, spasticity, and incontinence. Later after stroke, rehabilitative services may be provided in rehabilitation hospitals and wards, skilled nursing facilities, outpatient rehabilitation programs, or the home. While there is good evidence that coordinated multidisciplinary care improves outcome following stroke, there is little evidence that any specific program or services delivered in any specific setting are superior to any others.

REFERENCES

1. Bergen DC. The world-wide burden or neurologic disease Neurology 1996; 47:21–25.
2. Taylor TN, Davis PH, Torner JC, Holmes J, Meyer JW, Jacobson MF. Lifetime cost of stroke in the United States. Stroke 1996; 27:1459–1466.
3. Strand T, Asplund K, Eriksson S, Hegg E, Lithner F, Wester PO. A nonintensive stroke unit reduces functional disability and the need for long-term hospitalization. Stroke 1985; 16:29–34.
4. Kalra L, Dale P, Crome P. Improving stroke rehabilitation: a controlled study. Stroke 1993; 24:1462–1467.
5. Jorgensen HS, Nakayama H, Raaschou HO, Larsen K, Hubb P, Skyhoj Olsen T. The effect of a stroke unit: reductions in mortality, discharge rate to nursing home, length of hospital stay, and cost. Stroke 1995; 26:1178–1182.
6. Indredavik B, Bakke F, Solberg R, Rokseth R, Haheim LL, Holme I. Benefit of a stroke unit: randomized controlled trial. Stroke 1991; 22:1026–1031.
7. Indredavik B, Slordahl SA, Bakke F, Rokseth R, Haheim LL. Stroke unit treatment: long-term effects. Stroke 1997; 28:1861–1866.
8. Kalra L, Eade J. Role of stroke rehabilitation units in managing severe disability after stroke. Stroke 1995; 26:2031–2034.
9. Jozefczyk PB. Interdisciplinary team approach to rehabilitation. In: Good DC, Couch JR, eds. Handbook of Neurorehabilitation. New York: Marcel Dekker, 1994:153–163.
10. Lee AJ, Huber J, Stason WB. Poststroke rehabilitation in older americans. Med Care 1996; 34:811–825.
11. Kottke FJ. The effects of limitation of activity upon the human body. JAMA 1966; 196:825–830.
12. Halar EM, Bell KR. Contracture and other deleterious effects of immobility. In: Delisa JA, ed. Rehabilitation Medicine: Principles and Practice. 2d ed. Philadelphia: Lippincott, 1993:681–699.
13. Hoenig HM, Rubenstein LZ. Hospital-associated deconditioning and dysfunction. JAGS 1991; 39:220–222.
14. Kottke FJ. Deterioration of the bedfast patient: causes and effects. Public Health Rep 1965; 80:437–451.
15. Müller EA. Influence of training and inactivity on muscle strength. Arch Phys Med Rehabil 1970; 449–462.
16. Fiatarone MA, O'Neill EF, Ryan ND, et al. Exercise training and nutritional supplementation for physical frailty in very elderly people. N Engl J Med 1994; 330:1769–1775.
17. MacKay-Lyons M. Low-load, prolonged stretch in treatment of elbow flexion contractures secondary to head trauma: a case report. Phys Ther 1989; 69:292–296.
18. King TI. Plaster splinting as a means of reducing elbow flexor spasticity: a case study. Am J Occup Ther 1982; 36:671–673.

19. Booth BJ, Doyle M, Montgomery J. Serial casting for the management of spasticity in the head-injured adult. Phys Ther 1983; 63:1960–1966.
20. Keenan MAE. The orthopedic management of spasticity. J Head Trauma Rehabil 1987; 2:62–71.
21. Weiss A-PC, Sachar K. Soft tissue contractures about the elbow. Hand Clin 1994; 10:439–451.
22. Dobkin BH. Neuromedical complications in stroke patients transferred for rehabilitation before and after diagnostic related groups. J Neurol Rehab 1987; 1:3–7.
23. Couch JR. Medical complications in the rehabilitation patient. In: Good DC, Couch JR, eds. Handbook of Neurorehabilitation. New York: Marcel Dekker Inc., 1994:443–458.
24. Sioson E. Deep vein thrombosis in stroke patients: an overview. J Stroke Cerebrovasc Dis 1992; 2:74–79.
25. Wardlow C, Ogston D, Douglas AS. Venous thrombosis following stroke. Lancet 1972; 1:1305.
26. Wardlow C, Ogston D, Douglas AS. Deep vein thrombosis of legs after stroke: incidence and predisposing factors. Br Med J 1976; 1:1178–1183.
27. McCarthy ST, Turner J Robertson D, Hawkey CJ. Low dose heparin as a prophylaxis against DVT after acute stroke. Lancet 1977; 2:800–811.
28. McCarthy ST, Turner J. Low dose subcutaneous heparin in the prevention of deep vein thrombosis or pulmonary embolism following acute stroke. Age Ageing 1986; 15:84–88.
29. Cope C, Reyes TM, Skversky NJ. Phlebographic analysis of incidence of thrombosis in hemiplegia. Radiology 1973; 109:58–111.
30. Landi G, et al. Venous thromboembolism in acute stroke: prognostic importance of hypercoagulability. Arch Neurol 1992; 49:279–283.
31. Anderson FA Jr, Wheeler HB. Venous thromboembolism: risk factors and prophylaxis. Clin Chest Med 1995; 16:235–251.
32. Oczkowski WJ, Ginsberg JS, Shin A, Panju A. Venous thromboembolism in patients undergoing rehabilitation for stroke. Arch Phys Med Rehabil 1992; 73:712–716.
33. Weinmann EE, Salzman EW. Deep vein thrombosis. N Engl J Med 1994; 331:1630–1641.
34. Lensing AWA, Hirsh J, Buller HR. Diagnosis of venous thrombosis. In: Colman RW, Hirsh J, Marder VJ, Salzman EW, eds. Hemostasis and Thrombosis: Basic principles and Clinical Practice. 3d ed. Philadelphia: J. B. Lippincott, 1994:1297–1321.
35. Chaudhuri GX, Costa JL. Clinical findings associated with pulmonary embolism in a rehabilitation setting. Arch Phys Med Rehabil 1991; 72:671–673.
36. Verstraete M. The diagnosis and treatment of deep-vein thrombosis. N Engl J Med 1993; 329:1418–1420.
37. Collins R, Scrimgeour A, Yusuf S, Peto R. Reduction in fatal pulmonary embolism and venous thrombosis by perioperative administration of subcutaneous heparin: overview of results of randomized trials in general, orthopedic, and urologic surgery. N Engl J Med 1988; 318:1162–1173.

38. Hull R, Raskob G, Pineo G, et al. A comparison of subcutaneous low-molecular-weight heparin with warfarin sodium prophylaxis against deep-venous thrombosis after hip or knee implantation. N Engl J Med 1993; 329:1370–1376.
39. Hirsh J, Dalen JE, Deykin D, Poller L. Oral anticoagulants: mechanisms of action, clinical effectiveness, and optimal therapeutic range. Chest 1992; 102(suppl):312–326.
40. Hirsh J, Levine M. Confusion over the therapeutic range for monitoring oral anticoagulant therapy in North America. Thromb Haemost 1988; 59:129–132.
41. Fordyce MJF, Baker AS, Staddon GE. Efficacy of fixed minidose warfarin prophylaxis in total hip replacement. Br Med J 1991; 303:219–220.
42. Dale C, Gallus AS, Wycherly A, et al. Prevention of venous thrombosis with minidose warfarin after joint replacement. Br Med J 1991; 303:224.
43. Bern MM, Lokich JJ, Wallach SR, et al. Very low doses of warfarin can prevent thrombosis in central venous catheters. Ann Intern Med 1990; 112:423–428.
44. Antiplatelet Trialists' Collaboration. Collaborative overview of randomized trials of antiplatelet therapy. III. Reduction in venous thrombosis and pulmonary embolism by antiplatelet prophylaxis among surgical and medical patients. Br Med J 1994; 308:235–246.
45. Nicolaides AN, Fernandes E, Fernandes J, Pollock AV. Intermittent sequential pneumatic compression of the legs in the prevention of venous stasis and postoperative deep venous thrombosis. Surgery 1980; 87:69–76.
46. Hyers TM, Hull RD, Weg JG. Antithrombotic therapy for venous thromboembolic disease. Chest 1992; 102(suppl):408S–425S. (Erratum, Chest 1993; 103:1636.)
47. Brandjes DPM, Heijboer H, Buller HR, et al. Acenocoumaral and heparin compared with acenocoumaral alone in the treatment if proximal-vein thrombosis. N Engl J Med 1992; 327:1485–1489.
48. Hull RD, Raskob GE, Rosenbloom D, et al. Heparin for 5 days as compared with 10 days in the initial treatment of proximal venous thrombosis. N Engl J Med 1990; 322:1260–1264.
49. Harrison L, Johnston M, Massicotte MP, et al. Comparison of 5-mg and 10-mg loading doses in initiation of warfarin therapy. Ann Intern Med 1997; 126:133–136.
50. Wakefield TW, Greenfield LJ. Diagnostic approaches and surgical treatment of deep venous thrombosis and pulmonary embolism. Hematol Oncol Clin North Am 1993; 7:1251–1267.
51. Goldhaber SZ, Meyerovitz MF, Green D, et al. Randomized controlled trial of tissue plasminogen activator in proximal deep venous thrombosis. Am J Med 1990; 88:235–240.
52. Goldhaber SZ, Buring JE, Lipnick RJ, Hennekens CH. Pooled analyses of randomized trials of streptokinase and heparin in phlebographically documented acute deep venous thrombosis. Am J Med 1984; 76:393–397.
53. Ott P, Eldup E, Oxholm P, et al. Streptokinase therapy in the routine management of deep venous thrombosis in the lower extremities: a retrospective study of phlebographic results and therapeutic complications. Acta Med Scand 1986; 219:295–300.

54. Ballew KA, Philbrick JT, Becker DM. Vena cava filter devices. Clin Chest Med 1995; 16:295–305.
55. Holas MA, Depippo KL, Reding MJ. Aspiration and relative risk of medical complications following stroke. Arch Neurol 1994; 51:1052-1053.
56. Splaingard ML, Hutchins B, Sulton LD, Chaudhuri G. Aspiration in rehabilitation patients: videofluorscopy vs bedside clinical assessment. Arch Phys Med Rehabil 1988; 69:637–640.
57. Garon BR, Engle M, Ormiston C. Silent aspiration: results of 1,000 videofluorscopic evaluations. J Neurol Rehabil 1996; 10:121–126.
58. Veis SL, Logemann JA. Swallowing disorders in persons with cerebrovascular accident. Arch Phys Med Rehabil 1985; 66:372–375.
59. Robbins J, Levine RL. Swallowing after unilateral stroke of the cerebral cortex: preliminary experience. Dysphagia 1988; 3:11–17.
60. Horner J, Masey EW. Silent aspiration following stroke. Neurology 1988; 38:317–319.
61. Horner J, Massey EW, Riski JE, Lathrop DL, Chase KN. Aspiration following stroke: clinical correlates and outcome. Neurology 1988; 38:1359–1362.
62. Horner J, Massey EW, Brazer SR. Aspiration in bilateral stroke patients. Neurology 1990; 40:1686–1688.
63. Depippo KL, Holas MA, Reding MJ. The Burke dysphagia screening test: validation of its use in patients with stroke. Arch Phys Med Rehabil 1994; 75:1284–1286.
64. Brock RC. Lung Abscess. Oxford: Blackwell, 1952.
65. Bynum LJ, Pierce AK. Pulmonary aspiration of gastric contents. Am Rev Respir Dis 1976; 114:1129–1136.
66. Johanson WG Jr, Harris GD. Aspiration pneumonia, anaerobic infections, and lung abscess. Med Clin North Am 1980; 64:385–394.
67. Finegold S. Aspiration pneumonia. Rev Infect Dis 1991;13(suppl 9):S737–S742.
68. Dy RC, Kumar R, Scremin OU. Clinical outcomes of dysphagia in elderly patients with cerebrovascular accident. J Neurol Rehabil 1996; 10:217–222.
69. Logemann JA, Kahrilas PJ. Relearning to swallow after stroke—application of maneuvers and indirect biofeedback: a case study. Neurology 1990; 40:1136–1138.
70. Logemann JA, Kahrilas PJ, Kobara M, Vakil NB. The benefit of head rotation on pharyngoesophageal dysphagia. Arch Phys Med Rehabil 1989; 70:767–771.
71. Rasley A, Logemann JA, Kahrilas PJ, et al. Prevention of barium aspiration during videofluoroscopic swallowing studies: value of change in posture. Am J Radiol 1993; 160:1005–1009.
72. Hargrove R. Feeding the severely dysphagic patient. J Neurosurg Nurs 1980; 12:102–107.
73. Layne AL. Feeding strategies for the dysphagic patient: a nursing perspective. Dysphagia 1990; 5:84–88.
74. Shanahan TK, Logemann JA, Rademaker AW, Pauloski BR, Kahrilas PJ. Chin-down posture effect on aspiration in dysphagic patients. Arch Phys Med Rehabil 1993; 74:736–739.
75. Rosenbeck JC, Robbins J, Fishback B, Levine RL. Effects of thermal application on dysphagia after stroke. J Speech Hear Res 1991; 34:1257–1268.

76. Langmore SE, Miller RM. Behavioral treatment for adults with oropharyngeal dysphagia. Arch Phys Med Rehabil 1994; 75:1154–1160.
77. Martin AW. Dietary management of swallowing disorders. Dysphagia 1991; 6:129–134.
78. Pardoe EM. Development of a multistage diet for dysphagia. J Am Dietetic Assoc 1993; 93:568–571.
79. National Pressure Ulcer Advisory Panel. Pressure ulcers: incidence, economics, risk assessment. In: Consensus Development Conference Statement. Rockville, MD: National Pressure Ulcer Advisory Panel, 1989:5–6.
80. Reuler JB, Cooney TG. The pressure sore: pathophysiology and principles of management. Ann Intern Med 1981; 94:661–666.
81. Yarokony GM. Pressure ulcers: a review. Arch Phys Med Rehabil 1994; 75:908–917.
82. National Pressure Ulcer Advisory Panel. Pressure ulcers: incidence, economics, risk assessment. In: Consensus Development Conference Statement. West Dundee, IL: S-N Publications, 1989.
83. Allman RM, Goode PS, Patrick MM, et al. Pressure ulcer risk factors among hospitalized patients with activity limitation. JAMA 1995; 273:865–870.
84. Allman RM, Laprade CA, Noel LB, et al. Pressure sores among hospitalized patients. Ann Intern Med 1986; 105:37–42.
85. Allman RM, Walker JM, Hart MK, et al. Air-fluidized beds or conventional therapy for pressure ulcers: a randomized trial. Ann Intern Med 1987; 107:641–648.
86. Yarkony GM, Kirk PM, Carlson C, et al. Classification of pressure ulcers. Arch Dermatol 1990; 126:1218–1219.
87. Shea JD. Pressure sores: classification and management. Clin Orthop 175; 112:89–100.
88. Exton-Smith AN, Sherwin RW. The prevention of pressure sores: significance of spontaneous bodily movements. Lancet 1961; 2:1124–1126.
89. Carter DM, Balin AK. Dermatological aspects of aging. Med Clin North Am 1983; 67:531–543.
90. Kosiak M. Etiology and pathology of ischemic ulcers. Arch Phys Med Rehabil 1959; 40:62–69.
91. Dansereau JG, Conway H. Closure of decubiti in paraplegics. Plast Reconstr Surg 1964; 33:474–480.
92. Houle RJ. Evaluation of seat devices designed to prevent ischemic ulcers in paraplegic patients. Arch Phys Med Rehabil 1969; 50:587–594.
93. Lindan O. Etiology of decubitus ulcers: an experimental study. Arch Phys Med Rehabil 1961; 42:774–783.
94. Allman RM. Pressure ulcers among the elderly. N Engl J Med 1989; 320:850–853.
95. Hussain T. An experimental study of some pressure effects on tissues, with reference to the bed-sore problem. J Pathol Bacteriol 1953; 66:347–358.
96. Seiler WO, Stahelin HB. Decubitus ulcers: preventive techniques for the elderly patient. Geriatrics 1985; 40:53–60.
97. Andersen KE, Jensen O, Kvorning SA, Bach E. Decubitus prophylaxis: a prospec-

tive trial of the efficiency of alternating-pressure air-mattresses and water-mattresses. Acta Derm Venereol (Stockh) 1982; 63:227–230.
98. Argenta LC, Morykwas MJ. Vacuum-assisted closure: a new method for wound control and treatment: clinical experience. Ann Plast Surg 1997; 38:563–576.
99. Morykwas MJ, Argenta LC, Shelton-Brown E, McGuirt W. Vacuum-assisted closure: a new method for wound control and treatment: animal studies and basic foundation. Ann Plast Surg 1997; 38:553–562.
100. Taylor TV, Rimmer S, Day B, Butcher J, Dymock JW. Ascorbic acid supplementation in the treatment of pressure-sores. Lancet 1974; 2:544–546.
101. Pories WJ, Henzel JH, Rob CG, Strain WH. Acceleration of wound healing in man with zinc sulphate given by mouth. Lancet 1967; 1:121–124.
102. Hallbook T, Lanner E. Serum-zinc and healing of venous leg ulcers. Lancet 1972; 2:780–782.
103. Lance JW. Symposium synopsis. In: Feldman RG, Young RR, Koella WP, eds. Spasticity: Disordered Motor Control. Chicago: Year Book Medical, 1980.
104. Young RR. Spasticity: a review. Neurology 1994; 44(suppl 9):12–20.
105. Katz RT. Management of spastic hypertonia after stroke. J Neurol Rehabil 1991; 5:(suppl):5–12.
106. Young RR, Delwaide PJ. Drug therapy: spasticity. N Engl J Med 1981; 304:28–33, 96–99.
107. Nance PW, Shears AH, Nance DM. Reflex changes induced by clonidine in spinal cord injured patients. Paraplegia 1989; 27:296–301.
108. Young RR. Physiologic and pharmacologic approaches to spasticity. Neurol Clin North Am 1987; 5:529–539.
109. Dimitrijevic MR. Evaluation and treatment of spasticity. J Neurol Rehabil 1995; 9:97–110.
110. Hattab JR. Review of European clinical trials with baclofen. In: Feldman RG, Young RR, Koella WP, eds. Spasticity: Disordered Motor Control. Chicago: Year Book Medical, 1980.
111. Katz RT. Management of spasticity. Am J Phys Med Rehabil 1988 67:108–116.
112. Kerr WG. The use of diazepam (Valium) in the relief of spasticity. Paraplegia 1966; 4:149–154.
113. Glenn MB. Antispasticity medications in the patient with traumatic brain injury. J Head Trauma Rehabil 1986; 1:71–72.
114. Pinder RM, Brogden RN, Speight TM, Avery GS. Dantrolene sodium: a review of its pharmacological properties and therapeutic efficacy in spasticity. Drugs 1977; 13:3–23.
115. Ketel WB, Kolb ME. Long term treatment with dantrolene sodium of stroke patients with spasticity limiting the return of function. Curr Med Res Opin 1984; 9:161–169.
116. Bianchine JR. Drugs for Parkinsons disease, spasticity and acute muscle spasms. In: Gilman AG, Goodman LS, Rall PW, Murad F, eds. The Pharmacological Basis of Therapeutics. 7th ed. New York: Macmillan, 1985.
117. Coward DM. Tizanadine: neuropharmacology and mechanism of action. Neurology 1994; 44(suppl 9):S6–S11.

118. Hennues OL. A new skeletal muscle relaxant (DS 103-282) compared to diazepam in the treatment of muscle spasm of local origin. J Int Med Res 1981; 9:62–68.
119. Smolenski C, Muff S, Smolenski-Kantz S. A double-blind comparative trial of a new muscle relaxant, tizanadine (DS 103-282) and baclofen in the treatment of chronic spasticity in multiple sclerosis. Surr Med Res Opin 1981; 7:374–383.
120. Unnerstall JR, Kopajtic TA, Kuhar MJ. Distribution of alpha 2 agonist binding sites in the rat and human central nervous system: analysis of some functional, anatomic correlates of the pharmacologic effects of clonidine and related adrenergic agents. Brain Res 1984; 319:69–101.
121. Khahli AA, Betts HBB. Peripheral nerve block with phenol in the management of spasticity. JAMA 1967; 200:1155–1157.
122. Khahli AA. Physiatric management of spasticity by phenol nerve and motor point block. In: Ruskin AP, ed. Current Therapy in Physiatry. Philadelphia: W. B. Saunders, 1984.
123. Garland DE, Lucie RS, Waters RL. Current uses of open phenol nerve block for adult acquired spasticity. Clin Orthop Rel Res 1982; 165:217–222.
124. McComas AJ, Kereshi S, Manzano G. Multiple innervation of human muscle fibers. J Neurol Sci 1984; 64:55–64.
125. Mowery CA Gelberman RH, Rhoades CE. Upper extremity tendon transfers in cerebral palsy: electromyographic and functional analysis. J Pediatr Orthop 1985; 5:160–163.
126. Waters RL, Perry J, Garland DE. Surgical correction of gait abnormalities following stroke. Clin Orthop Rel Res 1978; 131:54–63.
127. Eggers GWN, Evans EB. Surgery in cerebral palsy. J Bone Joint Surg 1963; 45:1275–1305.
128. Sindou M, Abdennebi B, Sharkey P. Microsurgical selective procedures in peripheral nerves and the posterior root–spinal cord junction for spasticity. Appl Neurophysiol 1985; 48:97–104.
129. Burney TL, Senapati M, Desai S, et al. Effects of cerebrovascular accident on micturition. Urol Clin North Am 1996; 23:484–490.
130. Badlani GH, Vohara S, Motola JA. Detrusor behavior in patients with dominant hemispheric strokes. Neurourol Urodyn 1991; 10:119.
131. Taub NA, Wolfe CDA, Richardson E, et al. Predicting the disability of first-time stroke sufferers at one year: 12-month follow-up of a population-based cohort in southeast England. Stroke 1994; 25:352–357.
132. Wade DT, Hewer RL. Outlook after an acute stroke: urinary incontinence and loss of consciousness compared in 532 patients. Q J Med 1985; 56:601–608.
133. Hald T, Bradley WE. The nervous control of the urinary bladder. In: Hald T, Bradley WE, eds. The Urinary Bladder: Neurology and Urodynamics. Baltimore: Williams and Wilkins, 1982:48.
134. De Groat W. Anatomy and physiology of the lower urinary tract. Urol Clin North Am 1993; 20:383–401.
135. Borrie M, Campbell A, Caradoc-Davies TH, et al. Urinary incontinence after stroke: a prospective study. Age Ageing 1986; 15:177–181,

136. Gelber DA, Good DC, Laven LJ, Velhurst SJ. Causes of urinary incontinence after acute hemispheric stroke. Stroke 1993; 24:378–382.
137. Motola JA, Mascarenas B, Badlani GH. Cerebrovascular accidents: urodynamic and neuroanatomical findings. J Urol 1988; 139:512A.
138. Khan Z, Starer P, Wang WC, et al. Analysis of voiding disorders in patients with cerebrovascular accidents. Urology 1990; 35:265–270.
139. Adams M, Baron M, Caston MA. Urinary incontinence in the acute phase of cerebrovascular accident. Nurs Res 1966; 15:100–108.
140. Aruna BH, Badlani GH. Urologic problems in cerebrovascular accidents. Prob Urol 1993; 7:41.
141. Brocklehurst JC, Andrews K, Richards B, et al. Incidence and correlates of incontinence in stroke patients. J Am Geriatr Soc 1985; 33:540–542.
142. Bahita NN, Bradley WE. Neuroanatomy and physiology: innervation of the urinary tract. In: Raz S, ed. Female Urology. Philadelphia: WB Saunders, 1983:12.
143. Blaivas JG. The neurophysiology of micturition: a clinical study of 550 patients. J Urol 1982; 127:958–963.
144. Nishizawa O, Ebina K Sugaya K, et al. Effect of cerebellectomy on reflex micturition in the decerebrate dog as determined by urodynamic evaluation. Urol Int 1989; 44:152.
145. Khan Z, Hertanu J, Yang WC, et al. Predictive correlation of urodynamic dysfunction and brain injury after cerebrovascular accident. J Urol 1980; 126:86–88.
146. Dromerick A, Reding M. Medical and neurological complications during inpatient stroke rehabilitation. Stroke 1994; 25:358–361.
147. Coletta EM, Murphy JB. Physical and functional assessment of the elderly stroke patient. Am Fam Physician 1994; 49:1777–1785.
148. Fowler CF. Investigations of the neurogenic bladder. J Neurol Neurosurg Psych 1996; 60:6–13.
149. Dewire DM, Owens RS, Anderson GA, et al. A comparison of the urological complications associated with long-term management of quadraplegics with and without chronic indwelling catheters. J Urol 1992; 147:1069–1072.
150. Lum SK, Marshall VR. Results of prostatectomy in patients following a cerebrovascular accident. Br J Urol 1982; 54:186–189.
151. Schiller LR. Fecal incontinence. In: Sleisenger MH, Fordtran JS, eds. Gastrointestinal Disease. Philadelphia: WB Saunders, 1989:317–330.
152. Tobin GW, Brocklehurst JC. Faecal incontinence in residential homes for the elderly: prevalence, aetiology and management. Age Ageing 1986; 15:41–46.
153. Granger CV, Hamilton BB, Gresham GE, Kramer AA. The stroke rehabilitation outcome study. Part II. Relative merits of the total Barthel Index score and a four-item subscore in predicting patient outcomes. Arch Phys Med Rehabil 1989; 70:100–108.
154. Martelli H, Devroede G, Arhan P, Dugay C. Some parameters of large bowel motility in normal man. Gastroenterology 1978; 75:612.
155. King JC, Currie DM, Wright E. Bowel training in spina bifida: importance of education, patient compliance, age and anal reflexes. Arch Phys Med Rehabil 1994; 75:243–247.

156. Cardenas DD, Mayo ME, King JC. Urinary tract and bowel management. In: Braddom RL, ed. Physical Medicine and Rehabilitation. Philadelphia: WB Saunders, 1996:555–579.
157. Dikenson VA. Maintenance of anal continence—a review of pelvic floor physiology. Gut 1978; 19:1163–1174.
158. Longo WE, Ballantyne GH, Modlin IM. The colon, anorectum, and spinal cord patient. Dis Colon Rectum 1989; 32:261–267.
159. Cummings JH. Laxative abuse. Gut 1974; 15:758–766.
160. Smith B. Effect of irritant purgatives on the myenteric plexus in man and mouse. Gut 1968; 9:139–142.
161. Nudo R, Wise B, Sifuentes F, Milliken G. Neural substrates for the effects of rehabilitative training on motor recovery after ischemic infarct. Science 1996; 248:1791–1794.
162. Berspang B, Asplund K, Eriksson S, Fugl-Meyer AR. Motor and perceptual impairments in acute stroke patients: effects on self-care ability. Stroke 1987; 18:1081–1086.
163. Reding MJ, Potes E. Rehabilitation outcome following initial unilateral hemispheric stroke. Life table analysis approach. Stroke 1988; 19:1354–1358.
164. Kotila M, Waltimo O, Niemi M, Laaksonen R, Lempinen M. The profile of recovery from stroke and factors influencing outcome. Stroke 1984, 15:1039–1044.
165. Lincoln NB, Blackburn M, Ellis S, Jackson J, Edmans JA, Nouri EM, Walrer MF, Haworth H. An investigation of factors affecting progress of patients on a stroke unit. J Neurol Neurosurg Psychiatry 1989; 52:493–496.
166. Wade DT, Wood VA, Langton Hewer R. Recovery after stroke—the first 3 months. J Neurol Neurosurg Psychiatry 1985; 48:7–13.
167. Smith ME, Garraway WM, Smith DL, Akhtar AJ. Therapy impact on functional outcome in a controlled trial of stroke rehabilitation. Arch Phys Med Rehabil 1982; 63:21–24.
168. Shah S, Vanclay F, Cooper B. Predicting discharge status at commencement of stroke rehabilitation. Stroke 1989; 20;766–769.
169. Allen CMC. Predicting the outcome of acute stroke: a prognostic score. J Neurol Neurosurg Psychiatry 1984; 47:475–480.
170. Howard G, Till JS, Toole JF, Matthews C, Truscott BL. Factors influencing return to work following cerebral infarction. JAMA 1985; 253:226–232.
171. Shah S, Vanclay F, Cooper B. Efficiency, effectiveness, and duration of stroke rehabilitation. Stroke 1990; 21:241–246.
172. Kelly-Hayes M, Wolf PA, Kase CS, Gresham GE, Kannel WB, D'Agostino RB. Time course of functional recovery after stroke: the Framington Study. 40th Meeting of the American Academy of Neurology (1988, Cincinnati, OH). J Neurol Rehabil 1989; 3:65–70.
173. Hier DB, Edelstein G. Deriving clinical prediction rules from stroke outcome research. Stroke 1991; 22:1431–1436.
174. Granger CV, Sherwood CC, Greer DS. Functional status measures in a comprehensive stroke program. Arch Phys Med Rehabil 1977; 58:555–561.

175. Granger CV, Hamilton BB, Gresham GE. The stroke rehabilitation outcome study. Part I. General description. Arch Phys Med Rehabil 1988; 69:5–6–509.
176. Skilbeck CE, Wade DT, Langton-Hewer R, Wood VA. Recovery after stroke. J Neurol Neurosurg Psychiatry 1983; 46:5–8.
177. Fugl-Meyer AR, Jaasko L, Leyman L, Olsson S, Steglind S. The post-stroke hemiplegic patient. 1. A method for evaluation of physical performance. Scand J Rehabil Med 1975; 7:13–31.
178. Wade DT, Langton Hewer R, Wood VA, Skilbeck CE, Ismail IM. The hemiplegic arm after stroke: Measurement and recovery. J Neurol Neurosurg Psychiatry 1983; 46:521–524.
179. Heller A, Wade DT, Wood VA, Sunderland A, Langton Hewer R, Ward E. Arm function after stroke: measurement and recovery over the first three months. J Neurol Neurosurg Psychiatry 1987; 50:714–719.
180. McCulloch K, Cook EW III, Fleming WC, Novack TA, Nepomuceno CS, Taub E. A reliable test of upper extremity ADL function. Arch Phys Med Rehabil 1988; 69:755.
181. Nouri FM, Lincoln NB. An extended activities of daily living scale for stroke patients. Clin Rehabil 1987; 1:301–305.
182. Viitanen M, Fugl-Meyer KS, Bernspang B, Fugl-Meyer AR. Life satisfaction in long-term survivors after stroke. Scand J Rehabil Med 1988; 20:17–24.
183. Astrom M, Asplund K, Astrom T. Psychosocial function and life satisfaction after stroke. Stroke 1992; 23:527–531.
184. Santus G, Rezenigo A, Caregnato R, Inzoli MR. Social and family integration of hemiplegic elderly patients one year after stroke. Stroke 1990; 21:1019–1022.
185. Niemi M, Laaksonen MA, Kotila M, Waltimo O. Quality of life four years after stroke. Stroke 1988; 19:1101–1107.
186. Smith DL, Akhtar AJ, Garraway WM. Motor function after stroke. Age Ageing 1985; 14:46–48.
187. Bonita R, Beaglehole R. Recovery of motor function after stroke. Stroke 1988; 19:1497–1500.
188. Price SJ, Reding ML. Physical therapy philosophies and strategies. In: Good DC, Couch JR, eds. Handbook of Neurorehabilitation. New York: Marcel Dekker, 1994:181–196.
189. Bobath B. Adult hemiplegia: Evaluation and Treatment. London: William Heinmann Medical Books, 1970.
190. Carr JH, Shepherd RB. A Motor Relearning Programme for Stroke. London: William Heinemann Medical Books, 1987.
191. Erst E. A review of stroke rehabilitation and physiotherapy. Stroke 1990; 21:1081–1085.
192. Basmajian JV, Gowland CA, Finlayson AJ, Hall AL, Swanson LR, Stratford PW, Trotler JE, Branstater ME. Stroke treatment: comparison of integrated behavioral-physical therapy vs traditional therapy programs. Arch Phys Med Rehabil 1987; 68:267–272.
193. Dickstein R, Hocherman S, Pillar T, Shaham R. Stroke rehabilitation: three exercise therapy approaches. Phys Ther 1986; 66:1233–1238.

194. Wagenaar RC, Meijer OG, van Wieinrgen PCW, Kuik DJ, Hazenberg GJ, Lindeboom J, Wichers F, Rijswijk H. The functional recovery of stroke: a comparison between neurodevelopmental and the Brunnstrom method. Scand J Rehabil Med 1990; 22:1–8.
195. Wagenaar RC, Meijer OG. Effects of stroke rehabilitation (1). A critical review of the literature. J Rehabil Sci 1991; 4:61–73.
196. Taub E, Miller NE, Novack TA, Cook EW, Fleming WC, Nepomuceno CS, Connell JS, Crago JE. Technique to improve chronic motor deficit after stroke. Arch Phys Med Rehabil 1993; 74:347–354.
197. Taub E, Wolf SL. Constraint induced movement techniques to facilitate upper extremity use in stroke patients. Top Stroke Rehabil 1997; 3(4):38–61.
198. Hesse S, Bertelt C, Schaffrin A, Malezic M, Mauritz K-H. Restoration of gait in nonambulatory hemiparetic patients by treadmill training with partial body weight-support. Arch Phys Med Rehabil 1994; 75:1087–1093.
199. Hassid E, Rose D, Commisarow J, Guttry M, Dobkin BH. Improved gait symmetry in hemiparetic stroke patients induced during body weight-supported treadmill stepping. J Neurol Rehabil 1997; 11:21–26.
200. Laven L. Adaptive equipment. In: Good DC, Couch JR, eds. Handbook of Neurorehabilitation. New York: Marcel Dekker, 1994:317–341.
201. Good DC, Supan TJ. Basic principles of orthotics in neurologic disorders. In: Aiesen ML, ed. Orthotics in Neurologic Rehabilitation. New York: Demos, 1992:1–23.
202. Michael JW. Orthotic treatment of neurological deficits. In: Good DC, Couch JR, eds. Handbook of Neurorehabilitation. New York: Marcel Dekker, 1994:261–315.
203. Skilbeck CE, Wade DT, Langton Hewer R, Wood VA. Recovery after stroke. J Neurol Neurosurg Psychiatry 1983; 46:5–8.
204. Kertesz A. What do we learn from recovery from aphasia? Adv Neurol 1988; 47:277–292.
205. Lazar RB, Rubin SM. Speech therapy and communicative disorders in neurological rehabilitation. In: Good DC, Couch JR, eds. Handbook of Neurorehabilitation. New York: Marcel Dekker, 1994:219–241.
206. Albert ML, Helm-Estabrooks N. Diagnosis and treatment of aphasia. Part 2. JAMA 1988; 259:1205–1210.
207. Benson DF. Aphasia rehabiltation. Arch Neurol 1979; 36:187–189.
208. Fiedler RC, Granger CV. Uniform data system for medical rehabilitation. Report of first admissions for 1995. Am J Phys Med Rehabil 1997; 76:76–81.
209. Subacute Care: Policy Synthesis and Market Area Analysis. Submitted to: Department of Health and Human Services, Office of the Assistant Secretary for Planning and Evaluation, Washington, DC. Submitted by: Lewin-VHI, Inc., Nov. 1, 1995.
210. Scanlon WJ. Director, Health Financing and Systems Issues, Health, Education and Human Services Division. Testimony before the Committee on Finance, U.S. Senate, April 9, 1997. U.S. General Accounting Office. GAO/T-HEHS-97-106.
211. Keith RA, Wilson DB, Guitierrez P. Acute and subacute rehabilitation for stroke: a comparison. Arch Phys Med Rehabil 1995; 76:495–500.

212. Kramer AM, Steiner JF, Schlenker RE, Eilertsen TB, Hrincevich CA, Tropea DA, Ahmad LA, Eckhoff DG. Outcomes and costs after hip fracture and stroke. A comparison of rehabilitation settings. JAMA 1997; 277:396–404.
213. Wright RE, Rao N, Smith RM, Harvey RF. Risk factors for death and emergency transfer in acute and subacute inpatient rehabilitation. Arch Phys Med Rehabil 1996; 77:1049–1055.
214. Welch HG, Wennberg DE, Welch WP. The use of Medicare home health services. N Engl J Med 1996; 335:324–329.
215. Gladman JRF, Lincoln NB, Barer DH. A randomised controlled trial of domiciliary and hospital-based rehabilitation for stroke patients after discharge from hospital. J Neurol Neurosurg Psychiatry 1993; 56:960–966.

13

Pathophysiology of Ischemic Brain Damage

Shiva Sarraf-Yazdi, Daniel Laskowitz, and David S. Warner
Duke University Medical Center, Durham, North Carolina

INTRODUCTION

The brain is a complex organ which tolerates only minimal ischemic insult. Despite decades of intense research, the cerebral response to ischemia is only partially understood. This is reflected by the limited therapies available to patients presenting with stroke. With the exception of tissue plasminogen activator and in some countries nimodipine, there is little the clinician can offer other than diagnosis and supportive care.

Research has demonstrated that numerous critical events occur during the first few minutes of ischemia. Chief among these phenomena are energy failure, massive release of excitatory neurotransmitters, and the concomitant opening of ionic channels which perturb cellular homeostasis. Secondary events include cellular (cytotoxic) edema, production of free radicals, inhibition of protein synthesis, intracellular acidosis, repetitive spontaneous depolarizations, inflammation, initiation of apoptotic mechanisms, and disregulation of DNA repair.

These pathomechanisms, as defined in laboratory models of cerebral ischemia, will be reviewed in this chapter. When possible, correlations will be made with data derived from human studies, although that information is limited. Pharmacologic therapy of cerebral ischemia will be considered, with specific emphasis on the use of these agents as tools to define and test hypotheses concerning mechanisms of ischemic brain damage. Finally, two physiologic conditions known to profoundly affect ischemic outcome, temperature and glycemic state, will be considered in detail.

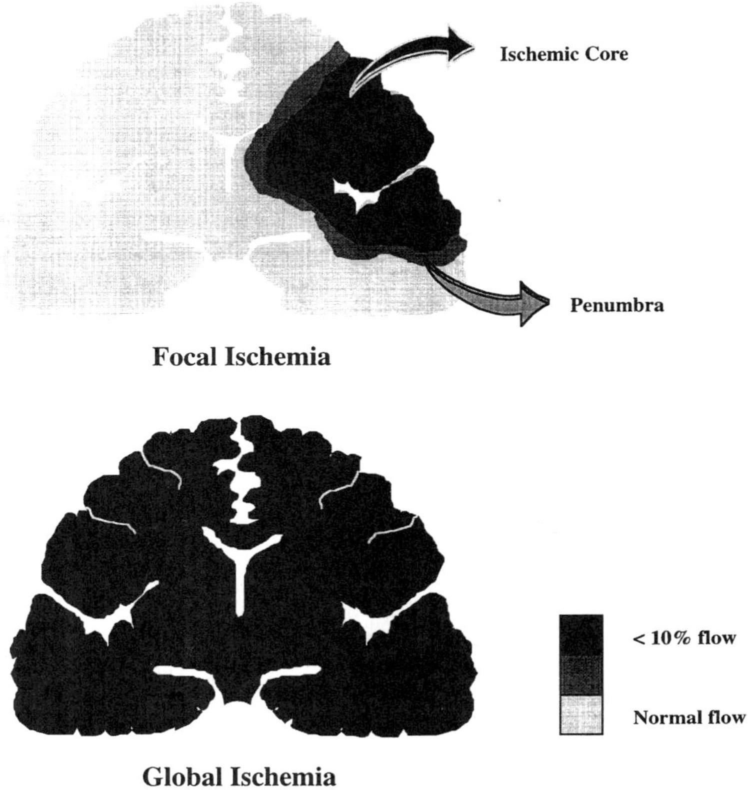

Figure 1 Global ischemia is classically associated with events such as cardiac arrest, resulting in hypoperfusion of the entire organ. A chief characteristic of global ischemia is absence of collateral flow to ischemic tissue. Focal ischemia represents occlusion of an artery distal to the Circle of Willis such as the middle cerebral artery. Because collateral flow from other vascular networks can be recruited, brain tissue sustains graded degrees of hypoperfusion, resulting in a densely ischemic core (pathophysiologically resembling global ischemia) surrounded by a penumbral zone. In the penumbra, the fate of neurons is precarious but presumably more salvageable than is the case for the ischemic core.

We will start with some definitions. *Cerebral ischemia* is a hemodynamic insult resulting in reduction of cerebral blood flow to values, which if sustained, will cause irreversible neuronal injury. *Outcome* from this insult can be quantified on either a histologic or neurologic (behavioral) basis. Two forms of ischemia are often discussed. *Global ischemia* is classically associated with events such as cardiac arrest resulting in hypoperfusion of the entire organ (Fig. 1). This term is also applied to states of regional hypoperfusion where there is no potential for recruitment of collateral flow (e.g., hemispheric ischemia). *Focal ischemia* represents occlusion of an artery distal to the circle of Willis such as the middle cerebral artery. Because collateral flow can occur, brain tissue sustains graded degrees of hypoperfusion, resulting in a densely *ischemic core* (pathophysiologically resembling global ischemia) surrounded by a *penumbral zone*. In the penumbra, the fate of neurons is precarious but presumably more salvageable than is the case for the ischemic core.

ENERGY FAILURE

The brain constitutes <5% of total body weight, yet may require up to 20% of cardiac output to maintain viability. This principally relates to delivery of oxygen and glucose, two metabolic substrates for which the brain has little storage capacity. Abrupt cessation of the delivery of either (e.g., anoxia or hypoglycemic shock) results in onset of electroencephalographic isoelectricity in seconds and total depletion of ATP within the first several minutes (Fig. 2). The implications of this energy failure are major.

Because neurons require energy for ionic homeostasis, ischemia results in rapid deterioration of ionic gradients. In particular, Ca^{2+} fluxes intracellularly (see below). However, loss of sodium ion gradients is also deleterious, the first manifestation of which is edema. Initially this edema is cytotoxic in nature, reflecting only a redistribution of water from the extracellular to intracellular compartments as sodium concentrations equilibrate across the cell membrane. Cytotoxic edema is rapidly reversible upon restoration of perfusion and is contrasted with vasogenic edema which occurs at a later stage of tissue injury. Vasogenic edema occurs only if the ischemic insult is severe enough to open the blood-brain barrier. Vasogenic edema is attributable to extravasation of proteins from plasma to interstitium, causing obligatory flow of free water into the extracellular space. Vasogenic edema resolves only after the infarct matures and undergoes necrosis.

Energy failure also results in loss of control of hydrogen ion homeostasis. Regulation of intracellular pH is energy dependent and involves an antiporter exchange with sodium ions. Loss of sodium ion homeostasis would serve to promote intracellular acidosis. This acidosis may inhibit several key enzymatic steps of glucose metabolism, enhance edema, and promote free-radical formation.

CALCIUM HOMEOSTASIS

Intracellular Ca^{2+} ion concentration is used to regulate numerous intracellular functions. Because the extracellular/intracellular Ca^{2+} concentration gradient is

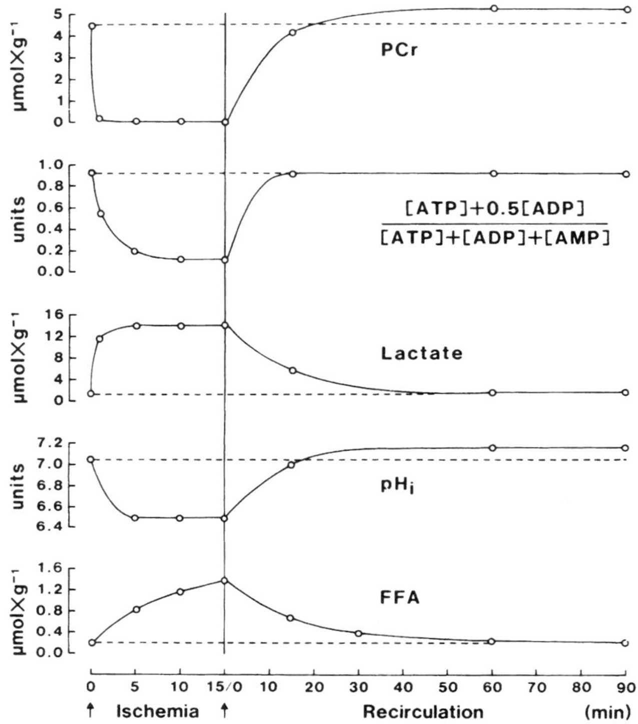

Figure 2 Changes in cerebral cortical concentrations of phosphocreatinine (Pcr), lactate, and free fatty acids (FFA), as well as in the adenylate energy charge and intracellular pH (pHi), during and following transient global ischemia. (From Ref. 2.)

normally 10,000:1, considerable energy is required to maintain homeostasis. The neuron has several mechanisms that regulate transport of Ca^{2+} into the cell (Fig. 3). Intracellular concentrations may also be controlled by binding with calmodulin and sequestration of Ca^{2+} into organelles. Finally, transport of Ca^{2+} out of the cell occurs via energy-dependent processes. It is clear that an overload of intracellular Ca^{2+} leads to irreversible injury of the neuron,[1] and this has been suggested to be the final common pathway of ischemically mediated neuronal death.[2,3]

Not surprisingly, attention has focused on interventions which inhibit entry of Ca^{2+} into the energy-deficient neuron. Ca^{2+} may enter via either voltage-sensitive Ca^{2+} channels, which are opened with neuronal depolarization (either physiologic or as a terminal event), or via agonist-operated channels, which are activated by release of excitatory neurotransmitters (i.e., glutamate or aspartate) from the presynaptic cell (Fig. 4).[3] Pharmacologic agents have been identified

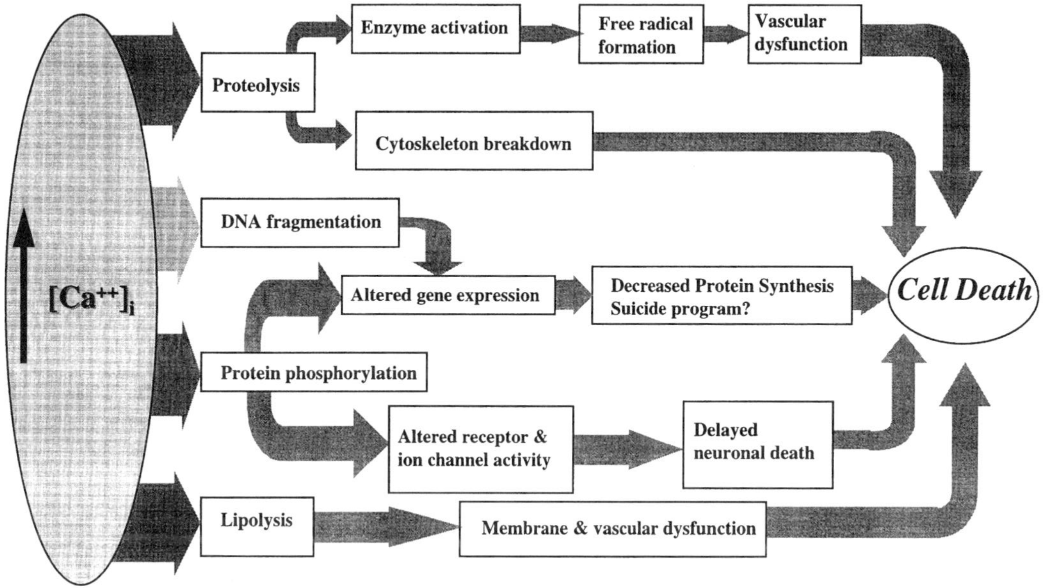

Figure 3 Intracellular Ca^{2+} concentration serves to regulate numerous intracellular functions and is therefore tightly regulated. Because the extracellular:intracellular Ca^{2+} gradient is approximately 10,000:1, energy failure allows massive influx of Ca^{2+}. Large increases in intracellular Ca^{2+} $[Ca^{2+}]_i$ initiate numerous cascades which may lead to cell death.

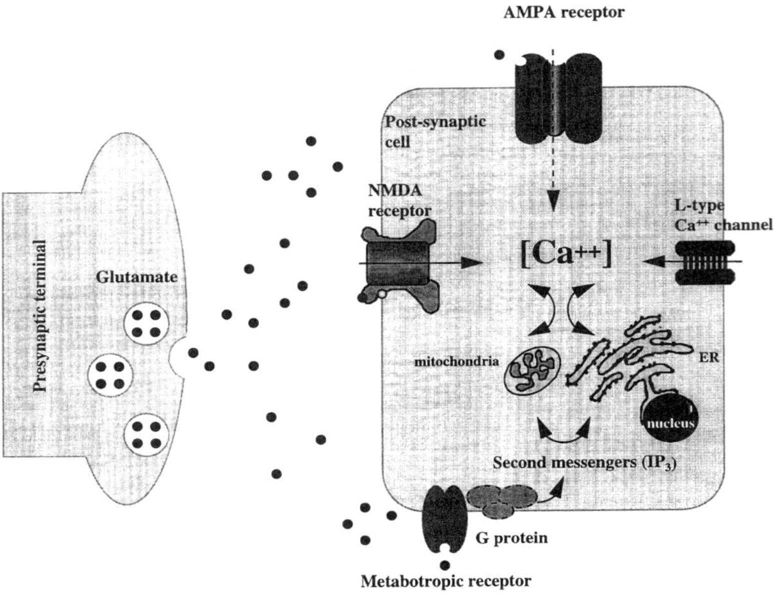

Figure 4 Intracellular Ca^{2+} can become increased by numerous mechanisms. High conductance influx is afforded by activation of the NMDA receptor which requires coagonism by glutamate and glycine and alleviation of a Mg^{2+} blockade during depolarization of the neuron. Depolarization also leads to opening of lower conductance L-type, voltage-dependent Ca^{2+} channels. Agonism of the metabotropic receptor by glutamate leads to release of intracellular stores of Ca^{2+}. The AMPA receptor is normally impermeable to Ca^{2+}. However, postischemic conformational change of the AMPA receptor subunits permits Ca^{2+} entry.

that inhibit Ca^{2+} influx through either portal of entry, and under some conditions these agents improve outcome from ischemic events.

A prototypical voltage-sensitive Ca^{2+} channel antagonist is the dihydropyridine compound nimodipine. This agent, which also exhibits preferential cerebrovascular dilatation,[4] has been evaluated for efficacy in treating humans with brain ischemia under several different conditions. With respect to global ischemia, Forsman et al. reported on the administration of nimodipine during out-of-hospital resuscitation from cardiac arrest.[5] Although treated patients exhibited a more rapid return to consciousness and greater cerebral blood flow during subsequent evaluation, no improvement in final neurologic status was observed when compared to those treated with placebo. This study was performed on a small group of patients. A larger, similar study was completed in Finland but again little benefit for nimodipine was observed.[6]

Nimodipine has also been evaluated in the context of focal ischemia in humans.[7–10] Most of these studies could be criticized on methodologic grounds (e.g., small sample sizes, delayed institution of therapy), but the trend suggests a modest improvement in outcome if nimodipine is administered.[11] None of the studies found administration of nimodipine to be detrimental; i.e., systemic vasodilatory effects were well tolerated.[12] Nimodipine has also been found to be mildly efficacious in the treatment of vasospasm caused by subarachnoid hemorrhage and has generally been accepted as a requisite therapy in the treatment of this disorder.[13,14] However, it remains unclear whether improved outcome is attributable to inhibition of neuronal Ca^{2+} influx or direct vascular effects of the drug. Nicardipine, an analog of nimodipine, has also been shown to reduce incidence of symptomatic vasospasm in patients with subarachnoid hemorrhage. Despite this, long-term neurologic outcome with nimodipine was not superior to treatment with hypertensive-hypervolemic therapy.[15,16]

Cumulatively, these studies indicate that the overall clinical effect of inhibition of Ca^{2+} entry via voltage-sensitive Ca^{2+} channels is weak. This may be attributable to the fact that antagonism of the voltage-sensitive Ca^{2+} channel does little to inhibit Ca^{2+} entry via agonist-operated channels which provide high conductivity for Ca^{2+} in the ischemic state. The role of agonist-operated Ca^{2+} channels will be considered under the topic of excitotoxicity.

EXCITOTOXICITY

Two concepts were appreciated in the mid-1980s. The first is selective vulnerability (Fig. 5). Selective vulnerability refers to a heterogeneous sensitivity of different brain regions to brief episodes of ischemia (similar to differential sensitivity of plants in a garden to the first autumn frost). Even within regions such as the hippocampus, a graded sensitivity by cell type can be observed.[17] Particularly sensitive are pyramidal cells in the CA1 sector. A standardized insult can result in near total obliteration of this population while pyramidal neurons in the CA3 sector (only micrometers away) are totally spared. This cannot be accounted for by differences in intraischemic blood flow.[18] What does distinguish these neurons is degree of glutamatergic afferentation, the CA1 sector by far having the richest supply. Similar findings are observed in the caudoputamen, layers III–V of the cortex, and Purkinje neurons of the cerebellum.

The second concept is that of delayed neuronal necrosis (Fig. 6). Neuropathologists have long known that if autopsy occurs immediately after cardiac arrest, little or no light microscopic changes in brain can be detected. However, modern cardiopulmonary resuscitation techniques have allowed individuals to survive severe global ischemic insults for extended durations after cardiac arrest. When autopsies are performed after several days of recovery,

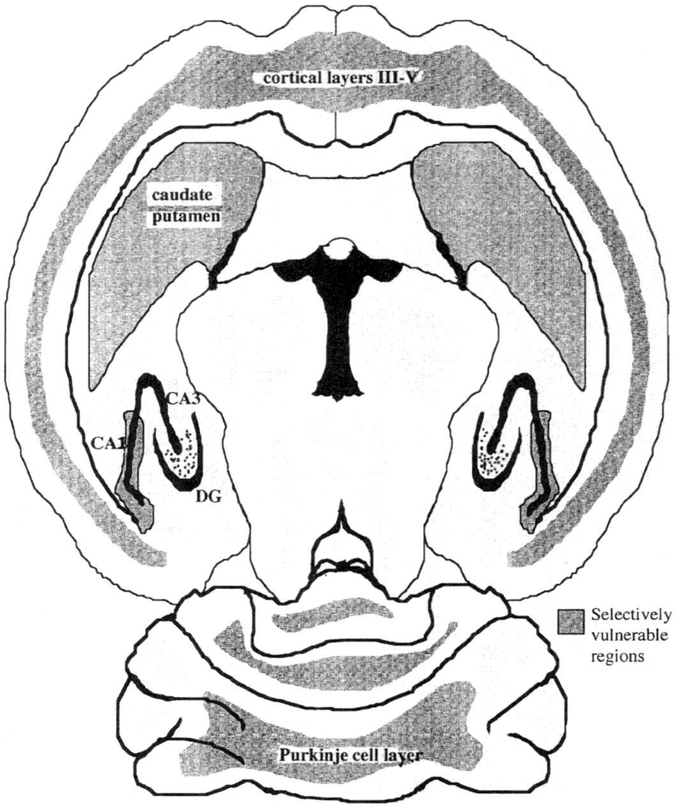

Figure 5 The brain exhibits differential regional sensitivity (selective vulnerability) to a global ischemic insult. Selectively vulnerable regions include the CA1 sector of the hippocampus, caudate and putamen, layers III–V of the cortex, and Purkinje neurons of the cerebellum.

neurohistologic changes not only become evident but are consistent with the phenomenon of selective vulnerability discussed above.[19] This correlates well with a documented impairment of memory in survivors of cardiac arrest.[20] Thus, the final extent of histologic damage cannot be observed until at least several days after the insult has occurred.

In the mid-1980s, major progress was made in the development of rodent models of ischemia which allowed prolonged recovery from the ischemic insult so as to routinely account for delayed neuronal necrosis.[21–23] The importance of delayed neuronal necrosis is enormous. Although resumption of ATP synthesis, correction of intracellular acidosis, and partial recovery of electroen-

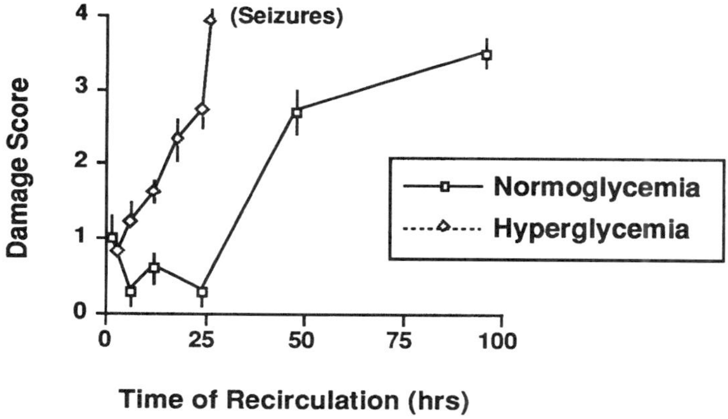

Figure 6 Rats recovering from 10 minutes of severe transient forebrain ischemia underwent histologic evaluation of extent of neuronal necrosis in selectively vulnerable regions at different intervals after reperfusion of the brain. In this case damage in the CA1 was sector of the hippocampus is depicted. A damage score of 0 indicates no histologic changes; a score of 4 indicates infarct. Delayed neuronal necrosis is evident in that histologic damage does not become manifest until the second day of recovery. Animals studied in parallel, which were infused with glucose prior to onset of ischemia, are also depicted. Note the accelerated rate of delayed neuronal necrosis and onset of seizures at approximately 24 hours postischemia in this group. (From Ref. 134.)

cephalographic activity occur within minutes after onset of reperfusion, it is clear that pathologic cascades are initiated by the ischemic insult which require time to result in cell death. The interval between reperfusion and cell death represents a potential therapeutic window. If the pathologic cascades can be identified, pharmacologic intervention seems possible even for the patient with delayed entry to medical care. There are also implications for laboratory studies of ischemia. Because it takes several days for final maturation of injury to become evident, outcome studies examining efficacy of a drug or physiologic intervention should permit sufficient recovery from the insult for delayed neuronal necrosis to be observed. Experiments using shorter recovery intervals should be considered inconclusive.

Several breakthroughs followed. It was shown with microdialysis studies that extracellular glutamate concentrations in the selectively vulnerable CA1 sector of the hippocampus become massively increased during ischemia and the immediate recirculation period (Fig. 7).[24,25] Ischemia also induces a surge of spontaneous neuronal activity in the same region, consistent with an abundance of excitatory neurotransmission.[26] In cell culture models, glutamate was shown to result in cell death when administered in concentrations similar to those found

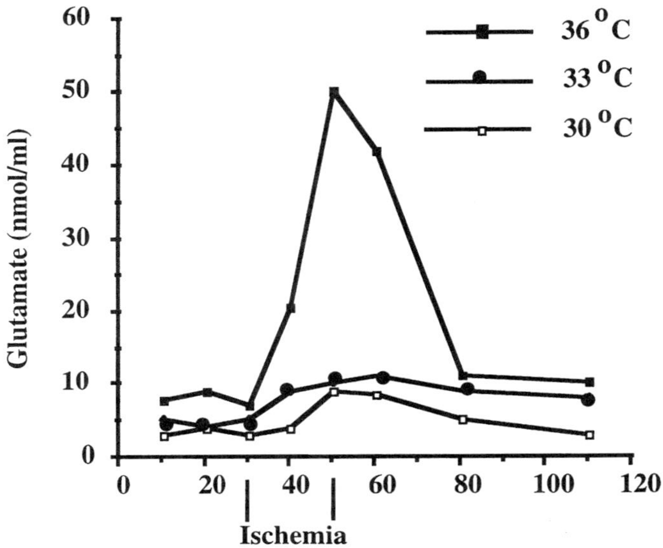

Figure 7 Extracellular glutamate, as measured by microdialysis, increases rapidly after onset of ischemia. Reperfusion allows return to normal concentrations. Note that modest reduction of brain temperature is effective in preventing this increase in extracellular glutamate. (From Ref. 114.)

in vivo during ischemia.[27] Finally, the extent of cell death was related to the concentration of extracellular Ca^{2+} in the culture medium.[28]

As stated above, Ca^{2+} may enter the cell via agonist-operated Ca^{2+} channels (Fig. 8). These channels are activated by glutamate. In fact, there are numerous postsynaptic glutamate receptor subtypes (e.g., NMDA, AMPA, t-ACPD), so named for the antagonists used to identify them. The most pertinent with respect to Ca^{2+} entry is the N-methyl-D-aspartate (NMDA) receptor. Agonism of the NMDA glutamate receptor is allosterically facilitated by the amino acid glycine which in and of itself is probably not a neurotransmitter but instead, a ubiquitous cofactor present in the synaptic cleft. When glycine and glutamate bind to the NMDA receptor complex during depolarization, a magnesium ion block is alleviated in the associated NMDA ionophore, and influx of Ca^{2+}, Na^{+}, and water ensues.[29,30] Thus antagonism of NMDA gated Ca^{2+} influx is possible by a variety of mechanisms including competitive antagonism of the glycine or glutamate receptors or noncompetitive antagonism of the NMDA ionophore.

The AMPA channel may become involved in ischemic injury in several ways. Activation of the AMPA receptor allows fast excitation, presumably being the focus of Na^{+} flux allowing depolarization which in turn contributes to

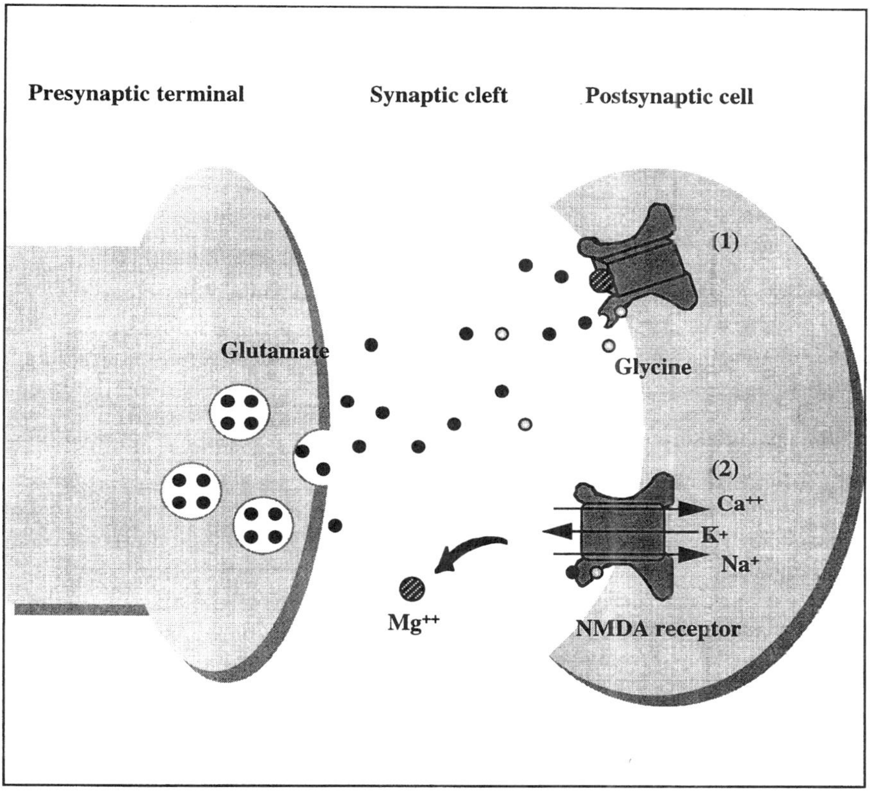

Figure 8 (1) Inactivated NMDA ionophore. Glutamate has not bound with the NMDA receptor. Glycine binding is requisite for channel activation but the glycine recognition site is often saturated by endogenous glycine present in the synaptic cleft. Magnesium ion causes a physical blockade of the Ca^{2+} channel. (2) Activated NMDA ionophore. The Mg^{2+} blockade is alleviated by depolarization of the neuron (via fast excitation at the AMPA receptor) in conjunction with binding of both glutamate and glycine to the NMDA receptor. Because all of these events must occur simultaneously, numerous potential sites exist for inhibition of Ca^{2+} influx via the NMDA ionophore. Competitive antagonists (e.g., selfotel) compete at the glutamate binding site. Noncompetitive antagonists (e.g., dizocilpine, ketamine, Mg^{2+}) act to physically block the Ca^{2+} channel. Glycine antagonists (e.g., ACEA 1021) competitively antagonize the glycine recognition site.

the release of Mg^{2+} blockade in the NMDA ionophore and opening of that channel to Ca^{2+}. Influx of Na^{+} through this ionophore may also enhance edema. The AMPA receptor associated ionophore is normally impermeable to divalent cations such as Ca^{2+}. However, ischemia may serve as a molecular trigger altering

AMPA receptor subunit assembly, resulting in Ca^{2+} permeability and enhanced toxicity of endogenous glutamate during the recovery interval.[31]

Finally, we consider the metabotropic receptor. This receptor does not operate by means of a transmembrane ion flux. In contrast, the metabotropic receptor stimulates synthesis of inositol triphosphate (via a G-protein-linked mechanism) which activates release of Ca^{2+} stores from intracellular organelles and effectively increases free intracellular Ca^{2+} concentration.[32]

Dramatic results have been achieved in focal ischemia with NMDA receptor antagonists. Both competitive antagonists such as selfotel (CGS 19755) and noncompetitive antagonists such as dizocilpine (MK-801) have been shown to reduce infarct volumes by ≈50% even if given at substantial intervals after onset of focal ischemia in laboratory animals.[33,34] However, these same compounds are entirely ineffective against global insults.[35] The reason for this is still unclear. One hypothesis is that with single-drug therapy, antagonism of agonist operated Ca^{2+} channels leaves Ca^{2+} flux unopposed through voltage-dependent Ca^{2+} channels and reconfigured AMPA channels.

Another theory has been proposed to explain the efficacy of NMDA antagonists in ameliorating focal ischemic injury which builds upon the concept of spontaneous depolarization (Fig. 9). Spontaneous depolarization is observed as an episodic and transient loss of direct-current potential within the marginally perfused focal ischemic penumbra.[36] Because some blood flow persists, the tissue may be able to repolarize but this state remains precarious leading to episodic depolarization and repolarization of the tissue. Most troublesome is the large increase in metabolic demand required for mass repolarization. In normal tissue, cerebral blood flow can be increased to meet this demand such as would occur during the electrophysiologically similar process of spreading depression. In contrast, collateral vessels in ischemic tissue are already maximally dilated and thus are incapable of providing an appropriate blood flow response. Consequently, tissue oxygen content episodically falls below critical levels causing repeated secondary insults to penumbral tissue.[37] The frequency of such insults presumably defines the eventual fate of that tissue. This theory is supported by observations that NMDA and AMPA receptor antagonists effectively block spontaneous depolarization, correlating with the known ameliorative effect of such compounds on infarct size.[38,39] In contrast, during global ischemia, spontaneous depolarizations have not been observed and hence under such conditions this mechanism of action may not be available to NMDA receptor antagonists.

There is some concern regarding the human importance of spontaneous depolarizations in focal ischemia. Such events have not been described in humans sustaining stroke. This may be due to invasive monitoring which is required to identify these depolarizations, thereby limiting examination on a widespread basis. Alternatively, such depolarizations may not exist. Spontaneous depolar-

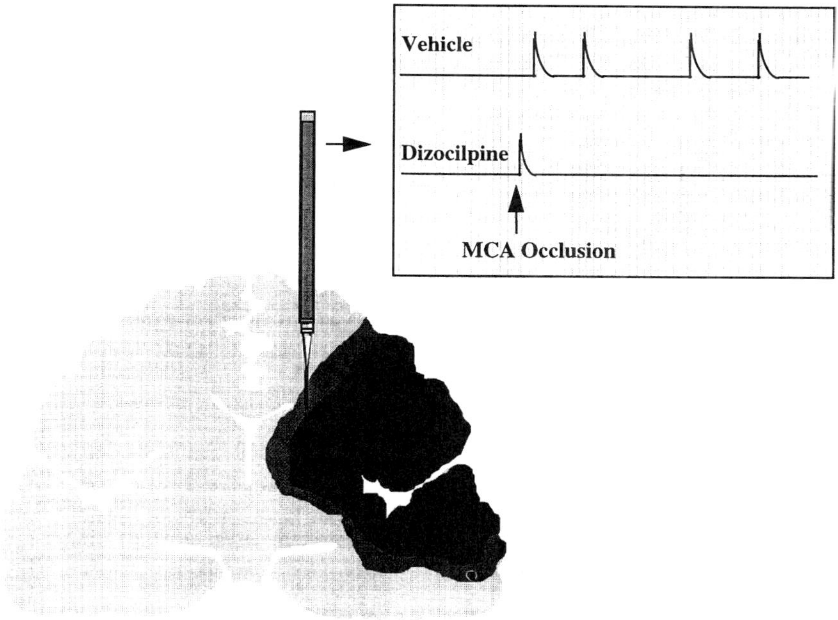

Figure 9 Placement of a direct-current recording microelectrode in the ischemic penumbra allows measurement of episodic waves of depolarization in marginally perfused tissue. Although repolarization frequently occurs, the depolarization and recovery place metabolic stress on the tissue. Concomitant measurement of tissue PO_2 and electrocortical activity reveals corresponding interval of tissue hypoxia sufficient to obliterate EEG activity. These secondary insults are believed to cause expansion of the infarct. Spontaneous depolarizations are inhibited by glutamate receptor antagonists (e.g., dizocilpine) and hypothermia, suggesting this to be a beneficial mechanism of action of these therapies in brain sustaining a focal ischemic insult.

ization waves have marked electrophysiologic similarity to spreading depression, which also has been difficult to identify in humans.[40] However, spontaneous depolarization is readily observed in brains of higher-order animals. Further, spontaneous depolarization waves have been observed in head trauma patients.[41] To date, therefore, inhibition of spontaneous depolarizations as a potential mechanism of glutamate antagonists during focal ischemic insults in humans remains speculative.

In contrast to NMDA receptor antagonists, compounds that antagonize glutamate at the AMPA receptor have been found to be protective against both focal and global ischemic injury.[42–46] The mechanism by which AMPA receptor antagonists ameliorate global injury is not clear. It is speculated that because fast excitation is inhibited by AMPA receptor antagonism neither the NMDA or voltage-dependent Ca^{2+} channels become activated. Others, however, have questioned the efficacy of AMPA receptor antagonists in global ischemia. Evidence has been presented that the predominant mechanism of action in these models is a non-specific prolonged reduction in brain temperature, which is sufficient in and of itself to be neuroprotective.[47]

Several AMPA receptor antagonists are in development which may have clinical utility. An additional advantage for this approach to therapy is absence of psychotomimetic side effects for this class of drug. Such problems have plagued clinical development of NMDA receptor antagonists which produce a hallucinatory mental state similar to that caused by ketamine.[48,49] Similarly, psychotomimetic effects seem to be absent for compounds which antagonize glutamatergic neurotransmission indirectly by competing with glycine at the NMDA recognition site. Glycine receptor antagonists have been found efficacious in animal models of focal (but not global) ischemia.[50,51]

FREE RADICAL FORMATION

Following ischemia onset, excessive glutamate release causes Ca^{2+} influx into ischemic neurons. Intracellular Ca^{2+} activates phospholipases, including phospholipase A2. This in turn, releases free fatty acids including arachidonic acid which is subsequently metabolized by cyclo-oxygenase and lipo-oxygenase to form vasoactive substances and reactive oxygen species.[52] These free radicals and reactive oxygen species abstract hydrogen from the polyunsaturated fatty acids to form free fatty acid radicals, which then react with other lipids to propagate the process of lipid peroxidation (Fig. 10). Although lipid peroxidation may occur anywhere in the body, the brain is uniquely vulnerable due to the high concentration of polyunsaturated fatty acids such as lineolic and arachidonic acids. Lactate accumulation caused by anaerobic metabolism in nonperfused tissue causes a local acidosis, which also favors this reaction.

Nitric oxide is also known to play a crucial role in free-radical formation.[53] Two isoforms of nitric oxide have been shown important. Endothelial nitric oxide serves as a vasodilator. Pharmacologic inhibition of endothelial nitric oxide synthase may present adverse effects if instituted during ischemia due to vasoconstriction and reduced cerebral blood flow. The formation of neuronal nitric oxide is stimulated by Ca^{2+} entry. Binding of Ca^{2+} to calmodulin serves to activate neuronal nitric oxide synthase. Nitric oxide itself is a weak free radical. However, when nitric oxide reacts with superoxide anion, peroxynitrite is formed which is highly reactive and thought to be a principle mediator of ischemia-in-

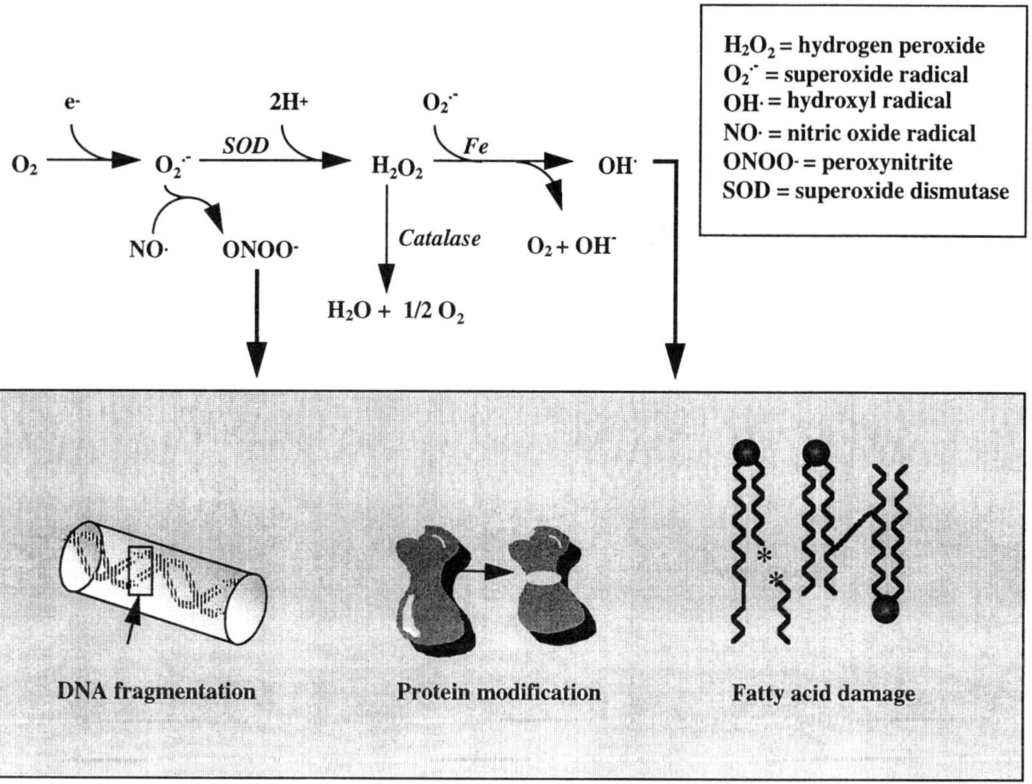

Figure 10 Free-radical cascades are initiated by both reperfusion and inflammatory mechanisms. Production of highly reactive species such as peroxynitrite and hydroxyl radical results in structural damage to numerous intracellular and cell membrane constituents. To some extent these processes are abated by natural free-radical scavengers, including superoxide dismutase and catalase.

duced free radical injury.[54] This predicts that interventions which serve to reduce availability of either neuronal nitric oxide or superoxide will retard formation of peroxynitrite and thereby reduce ischemic injury.

The importance of these events to outcome has been documented by use of both pharmacologic agents and genetically engineered mice. Both neuronal nitric oxide synthase antagonists and superoxide dismutase itself reduce ischemic injury in laboratory models. Mice that carry transgenes allowing overexpression of superoxide dismutase have reduced injury from both focal and global ischemia.[55,56] Similarly, targeted disruption of the DNA coding sequence for neuronal nitric oxide synthase also reduces the size of focal ischemic lesions.[57] Conversely, targeted disruption of superoxide dismutase DNA coding sequences causes increased edema and enlarged infarcts after focal ischemia.[58]

INFLAMMATION

Although the histological progression of postischemic inflammation has been understood for some time, there has been considerable advancement in our understanding of the biochemical pathways associated with inflammation and how this has the potential to exacerbate tissue injury. Recent data suggest that this inflammatory reaction may contribute to immediate and delayed tissue injury after stroke, causing interest in the possibility of therapeutically manipulating the inflammatory cascade to ameliorate ischemic injury.

Inflammatory events following focal ischemia have been described in detail in both primates and rodents. The earliest evidence of inflammation after focal ischemia in rats occurs at 6 hours, when neutrophils begin to invade the ischemic parenchyma. After 3 days, there is a heavy neutrophil-predominant infiltrate in the injured tissue. From 5 to 15 days, there is evidence of reactive gliosis, neovascularization, and connective tissue matrix formation. During this period, the inflammatory infiltrate slowly changes from polymorphonuclear cells to mononuclear cells, and by 15 days, neutrophils are essentially absent.[59] The chronic lesion is characterized by cavitation, continued removal of necrotic and connective tissue by macrophages, and formation of a glial scar. It is worth noting that this time course may be significantly delayed in models of permanent focal ischemia, and neutrophil infiltration occurs sooner and to a greater extent in reperfused tissues than in permanently ischemic tissues.[60] This difference in the evolution of the inflammatory response between permanent ischemia and ischemia with reperfusion may assume increased clinical relevance with the trend toward early use of thrombolytic agents in acute stroke.

Understanding molecular mechanisms of this inflammatory reaction has led to novel therapeutic strategies. The hallmark of the acute inflammatory reaction is invasion of neutrophils which release proteases and participate in the formation of free radicals such as superoxide anion. Neutrophil migration is regulated by adhesive interactions between circulating leukocytes and the vascular endothelium (Fig. 11). The primary molecular species responsible for this interaction are integrins on the leukocyte cell surface (primarily CD11/CD18), and adhesion molecules expressed by the vascular endothelium. These adhesion molecules are rapidly expressed after exposure to inflammatory cytokines such as IL-1β and TNFα. Several studies have demonstrated that post-ischemic neurologic deficit is reduced when animals are pretreated with antibodies that functionally block these molecules.[61–64] In other models of permanent occlusion, there has been minimal beneficial effect, indicating a disparity between transient ischemia/reperfusion and permanent ischemia.[65]

Inflammatory cytokines such as TNFα, IL-6, and IL-1β are upregulated following ischemia, and may also play an important role in regulating the postischemic inflammatory process. Within the central nervous system, TNFα is produced primarily by microglia, although neuronal upregulation has been demonstrated shortly after ischemia as well. As mentioned previously, TNFα contributes to the propagation of the inflammatory response by upregulating expression of adhesion molecules by endothelial cells. TNFα is also associated with microglial activation and blood-brain barrier disruption. Although clearly contributing to the inflammatory cascade, it is likely that TNFα may also serve a protective function. Mice genetically engineered not to express the receptor for this protein actually have larger infarcts following focal ischemia than do controls.[66] Platelet activating factor is also increased acutely after injury, and has been suggested to be an important mediator of the early inflammatory reaction to ischemia. In addition to increasing blood-brain barrier permeability and vasoconstriction, platelet-activating factor may have a direct cytotoxic effect on neuronal cells.[67,68] Transforming growth factor beta-1 (TGF-β1) is a cytokine that opposes many of the inflammatory effects of pro-inflammatory cytokines such as IL-6, TNFα, and IL-1β. TGF-β is also upregulated by neurons following ischemia.[69] Preliminary observations suggest that TGF-β reduces infarct volume in a rabbit model of embolic stroke.[70]

A more thorough understanding of the role of inflammatory cytokines in modulating the response of brain to ischemic injury may lead to new pharmacologic strategies for minimizing brain injury after stroke. Preliminary work suggests a protective role for IL-1 receptor and platelet-activating factor antagonists in animal models.[67,68,71,72] Measurement of inflammatory cytokines may also have the potential for providing diagnostic and prognostic information, and may help identify patients with early stroke. In particular, recent observations suggest that early production of IL-6, which may be detectable in the cerebrospinal fluid and plasma, correlates with the eventual infarct size after acute stroke in humans.[73,74]

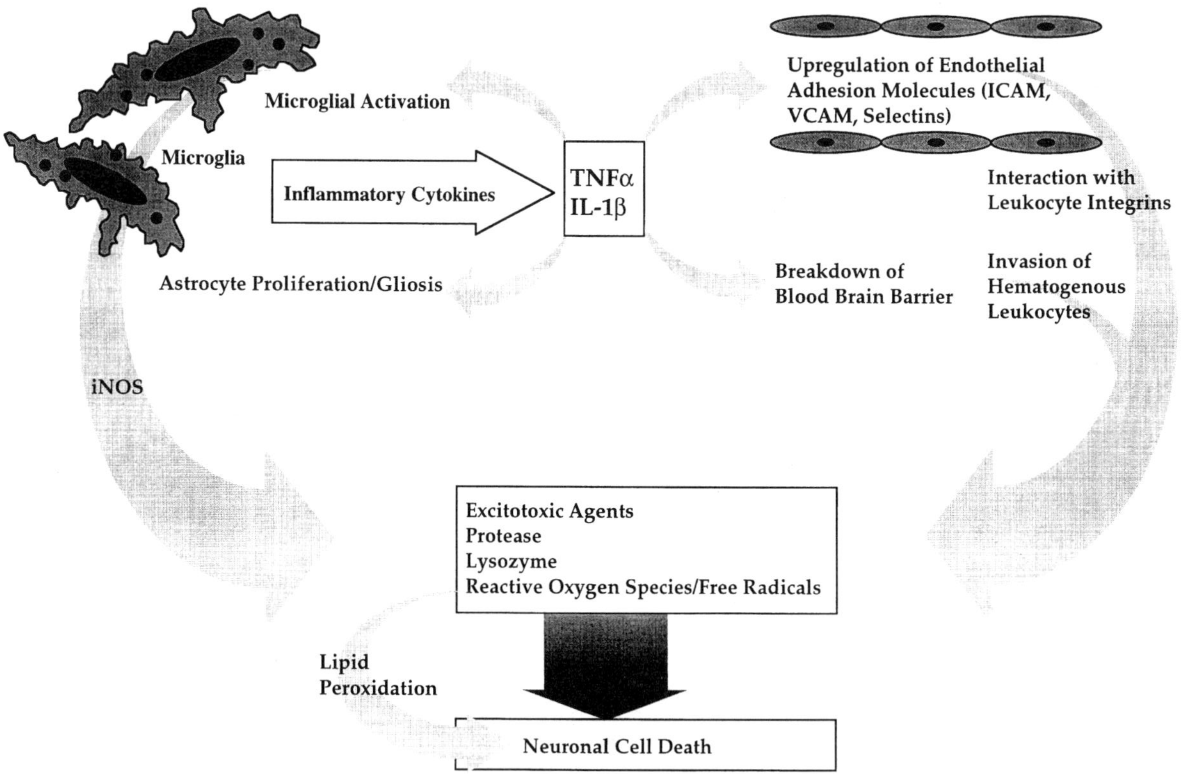

Figure 11 Recruitment of neutrophils and activation of microglial result in initiation of degradative inflammatory cascades in postischemic brain.

APOPTOSIS AND DISREGULATION OF DNA REPAIR

Because ischemia induces an injurious disregulation of many intracellular functions, it seems ironic that ischemia may also induce a highly regulated sequence of DNA transcriptional events which teleologically were designed to aid in development of the organism. Clues to involvement of native genetic code in the response to ischemia were found in studies that identified upregulation of immediate early genes and heat shock proteins.[75,76] Although these events can be classified as stress responses to ischemia, the concept that genetic code could mount an organized response to ischemia was revolutionary.

Further evidence was found in the field of apoptosis.[77] During development and maturity, homeostasis is maintained through a balance of cell proliferation and cell death. Two distinct processes of cell death can be recognized. Necrosis results from exogenous events causing passive cellular injury. Apoptosis is an active, gene-directed form of cell death. Apoptosis is strictly regulated and provides a mechanism for the removal of unnecessary or damaged cells. The histologic hallmarks of these two processes are blurred, making distinction sometimes difficult. As a result, controversy persists regarding the relative importance of these two mechanisms in ischemic cell death.

Evidence for apoptosis is largely derived from examination of proteins thought to represent apoptotic mechanisms. For example, the Bcl-2 protein is a known regulator of apoptosis during development. Bcl-2 suppresses apoptotic mechanisms that might otherwise respond to exogenous stimuli. Mutant mice overexpressing Bcl-2 have markedly reduced infarct volumes after focal ischemia when compared to normal animals.[78] Bcl-2 protein expression is also upregulated after global ischemia in the rat in structures resistant to ischemia.[79] In contrast, bax, a pro-apoptotic protein, was found to be upregulated in selectively vulnerable structures while expression of Bcl-2 was reduced. Besides suggesting an alternative mechanism for selective vulnerability, this work provides evidence that apoptotic mechanisms are active in the response to ischemia.

Perhaps the strongest support for an apoptotic mechanism of ischemic injury was provided in an experiment examining focal ischemia in the rat.[80] Animals were subjected to either 30 or 90 minutes of middle cerebral artery occlusion. Twenty-four hours after ischemia, large infarcts were found in the 90-minute group but little or no damage was seen in the 30 minute group. At 2 weeks postischemia, however, infarct size resulting from either duration of insult was large. This suggests initiation of apoptosis in the 30-minute group, which required a prolonged interval to result in tissue damage. Development of infarcts over the 2-week interval in the 30-minute group was inhibited by cycloheximide, a protein synthesis inhibitor, which presumably interfered with expression of pro-apoptotic proteins.

However, others have also examined rat brain after ischemia and found conflicting results. A prime mechanism of apoptosis is DNA fragmentation prior to cell death. When postischemic brains were sequentially analyzed at different intervals after ischemia, in most cases DNA fragmentation was evident only after other hallmarks of cell death had become evident, indicating a more important role for necrosis than apoptosis.[81]

The cell also possesses mechanisms to repair damaged DNA (such as what might result from free-radical production). Poly(ADP-ribose) polymerase (PARP) is an energy-dependent repair enzyme which is activated by DNA fragments (Fig. 12). The pivotal role of PARP in mediating ischemic death has been examined in mutant mice having targeted deletion of the genetic code for this protein.[82,83] PARP-deficient mice have a marked resistance to focal cerebral ischemia. Cell cultures made from brains of these PARP-deficient mice are also resistant to both NMDA and nitric oxide toxicity, indicating that PARP plays a role far downstream from Ca^{2+}-regulated mechanisms. Support for these findings was provided by studies which examined effects of pharmacologic antagonism of PARP synthesis in the rat.[84] Treated animals had markedly smaller infarcts after focal ischemia than did vehicle-treated controls. The presumed mechanism of injury to the neuron by PARP relates to its dependence on NAD for function. If ischemia induces massive upregulation of PARP activity, ATP will be depleted in the course of NAD synthesis, leading to generalized energy failure and delayed cell death.

HYPERGLYCEMIA

Laboratory research has presented a paradox to those dealing with cerebral ischemia. Although normal brain depends almost totally on a continuous delivery of exogenous glucose to maintain cellular energy requirements, ischemic or hypoxic brain finds continued glucose availability to be detrimental. Pursuit of an explanation has yielded a large body of information, some of which has considerable clinical relevance.

The initial observation that glucose infusion worsens ischemic outcome was serendipitous. Myers and Yamaguchi designed an experiment to assess the effects of brief cardiac arrest on learned visual tasks in fasted primates.[85] They recognized that successful cardiac resuscitation could be enhanced by prearrest intravenous volume loading. However, the investigators were inconsistent with the types of fluids administered. Most animals recovered from the cardiac arrest and had visual cortical function assessed, but two monkeys developed seizures and died early after reperfusion. In retrospect, the investigators recognized that those two monkeys had received dextrose in their fluid bolus, whereas those that survived had not. This association between glucose infusion and worsened out-

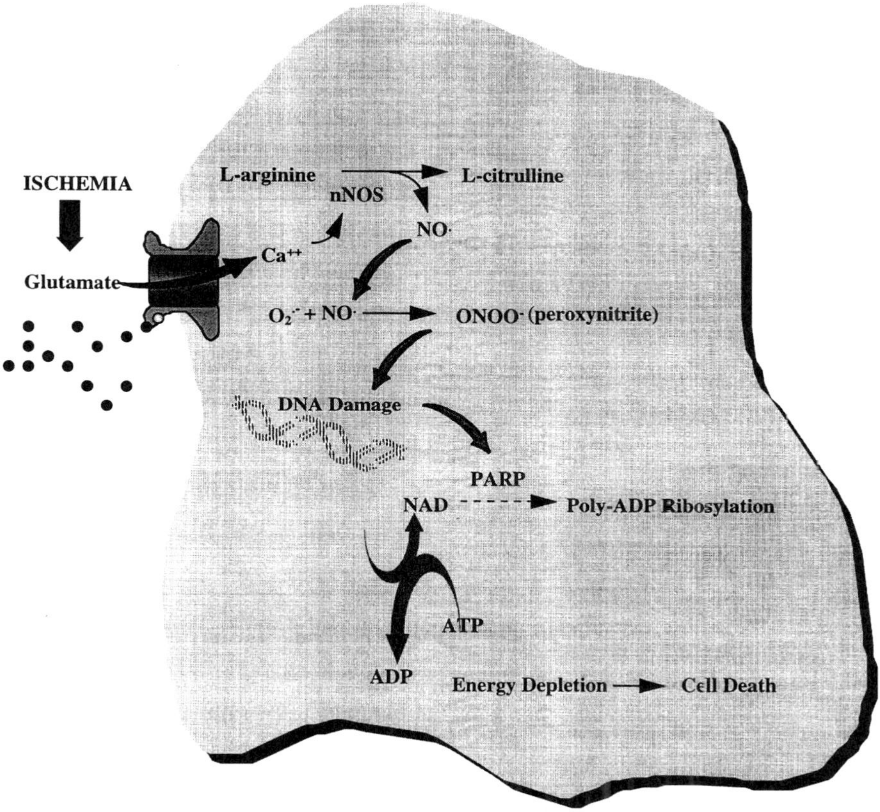

Figure 12 Experimental work using both transgenic mice and cell culture models has determined that poly(ADP-ribose) polymerase (PARP) becomes activated in postischemic brain. This enzyme, which serves to repair damage DNA, requires substantial energy derived from NAD to function. Overactivation of PARP by ischemia is believed to result in sufficient expenditure of energy to deplete reserves, resulting in cell death.

come from global ischemia was soon validated under more controlled conditions in the same laboratory, and has subsequently been repeated with remarkable consistency in numerous models, species, and research centers (Fig. 13).

Other investigators had suggested an unfavorable relationship between cerebral acidosis and ischemic injury.[86] It was not long until such acidosis was linked to glucose administration.[87] In the absence of sufficient oxygen supply, cellular energy requirements may be partially supported by anaerobic glycolysis. Under conditions of hypoxemia or ischemia, hyperglycemia would be expected to allow a disproportionate delivery of glucose and some ATP produc-

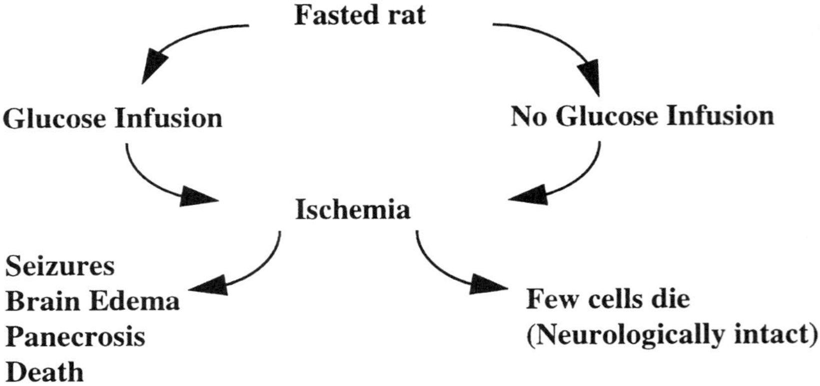

Figure 13 Pre-ischemic intravenous glucose infusion can have dramatic effects on outcome from global ischemia. An insult that causes only minor selective neuronal necrosis in fasted animals is lethal to animals made hyperglycemic prior to ischemia.

tion at the cost of an enhanced accumulation of lactate, the end product of glycolysis. Lactate has a pKa of 3.83; i.e., at physiologic pH virtually all of it is ionized. The predicted effect of preischemic glucose infusion would therefore be an intracellular acidosis. This acidosis is believed to be the cause of worsened outcome.[88]

Although investigative work has provided a very consistent series of outcome results, clinicians may still be uncertain as to how this information should guide their practice. It can be argued that many laboratory protocols were designed to produce maximal effects—i.e., the animals were rendered severely hyperglycemic. Does this correlate with a modest glucose infusion, such as occurs with 1 L of dextrose-containing solution? Lanier et al. addressed this question by administering D_5W (in a volume equivalent to giving 1 L of the same solution to a human weighing 70 kg) to monkeys before inducing a reversible global ischemic insult.[89] Neurologic outcome in those monkeys was compared to a group that had instead received the same volume of normal saline solution. A significantly worsened neurologic outcome was observed in the animals receiving dextrose. Thus, as far as this primate model can predict, modest doses of glucose may predispose patients to a worsened outcome when exposed to a global ischemic insult.

In the case of focal ischemia, the effect of glucose administration on outcome is not quite as clear. There have been mixed experimental results, although the preponderance of data indicates a worsened outcome. It has been speculated that these discrepancies are attributable to variations in collateral flow to the ischemic penumbra within different ischemic models.[90]

In an effort to determine if animal investigations are relevant to the human condition, numerous investigators have examined the relationship between blood glucose concentration at the time of hospital admission and outcome from stroke.[91–95] The majority of those studies did find a relationship: patients who fared the worst neurologically also had the highest admission glucose values. Although this is consistent with the preponderance of animal studies, it has not been definitively determined whether the elevated glucose values in stroke patients represent a reactive stress hyperglycemia, or rather are coincident and truly cause a worsened outcome.

Although exceptions have been documented, evidence derived not only from stroke patients but also from patients recovering from head trauma, drowning, cardiac arrest, and cardiopulmonary bypass, supports aggressive management of the glycemic state during central nervous system insults. As presented above, only modest preischemic infusion of dextrose may predispose primates to markedly worsened outcome from ischemia. However, other work has indicated that postischemic hyperglycemia is unlikely to worsen outcome, at least in the case of global ischemia.[96] The extent to which glucose is withheld in patients with new-onset stroke remains a matter of clinical judgment.

Also undefined in humans is the value of administering insulin to reduce hyperglycemia if a stroke is believed to be in evolution. Several animal studies have documented clear benefit from insulin administration.[97,98] This may be attributable either to the effect of insulin on glucose availability or to the nerve growth hormone-like effect of insulin which may be protective independent of any hypoglycemic effect.[99] Studies of human brain injury correlate closely with animal studies in defining a step function of blood glucose concentrations on ischemic outcome. Subjects with glucose values greater than 180 mg/dL consistently have worsened outcome.[100,101] Because no human trials on efficacy of insulin therapy have been performed, the clinician can only assume that use of insulin to reduce glucose concentrations <180 mg/mL will be beneficial. These efforts might be best applied during surgical procedures, when ischemic insults can be anticipated (e.g., cerebral aneurysm clipping with temporary vascular occlusion).

HYPOTHERMIA

Development of rodent models of cerebral ischemia was crucial to understanding the importance of temperature in response of brain to ischemia. Those models provided opportunity for thorough examination of factors influencing ischemic outcome using disease free, genetically consistent, and low-cost subjects. Dramatic reduction in neural injury was observed when brain temperature was reduced by only 3–5°C during the ischemic insult in models of focal ischemia,[102–104] global ischemia,[105,106] brain trauma,[107,108] or status epilepticus.[109]

Mild hypothermia may also be neuroprotective when instituted after the ischemic insult under certain conditions. Original work suggested that the therapeutic window (i.e., interval until onset of hypothermia) may persist for only 30 minutes after reperfusion of the brain.[110] Later work indicated that the therapeutic window may extend up to 12 hours after reperfusion.[111] However, there is also evidence that hypothermia initiated after ischemia only delays the cascade of pathophysiologic events, which ultimately results in an outcome similar to that observed for normothermic comparators. Indeed, the majority of laboratory studies examining hypothermic protection have examined outcome only several days after the ischemic event. When animals were examined at weeks to months after ischemia, histologic evidence of postischemic hypothermic intervention was markedly diminished, particularly if the duration of hypothermia was 12 hours or less.[111,112] In contrast, when gerbils with appropriate monitoring of brain temperature were exposed to mild hypothermia for 24 hours after global ischemia, examination of histologic and neurologic changes at 6 months revealed a persistent benefit from hypothermia.[113] The human relevance of these studies has not been defined in clinical trials. The data suggest, however, that should postischemic hypothermia be employed, prolonged intervals (up to 24 hours) may be required to obtain lasting benefit.

For several decades it was thought that the predominant mechanism by which hypothermia caused protection was by virtue of its effects on cerebral metabolic rate. This is derived from observations that deep hypothermia is profoundly protective and that it also causes major reduction in cerebral metabolic rate. This has been called into question because mild hypothermia offers potent neuroprotection although cerebral metabolic rate is only minimally reduced. Other cellular and biochemical effects better explain how mild hypothermia protects. As stated above, extracellular concentrations of glutamate become massively increased during ischemia. Mild hypothermia effectively blocks this increase in glutamate (Fig. 7).[114–116] The mechanism for this is unknown. Postsynaptic consequences may also be important. Energy failure is associated with a large Ca^{2+} influx. In vitro studies have shown that mild hypothermia reduces Ca^{2+} influx.[117,118] Presumably, this decreases opportunity for intracellular Ca^{2+} to accumulate to concentrations sufficient to exert toxic effects.

Undoubtedly there are also numerous generalized effects of hypothermia on intracellular enzymatic activity. Mild reductions in brain temperature, while having no effect during the early recirculation interval,[119] hasten recovery of protein synthesis after reperfusion.[120] However, specific molecular effects are also being defined. Protein kinase C (PKC), an enzyme involved in regulating neuronal excitability and neurotransmitter release, is activated in response to an increase in cytosolic Ca^{2+}. Hypothermia has been demonstrated to diminish membrane-bound PKC activity in selectively vulnerable regions of the postischemic brain.[121]

Hypothermia also influences free-radical formation. Nitric oxide synthase activity in ischemic brain is suppressed by hypothermia.[122] Hypothermia also reduces accumulation of lipid peroxidation products and the consumption of free radical scavengers in ischemic brain.[123,124] Using two different models of brain injury (global ischemia or traumatic brain injury), Globus et al. demonstrated that free-radical production persists for at least several hours after reperfusion.[125, 126] The quantity of ischemia-induced free radical generation is reduced to almost preischemic baseline values by moderate hypothermia.

The electrophysiologic effects of hypothermia during focal ischemia are also of potential importance. As stated above, tissue in the ischemic penumbra shows recurrent episodes of depolarization which have been associated with transient intervals of tissue hypoxia and depression of electrical activity.[37] Hypothermia greatly diminishes the frequency of such depolarizations.[127]

It seems, therefore, that mild hypothermia involves a multiplicity of mechanisms, which in concert provide protection that to date is unparalleled by pharmacologic therapy. Unfortunately, with the exception of use in some intraoperative and intensive care settings, logistical issues, cost, and adverse effects of hypothermia have limited application of this therapy.

HYPERTHERMIA

Another series of laboratory-based observations have consistently shown hyperthermia to adversely affect both pathophysiologic processes and histologic/neurologic outcome from brain ischemia or trauma. The first observation was made by Busto et al., who showed that increasing brain temperature from 36°C to 39°C in the rat during global ischemia caused an ≈50% increase in neuronal injury.[105] This observation has been repeated by others.[128] Perhaps the most convincing data come from a canine study conducted by Wass et al.[129] Dogs were subjected to transient global ischemia with brain temperature held at 37.0, 38.0, or 39.0°C. Normothermic animals (37.°0C) were left essentially neurologically normal by the ischemic insult. In contrast, hyperthermic animals (39.0°C) either were comatose or died.

With respect to focal ischemia a similar pattern emerges. Infarct volumes in rats undergoing transient middle cerebral artery occlusion were almost tripled when brain temperature was increased from 37.0°C to 40.0°C.[127] Other investigators have demonstrated that an increase in brain temperature by as little as 1.2°C from normothermic values is also sufficient to triple the size of cortical infarct (Fig. 14).[130]

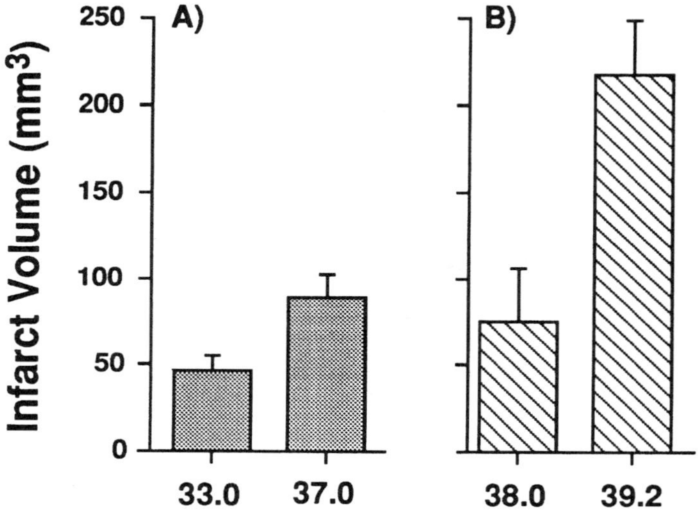

Figure 14 Brain temperature can have major effects on outcome from focal cerebral ischemia in the rat. (A) Rats were subjected to 60 minutes of transcranial temporary middle cerebral artery occlusion and 4 days recovery with pericranial temperature maintained at either 33.0 or 37.0°C during the ischemic insult. Mild hypothermia reduced infarct size by 48%.[103] (B) Rats were subjected to 90 minutes of filament occlusion of the middle cerebral artery and 4 days' recovery with pericranial temperature maintained at either 38.0 or 39.2°C during the ischemic insult. An increase of pericranial temperature by 1.2°C nearly tripled infarct size.[130]

The mechanistic basis for the potent adverse effect of hyperthermia is not entirely defined but some clues have been provided. Glutamate release in the penumbra of a rat focal ischemic lesion is increased by ≈10-fold when brain temperature is increased from 37.0°C to 39.0°C.[131] The frequency of spontaneous depolarizations occurring in the ischemic penumbra is markedly increased during mild hyperthermia. It has also been shown in both head injury and ischemia models that mild hyperthermia increases the rate of free-radical formation.[125,126]

In conclusion, there is overwhelming laboratory evidence that brain temperature is crucial in defining outcome from an ischemic insult. The mechanisms for this action are multifactorial. Direct human evidence for such effects is lacking in patients with stroke. However, results of laboratory studies are consistent with observations that surgical patients subjected to deep hypothermia are markedly protected from ischemia and that head trauma patients may have improved outcome resulting from sustained, mild hypothermic therapy.[132,133] Extrapolation of these findings to the patient who presents with new-onset stroke at hospital admission has been inadequately investigated. Because hypothermic therapy is substantially invasive (e.g., heavy sedation, neuromuscular blockade to prevent shivering, mechanical ventilation), carefully controlled trials are required to prove safety and efficacy. However, given lack of any evidence that hyperthermia may be of benefit in ischemia, aggressive treatment of fever in patients with stroke would seem justified given the consistent demonstration of the adverse effect of hyperthermia in models of central nervous system injury.

REFERENCES

1. Uematsu D, Greenberg J, Reivich M, et al. Direct evidence for calcium-induced ischemic and reperfusion injury. Ann Neurol 1989; 26:280–283.
2. Siesjö B. Cerebral circulation and metabolism. J Neurosurg 1984; 60:883–908.
3. Siesjö B, Bengtsson F. Calcium fluxes, calcium antagonists, and calcium-related pathology in brain ischemia, hypoglycemia, and spreading depression: a unifying hypothesis. J Cereb Blood Flow Metab 1989; 9:127–140.
4. Auer L. Pial arterial vasodilation by intravenous nimodipine in cats. Arzneim Forsch Drug Res 1981; 31:1423–1425.
5. Forsman M, Aarseth H, Nordby H, et al. Effects of nimodipine on cerebral blood flow and cerebrospinal fluid pressure after cardiac arrest: correlation with neurologic outcome. Anesth Analg 1989; 68:436–443.
6. Roine R, Kaste M, Kinnunen A, et al. Nimodipine after resuscitation from out-of-hospital ventricular fibrillation. JAMA 1990; 264:3171–3177.
7. Bogousslavsky J, Regli F, Zumstein V, et al. Double-blind study of nimodipine in non-severe stroke. Eur Neurol 1990; 30:23–26.
8. Gelmers H, Gorter K, De Weerdt C, et al. A controlled trial of nimodipine in acute ischemic stroke. N Engl J Med 1988; 318:203–207.
9. Paci A, Ottaviano P, Trenta A, et al. Nimodipine in acute ischemic stroke: a double-blind controlled study. Acta Neurol Scand 1989; 80:282–286.
10. Martinezvila E, Guillen F, Villanueva J, et al. Placebo-controlled trial of nimodipine in the treatment of acute ischemic cerebral infarction. Stroke 1990; 21:1023–1028.
11. Gelmers H, Hennerici M. Effect of nimodipine on acute ischemic stroke pooled results from five randomized trials. Stroke 1990; 21:IV81–IV84.
12. Fagan S, Gengo F, Bates V, et al. Effect of nimodipine on blood pressure in acute ischemic stroke in humans. Stroke 1988; 19:401–402.
13. Ohman J, Servo A, Heiskanen O. Long-term effects of nimodipine on cerebral infarcts and outcome after aneurysmal subarachnoid hemorrhage and surgery. J Neurosurg 1991; 74:8–13.
14. Allen G, Ahn H, Preziosi T, et al. Cerebral arterial spasm—a controlled trial of nimodipine in patients with subarachnoid hemorrhage. N Engl J Med 1983; 308:619–624.
15. Haley E, Kassell N, Torner J. A randomized controlled trial of high-dose intravenous nicardipine in aneurysmal subarachnoid hemorrhage. J Neurosurg 1993; 78:537–547.

16. Haley EC, et al. A randomized trial of two doses of nicardipine in aneurysmal subarachnoid hemorrhage. J Neurosurg 1994; 80:788–796.
17. Kirino T, Sano K. Selective vulnerability in the gerbil hippocampus following transient ischemia. Acta Neuropathol 1984; 62:201–208.
18. Smith M-L, Auer R, Siesjö B. The density and distribution of ischemic brain injury in the rat following 2–10 min of forebrain ischemia. Acta Neuropathol 1984; 64:319–332.
19. Petito CK, Feldman E, Pulsinelli WA, et al. Delayed hippocampal damage in humans following cardiorespiratory arrest. Neurology 1987; 37:1281–1286.
20. Grubb N, O'Carroll R, Cobbe S, et al. Chronic memory impairment after cardiac arrest outside hospital. Br Med J 1996; 313:143–146.
21. Kirino T, Tamura A, Sano K. Delayed neuronal death in the rat hippocampus following transient forebrain ischemia. Acta Neuropathol 1984; 64:139–147.
22. Pulsinelli W, Brierley J, Plum F. Temporal profile of neuronal damage in model of transient forebrain ischemia. Ann Neurol 1982; 11:491–498.
23. Smith M, Bendek G, Dahlgren N, et al. Models for studying long-term recovery following forebrain ischemia in the rat. 2. A 2-vessel occlusion model. Acta Neurol Scand 1984; 69:385–401.
24. Benveniste H, Drejer J, Schousboe A, et al. Elevation of the extracellular concentrations of glutamate and aspartate in rat hippocampus during transient cerebral ischemia monitored by intracerebral microdialysis. J Neurochem 1984; 43:1369–1374.
25. Benveniste H, Jorgensen M, Sandberg M, et al. Ischemic damage in hippocampal CA1 is dependent on glutamate release and intact innervation from CA3. J Cereb Blood Flow Metab 1989; 9:629–639.
26. Suzuki R, Yamaguchi T, Li C, et al. The effects of 5–minute ischemia in Mongolian gerbils. II. Changes of spontaneous neuronal activity in cerebral cortex and CA1 sector of hippocampus. Acta Neuropathol 1983; 60:217–222.
27. Choi D, Maulucci-Gedde M, Kriegstein A. Glutamate neurotoxicity in cortical cell culture. J Neurosci 1987; 7:357–368.
28. Choi D. Ionic dependence of glutamate neurotoxicity in cortical cell culture. J Neurosci 1987; 7:369–379.
29. Mayer M, Westbrook G, Guthrie P. Voltage-dependent block by Mg^{2+} of NMDA responses in spinal cord neurons. Nature 1984; 309:261–263.
30. Nowak L, Bregestovski P, Ascher P, et al. Magnesium gates glutamate-activated channels in mouse central neurons. Nature 1984; 307:462–465.
31. PellegriniGiampietro DE, Gorter JA, Bennett MVL, et al. The GLuR2 (GLuR-B) hypothesis: Ca^{2+} permeable AMPA receptors in neurological disorders [Review]. Trends Neurosci 1997; 20:464–470.
32. Baskys A. Metabotropic receptors and 'slow' excitatory actions of glutamate agonists in the hippocampus. TINS 1992; 15:92–96.
33. Simon R, Shiraishi K. N-Methyl-D-aspartate antagonist reduces stroke size and regional glucose metabolism. Ann Neurol 1990; 27:606–611.
34. Park CK, Nehls DG, Graham DI, et al. Focal cerebral ischaemia in the cat: treatment with the glutamate antagonist MK-801 after induction of ischaemia. J Cereb Blood Flow Metab 1988; 8:757–762.

35. Lanier W, Perkins W, Karlsson B, et al. The effects of dizocilpine maleate (MK-801), an antagonist of the N-methyl-D-aspartate receptor, on neurologic recovery and histopathology following complete cerebral ischemia in primates. J Cereb Blood Flow Metab 1990; 10:252–261.
36. Nedergaard M, Hansen A. Characterization of cortical depolarizations evoked in focal cerebral ischemia. J Cereb Blood Flow Metab 1993; 13 568–574.
37. Back T, Kohno K, Hossman K-A. Cortical negative DC deflections following middle cerebral artery occlusion and KCl-induced spreading depression: effect on blood flow, tissue oxygenation, and electroencephalogram. J Cereb Blood Flow Metab 1994; 14:12–19.
38. Iijima T, Mies G, Hossman K. Repeated negative DC deflections in rat cortex following middle cerebral artery occlusion are abolished by MK-801—effect on volume of ischemic injury. J Cereb Blood Flow Metab 1992; 12:727–733.
39. Mies G, Kohno K, Hossmann KA. Prevention of periinfarct direct current shifts with glutamate antagonist NBQX following occlusion of the middle cerebral artery in the rat. J Cereb Blood Flow Metab 1994; 14:802–807.
40. McLachlan R, Girvin J. Spreading depression of Leão in rodent and human cortex. Brain Res 1994; 666:133–136.
41. Mayevsky A, Doron A, Manor T, et al. Cortical spreading depression recorded from the human brain using a multiparametric monitoring system. Brain Res 1997; 740:268–274.
42. Buchan A, Xue D, Huang Z, et al. Delayed AMPA receptor blockade reduces cerebral infarction induced by focal ischemia. NeuroReport 1991; 2:473–476.
43. Buchan A, Li H, Pulsinelli W. The N-methyl-D-aspartate antagonist, MK-801, fails to protect against neuronal damage caused by transient, severe forebrain ischemia in adult rats. J Neurosci 1991; 11:1049–1056.
44. Nellgård B, Wieloch T. Postischemic blockade of AMPA but not NMDA receptors mitigates neuronal damage in the rat brain following transient severe cerebral ischemia. J Cereb Blood Flow Metab 1992; 12:2–11.
45. Le Peillet E, Arvin B, Moncada C, et al. The non-NMDA antagonists, NBQX and GYKI 52466, protect against cortical and striatal cell loss following transient global ischaemia in the rat. Brain Res 1992; 571:115–120.
46. Gill R, Nordholm L, Lodge D. The neuroprotective actions of 2,3-dihydroxy-6-nitro-7-sulfamoyl-benzo(F)quinoxaline (NBQX) in a rat focal ischaemia model. Brain Res 1992; 580:35–43.
47. Nurse S, Corbett D. Neuroprotection after several days of mild, drug-induced hypothermia. J Cereb Blood Flow Metab 1996; 16:474–480.
48. Willetts J, Balster R, Leander J. The behavioral pharmacology of NMDA receptor antagonists. Trends Pharm Sci 1990; 11:423–428.
49. Davis S, Albers G, Diener H, et al. Termination of acute stroke studies involving selfotel treatment. Lancet 1997; 329:32.
50. Warner DS, Martin HJ, Ludwig P, et al. In vivo models of cerebral ischemia: effects of parenterally administered NMDA receptor glycine site antagonists. J Cereb Blood Flow Metab 1995; 15:188–196.
51. Takaoka S, Bart RD, Pearlstein R, et al. Neuroprotective effect of NMDA recep-

tor glycine recognition site antagonism persists when brain temperature is controlled. J Cereb Blood Flow Metab 1997; 17:161–167.
52. Siesjö B, Agardh C-D, Bengtsson F. Free radicals and brain damage. Cerebrovasc Brain Metab Rev 1989; 1:165–211.
53. Dawson D. Nitric oxide and focal cerebral ischemia: multiplicity of actions and diverse outcome. Cerebrovasc Brain Metab Rev 1994; 6:299–324.
54. Crow JP, Beckman JS. The importance of superoxide in nitric oxide–dependent toxicity; evidence for peroxynitrite-mediated injury. Adv Exp Med Biol 1996; 387:147–161.
55. Yang G, Chan PH, Chen J, et al. Human copper-zinc superoxide dismutase transgenic mice are highly resistant to reperfusion injury after focal cerebral ischemia. Stroke 1994; 25:165–170.
56. Murakami K, Kondo T, Epstein C, et al. Overexpression of CuZn-superoxide dismutase reduces hippocampal injury after global ischemia in transgenic mice. Stroke 1997; 28:1797–1804.
57. Hara H, Huang P, Panahian N, et al. Reduced brain edema and infarction volume in mice lacking the neuronal isoform of nitric oxide synthase after transient MCA occlusion. J Cereb Blood Flow Metab 1996; 16:605–611.
58. Kondo T, Reaume AG, Huang TT, et al. Reduction of CuZn-superoxide dismutase activity exacerbates neuronal cell injury and edema formation after transient focal cerebral ischemia. J Neurosci 1997; 17:4180–4189.
59. Clark RK, Lee EV, White RF, et al. Reperfusion following focal stroke hastens inflammation and resolution of ischemic injured tissue. Brain Res Bull 1994; 35:387–392.
60. Clark RK, Lee EV, Fish CJ, et al. Development of tissue damage, inflammation and resolution following stroke: an immunohistochemical and quantitative planimetric study. Brain Res Bull 1993; 31:565–572.
61. Clark WM, Madden KP, Rothlein R, et al. Reduction of central nervous system ischemic injury by monoclonal antibody to intercellular adhesion molecule. 1991; 75:623–627.
62. Clark WM, Madden KP, Rothlein R, et al. Reduction of central nervous system ischemic injury in rabbits using leucocyte adhesion antibody treatment. Stroke 1991; 22:877–883.
63. Zhang R, Chopp M, Li Y. Anti ICAM-1 antibody reduces ischemic cell damage after transient middle cerebral artery occlusion in the rat. Neurology 1994; 44:1747–1751.
64. Chen H, Chopp M, Zhang RL, et al. Anti-CD11b monoclonal antibody reduces ischemic cell damage after transient focal cerebral ischemia in rat. Ann Neurol 1994; 35:458–463.
65. Takeshima R, Kirsch JR, Koehler RC, et al. Monoclonal leukocyte antibody does not decrease injury of transient focal cerebral ischemia in cats. Stroke 1992; 23:247–252.
66. Bruce A, Boling W, Kindy M, et al. Altered neuronal and microglial responses to excitotoxic and ischemic brain injury in mice lacking TNF receptors. Nature Med 1996; 2:788–794.

67. Frerichs K, Feuerstein G. Platelet-activating factor-key mediator in neuroinjury? Cerebrovasc Brain Metab Rev 1990; 2:148–160.
68. Lindsberg PJ, Yue TL, Frerichs KU, et al. Evidence for platelet activating factor as a novel mediator in experimental stroke in rabbits. Stroke 1990; 21:1452–1457.
69. Lehrmann E, Kiefer R, Finsen B, et al. Cytokines in cerebral ischemia: expression of transforming growth factor beta-1 (TGF-b1) mRNA in the postischemic adult rat hippocampus. Exp Neurol 1995; 131:114–123.
70. Gross C, Bednar M, Howard D, et al. Transforming growth factor-beta 1 reduces infarct size after experimental ischemia in a rabbit model. Stroke 1993; 24:558–562.
71. Relton J, Martin D, Thompson R, et al. Peripheral administration of interleukin-1 receptor antagonist inhibits brain damage after focal cerebral ischemia in the rat. Exp Neurol 1996; 138:206–213.
72. Betz A. Attenuation of stroke size in rats using an adenoviral vector to induce overexpression of interleukin-1 receptor antagonist in brain. J Cereb Blood Flow Metab 1995; 15:547–551.
73. Tarkowski E, Rosengren L, Blomstrand C, et al. Early intrathecal production of interleukin-6 predicts the size of the brain lesion in stroke. Stroke 1995; 26:1393–1398.
74. Fassbender K, Rossol S, Kammer T, et al. Proinflammatory cytokines in serum of patients with acute cerebral ischemia: kinetics of secretion and relation to the extent of brain damage and outcome of disease. J Neurol Sci 1994; 122:135–139.
75. Kamme F, Campbell K, Wieloch T. Biphasic expression of the Fos and Jun families of transcription factors following transient forebrain ischemia in the rat. Eur J Neurosci 1995; 7:2007–2016.
76. Sharp F, Kinouchi H, Kolstinaho J. HSP70 heat shock gene regulation during ischemia. Stroke 1993; 24:172–175.
77. Choi D. Ischemia-induced neuronal apoptosis. Curr Opin Neurobiol 1996; 6:667–672.
78. Martinou J-C, Dubois-Dauphin M, Staple JK, et al. Overexpression of bcl-2 in transgenic mice protects neurons from naturally occurring cell death and experimental ischemia. Neuron 1994; 13:1017–1030.
79. Krajewski S, Mai J, Krajewska M, et al. Upregulation of bax protein levels in neurons following cerebral ischemia. J Neurosci 1995; 15:6364–6376.
80. Du C, Hu R, Csernansky CA, et al. Very delayed infarction after mild focal cerebral ischemia: a role for apoptosis? J Cereb Blood Flow Metab 1996; 16:195–201.
81. Petito CK, Torres-Munoz J, Roberts B, et al. DNA fragmentation follows delayed neuronal death in CA1 neurons exposed to transient global ischemia in the rat. J Cereb Blood Flow Metab 1997; 17:967–976.
82. Eliasson MJL, Sampei K, Mandir AS, et al. Poly(ADP-ribose) polymerase gene disruption renders mice resistant to cerebral ischemia. Nature Med 1997; 3:1089–1095.
83. Endres M, Wang ZQ, Namura S, et al. Ischemic brain injury is mediated by the activation of poly(ADP-ribose) polymerase. J Cereb Blood Flow Metab 1997; 17:1143–1151.

84. Takahashi K, Greenberg JH, Jackson P, et al. Neuroprotective effects of inhibiting poly(ADP-ribose) synthetase on focal cerebral ischemia in rats. J Cereb Blood Flow Metab 1997; 17:1137–1142.
85. Myers RE, Yamaguchi S. Nervous system effects of cardiac arrest in monkeys. Preservation of vision. Arch Neurol 1977; 34:65–74.
86. Swanson P. Acidosis and some metabolic properties of isolated cerebral tissues. Arch Neurol 1969; 20:653–663.
87. Rehncrona S, Rosen I, Siesjö B. Brain lactic acidosis and ischemic cell damage. 1. Biochemistry and neurophysiology. J Cereb Blood Flow Metab 1981; 1:297–311.
88. Siesjö B, Smith M, Warner D. Acidosis and ischemic brain damage. In: Raichle E, Powers WJ, eds. Cerebrovascular Diseases. New York: Raven, 1987; 83–95.
89. Lanier W, Stangland K, Scheithauer B, et al. The effects of dextrose infusion and head position on neurologic outcome after complete cerebral ischemia in primates: examination of a model. Anesthesiology 1987; 66:39–48.
90. Ginsberg M. Glycolytic metabolism in brain ischemia. In: Weinstein PR, Faden AI, eds. Protection of the brain from ischemia, Baltimore: Williams and Wilkins, 1990; 37–48.
91. Adams HP, Olinger CP, Marler JR, et al. Comparison of admission serum glucose concentration with neurologic outcome in acute cerebral infarction. A study in patients given naloxone. Stroke 1988; 19:455–458.
92. Berger L, Hakim A. The association of hyperglycemia with cerebral edema in stroke. Stroke 1986; 17:865–871.
93. Candelise L, Landi G, Orazio E, et al. Prognostic significance of hyperglycemia in acute stroke. Arch Neurol 1985; 42:661–663.
94. Pulsinelli WA, Levy DE, Sigsbee B, et al. Increased damage after ischemic stroke in patients with hyperglycemia with or without established diabetes mellitus. Am J Med 1983; 74:540–544.
95. Schneider S, Tomasi L, Thompson J. Prognostic implications of hyperglycemia and reduced cerebral blood flow in childhood near-drowning. Neurology 1990; 40:820–823.
96. Pulsinelli W, Waldman S, Rawlinson D, et al. Moderate hyperglycemia augments ischemic brain damage: A neuropathologic study in the rat. Neurology 1982; 32:1239–1246.
97. Warner D, Gionet T, Todd M, et al. Insulin-induced normoglycemia improves ischemic outcome in hyperglycemic rats. Stroke 1992; 23:1775–1781.
98. Hamilton M, Tranmer B, Auer R. Insulin reduction of cerebral infarction due to transient focal ischemia. J Neurosurg 1995; 82:262–268.
99. Voll C, Auer R. Insulin attenuates ischemic brain damage independent of its hypoglycemic effect. J Cereb Blood Flow Metab 1991; 11:1006–1014.
100. Lam A, Winn H, Cullen B, et al. Hyperglycemia and neurological outcome in patients with head injury. J Neurosurg 1991; 75:545–551.
101. Li P-A, Shamloo M, Smith M-L, et al. The influence of plasma glucose concentrations on ischemic brain damage is a threshold function. Neurosci Lett 1994; 177:63–65.

102. Onesti S, Baker C, Sun P, et al. Transient hypothermia reduces focal ischemic brain damage in the rat. Neurosurgery 1991; 29:369–373.
103. Ridenour T, Warner D, Todd M, et al. Mild hypothermia reduces infarct size resulting from temporary but not permanent focal ischemia in the rat. Stroke 1992; 23:733–738.
104. Chen H, Chopp M, Zhang Z, et al. The effect of hypothermia on transient middle cerebral artery occlusion in the rat. J Cereb Blood Flow Metab 1992; 12:621–628.
105. Busto R, Dietrich W, Globus M, et al. Small differences in intraischemic brain temperature critically determine the extent of neuronal injury. J Cereb Blood Flow Metab 1987; 7:729–738.
106. Sano T, Drummond J, Patel P, et al. A comparison of the cerebral protective effects of isoflurane and mild hypothermia in a model of incomplete forebrain ischemia in the rat. Anesthesiology 1992; 76:221–228.
107. Clifton G, Jiang J, Lyeth B, et al. Marked protection by moderate hypothermia after experimental traumatic brain injury. J Cereb Blood Flow Metab 1991; 11:114–121.
108. Dietrich W, Alonso O, Busto R, et al. Post-traumatic brain hypothermia reduces histopathological damage following concussive brain injury in the rat. Acta Neuropathol 1994; 87:250–258.
109. Lundgren J, Smith M-L, Blennow G, et al. Hyperthermia aggravates and hypothermia ameliorates epileptic brain damage. Exp Brain Res 1994; 99:43–55.
110. Busto R, Dietrich W, Globus M, et al. Postichemic moderate hypothermia inhibits CA1 hippocampal ischemic neuronal injury. Neurosci Lett 1989; 101:299–304.
111. Colbourne F, Corbett D. Delayed and prolonged post-ischemic hypothermia is neuroprotective in the gerbil. Brain Res 1994; 654:265–272.
112. Dietrich W, Busto R, Alonso O, et al. Intraischemic but not postischemic brain hypothermia protects chronically following global forebrain ischemia in rats. J Cereb Blood Flow Metab 1993; 13:541–549.
113. Colbourne F, Corbett D. Delayed postischemic hypothermia: a six month survival study using behavioral and histologic assessments of neuroprotection. J Neurosci 1995; 15:7250–7260.
114. Busto R, Globus MY-T, Dietrich WD, et al. Effect of mild hypothermia on ischemia-induced release of neurotransmitters and free fatty acids in rat brain. Stroke 1989; 20:904–910.
115. Patel P, Drummond J, Cole D, et al. Differential temperature sensitivity of ischemia-induced glutamate release and eicosanoid production in rats. Brain Res 1994; 650:205–211.
116. Illievich U, Zornow M, Choi K, et al. Effects of hypothermia or anesthetics on hippocampal glutamate and glycine concentrations after repeated transient global cerebral ischemia. Anesthesiology 1994; 80:177–186.
117. Bickler P, Buck L, Hansen B. Effects of isoflurane and hypothermia on glutamate receptor-mediated calcium influx in brain slices. Anesthesiology 1994; 81:1461–1469.
118. Arai H, Uto A, Ogawa Y, et al. Effect of low temperature on glutamate-induced

intracellular calcium accumulation and cell death in cultured hippocampal neurons. Neurosci Lett 1993; 163:132–134.
119. Bergstedt K, Hu B, Wieloch T. Postischaemic changes in protein synthesis in the rat brain: effects of hypothermia. Exp Brain Res 1993; 95:91–99.
120. Widmann R, Miyazawa T, Hossmann K. Protective effect of hypothermia on hippocampal injury after 30 minutes of forebrain ischemia in rats is mediated by postischemic recovery of protein synthesis. J Neurochem 1993; 61:200–209.
121. Busto R, Globus M, Neary J, et al. Regional alterations of protein kinase C activity following transient cerebral ischemia: Effects of intraischemic brain temperature modulation. J Neurochem 1994; 63:1095–1103.
122. Kader A, Frazzini V, Baker C, et al. Effect of mild hypothermia on nitric oxide synthesis during focal cerebral ischemia. Neurosurgery 1994; 35:272–277.
123. Baiping L, Xiujuan T, Hongwei C, et al. Effect of moderate hypothermia on lipid peroxidation in canine brain tissue after cardiac arrest and resuscitation. Stroke 1994; 25:147–150.
124. Karibe H, Chen S, Zarow G, et al. Mild intraischemic hypothermia suppresses consumption of endogenous antioxidants after temporary focal ischemia in rats. Brain Res 1994; 649:12–18.
125. Globus M, Busto R, Lin B, et al. Detection of free radical activity during transient global ischemia and recirculation: effects of intraischemic brain temperature modulation. J Neurochem 1995; 65:1250–1256.
126. Globus M, Alonso O, Dietrich W, et al. Glutamate release and free radical production following brain injury: effects of posttraumatic hypothermia. J Neurochem 1995; 65:1704–1712.
127. Chen Q, Chopp M, Bodzin G, et al. Temperature modulation of cerebral depolarization during focal cerebral ischemia in rats: correlation with ischemic injury. J Cereb Blood Flow Metab 1993; 13:389–394.
128. Minamisawa H, Smith M, Siesjö B. The effect of mild hyperthermia and hypothermia on brain damage following 5, 10, and 15 minutes of forebrain ischemia. Ann Neurol 1990; 28:26–33.
129. Wass C, Lanier W, Hofer R, et al. Temperature changes of ≥1°C alter functional neurologic outcome and histopathology in a canine model of complete cerebral ischemia. Anesthesiology 1995; 83:325–335.
130. Warner DS, McFarlane C, Todd MM, et al. Sevoflurane and halothane reduce focal ischemic brain damage in the rat: possible influence on thermoregulation. Anesthesiology 1993; 79:985–992.
131. Takagi K, Ginsberg M, Globus MY-T, et al. Effect of hyperthermia on glutamate release in ischemic penumbra after middle cerebral artery occlusion in rats. Am J Physiol 1994; 266:H1770–H1776.
132. Silverberg GD, Reitz BA, Ream AK. Hypothermia and cardiac arrest in the treatment of giant aneurysms of the cerebral circulation and hemangioblastoma of the medulla. J Neurosurg 1981; 55:337–346.

133. Marion DW, Penrod LE, Kelsey SF, et al. Treatment of traumatic brain injury with moderate hypothermia. N Engl J Med 1997; 336:540–546.
134. Smith ML, Kalimo H, Warner DS, et al. Morphologic lesions in the brain preceding the development of post-ischemic seizures. Acta Neuropathol 1988; 76:253–264.

14
Heparin and Antiplatelets in Acute Cerebral Ischemia

Jeffrey Minuk and Robert Côté
McGill University, Montreal, Quebec, Canada

HEPARIN

Clinical Chemistry and Pharmacology

Heparin is a glycosaminoglycan consisting of alternating residues of uronic acid and D-glucosamine. In its unfractionated form, it is an admixture of molecules ranging from 3,000 to 30,000 daltons, with a mean molecular weight of 15,000 daltons.[1] Heparin's anticoagulant effect is mediated primarily by its interaction with antithrombin III (ATIII) as it acts as a template on which the inactivation of thrombin by ATIII is accelerated. The heparin/ATIII complex can also inactivate coagulation factor Xa. Heparin can also inactivate thrombin by an ATIII-independent fashion via a plasma cofactor called heparin cofactor II. This latter mechanism requires very high doses of heparin and is responsible for heparin's partial effectiveness in ATIII-deficient individuals. Other effects include inhibiting the activation of factors V and VIII. Heparin also variably effects platelet aggregation, having been reported to both promote and inhibit platelet aggregation,[2,3] and it has also been reported to increase vessel permeability experimentally.[4]

The anticoagulant effect of heparin is monitored by using the activated partial thromboplastin time (APTT). This test is sensitive to the inhibitory effect of heparin on thrombin and factor Xa. The APTT correlates well with heparin concentrations required in the treatment of deep venous thrombosis (DVT), pulmonary thromboembolus (PTE), acute myocardial infarction (AMI), and unstable angina.[5,6] Both animal and human studies indicate that for therapeutic purposes, sufficient heparin should be given to increase the APTT 1.5 to 2.0 times control values.

Initiation of Heparin Therapy

In most instances of acute ischemic events, heparin will be administered by continuous intravenous infusion. Intravenous heparin is usually administered with a bolus injection of 5,000 to 10,000 units followed by 1,000 units per hour. The bolus injection of heparin will rapidly saturate the bindings sites involved in its clearance and allow the subsequent initial maintenance doses of heparin to have a rapid therapeutic effect.[2,7] In some situations (see below), the bolus may be withheld. The APTT is not altered in patients receiving intermittent fixed doses of subcutaneous heparin and therefore does not need to be monitored.

Use of Heparin

Heparin has been used in the treatment of a wide variety of venous and arterial occlusive disorders including DVT, PTE, AMI, unstable angina, postpercutaneous transluminal coronary angioplasty (PTCA), maintenance of vascular graft patency, and ischemic cerebrovascular conditions. Heparin has been clearly shown to be effective in the treatment of both DVT and PTE.[8–11] Heparin has also be shown to be effective in DVT prevention in high-risk surgical patients[12] and in patients undergoing major orthopedic interventions (e.g., total hip replacement).[13] Heparin has also been shown to reduce the incidence of venous thromboembolism in patients with acute myocardial infarction.[14,15] Summaries on the use of heparin in venous occlusive disease have been previously published.[16]

The precise indications for heparin in the setting of transient ischemic attacks (TIA) and acute ischemic stroke remain to be defined. Presently, there is no consensus on when and in which stroke types heparin should be used. Treatment with heparin has been reported in patients presenting with acute ischemic stroke, cardioembolic strokes, acute partial stable strokes, progressing strokes, and TIAs. However, generally, these studies, up until recently, were performed in the pre-CT era and have suffered from several methodological limitations including small numbers of patients and rarely being randomized, controlled, or blinded. The use of heparin in these various acute cerebral ischemic presentations is discussed below.

ACUTE ISCHEMIC STROKE

The efficacy of heparin in the setting of acute ischemic stroke has been investigated in the recently completed International Stroke Trial (IST).[17] In this open trial of 19,435 patients, half were randomized to receive subcutaneous unfractionated heparin (one-quarter 5,000 units twice daily, and one quarter 12,500 units twice daily), and half were to "avoid heparin." In this 3 × 2 factorial design, half were randomized to receive acetylsalicylic acid (ASA), 300 mg/day, and half were to "avoid ASA." Patients were randomized within 48 hours of acute stroke symptoms. Primary outcomes of efficacy were death from any cause within 14 days and death or dependency at 6 months. Secondary outcomes at 14 days were recurrent strokes, intracranial hemorrhage (from either recurrent hemorrhagic stroke or hemorrhagic transformation of the original stroke), pulmonary emboli, and extracerebral hemorrhages requiring transfusion. Secondary outcomes at 6 months were death from any cause, proportion of patients with full recovery, and number of patients living at home.

Heparin at either dose had no significant effect on mortality within 14 days. At 6 months, there was no difference in the number of dead or dependent between those who received heparin and those who did not receive heparin. Heparin was associated with a significant reduction in recurrent ischemic strokes within 14 days, but this benefit was offset by a proportionate increase in hemorrhagic stroke. Heparin was also associated with an excess of nine transfused or fatal extracranial hemorrhages per 1,000 patients. Compared with 10,000 units of heparin per day, 25,000 units was associated with significantly more transfused or fatal extracranial hemorrhages, more hemorrhagic strokes, and excess of deaths or nonfatal recurrent strokes within 14 days. Furthermore, heparin was associated with only a marginally significant reduction in pulmonary embolism.

Several criticisms, from a methodological point of view, have been put forward after the publication of the IST results.[18] Computer tomography (CT) was not absolutely required at randomization, so patients with hemorrhagic strokes may have been included. The absence of blinding and placebo control may have allowed for increased attention to bleeding in those treated with heparin. Furthermore, there was no systematic coagulation monitoring. The methodology of IST differs considerably from the usual North American practice of administering heparin intravenously according to the APTT within a few hours of stroke onset and after the completion of a CT. All of these factors could have lead to a systematic bias against heparin.

CARDIOEMBOLIC STROKE

It is estimated that about 15% of all ischemic strokes are cardioembolic.[19] Certain clinical features are said to be suggestive of a cardioembolic stroke. These include the presence of certain cardiac conditions, maximum deficit at the onset, stroke heralded by seizure, absence of preceding TIA, and presence of isolated branch vessel occlusion syndromes (isolated expressive aphasia, monoplegias, global aphasia without hemiparesis).[20] However, the degree of reliability of these features is uncertain, and in a substantial number of cases the cause of the ischemic event may be due to concomitant atherothrombotic disease affecting the cervicocerebral vasculature. Regardless, various cardiac disorders may be more closely associated with ischemic stroke. These include atrial fibrillation, valvular heart disease (with or without atrial fibrillation), presence of prosthetic heart valves, acute myocardial infarction, and septal deffects.[20] The most common cardiac disorders associated with cardioembolic stroke are discussed below.

ATRIAL FIBRILLATION

The risk of stroke in patients with atrial fibrillation (AF) is about six times higher than in patients without AF, in long-term prospective studies.[21,22] The relative risk of stroke is about 17 times higher when AF is present in the setting of valvular disease.[21,22] The presence of additional clinical disease (e.g., hypertension, previous cerebral ischemic events, congestive heart failure, or diabetes) or of electrocardiographically proven structural heart disease (e.g., enlarged left atrium or valvular disease—see below) will further increase the risk of ischemic events in patients with AF.[23,24] Although several recent studies have confirmed the efficacy of long-term oral anticoagulation for both primary and secondary prevention of stroke in patients with AF,[25–31] less information is available about the efficacy of heparin in the acute setting.

Nonvalvular Atrial Fibrillation

The risk of early stroke recurrence probably differs for patients with valvular and nonvalvular atrial fibrillation (NVAF). For NVAF, earlier retrospective studies suggested a high rate of stroke recurrence—between 12% and 15% within the first 2 weeks.[20,32–42] More recent prospective studies, however, indicate that this may not be the case. The risk of stroke recurrence in these patients within the first 2 weeks based on these studies is closer to 4% to 5%, similar to patients who present with normal sinus rhythm.[17,43–47] Notwithstanding the apparent safety of early anticoagulation in the poststroke period for most patients, the low risk of early stroke recurrence in NVAF and the increased risk of hemorrhagic transformation leave little justification for immediate and routine anticoagulation in this setting.

In the recently completed IST (see above), more than 3,000 patients with atrial fibrillation were entered. Within the first 14 days after a stroke, heparin-treated patients had 21 fewer recurrent ischemic strokes per 1,000 patients but this was offset by an increase of 16 hemorrhagic strokes per 1,000 patients.

Valvular Atrial Fibrillation

In the past, atrial fibrillation occurred most often in the setting of rheumatic valve disease, particularly rheumatic mitral stenosis. Other valvular diseases associated with atrial fibrillation include rheumatic mitral regurgitation, congenital mitral stenosis, and mitral annular calcification. Aortic valve disease is usually not associated with atrial fibrillation except in the setting of concomitant mitral valve disease or ischemic heart disease.

Through recurrence rates for patients with valvular AF are not available for the first 2 weeks, early studies indicate that between 20% and 60% of such patients have a stroke recurrence, and that most of the recurrences occurred in the first 6 months.[48–50] As well, the overall stroke risk is three times higher for patients with valvular AF that for patients with NVAF.[48–50] As the risk of early stroke recurrence may be higher in patients with valvular AF than in those with NVAF, early anticogulation (within 48 hours) should be considered if no contraindications exist (see below).

Prosthetic Heart Valves

Prosthetic heart valves may be either mechanical or bioprosthetic. Mechanical valves have the highest risk of systemic embolization. Patients with mechanical valves, whether in atrial fibrillation or not, require lifelong oral anticoagulation. Patients with bioprosthetic valves are generally treated with oral anticoagulants for the first 3 months after valve replacement, and thereafter with antiplatelet agents.[51–55]

If an ischemic stroke occurs in a patient with a prosthetic valve, oral anticoagulation should be discontinued for at least 72 hours.[56] The patient could, thereafter, be treated temporarily with intravenous heparin if there is no evidence of intracerebral hemorrhage on a cerebral CT scan repeated at that time and subsequently restarted on oral anticoagulation. If a hemorrhagic process is present on either the initial or subsequent CT scans or if the infarct is massive, anticoagulation may be withheld for 7 to 10 days.

Acute Myocardial Infarction

The risk of ischemic stroke in the setting of acute myocardial infarction (AMI) is between 1% and 3%. This risk is doubled in the setting of an anterior AMI.[57,58]

Left ventricular thrombus may be seen in up to 40% of all AMI.[59,60] The presence of a left ventricular aneurysm, atrial fibrillation, or congestive heart failure increases the risk of thrombus formation. Most thrombi occur within the first 48 hours after AMI, and the presence of a left ventricular thrombus increases the risk of systemic embolism. Anticoagulation with heparin has been shown to reduce the incidence of mural thrombus and cardioembolic stroke.[61] It is therefore recommended that heparin be administered as soon as the diagnosis of anterior AMI is made. Heparin should also be administered in the setting of any AMI complicated by severe left ventricular dysfunction, echocardiographic evidence of a mural thrombus, or atrial fibrillation. Oral anticoagulation should follow for at least 3 months in the setting of atrial fibrillation.[62]

Endocarditis

Neurologic complications occur in about 30% of patients with infective endocarditis.[63–65] Stroke and encephalopathy are among the commonest of these neurologic complications. Heparin therapy is generally not indicated in patients with infective endocarditis who are in normal sinus rhythm with either a native or bioprosthetic valve.[66,67] Heparin may, however, be indicated when a cerebral embolic event occurs during the course of antibiotic treatment for infective endocarditis, particularly if the patient has AF, a large atrial appendage, or large valvular vegetations.[54] However, adequate antibiotic therapy is crucial and is more important than anticoagulation in preventing neurologic complications.[67] If patients are already an oral anticoagulation (for AF and/or mechanical valve), this should probably be continued throughout the period of antibiotic treatment or else temporarily replaced with intravenous heparin. However, if an ischemic cerebrovascular complication occurs in a patient already taking oral anticoagulants, this should be withheld for at least 72 hours. If a cerebral CT at that time shows no sign of hemorrhage, intravenous heparin followed by oral anticoagulation could then be administered. In patients who present with a focal neurological event during their treatment, consideration should be given to cerebral angiography to exclude a mycotic aneurysm.[68–70]

Nonbacterial thrombotic endocarditis is associated with a high incidence of systemic embolization and disseminated intravascular coagulation.[71,72] These patients should be strongly considered for short-term heparin therapy.[71,72]

Immediate Anticoagulation in Cardioembolic Stroke

The Cerebral Embolism Study Group reported a randomized trial on immediate anticoagulation with heparin of ischemic strokes presumed to be of cardiac origin.[32] The study was terminated early, with only 63 of the 140 patients targeted to be enrolled. The data were not statistically significant but they did report a trend toward reduction of recurrent embolism in patients given early anticoagulation. However, only two recurrences were reported in 21 patients who did not receive early anticoagulation (one of these patients had a left ventricular aneurysm with the sick sinus syndrome, and the other had an acute myocardial infarction). The study population was very heterogeneous and included not only patients with NVAF but also those with an AMI and valvular and postoperative AF. None of the patients who had received early anticoagulation had hemorrhagic transformation of their infarcts. Therefore this study did not have the power to demonstrate a clear, beneficial effect of heparin in stroke recurrence after a presumed cardioembolic stroke. The early administration of heparin, however, was not detrimental. The relative safety of early anticoagulation with heparin after cardioembolic stroke has also been supported in a more recent retrospective study.[43]

Recommendations for Anticoagulation in Acute Cardioembolic Stroke

Often patients with an acute ischemic stroke presumed to be of cardioembolic origin will be treated immediately with heparin. Such groups of patients include those with acute ischemic stroke in the setting of rheumatic heart disease, intramural or mural thrombi, prosthetic heart valves, and some cases of NVAF. When considering the use of heparin in the immediate poststroke period, presumed to be of cardiac origin, the risk of heparin-induced hemorrhage must be weighed against the risk of early stroke recurrence and the potential protective effect of heparin in reducing this risk.

Treatment with heparin could be considered in those nonacutely hypertensive patients who have suffered a small or moderate-size stroke and whose initial CT scan of the brain shows no evidence of hemorrhage. In these cases a second CT scan should probably be performed 48 to 72 hours after initiation of therapy to document any hemorrhagic transformation. Some reports, however, suggest that early anticoagulation is not necessarily associated with hemorrhagic transformation and that even if hemorrhagic transformation occurs, clinical deterioration is not always observed.[43,73,74] At the present time, however, it appears more prudent to withhold heparin in the setting of a hemorrhagic infarction or transformation. An alternative approach in some cases, such as NVAF, would be to avoid anticoagulation with heparin and simply begin oral anticoagulation following a repeat CT scan done 48 to 72 hours after the cerebral ischemic event if no blood is detected.[75]

Conversely, we recommend that anticoagulation be withheld in patients with large strokes or uncontrolled hypertension because of the potential for hemorrhagic transformation and subsequent clinical deterioration. There is, however, no rigorous data which address the question of the level of blood pressure and increased risk of anticoagulation with heparin. However, some investigators have suggested that anticoagulation should be withheld when blood pressure is > 180/90.[32]

Severe strokes as judged clinically (dense hemiplegia, somnolence, hemianopsia, gaze preference with or without aphasia) should not be given immediate anticoagulation. A CT scan with a hyperdense middle cerebral artery sign or a CT scan showing loss of the insular ribbon along with attenuation of the lentiform nuclei and hemispheric sulcal effacement are predictive of large infarcts.[76] Anticoagulation should therefore be withheld in patients whose CT scan of the brain shows either a hyperdense middle cerebral artery (usually indicative of occlusion) or a combination of the above-mentioned three parenchymal signs. These patients should be prescribed compression stockings and could be considered for subcutaneous unfractionated heparin (5,000 units every 12 hours) for prophylaxis against DVT or pulmonary embolism.[77,78]

Risk of Hemorrhagic Transformation with Acute Anticoagulation

Spontaneous hemorrhagic transformation of an acute ischemic stroke is said to occur as early as 6 hours and generally before 48 hours after the initial event.[73,79] The risk is greatest with large infarcts and infarcts presumed to be of cardioembolic origin.[73,74] Hemorrhage is seen in about 3% to 5% of initial CT scans of nonanticoagulated cardioembolic stroke patients.[32] However, with sequential CT scanning, hemorrhage is seen in 13% to 25% of cases.[36,80,81] Furthermore, patients already taking oral anticoagulants are at increased risk of hemorrhagic complications in the setting of an acute ischemic stroke.[32]

The Cerebral Embolism Study Group reported no association between hemorrhagic transformation and the age of the patient, presence of hypertension, or degree of anticoagulation (as assessed by the APTT). Only the presence of a "large" infarct and perhaps the administration of a "bolus" dose of heparin were associated with an increased risk of hemorrhagic transformation.[74] Recent studies report that between 0% and 24% of patients will experience clinical worsening due to hemorrhagic transformation after immediate anticoagulation, but that most patients with hemorrhagic transformation will be asymptomatic.[32,74]

STROKE IN PROGRESSION

Stroke in progression, sometimes referred to as progressing stroke or stroke in evolution, has been defined in many ways.[82] In practical terms, stroke in progression may be defined as an increasing neurological deficit observed since the patient's admission to hospital. Ideally, this diagnosis should be made after repeated examinations performed by the same examiner. Occasionally, a history of progressing or fluctuating deficit will be obtained from the patient or family. Studies indicate that between 20% and 40% of patients will have progression of their ischemic strokes after admission to the hospital. This progression generally takes place within the first 24 to 48 hours but can occasionally be delayed.[83–85]

The biological factors underlying stroke in progression remain incompletely understood. It is often assumed that progression of deficits is due to further propagation of an arterial thrombus or distal embolization. Consequently, it is rationalized that antithrombotic agents such as heparin may be of benefit. However, other mechanisms may be responsible for progression of the neurological deficit. These include local edema or hemorrhage within the ischemic territory, metabolic disturbances (hyperglycemia, hypoglycemia, hyponatremia), hypoxia, release of neurotransmitters, or intercurrent infection.[86] Heparin would not be expected to have a beneficial impact on these factors.

In a recent survey on the use of antithrombotic agents by American neurologists, 70% of the respondents felt that stroke in progression was an indication for the use of heparin.[87] Early studies did in fact suggest that treatment with heparin could reduce the likelihood of stroke progression.[88–91] However, these studies were poorly designed, nonblinded, and nonrandomized, and they predated the use of CT. Duke et al. have reported the only randomized, double-blinded, placebo-controlled study on the use of heparin in the prevention of stroke progression.[92] All patients studied (n = 225 patients) had an acute partial stroke within the preceding 48 hours and had a deficit that remained stable for at least 1 hour. One group received intravenous heparin, adjusted to maintain the APTT between 50 and 70 seconds. The other group received placebo. There was no statistically significant difference in stroke progression rates between the two groups. This study therefore did not support the use of intravenous heparin in acute ischemic stroke. Until more data are available, the use of heparin in this clinical context remains a matter of preference based on the treating physician's judgment.

ACUTE TIA

After a TIA, the risk of stroke is estimated to be about 4% to 8% in the first month and about 12% to 13% in the first year.[93,94] Furthermore, approximately 40% of patients with a stroke have had at least one preceding TIA.[94] Therefore TIAs must be considered important predictors for ischemic stroke, and treatment of TIAs may thus reduce the risk of subsequent ischemic stroke.

TIAs, either single or recurrent, are at times treated with heparin, with the view to prevent impending stroke and/or to allow sufficient time for investigations, including appropriate carotid imaging studies, to be performed. Until 1988, there were no randomized controlled studies on the use of heparin in TIAs, and previous nonrandomized studies showed no benefit of heparin in the prevention of recurrent TIA or stroke.[95] The only randomized study on the use of heparin in acute TIA compared its use against ASA in the prevention of recurrent TIAs or stroke.[96] No difference between treatments was reported; however, the numbers were small and the power of the study inadequate. Therefore, the routine use of heparin in the context of a single or recurrent TIA cannot be recommended because of the lack of supporting evidence. We would suggest the use of appropriate antiplatelet therapy and prompt investigation to determine the cause of these events.

Crescendo TIAs may be defined as recurrent, transient cerebral or retinal ischemic episodes characterized by an increased frequency, duration, and severity of events in a short period of time, usually hours or days. Such TIAs are associated with a significantly increased risk of cerebral infarction and often high-grade ipsilateral internal carotid artery atherosclerotic stenosis.[97,98] Though never studied in a normal fashion, it would be acceptable to anticoagulate with heparin those presenting with this symptomatology and more so if they are already receiving antiplatelet agents. If the appropriate investigations revealed significant ipsilateral internal carotid stenosis (≥70%) and if the patient was an acceptable surgical risk, anticoagulation could be continued until carotid endarterectomy could be scheduled.

OVERVIEW OF HEPARIN IN ACUTE STROKE

In 1993, Sandercock and colleagues published a review on the use of antithrombotics in acute ischemic stroke.[99] This included 10 controlled trials reporting on the use of heparin in acute ischemic stroke (six trials with standard unfractionated heparin and four with low-molecular-weight heparin). Overall, heparin therapy was associated with a highly significant 81% reduction in the odds of DVT. There was also a trend for fewer pulmonary emboli. There were also fewer deaths recorded in the heparin-treated group, but this did not reach statistical significance. However, a trend existed toward increased risk of hemorrhagic transformation of the infarct in the heparin-treated patients. Even when these data are combined with results from the IST and notwithstanding the criticisms of the IST in regard to heparin (see above), there are insufficient data to conclude about any benefit of heparin on neurological or functional outcome in either the short or long term.

OTHER ACUTE CEREBROVASCULAR DISORDERS

Cerebral Venous Thrombosis (CVT)

The clinical presentation, predisposing factors, and morbid anatomy of CVT have been reviewed elsewhere.[100] Recent studies on CVT have implicated, for some patients at least, a hereditary prothrombotic state in its pathogenesis—namely, resistance to activated protein C.[101,102]

The optimal treatment of CVT has remained controversial up until recently. The use of heparin has been traditionally discouraged because of the risk of hemorrhagic complications. However, in 1991, Einhaupl and colleagues reported the first randomized, double-blinded, placebo-controlled trial on the use of heparin in CVT.[103] Although they reported a beneficial effect of heparin, this study had many methodological limitations including a small number of enrolled patients (20), and the use of a nonvalidated neurological scale. Patients who received heparin therapy had improved neurologic outcome at 3 days and 3 months and a lower mortality rate than patients who received placebo. In this group of 20 patients, there was no significant difference in the number of intracranial hemorrhages between the two groups. These same authors reported, as well, a retrospective analysis on the occurrence of intracranial hemorrhage in 112 patients with CVT (77 received heparin and 35 did not). The intracranial hemorrhagic rate was higher in the group that did not receive heparin, but this may simply reflect a selection bias in the group not treated with heparin which may have been more ill than the treated group and therefore more likely to develop intracranial hemorrhage. However, heparin did not appear to worsen the clinical outcome in patients with intracranial hemorrhage.

In view of these data, we recommend consideration of intravenous heparin in the context of CVT if no contraindications to its use are present. In these cases, heparin may be used in conjunction with other treatment modalities, particularly those aimed at reducing intracranial pressure and control of seizures. We would not, however, recommend heparin if a hemorrhagic process is present on cerebral CT scan.

Stroke Secondary to Prothrombotic States

The commonest prothrombotic states are ATIII deficiency, protein C deficiency, protein S deficiency, resistance to activated protein C, and the antiphospholipid antibody syndrome.[104] Of those, the last has been especially associated with cerebral arterial ischemic phenomena. The other conditions are usually associated with venous thromboembolic disease including CVT. Prothrombotic states should be considered in all young patients with ischemic cerebrovascular disease, in those without risk factors for atherosclerosis, and in those with a family history of venous occlusive disease. Though there is some general consensus that patients with these prothrombotic states should be treated with long-term oral anticoagulation,[104] there are no specific data supporting the benefit of heparin in the acute period. Blood for appropriate investigation of these coagulation disorders should be drawn prior to the initiation of anticoagulation therapy.

COMPLICATIONS OF HEPARIN THERAPY

The most common complications of heparin therapy given in the context of acute cerebral ischemia are heparin-induced hemorrhages and heparin-induced thrombocytopenia (HIT).

Hemorrhagic Complications

Heparin therapy can be associated with both major and minor hemorrhagic complications. The major complications are intracranial hemorrhage, retroperitoneal hemorrhage, and hemorrhage leading to hospitalization, transfusion, and death. Although heparin can induce hemorrhage by several possible mechanisms (inhibiting coagulation, inhibiting platelet function, thrombocytopenia, or increasing vessel wall permeability), its anticoagulant effect is thought to be the factor most often responsible for its hemorrhagic effects.[1,7]

Factors Associated with Increased Risk of Hemorrhage

In general, the risk of heparin-induced hemorrhages is influenced by several factors including the dosage used, the route of administration, and the concomitant use of antiplatelet or thrombolytic agents. The age of the patient and the presence of comorbid conditions (see below) are also important factors.

The overall risk of major bleeding during heparin therapy varies from 1% to 33% based on several studies reported in the 1970s and 1980s.[105–110] More recent studies indicate that major bleeding rates during intravenous heparin therapy are < 5%.[7,111] Although bleeding can still occur when the anticoagulant effect of heparin is in the therapeutic range, there is a positive correlation between the risk of bleeding and the total daily dosage of heparin administered as well.[112]

Information stemming from several studies comparing methods of administration have shown that intermittent intravenous heparin is associated with a greater risk of bleeding than continuous infusions.[105–110] This difference may be explained by the higher doses generally used in the intermittent intravenous dosing regimen. On the other hand, bleeding risks do not appear to differ greatly between intravenous administration and subcutaneous injection (about 5.2% and

4.1%, respectively).[113] The risk of bleeding complications (including intracranial hemorrhage) with heparin is increased by the concomitant use of thrombolytic agents such as streptokinase or tissue plasminogen activator.[114–117] In one of these studies, the risk of intracranial hemorrhage correlated with an increased APTT.[117] The concomitant use of ASA also increases the risk of heparin-induced bleeding.[118,119] Certain comorbid clinical situations such as recent trauma, surgery, or renal failure all appear to increase the risk of bleeding complications.[112,120] Finally, some studies have indicated that older patients are at higher risk of heparin-associated hemorrhage.[121,122]

Intracranial Hemorrhage

Intracranial hemorrhage (ICH) is the most serious complication of heparin therapy. There are limited data on the risk of ICH when heparin is used in acute ischemic or cardioembolic stroke. Most studies did not perform routine CT scans of the brain both prior to and at a fixed time after intravenous anticoagulation. Sandercock et al. reported on the combined incidence of ICH in several studies utilizing standard unfractionated heparin or low-molecular-weight heparin.[99] In the studies in which repeat CT scans of the brain were performed only when there was clinical deterioration, treatment with heparin was associated with an excess of ICH. The overall incidence of ICH in the treatment arms of these studies was about 1.5%. In studies that performed CT scans of the brain routinely at the end of the study, the incidence of ICH was about 7.4% in the treatment group and about 6.9% in the control group. None of these results were statistically significant. However, most patients with ICH associated with heparin therapy remain asymptomatic (see above).[32,74]

Heparin-Induced Thrombocytopenia

Two types of heparin-induced thrombocytopenia (HIT) have been recognized.[123] Type I is the commonest form, and is said to occur to some extent in nearly all patients receiving unfractionated heparin.[124] Thrombocytopenia typically occurs within 1 to 5 days of initiation of treatment, but platelet counts rarely drop below 50,000. Discontinuation of heparin is generally not required. Type I HIT is not associated with thromboembolic events. Heparin-induced platelet activation and aggregation and the failure of electronic counters to distinguish these aggregates are likely responsible for the apparent thrombocytopenia.[125–127]

Type II HIT is the more serious form and is often associated with thromboembolic events. Type II HIT generally begins during the second week of treatment. Platelet counts frequently drop below 50,000 and often below 10,000. Thromboembolic events including major arterial occlusions and stroke occur in about 1% to 2% of patients.[123] Type II HIT is mediated by platelet aggregating

IgG antibodies.[128,129] Treatment of Type II HIT includes discontinuation of heparin, and may include platelet transfusions or the administration of antiplatelet agents (ASA or nonsteroidal anti-inflammatory drugs).[123] The use of heparinoids in the management of this complication has also been suggested by some.[130]

Although there has been some debate as to the value of routine platelet count monitoring, most investigators recommend that platelet counts be performed at the initiation of heparin therapy and periodically thereafter, perhaps every 2 to 3 days.[123]

ANTIPLATELET AGENTS

Mechanism of Action and Clinical Pharmacology of ASA

ASA acetylates the enzyme prostaglandin H/G synthetase, thereby interfering with its cyclo-oxygenase activity, and in turn leads to diminished prostaglandin synthesis.[131–133] Cyclo-oxygenase converts arachidonic acid to prostaglandin H2. Platelets and vascular endothelial cells in turn convert prostaglandin H2 to thromboxane A2 (TXA2) and prostacyclin (PGI2), respectively.[134] TXA2 induces platelet aggregation and causes vasoconstriction, while PGI2 has opposite effects. The antithrombotic effect of ASA is potentially mediated by several different mechanisms, but interference with the production of TXA2 is thought to be the most clinically relevant mechanism.[135]

ASA inhibits platelet function within 1 hour of its ingestion.[136–138] Although its half-life is only about 20 to 30 minutes, its effect on platelets is irreversible, making the duration of the effect of ASA equal to the life span of platelets, approximately 10 days. Because of its rapid onset of full biological activity, ASA has a potential role to play in the setting of acute cerebral ischemia. This notion is further strengthened by some studies which have shown increased thromboxane production, which is ASA suppressible, in the early phases of an acute ischemic stroke.[139]

Optimal Dose of ASA

The optimal dose of ASA in the management of ischemic cerebrovascular disease remains a topic of great controversy.[140–142] Low (75 to 80 mg), intermediate (325 to 650 mg), and high (975 to 1,300 mg) daily doses have all been advocated. The minimal dose required to significantly reduce thromboxane-dependent platelet aggregation is 20 mg/day in healthy subjects.[143,144] Somewhat higher doses, however, may be required to significantly inhibit TXA2 release in patients who have previously suffered a stroke (at least 40 mg/day).[145] The most widely tested doses for the prevention of ischemic cerebrovascular disease are between 75 and 325 mg.[146]

ASA IN ACUTE ISCHEMIC STROKE

Though the role of ASA is firmly established for the secondary prevention of ischemic coronary and cerebrovascular syndromes, its role in the setting of acute cerebral ischemia remains to be fully defined.

The first randomized trial of ASA in the setting of recent transient ischemic attacks was reported in 1989.[96] In this trial 55 patients were randomized to receive either intravenous dose-adjusted heparin or ASA, 1,300 mg/day within 7 days of a transient ischemic attacks. There was no placebo group. There was no statistically significant difference in TIA recurrence rates between the groups (29.7% in the heparin group, and 25% in the ASA group). One of 27 heparin-treated patients had a cerebral infarction, while 4 of 28 ASA-treated patients had such an event. This study suggested that there was no significant differences between ASA and heparin in the setting of recent transient ischemic attacks. However, the number of patients was small and no firm conclusions could be drawn.

In the Multicentre Acute Stroke Trial–Italy (MAST-I),[147] patients were randomized to receive either intravenous streptokinase, streptokinase plus ASA, ASA alone, or neither drug within 6 hours of an ischemic stroke. A total of 309 patients were randomized to the ASA groups, and of these, 153 patients received ASA alone. ASA treatment was associated with a reduction in the short-term (10-day) and long-term (6-month) case fatality rate, but this did not attain statistical significance. These data, however, do suggest a possible role for ASA in the setting of acute cerebral ischemia.

The efficacy of ASA in the setting of acute ischemic stroke has been further investigated in two recently completed large, randomized trials—the International Stroke Trial (IST)[17,99,148] and the Chinese Acute Stroke Trial (CAST).[149]

Of 19,435 patients entered into the IST, half were randomized to receive subcutaneous unfractionated heparin (one-quarter 5,000 units twice daily and one-quarter 12,500 units twice daily), and half were to "avoid heparin." In this 3×2 factorial design, half were randomized to receive ASA (300 mg/day) and half were to "avoid ASA." Patients were randomized within 48 hours of acute stroke symptoms. Primary outcomes of efficacy were death from any cause within 14 days, and death or dependency at 6 months. Secondary outcomes at 14 days were recurrent strokes, intracranial hemorrhage (from either recurrent hemorrhagic stroke or hemorrhagic transformation of the original stroke), pulmonary emboli, and extracerebral hemorrhages requiring transfusion. Secondary outcomes at 6 months were death from any cause, proportion of patients with full recovery, and number of patients living at home.

At 14 days, ASA had no significant effect on mortality but was associated with significantly fewer recurrent ischemic strokes. ASA had no significant effect on death or dependency at 6 months.

In the CAST, 21,106 patients were randomized to receive either ASA (160 mg/day) or placebo within 48 hours of acute ischemic stroke. Primary comparisons were death from any cause during the treatment period (up to 4 weeks). Secondary comparisons were fatal or nonfatal recurrent stroke, death or nonfatal stroke, transfused or fatal extracranial hemorrhage, and pulmonary embolism during the treatment period.

ASA was associated with a 14% proportionate reduction in mortality during the treatment period. ASA-treated patients had significantly fewer recurrent ischemic strokes but also a nonsignificant slight excess of hemorrhagic stroke. ASA was associated with a small but significant excess of transfused or fatal extracranial hemorrhages. The numbers of nonfatal pulmonary emboli did not differ in either treatment group.

When data from the IST and CAST are combined, ASA, when begun early in the setting of acute ischemic stroke, is responsible for nine fewer deaths or nonfatal strokes per 1,000 patients in the first few weeks. Early ASA treatment is also associated with 13 fewer dead or dependent per 1,000 patients several weeks or months following acute ischemic stroke.

OTHER ANTIPLATELET AGENTS

Although other antiplatelet agents such as ticlopidine,[150,151] clopidogrel,[152] and dipyridamole[153] have the potential to be beneficial in the long-term prevention of cerebral ischemia, none has been specifically compared to ASA in the acute setting. However, for some of these drugs, such as ticlopidine and clopidogrel, the full antiaggregant effect is established only after several days,[154,155] which makes it unlikely that these agents would be useful in the management of acute cerebral ischemia.

Over the past few years several newer antiplatelet agents have been developed that may have greater promise because their antithrombotic effect is much more rapid. These include antagonists of the platelet-bound fibrinogen receptor GPIIb-IIIa, inhibitors of platelet adhesion, inhibitors of the enzyme thromboxane synthetase, inhibitors of thrombin, and inhibitors of factor Xa. Many of these agents have been studied in experimental animal models.[156–160] Only GPIIb-IIIa antagonists and direct thrombin inhibitors have been studied in humans, specifically in the settings of unstable angina,[161–162] deep venous thrombosis prophylaxis,[163,164] or as adjuvant therapy during coronary thrombolysis[165–168] or angioplasty.[169,170] Studies in the setting of acute cerebral ischemia are ongoing.

COMPLICATIONS OF ASA THERAPY

The main complications of ASA therapy are gastric.[136] ASA can produce both short-term and long-term complications. The short-term complications include gastric erosions and gastric hemorrhage, while long-term complications include anemia and gastric ulceration. ASA treatment is not usually associated with duodenal ulceration.[171] Both short-term and long-term ASA use are associated with a dose-dependent increase in gastrointestinal bleeding.[171–173] Although the pathophysiology of ASA-related gastric erosions is not precisely known, several different mechanisms have been proposed. These include the inhibition of gastric mucosal prostaglandin synthesis,[171] inhibition of gastric mucosal cell regeneration,[174] an antihemostatic effect,[175] and impairment of mucus formation.[176]

Gastric side effects can be minimized by the use of lower doses of ASA, the concomitant use of antacids,[173] cimetidine,[172] histamine H_2-receptor antagonists,[177,178] or the use of either buffered or enteric-coated preparations.[179]

CONCLUSIONS

Both heparin and ASA are commonly prescribed in the setting of acute cerebral ischemia. Other than the use of low-dose heparin for prophylaxis against DVT or pulmonary embolism, there is little evidence to date that heparin is otherwise of benefit in acute ischemic stroke; it may be even harmful. ASA, on the other hand, has a small but significant benefit and should be prescribed as soon as possible to most patients after acute ischemic stroke. Newer antiplatelet agents, however, such as GPIIb/IIIa antagonists and direct thrombin inhibitors may prove to be of greater benefit in this context.

REFERENCES

1. Hirsh J. Heparin. N Engl J Med 1991; 324:1565–1574.
2. Eika C. Inhibition of thrombin-induced aggregation of human platelets by heparin. Scand J Haematol 1971; 8:216–222.
3. Kelton JG, Hirsh J. Bleeding associated with antithrombotic therapy. Sem Hematol 1980; 17:259–291.
4. Blajchman MA, Young E, Ofosu FA. Effects of unfractionated heparin, dermatan sulfate and low molecular weight heparin on vessel wall permeability in rabbits. Ann NY Acad Sci 1989; 556:245–254.
5. Chiu HM, Hirsh J, Yung WL, Regoeczi E, Gent M. Relationship between anticoagulant and antithrombotic effects of heparin. Blood 1987; 49:171–184.
6. Levine M, Hirsh J, Gent M, et al. A randomized trial comparing activated partial

thromboplastin time with heparin assay in patients with acute venous thromboembolism requiring large daily doses of heparin. Arch Intern Med 1994; 154:49–56.
7. Hirsh J, Raschke R, Warketin TE, Dalen JE, Deykin D, Poller L. Heparin: mechanism of action, pharmacokinetics, dosing considerations, monitoring, efficacy, and safety. Chest 1995; 108(suppl):258S–275S.
8. Barrit DW, Jordan SC. Anticoagulant drugs in the treatment of pulmonary embolism: a controlled clinical trial. Lancet 1960; 1:1309–1312.
9. Kernohan RJ, Todd C. Heparin therapy in thromboembolic disease. Lancet 1966; 1:621–623.
10. Hull RD, Raskob GE, Hirsh J, et al. Continuous intravenous heparin compared with intermittent subcutaneous heparin in the initial treatment of proximal-vein thrombosis. N Engl J Med 1986; 315:1109–1114.
11. Brandjes DPM, Heijboer H, Buller HR, de Rijk M, Jagt M, ten Cate JW. Acenocoumarol and heparin compared with acenocoumarol alone in the initial treatment of proximal vein thrombosis. N Engl J Med 1992; 327:1485–1489.
12. Nurmohamed MT, Rosendaal RB, Buller HR, et al. Low-molecular weight heparin versus standard heparin in general and orthopedic surgery: a meta-analysis. Lancet 1992; 340:152–155.
13. Imperiale TF, Speroff T. A meta-analysis of methods to prevent venous thromboembolism following total hip replacement. JAMA 1994; 71:1780-1785.
14. Marks P, Teather D. Subcutaneous heparin: a logical prophylaxis for deep venous thrombosis after myocardial infarction. Practitioner 1978; 220:425–435.
15. Warlow C, Terry G, Kenmure AC, Beattie AG, Ogston D, Douglas AS. A double-blinded trial of low doses of subcutaneous heparin in the prevention of deep-vein thrombosis after myocardial infarction. Lancet 1973; 2:934–940.
16. Fourth ACCP Consensus Conference on Antithrombotic Therapy. Dalen JE, Hirsh J, eds. Chest 1995; 108:225S–522S.
17. International Stroke Trial Collaborative Group. The International Stroke Trial (IST): a randomised trials of aspirin, subcutaneous heparin, both, or neither among 19,435 patients with acute ischaemic stroke. Lancet 1997; 349:1569–1581.
18. Bousser M-G. Aspirin or heparin immediately after a stroke? Commentary. Lancet 1997; 349:1564–1565.
19. Cerebral Embolism Task Force. Cardiogenic brain embolism. Arch Neurol 1986; 43:71–84.
20. Second Report of the Cerebral Embolism Task Force. Cardiogenic brain embolism. Arch Neurol 1989; 46:727–743.
21. Wolf PA, Abbot RD, Kannel WB. Atrial fibrillation as an independent risk factor for stroke: the Framingham study. Stroke 1991; 22:983–988.
22. Wolfe PA, Dawber TR, Thomas HE, Kannel WB. Epidemiologic assessment of chronic atrial fibrillation and risk of stroke: the Framingham study. Neurology 1978; 28:973–977.
23. Atrial Fibrillation Investigators. Risk factors for stroke and efficacy of antithrombotic therapy in atrial fibrillation: analysis of pooled data from five randomized controlled trials. Arch Intern Med 1994; 154:1449–1457.
24. Stroke Prevention in Atrial Fibrillation Investigators. Predictors of thromboem-

bolism in atrial fibrillation: echocardiographic features of patients at risk. Ann Intern Med 1992; 116:6–12.
25. Peterson P, Boysen G, Godtfredsen J, Anderson E, Anderson B. Placebo-controlled, randomized trial of warfarin and aspirin for prevention of thromboembolic complications in chronic atrial fibrillation: the Copenhagen AFASAK study. Lancet 1989; 1:175–179.
26. Boston Area Anticoagulation Trial for Atrial Fibrillation Investigators. The effect of low-dose warfarin on the risk of stroke in patients with nonrheumatic atrial fibrillation. N Engl J Med 1990; 323:1505–1511.
27. Stroke Prevention in Atrial Fibrillation Investigators. The stroke prevention in atrial fibrillation study: final results. Circulation 1991; 84:527–539.
28. Connolly S, Laupacis A, Gent M. Canadian atrial fibrillation anticoagulation (CAFA) study. J AM Coll Cardiol 1991; 18:349–355.
29. Ezekowitz MD, Ridgers S, James K, et al. VA cooperative study of warfarin in the prevention of stroke associated with nonrheumatic atrial fibrillation. N Engl J Med 1992; 327:1406–1412.
30. European Atrial Fibrillation Trial Study Group. Secondary prevention in nonrheumatic atrial fibrillation after transient ischemic attack or minor stroke. Lancet 1993; 342:1255–1262.
31. Stroke Prevention in Atrial Fibrillation Investigators. Warfarin versus aspirin for prevention of thromboembolism in atrial fibrillation: Stroke Prevention in Atrial Fibrillation II study. Lancet 1994; 343:687–691.
32. Cerebral Embolism Study Group. Immediate anticoagulation of embolic stroke: a randomized trial. Stroke 1983; 14:668–676.
33. Furlan AJ, Cavalier SJ, Hobbs RE, Weinstein MA, Modic MI. Hemorrhage and anticoagulation after nonseptic embolic brain infarction. Neurology 1982; 32:280–282.
34. Koller RL. Recurrent embolic cerebral infarction and anticoagulation. Neurology 1982; 32:283–285.
35. Hart RG, Coull BM, Hart PD. Early recurrent embolism associated with nonvalvular atrial fibrillation. Stroke 1983; 14:688–693.
36. Lodder J, van der Lugt PM. Evaluation of the risk of immediate anticoagulant treatment in patients with embolic stroke of cardiac origin. Stroke 1983; 14:42–46.
37. Darling RC, Austen WG, Linton RR. Arterial embolism. Surg Gynecol Obstet 1967; 124:106–114.
38. Daly R, Mattingly TW, Holt CT, et al. Systemic arterial embolism in rheumatic heart disease. Am Heart J 1954; 42:566–581.
39. Fisher CM. Reducing risks of cerebral embolism. Geriatrics 1979; 34:59–66.
40. Shields RW Jr, Laureno R, Lachman T, Victor M. Anticoagulant-induced hemorrhage in acute cerebral embolism. Stroke 1984; 15:426–437.
41. Bass E. Anticoagulation in cerebral embolism. Can J Neurol Sci 1983; 10:32–36.
42. Fleming HA, Bailey SM. Mitral valve disease, systemic embolism and anticoagulation. Postgrad Med 1971; 47:599–604.
43. Chamorro A, Vila N, Saiz A, Alday M, Tolosa E. Early anticoagulation after large cerebral embolic infarction: a safety study. Neurology 1995; 45:861–865.

44. Rothrock JF, Dittrich HC, McAllen S, Taft BJ, Lyden PD. Acute anticoagulation following cardioembolic stroke. Stroke 1989; 20:730–734.
45. Sacco RL, Foulkes MA, Mohr JP, Wolf PA, Hier DB, Price TR. Determinants of early recurrence of cerebral infarction: the Stroke Data Bank. Stroke 1989; 20:983–989.
46. Yasaka M, Yamaguchi T, Oita J, Sawada T, Shichiri M, Omae T. Clinical features of recurrent embolization in acute cardioembolic stroke. Stroke 1993; 24:1681–1685.
47. Bogousslavsy J, Van Meele G, Regli F, Kappenberger L. Pathogenesis of anterior circulation stroke in patients with nonvalvular atrial fibrillation: the Lausanne Stroke Registry. Neurology 1990; 40:1046–1050.
48. Szekely P. Systemic embolism and anticoagulation prophylaxis in rheumatic heart disease. BMJ 1964; 1:209–212.
49. Levine HJ. Which atrial fibrillation patients should be on chronic anticoagulation. J Cardiovasc Med 1981; 6:483–487.
50. Carter AB. Prognosis of cerebral embolism. Lancet 1965; 2:514–519.
51. Cannegieter SC, Rosendaal FR, Briet E. Thromboembolic and bleeding complications in patients with mechanical valve prosthesis. Circulation 1994; 89:635–641.
52. Cannegieter SC, Rosendaal FR, Wintzen AR, van der Meer FJ, Vanderbroucke JP, Briet E. Optimal oral anticoagulant therapy in patients with mechanical heart valves. N Engl J Med 1995; 333:11–17.
53. Burchfiel CM, Hammermeister KE, Krause-Steinrauf H, et al. Left atrial dimensions and risk of systemic embolism in patients with a prosthetic heart valve. J Am Coll Cardiol 1990; 15:32–41.
54. Stein PD, Alpert JS, Copeland J, Dalen JE, Goldman S, Turpie AGG. Antithrombotic therapy in patients with mechanical and biological prosthetic heart valves. Chest 1995; 108(suppl):371S–379S.
55. Vongpatanasin W, Hillis LD, Lange RA. Prosthetic heart valves. N Engl J Med 1996; 335:407–416.
56. Sherman DG. Cardiac embolism: the neurologist's perspective. Am J Cardiol 1990; 65:32C–37C.
57. Vaitkus PT, Berlin JA, Schwartz JS, Barnathan ES. Stroke complicating acute myocardial infarction: a meta-analysis of risk modification by anticoagulation and thrombolytic therapy. Arch Intern Med 1992; 192:2020–2024.
58. Komrad MS, Coffey CE, Coffey KS, Mckinnis R, Massey EW, Califf RM. Myocardial infarction and stroke. Neurology 1984; 34:1403–1409.
59. Asinger RW, Mikkel FI, Elsperger J, Hodges M. Incidence of left-ventricular thrombosis after acute transmural myocardial infarction: serial evaluation by two-dimensional echocardiography. N Engl J Med 1981; 305:297–302.
60. Spirito P, Belloti P, Chiarelli F, Domenicucci S, Sementa A, Vecchio C. Prognostic significance and natural history of left ventricular thrombi in patients with acute anterior myocardial infarction: a two-dimensional echocardiographic study. Circulation 1985; 72:774–780.
61. Vaitkus PT, Barnathan ES. Embolic potential, prevention and management of

mural thrombus complicating acute anterior myocardial infarction: a meta-analysis. J Am Coll Cardiol 1993; 22:1004–1009.
62. Cairns JA, Lewis D Jr, Meade TW, Sutton GC, Theroux P. Antithrombotic agents n coronary artery disease. Chest 1995; 108(suppl):380S–400S.
63. Lones HR, Siekert RG, Geraci JE. Neurologic manifestations of bacterial endocarditis. Ann Intern Med 1969; 71:21–28.
64. Pruitt AA. Rubin RH, Karchmer AW, Duncan GW. Neurologic complications of bacterial endocarditis. Medicine 1978; 57:329–343.
65. Salgado AV, Furlan AJ, Keys TF, Nichols TR, Beck GJ. Neurologic complications of endocarditis: a 12-year experience. Neurology 1989; 39:173–179.
66. Paschalis C, Pugsley W, John R, Harrison MJ. Rate of cerebral embolic events in relation to antibiotic and anticoagulant therapy in patients with bacterial endocarditis. Eur Neurol 1990; 30:87–89.
67. Davenport J, Hart RG. Prosthetic valve endocarditis 1976–1987: antibiotics, anticoagulation and stroke. Stroke 1990; 21:993–999.
68. Salgado AV, Furlan AJ, Keys TF. Mycotic aneurysms, subarachnoid hemorrhage and indications for cerebral angiography in infective endocarditis. Stroke 1987; 18:1057–1060.
69. Tunkel AE, Kaye D. Neurologic complications of infective endocarditis. Neurol Clin 1993; 11:419–440.
70. Gillinov AM, Shah RV, Curtis WE, et al. Valve replacement in patients with endocarditis and acute neurologic deficit. Ann Thorac Surg 1996; 61:1125–1129.
71. Lopez JA, Ross RS, Fishbein MC, Siegel RJ. Non-bacterial thrombotic endocarditis: a review. Am Heart J 1987; 113:773–784.
72. Sach GH, Levin J, Bell WR. Trousseau's syndrome and other manifestations of chronic disseminated coagulopathy in patients with neoplasms: clinical, pathophysiologic and therapeutic features. Medicine 1977; 56:1–37.
73. Hakim AM, Ryder-Cook A, Melanson D. Sequential computerized tomographic appearance of strokes. Stroke 1983; 14:893–897.
74. Cerebral Embolism Study Group. Immediate anticoagulation of embolic stroke: brain hemorrhage and management options. Stroke 1984; 15:779–789.
75. Sherman DG, Dyken ML Jr, Gent M, Harrison MJG, Hart RG, Mohr JP. Antithrombotic therapy for cerebrovascular disorders: an update. Chest 1995; 108(suppl):444S–456S.
76. Moulin T, Cattin F, Crepin-Leblond T, et al. Early CT signs in acute middle cerebral artery infarction: predictive value for subsequent infarct locations and outcome. Neurology 1996; 47:366–375.
77. Turpie AGG, Gent M, Côté R, et al. A low-molecular-weight heparinoid compared with unfractionated heparin in the prevention of deep vein thrombosis in patients with acute ischemic stroke. A randomized, double-blind study. Ann Intern Med 1992; 117:353–357.
78. Turpie AGG, Levin MN, Carter GJ, et al. A double-blind randomized trial of ORG 10172 low molecular weight heparinoid in the prevention of deep vein thrombosis in thrombotic stroke. Lancet 1987; 1:523–526.

79. Miller VT, Hart RG. Heparin anticoagulation in acute brain ischemia. Stroke 1998; 19:403–406.
80. Kelly RG, Berger JR, Alter M, Kovacs AG. Cerebral ischemia and atrial fibrillation: prospective study. Neurology 1984; 34:1285–1291.
81. Hayman LA, Evans RA, Bastian FO, Hinck VC. Delayed high dose contrast CT: identifying patients at risk of massive hemorrhagic infarction. AJR 1981; 136:1151–1159.
82. Gautier JC. Stroke-in-progression. Stroke 1985; 16:729–733.
83. Millikan CH, McDowell FH. Treatment of progressing stroke. Stroke 1981; 12:397–409.
84. Britton M, Roden A. Progression of stroke after arrival at hospital. Stroke 1985; 16:629–632.
85. Davalos A, Cendra E, Tervel J, Martinez M, Genis D. Deteriorating ischemic stroke: risk factors and prognosis. Neurology 1990; 40:1865–1869.
86. Fisher M, Garcia JH. Evolving stroke and the ischemic penumbra. Neurology 1996; 47:884–888.
87. Marsh lll EE, Adams HP, Biller J, et al. Use of antithrombotic drugs in the treatment of acute ischemic stroke: a survey of neurologists in practice in the United States. Neurology 1989; 39:1631–1634.
88. Fisher CM. Use of anticoagulants in cerebral thrombosis. Neurology 1958; 8:311–332.
89. Carter AB. Anticoagulant treatment in progressing stroke. BMJ 1961; 2:70–73.
90. Fisher CM. Anticoagulant therapy in cerebral thrombosis and cerebral embolism: a national cooperative study. Interim report. Neurology 1961; 11:132–138.
91. Baker RN, Broward JA, Fong HC, et al. Anticoagulant therapy in cerebral infarction. Neurology 1962; 12:823–835.
92. Duke RJ, Bloch RF, Turpie AGG, Trebilcock R, Bayer N. Intravenous heparin for the prevention of stroke progression in acute partial stable stroke: a randomized controlled trial. Ann Intern Med 1986; 105:825–828.
93. Feinberg WM, Albers GW, Barnett HJM, et al. Guidelines for the management of transient ischemic attacks. From the ad hoc committee on guidelines for the management of transient ischemic attacks of the Stroke Council of the American Heart Association. Stroke 1994; 25:1320–1335.
94. Wolf PA, Kannel WB, Verter J. Current status of risk factors for stroke. Neurol Clin 1983; 1:317–343.
95. Keith DS, Phillips SJ, Whisnant JP, Nishimaru K, O'Fallon WM. Heparin therapy for recent transient focal cerebral ischemia. Mayo Clin Proc 1987; 62:1101–1106.
96. Biller J, Bruno A, Adams HP, et al. A randomized trial of aspirin or heparin in hospitalized patients with recent transient ischemic attacks: a pilot study. Stroke 1989; 20:441–447.
97. Wilson SE, Mayberg MR, Yatsu F, Weiss DG. Crescendo transient ischemic attacks: a surgical imperative. J Vasc Surg 1993 17:249–256.
98. Bruno A, Jeffries L, Lakind E, Qualls C. Predictors of cerebral infarction following transient ischemic attacks. J Stroke Cerebrovasc Dis 1993; 3:23–28.
99. Sandercock PAG, van den Belt AGM, Lindley RJ, Slattery J. Antithrombotic

therapy in acute ischaemic stroke: an overview of the completed randomized trials. J Neurol Neurosurg Psychiatry 1993; 56:17–25.
100. McIlraith DM, Cote R. Cerebral venous thrombosis. In: Leclerc JR, ed. Thromboembolic Disorders. Philadelphia: Lea & Febiger, 1990:382–399.
101. Zuber M, Toulon P, Marnet L, Mas J-L. Factor V Leiden mutation in cerebral venous thrombosis. Stroke 1996; 27:1721–1723.
102. Deschiens M-A, Conard J, Horellou MH, et al. Coagulation studies, Factor V Leiden and anticardiolipin antibodies in 40 cases of cerebral venous thrombosis. Stroke 1996; 27:1724–1730.
103. Einhaupl KM, Villringer A, Meister W, et al. Heparin treatment in sinus venous thrombosis. Lancet 1991; 338:597–600.
104. De Stefano V, Finazzi G, Mannucci PM. Inherited thrombophilia: pathogenesis, clinical syndromes and management. Blood 1996; 87:3531–3544.
105. Salzman EW, Deykin D, Shapiro RM, Rosenberg R. Management of heparin therapy: controlled prospective trial. N Engl J Med 1975; 292:1046–1050.
106. Glazier RL, Corwell EB. Randomized prospective trial of continuous vs intermittent heparin therapy. JAMA 1976; 236:1365–1367.
107. Mant MJ, O'Brien BD, Thong KL, Hammond GW, Birtwhistle RV, Grace MG. Haemorrhagic complications of heparin therapy. Lancet 1977; 1:1133–1135.
108. Wilson JR, Lampman J. Heparin therapy: a randomized prospective study Am Heart J 1979; 97:155–158.
109. Fagher B, Lundh B. Heparin treatment of deep vein thrombosis. Acta Med Scand 1981; 210:357–361.
110. Wilson JE, Bynum LJ, Parkey RW. Heparin therapy in venous thromboembolism. Am J Med 1981; 70:808–816.
111. Raschke RA, Reilly BM, Guidry J, Fontana JR, Srinivas S. The weight-based heparin nomogram compared with a 'standard care' nomogram: a randomized controlled trial. Ann Intern Med 1993; 119:874–811.
112. Levine MN, Hirsh J, Kelton JG. Heparin induced bleeding. In: Lane DA, Lindahl U, eds. Heparin: Chemical and Biological Properties, Clinical Applications. London: Edward Arnold, 1989:517–532.
113. Hommes DW, Bura A, Mazzolai L, Buller HR, ten Cate JW. Subcutaneous heparin compared with continuous intravenous heparin administration in the initial treatment of deep vein thrombosis: a meta-analysis. Ann Intern Med 1992; 116:279–284.
114. SCATI Group. Randomized controlled trial of subcutaneous calcium-heparin in acute myocardial infarction. Lancet 1989; 2:182–185.
115. Gruppo Italiano per lo Studo della Supravvivenza nell'Infarto Miocardico. GISSI-2. A factorial randomized trial of alteplase versus streptokinase and heparin versus no heparin among 12,490 patients with acute myocardial infarction. Lancet 1990; 2:65–70.
116. Bleich SD, Nichols T, Schumacher R, et al. The role of heparin following coronary thrombolysis with tissue plasminogen activator. Circulation 1989; 80(suppl):113.
117. Global Use of Strategies to Open Occluded Coronary Arteries (GUSTO) IIa In-

vestigators. Randomized trial of intravenous heparin versus recombinant hirudin for acute coronary syndromes. Circulation 1994; 90:1631–1637.
118. Yett HS, Skillman JJ, Salzman EW. The hazards of heparin plus aspirin (letter). N Engl J Med 1978; 248:1092.
119. Sethi GK, Copeland JG, Goldman S, Moritz T, Zadina K, Henderson WG. Implications of preoperative administration of aspirin in patients undergoing coronary artery bypass grafting. J Am Coll Cardiol 1990; 15:15–20.
120. Hull RD, Raskob GE, Rosenbloom D, et al. Heparin for 5 days versus for 10 days in the initial treatment of proximal venous thrombosis. N Engl J Med 1990; 322:1260–1264.
121. Jick H, Slone D, Borda IT, Shapiro S. Efficacy and toxicity of heparin in relation to age and sex. N Engl J Med 1968; 279:284–286.
122. Basu D, Gallus A, Hirsh J, Cade J. A prospective study of the value of monitoring heparin treatment with the activated partial thromboplastin time. N Engl J Med 1972; 287:324–327.
123. Becker PS, Miller VT. Heparin-induced thrombocytopenia. Stroke 1989; 20:1449–1459.
124. Kelton JG, Murphy WG. Acute thrombocytopenia and thrombosis. Heparin-induced thrombocytopenia and thrombotic thrombocytopenic purpura. Ann NY Acad Sci 1987; 509:205–221.
125. Green D. Heparin-induced thrombocytopenia. Med J Aust 1986; 144:HS37–HS39.
126. Nelson JC, Lerner RG, Goldstein R, Cagin NA. Heparin-induced thrombocytopenia. Arch Intern Med 1978; 138:548–552.
127. Chong BH, Ismail F. The mechanism of heparin-induced platelet aggregation. Eur J Haematol 1989; 43:245–251.
128. Kelton JG, Sheridan D, Santos A, et al. Heparin-associated thrombocytopenia: laboratory studies. Blood 1988; 72:925–930.
129. Chong BH, Fawaz I, Chesterman CN, Berndt MC. Heparin-induced thrombocytopenia: mechanism of interaction of the heparin-dependent antibody with platelets. Br J Haematol 1989; 73:235–240.
130. Magnani HN. Heparin-induced thrombocytopenia (HIT): an overview of 230 patients treated with Orgaran (Org 10172). Thromb Haemost 1993; 70:554–561.
131. Roth GJ, Stanford N, Majerus PW. Actylation of prostaglandin synthase by aspirin. Pro Natl Acad Sci USA 1975; 72:3073–3077.
132. Moncada S, Vane JR. Pharmacology and exogenous roles of prostaglandin endoperoxides, thromboxane-A2 and prostacyclin. Pharmacol Rev 1978; 30:291–331.
133. Patrono C, Ciabattoni G, Patrignani P, et al. Clinical pharmacology of platelet cyclo-oxygenase inhibition. Circulation 1985; 72:1177–1184.
134. Weksler BB, Prett SB, Alonso D, et al. Differential inhibition by aspirin of vascular and platelet prostaglandin synthesis in atherosclerotic patients. N Engl J Med 1983; 308:800–805.
135. Patrono C. Aspirin as an antiplatelet drug. N Engl J Med 1994; 330:1287–1294.
136. Hirsh J, Dalen JE, Fuster V, Harker LB, Patrono C, Roth G. Aspirin and other platelet active drugs. The relationship among dose, effectiveness, and side effects. Chest 1995; 108(suppl):247S–257S.

137. AHFS Drug Information 92. Bethesda, MD: American Society of Hospital Pharnacists, 1992:1055.
138. Pederson AK, FitzGerald GA. Dose-related kinetics of aspirin: presystemic acetylation of platelet cyclooxygenase. N Engl J Med 1984; 311:1206–1211.
139. Koudstaal PJ, Ciabattoni G, van Gijn J, et al. Increased thromboxane biosynthesis in patients with acute cerebral ischemia. Stroke 1993; 24:219–223.
140. Hart RG, Harrison MJG. Aspirin wars: the optimal dose of aspirin to prevent stroke. Stroke 1996; 27:585–587.
141. Barnett HJM, Kaste M, Meldrum H, Eliasziw M. Aspirin dose in stroke prevention: beautiful hypothesis slain by ugly facts. Stroke 1996; 27:588–592.
142. Patrono C, Roth GJ. Aspirin in ischemic cerebrovascular disease: how strong is the case for a different dosing regimen. Stroke 1996; 27:756–760.
143. FitzGerald GA, Oates JA, Hawiger J, et al. Endogenous biosynthesis of prostacyclin and thromboxane and platelet function during chronic administration of aspirin in man. J Clin Invest 1983; 71:676–688.
144. De Caterina R, Giannessi D, Boem A, et al. Equal antiplatelet effects of aspirin 50 or 324 mg/day in patients after acute myocardial infarction. Throm Haemost 1985; 54:528–532.
145. Tohgi H, Konno S, Tamura K, Kimura B, Kawano K. Effects of low-to-high doses of aspirin on platelet aggregability and metabolites of thromboxane A2 and prostacyclin. Stroke 1992; 23:1400–1403.
146. Antiplatelet Trialists' Collaboration. Collaborative overview of randomised trials of antiplatelet therapy. 1. Prevention of death, myocardial infarction, and stroke by prolonged antiplatelet therapy in various categories of patients. BMJ 1994; 308:81–106.
147. Multicentre Acute Stroke Trial—Italy (MAST-I) Group. Randomised controlled trial of streptokinase, aspirin, and the combination of both in the treatment of acute ischaemic stroke. Lancet 1995; 346:1509–1514.
148. International Stroke Trial Pilot Study Collaborative Group. Study design of the International Stroke Trial (IST), baseline data, and outcome in 984 randomised patients in the pilot study. J Neurol Neurosurg Psychiatry 1996; 60:371–376.
149. CAST (Chinese Acute Stroke Trial) Collaborative Group. CAST: randomised placebo-controlled trial of early aspirin use in 20,000 patients with acute ischaemic stroke. Lancet 1997; 349:1641–1649.
150. Hass WK, Easton JD, Adams HP, et al. A randomized trial comparing ticlopidine hydrochloride with aspirin for the prevention of strokes in high-risk patients. N Engl J Med 1989; 321:501–507.
151. Gent M, Blakely JA, Easton JD, et al. The Canadian American Ticlopidine Study (CATS) in thromboembolic stroke. Lancet 1989; 1:1215–1220.
152. Caprie Steering Committee. A randomised, blinded, trial of clopidogrel versus aspirin in patients at risk of ischaemic events (CAPRIE). Lancet 1996; 1329–1339.
153. Diener HC, Cunha L, Forbes C, Sivenius J, Smets P, Lowenthal A. European Stroke Prevention Study 2. Dipyridamole and acetylsalicylic acid in the secondary prevention of stroke. J Neurol Sci 1996; 143:1–13.
154. Herbert JM, Frehel D, Vallee E, Kieffer G, Gouy D, Berger Y, Necciari J, Defreyn

G, Maffrand JP. Clopidogrel, a novel antiplatelet and antithrombotic agent. Cardiovasc Drug Rev 1993; 11:180–198.

155. Di Minno G, Cerbone AM, Mattioli PL, Turco S, Iovine C, Mancini M. Functionally thrombasthenic state in normal platelets following the administration of ticlopidine. J Clin Invest 1985; 75:328–338.

156. Haskel EJ, Prager NA, Sobel BE, Abendschein CR. Relative efficacy of antithrombin compared with antiplatelet agents in accelerating coronary thrombolysis and preventing early reocclusion. Circulation 1991; 83:1048–1056.

157. Heras M, Chesebro JH, Penny WJ, Bailey KA, Badimon L, Fuster V. Effects of thrombin inhibition on the development acute platelet-thrombus deposition during angioplasty in pigs: heparin versus recombinant hirudin, a specific thrombin inhibitor. Circulation 1989; 79:657–665.

158. Klement P, Borm A, Hirsh J, Maraganore J, Wilson G, Weitz J. Thrombin inhibitors on tissue plasminogen activator induced thrombolysis in a rat model. Thromb Haemost 1992; 68:64–68.

159. Kelly AB, Marzec UM, Krupski W, et al. Hirudin interruption of heparin-resistant arterial thrombus formation in baboons. Blood 1991; 77:1006–1012.

160. Bagdy D, Barabas E, Szabo G, Bajusz S, Szell E. In vivo anticoagulant and antiplatelet effects of D-PheProArgH and D-MePhe-Pro-Arg-H. Thromb Haemost 1992; 67:357–365.

161. Schulman SP, Goldschmidt-Clermont PJ, Navetta FI, et al. Integrelin in unstable angina: a double-blind randomized trial (abstract). Circulation 1993; 88(suppl 1):608.

162. Topol EJ, Fuster V, Harrington RA, et al. Recombinant hirudin for unstable angina pectoris: a multicenter, randomized angiographic study. Circulation 1994; 89:1557–1566.

163. Ginsberg JS, Nurmohamed MT, Gent M, et al. Use of hirulog in the prevention venous thrombosis after major hip or knee surgery. Circulation 1994; 90:2385–2389.

164. Eriksson BI, Ekman S, Kalebo P, Zachrisson B, Bach D, Close P. Prevention of deep-vein thrombosis after total hip replacement: direct thrombin inhibition with recombinant hirudin, CGP 39393. Lancet 1996; 347:635–639.

165. Lidon RM, Theroux P, Bonan R, et al. A pilot early angiographic patency study using a direct thrombin inhibitor as adjunctive therapy to streptokinase in acute myocardial infarction. Circulation 1994; 89:1567–1572.

166. Theroux P, Perez-Villa F, Waters D, Lesperance J, Shabani F, Bonan R. A randomized double-blind comparison of two doses of hirulog or heparin as adjunctive therapy to streptokinase to promote early patency of the infarct-related artery in acute myocardial infarction. Circulation 1995; 91:2132–2139.

167. Cannon CP, McCabe CH, Henry TD, et al. A pilot trial of recombinant desulfatohirudin compared with heparin in conjunction with tissue-type plasminogen activator and aspirin for acute myocardial infarction: results of the Thrombolysis in Myocardial Infarction (TIMI) 5 trial. J Am Coll Cardiol 1994; 23:993–1003.

168. Antman EM, for the TIMI 9A Investigators. Hirudin in acute myocardial infarc-

tion: safety report from the thrombolysis and thrombin inhibition in myocardial infarction (TIMI) 9A trial. Circulation 1994; 90:1624–1630.
169. EPIC Investigators. Use of a monoclonal antibody directed against the platelet glycoprotein IIb/IIIa receptor in high-risk coronary angioplasty. N Engl J Med 1994; 330:956–961.
170. Teheng JE, Harrington RA, Kottke-Marchant K, et al. Multicenter, randomized, double-blind placebo-controlled trial of the platelet integrin glycoprotein IIb/IIIa blocker Integrelin in elective coronary intervention. Impact investigators. Circulation 1995; 91:2151–2157.
171. Pirchard PJ, Kitchingman GK, Walt RP, Daneshmend TK, Hawkey CJ. Human gastric mucosal bleeding induced by low dose aspirin, but not warfarin. BMJ 1989; 298:493–496.
172. Hawkey CJ, Somerville KW, Marshall S. Prophylaxis of aspirin induced gastric mucosal bleeding with ranitidine. Aliment Pharmacol Ther 1988; 2:245–252.
173. Prichard PJ, Kitchingman GK, Hawkey CJ. Gastric mucosal bleeding: what dose of ASA is safe? Gut 1987; 28:A1401.
174. Penney AG, Malcontenti-Wilson C, O'Brien PE, Andrews FJ. NSAID-induced delay in gastric ulcer healing is not associated with decreased epithelial cell proliferation in rats. Dig Dis Sci 1995; 40:2684–2693.
175. Hawkey CJ. Review article: aspirin and gastrointestinal bleeding. Aliment Pharmacol Ther 1994; 8:141–146.
176. Langman MJ, Brooks P, Hawkey CL, Silverstein F, Yeomans N. Non-steroidal anti-inflammatory drug associated ulcer: epidemiology, causation and treatment. J Gastro Hepatol 1991; 6:442–449.
177. Taha AS, Hudson N, Hawkey CJ, et al. Famotidine for the prevention of gastric and duodenal ulcers caused by nonsteroidal antiinflammatory drugs. N Engl J Med 1996; 334:1435–1439.
178. Bank S, Blumstein M, Greenberg RE, Magier D, Lavin PT. Relative efficacy of famotidine in the healing of active benign ulceration: comparison of nonsteroidal anti-inflammatory- or aspirin-induced gastric ulcer and idiopathic gastric ulceration. Long Island Jewish Medical Center Acid-Peptic Study Group. Clin Ther 1993; 15:36–45.
179. Mielants H, Veys EM, Verbruggen G, Schelstraete K, Veys EM. Salicylate-induced gastrointestinal bleeding: comparison between soluble buffered, enteric-coated and intravenous administration. J Rheumatol 1979; 6:210–218.

15

Use of Low-Molecular-Weight Heparin and Heparinoid in Acute Stroke

Richard Kay and Ka Sing Wong
The Chinese University of Hong Kong, Shatin, Hong Kong, China

Alexander G. G. Turpie
McMaster University, Hamilton, Ontario, Canada

INTRODUCTION

Heparin is a heterogeneous mixture of sulfated polysaccharides with an average molecular weight of 15,000 daltons. Low-molecular-weight heparins (LMWHs) are produced from standard heparin (SH) by chemical or enzymatic depolymerization to yield components that are about one-third in molecular weight of SH. Interests in LMWH came from observations in the 1970s that fractions of SH progressively lose their ability with reduction of molecular weight to prolong the activated partial thromboplastin time (APTT) while retaining their ability to inhibit activated factor X (factor Xa).[1,2] To understand the rationale for using LMWH in acute stroke, it would be useful first to discuss the relative properties of heparin and LMWH, and to review the experience gained from the use of LMWH in other thromboembolic conditions.

ACTION OF HEPARIN AND LMWH

Heparin has five main effects on hemostasis. First, it interacts with antithrombin III (AT III), a naturally occurring anticoagulant protein, to produce a conformational change in the AT III molecule that accelerates its ability to inhibit the activated coagulation enzymes, thrombin and factors Xa and IXa. Of these enzymes, thrombin is most sensitive to the action of heparin, but heparin molecules with fewer than 18 saccharides (MW < 5,400) are unable to bind thrombin and AT III simultaneously. However, they retain their ability to catalyze the inhibition of factor Xa by AT III. Second, at high concentrations only, heparin binds to heparin cofactor II, another naturally occurring protein, to inhibit thrombin specifically. Third, heparin interferes with the interaction of coagulation factors on the surface of platelets, which form the main template for activation of the coagulation cascade. Fourth, heparin inhibits platelet aggregation, and fifth, it increases vessel wall permeability. All of these five effects can lead to bleeding, whereas it is the first effect, the inhibitory effect on activated coagulation enzymes, that is responsible for heparin's antithrombotic action.

Depolymerization of heparin to LMWH reduces its ability to catalyze thrombin inhibition without substantially affecting its ability to catalyze the inhibition of factor Xa. Compared with SH, LMWH has a modest effect in prolonging global tests of coagulation even at high concentrations (Fig. 1). Another major difference between the two compounds is their effect on platelet function. At a low concentration SH will completely inhibit collagen-induced platelet aggregation. For LMWH to have the same effect, a concentration that is 100 times

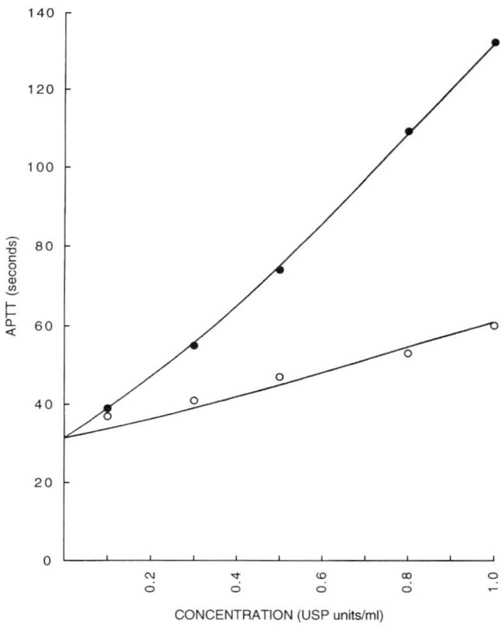

Figure 1 Comparative effects of standard heparin (closed circles) and low-molecular-weight heparin (open circles) on APTT. (From Ref. 25.)

greater would be required. The potential of LMWH for causing microvascular bleeding is thus greatly reduced.

Despite these major differences, LMWH retains marked antithrombotic activity that cannot be measured by standard coagulation tests (and many physicians are uncomfortable about this). In animal models of thrombosis, LMWH at a low concentration will effectively inhibit thrombus growth and at the same time cause less bleeding than an equivalent dose of heparin.[3]

PHARMACOKINETIC PROPERTIES OF HEPARIN AND LMWH

Heparin has two mechanisms of clearance: (1) a saturable mechanism of binding to plasma proteins and vascular endothelium, and (2) renal excretion. It has little antithrombotic activity until the binding capacity of the plasma proteins and vascular endothelium is overcome. Only then does free heparin exhibits its antithrombotic activity. The binding capacity for heparin varies markedly from one patient to another and within an individual patient, depending on the health of that individual, because the heparin-binding proteins are acute-phase proteins that increase in concentration during periods of illness. Thus, the binding capacity in any given patient cannot be estimated and, for this reason, coagulation must be monitored to adjust the dose of heparin to be given.

In contrast to SH, LMWH has a much lower affinity for the plasma proteins and vascular endothelium. In addition, it is rapidly and completely absorbed from the subcutaneous tissue, unlike SH, which often has a poor rate of absorption following subcutaneous administration. As a result of these properties, the bioavailability of LMWH is very good even when injected at low doses subcutaneously and the anticoagulant response to fixed dosages of LMWH is much more predictable.

Since the clearance of LMWH does not have a rapid saturable phase, its plasma half-life is up to four times longer than that of SH. LMWH is cleared principally by the renal route, and its biological half-life is increased in renal failure.

CLINICAL ADVANTAGES OF LMWH

The greater bioavailability and longer half-life of LMWH over SH allow LMWH to be given subcutaneously once or twice daily, while the more predictable anticoagulant response to fixed doses permits LMWH to be administered without laboratory monitoring. Furthermore, the relative lack of hemorrhagic potential allows LMWH to be given in doses that achieve anti–factor Xa levels several times higher than those achieved by SH. In a study of a LMWH in the treatment of venous thrombosis, the plasma anti–factor Xa level that was achieved was approximately 0.9 unit/mL.[4] If SH is given instead, to prolong the APTT to 1.5 to 2.5 times control, the anti–factor Xa level will be about 0.2 to 0.3 unit/mL. If one gives SH to achieve an anti–factor Xa level of 0.9 unit/mL, standard coagulation tests will be unmeasurable, and the associated bleeding would not be acceptable. Thus, with LMWH, three to four times as much antithrombotic activity can be given without increasing the risk of bleeding.

Many LMWHs have been developed for clinical use, and some have been studied extensively in clinical trials in Europe and North America (Table 1). In the United States, enoxaparin and dalteparin are currently approved for clinical use. In Canada and Europe, a greater number of LMWHs are available. A low-molecular-weight heparinoid, danaparoid, consisting mainly of heparan sulfate with a small quantity of dermatan sulfate and chondroitin sulfate, has also been developed for clinical use. Table 2 lists the potential advantages of LMWH and heparinoid in the clinical setting.

Prevention of Venous Thrombosis in Surgical Patients

The initial clinical trials performed with LMWH were centered upon the prevention of deep-vein thrombosis (DVT) in patients undergoing general or orthopedic surgery. Pooled analysis of randomized studies comparing LMWH with SH showed a significant reduction (relative risk 0.74; 95% confidence interval [CI] 0.64–0.84) in DVT in the LMWH group with no significant difference in bleeding rates.[5] In total hip arthroplasty, where the risk of developing DVT is particularly high, a meta-analysis comparing LMWH with SH showed a significant reduction (odds ratio 0.40; 95% CI 0.28–0.59) in proximal DVT in the LMWH group with no significant difference in the rates of distal DVT or bleeding between the two groups.[6]

Table 1 Commonly Used Low-Molecular-Weight Heparins

Dalteparin	(Fragmin)
Danaparoid[a]	(Orgaran)
Enoxaparin	(Lovenox)
Nadroparin	(Fraxiparine)
Tinzaparin	(Logiparin)

[a]Heparinoid.
Trade names in parentheses.

Table 2 Potential Advantages of LMWH

Good and rapid absorption when given subcutaneously
Lack of binding to plasma proteins: Good bioavailability at low doses
Long half-life: Can be given once or twice daily
Stable dose response: Can be given in fixed doses without monitoring
Lack of effect on platelets: Less bleeding compared with heparin
Resistance does not develop

Prevention of Venous Thrombosis in Stroke Patients

Venous thromboembolism is a common complication in patients with acute stroke. In addition to systemic risk factors such as age and concurrent infections, venous stasis in the paretic lower limb increases the risk of DVT. Although prophylaxis with low-dose heparin or LMWH is widely accepted for other high-risk patients, there is still great reluctance among physicians to use any antithrombotic therapy in stroke patients for fear of bleeding into the infarcted brain.

Estimates of the frequency of DVT in untreated stroke patients range from 20% to 75%.[7] The reported frequency depends on the method used to detect DVT and, importantly, on the degree of lower limb paresis. Most of the thrombi will occur in the paretic limb in which the frequency ranges from 50% to 75%.[8] Methods in preventing DVT in high-risk stroke patients include low-dose heparin, LMWH, and graduated compression stockings. Of these, low-dose subcutaneous heparin has been the most evaluated. In two randomized trials, low-dose heparin given subcutaneously in doses of 5,000 units every 8 hours was compared with placebo. In the first study,[9] the frequency of DVT was reduced from 12 of 16 patients given placebo to 2 of 16 patients given low-dose heparin. In the second study,[10] the frequency of DVT was reduced from 117 to 161 patients (73%) to 32 of 144 patients (22%).

There have been two small studies using LMWH for the prevention of DVT in patients with ischemic stroke. The results were inconsistent. The first study[11] compared LMWH in a dose of 2,500 anti–factor Xa units twice daily with placebo and demonstrated a reduction in the rate of DVT from 15 of 30 (50%) patients to 6 of 27 (22%) patients. In the second study,[12] LMWH was given in weight-adjusted doses once daily (3,000 to 5,500 anti–factor Xa units daily). In contrast to the first study, there was no difference in the frequency of DVT between 42 LMWH-treated patients (36%) and 50 placebo-treated patients (34%).

The low-molecular-weight heparinoid danaparoid, which is a chemically distinct from heparin, has been evaluated for the prevention of DVT in patients with ischemic stroke in two studies by Turpie et al. In the first study,[13] 50 patients received danaparoid for 14 days and 25 patients received placebo. Patients were screened for DVT using ^{125}iodine-labeled fibrinogen leg scanning and impedance plethysmography, and diagnosis of DVT was confirmed by venography.

Two of 50 patients (4%) in the heparinoid group and 7 of 25 (28%) in the placebo group developed DVT ($P = .005$). There was one major hemorrhage in the treatment group and one minor hemorrhage in the placebo group. However, in this study, computed tomography of the brain was not repeated after treatment; hence, the rates of hemorrhagic transformation of the infarct (HTI) could not be determined. In the second study,[14] 45 patients with lower-limb paresis were randomized to receive danaparoid in a dose of 750 anti–factor Xa units subcutaneously every 12 hours, while 42 patients were given SH 5,000 units subcutaneously every 12 hours. Treatment was started on average 5 days after the onset of stroke and continued for 14 days. DVT was detected in 9% of the danaparoid group and 31% of the heparin group ($P = .01$). CT of the brain was repeated at the end of the treatment period. The frequency of HTI was 9.3% in the danaparoid group and 5.6% in the heparin group ($P > .10$).

An overview suggests that, compared with placebo-treated patients, there is a significant 87% (standard deviation 16%) reduction in the odds of DVT in stroke patients treated with LMWH or heparinoid.[15] Furthermore, there is a nonsignificant trend toward the reduction of pulmonary embolism. Preliminary data also suggest that treatment of stroke patients with these agents is not associated with an excess risk of HTI.

Treatment of Venous Thrombosis

For the treatment of established venous thrombosis, there is increasing evidence that subcutaneous LMWH is an effective alternative to intravenous SH. A meta-analysis of nine randomized trials[16] comparing subcutaneous fixed-dose LMWH with intravenous adjusted-dose heparin in the treatment of proximal-vein thrombosis showed a reduced risk of recurrent venous thromboembolism, a reduction in major bleeding, and a decrease in mortality with LMWH, all of which were clinically important and statistically significant (Table 3). The biological reason for the reduction in mortality is not clear, but it is an important observation that requires further investigation.

Table 3 Treatment of DVT with LMWH: A Meta-Analysis

	LMWH	Heparin	RRR[a]	(95% CI)	*P*
Recurrent DVT	3.1%	6.6%	53%	(18–73)	< .01
Major bleeding	0.9%	3.2%	68%	(31–85)	< .005
Mortality	3.9%	7.1%	47%	(10–69)	< .04

[a]RRR = Relative risk reduction.
Source: Ref. 16.

LMWH IN ISCHEMIC HEART DISEASE

Unit recently, aspirin was the mainstay of treatment of patients with unstable angina. Heparin was shown to be more effective in a Canadian study which randomized 484 patients to receive either aspirin 325 mg twice daily or intravenous heparin adjusted to prolong the APTT to 1.5 to 2.5 times control.[17] Myocardial infarction occurred in 3.7% of patients assigned to aspirin and 0.8% of patients assigned to heparin (P = .035). Moreover, in patients treated with aspirin plus anticoagulation (heparin followed by warfarin), there was a 46% reduction in the risk of recurrent angina, myocardial infarction, or death compared with patients treated with aspirin alone.[18] Thus, a combination of an antiplatelet agent and an anticoagulant may be the treatment of choice for arterial thrombosis, at least in the coronary circulation.

The first published study of LMWH for the treatment of unstable angina came from an open trial comparing aspirin, aspirin plus adjusted-dose intravenous heparin, and aspirin plus fixed-dose subcutaneous nadroparin.[19] Nonfatal myocardial infarction occurred in 7 of 73 patients in the aspirin group, 4 of 70 patients in the aspirin plus heparin group, and none of 68 patients in the aspirin plus LMWH group. A larger, double-blind trial showed that the addition of dalteparin to a regimen of aspirin and antianginal drugs reduced the risk of death or myocardial infarction in patients with unstable angina from 4.8% to 1.8% at 6 days (P = .001).[20] Finally, subcutaneous enoxaparin plus aspirin was shown to reduce the risk of recurrent angina, myocardial infarction, or death by 16% (P = .019) compared with intravenous heparin plus aspirin.[21] In all three studies, the use of LMWH was not associated with an excess of major hemorrhage.

LMWH IN ACUTE ISCHEMIC STROKE

Since 1995, three randomized placebo-controlled trials using a LMWH or heparinoid for the treatment of acute ischemic stroke have been reported.[22–24] The results were conflicting (Table 4). The first of these trials, known as "Fraxiparine in Ischemic Stroke Study" (FISS),[22] was performed entirely on Chinese patients in Hong Kong. It compared two dosages of nadroparin (Fraxiparine) versus placebo in patients whose onset of stroke was within 48 hours of randomization (Table 5). Treatment was given for 10 days, after which oral aspirin, 100 mg daily, was prescribed to all patients. The primary outcome measure was "poor outcome", a composite of death from any cause or dependency with respect to activities of daily living, at 6 months after the stroke. The FISS trial screened 2,750 patients in 20 months and randomized 312 patients. Four randomized patients were excluded from analysis because of entry ineligibility. At the 6-month follow-up, which was 99.4% complete, patients in the high-dose group had significantly

Table 4 Trials of LMWH for the Treatment of Acute Ischemic Stroke

	FISS	FISS bis	TOAST
Patients randomized	308	767	1281
Time window	48 h	24 h	24 h
Main outcome measure	death or "dependency"	death or Barthel < 85	"favorable outcome"[a]
Interim follow-up	3 months	3 months	7 days
Treatment group 1	high-dose = 53%	high-dose = 65%	59%
Treatment group 2	low-dose = 60%	low-dose = 62%	—
Placebo group	64%	61%	54%
P value	.12	.41	.07
Final follow-up	6 months	6 months	3 months
Treatment group 1	high-dose = 45%	high-dose = 59%	75%
Treatment group 2	low-dose = 52%	low dose = 57%	—
Placebo group	65%	57%	74%
P value	.005	.62	.49
Main safety measure	any HTI	all bleeds[b]	serious ICH
Measured at	10 days	6 months	10 days
Treatment group 1	high-dose = 6.2%	high-dose = 32%	2.4%
Treatment group 2	low-dose = 8.6%	low-dose = 16%	—
Placebo group	12%	15%	0.8%
P value	.19	.01	.05

[a]Combination of Glasgow Outcome Scale of I or II and Modified Barthel Index of 12 or greater.
[b]Except asymptomatic ICH.
HTI = hemorrhagic transformation of the infarct; ICH = intracranial hemorrhage.

fewer poor outcomes than patients in the placebo group (Fig. 2). The relative risk reduction was 31% (95% CI 10% to 46%) and the number of patients needed to be treated to prevent one poor outcome was 5 (95% CI 3 to 18). However, the difference in poor outcomes between the low-dose group and the placebo group did not reach statistical significance at 6 months, nor did that between the high-dose group and the placebo group at 3 months. The frequency of HTI, measured at the end of the treatment period of 10 days, was not statistically different between patients who received nadroparin and patients who received placebo.

Based on the experience of the first FISS trial, a second "FISS bis" trial was conducted mainly in Europe,[23] with some contribution from Canada and Hong Kong. The major changes in design for FISS bis were a shorter time window (24 hours), a weight-adjusted dosage (on average 50% higher), exclusion of patients without significant paresis, and the replacement of "dependency" by the Barthel index (<85) in the definition of poor outcome. A total of 767 patients were randomized within 1 year. At the 6-month follow-up, 59% of patients in

Table 5 Study Design of the FISS Trial

Inclusion criteria	
Onset of stroke ≤ 48 hours	
Written informed consent	
Exclusion criteria	
Age > 80 years	
CT evidence of intracranial hemorrhage	
Transient neurologic deficits	
Blood pressure > 180/120 mm Hg	
Major confounding illness	
Recent major operation	
Known tendency toward bleeding	
Current anticoagulant therapy	
Valvular heart disease	
Known adverse reaction to heparin	
Treatment schedule	(subcutaneously for 10 days)
High-dose group:	Fraxiparine 0.4 mL q12h
Low-dose group:	Fraxiparine alternating with placebo 0.4 mL q12h
Placebo group:	Placebo 0.4 mL q12h
Primary outcome	
Death or dependency 6 months after stroke	

Source: Ref. 22.

the high-dose group, 57% of patients in the low-dose group, and 57% patients in the placebo group had a poor outcome ($P = .62$). The proportion of patients with any bleeding episode (excluding asymptomatic HTI) during the 6-month observation period reached 32% for the high-dose group, 16% for the low-dose group, and 15% for the placebo group ($P = .01$). Thus it was concluded that there were no overall benefits in the primary endpoint at either dose. Of the secondary endpoints, there was a significantly lower rate of pulmonary embolism with both doses. Compared with placebo, there were significantly more bleeds with high-dose nadroparin but no more with low-dose nadroparin.

In the United States, an NIH-sponsored trial known as "Trial of ORG 10172 in Acute Stroke Treatment" (TOAST) was conducted over a 6-year period using the heparinoid danaparoid (Orgaran), which was given within 24 hours of stroke by intravenous infusion for 7 days.[24] The primary outcome measure was "favorable outcome," which is a combination of a Glasgow Outcome Scale score of I or II and a modified Barthel index of 12 or greater (on a 0 to 20 scale), at 3 months or 7 days after the stroke. The TOAST trial screened 25,624 patients and randomized 1,281 patients. At the 3-month follow-up, 75.2% of patients treated with

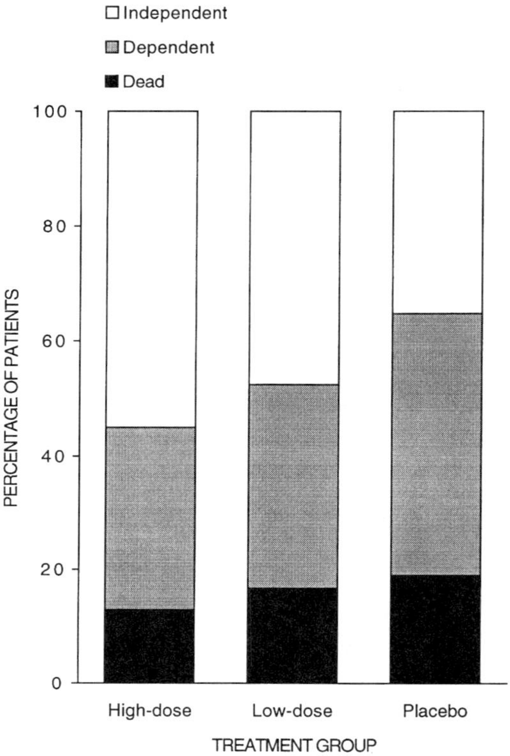

Figure 2 The FISS trial demonstrated a significant (P = .005), dose-dependent reduction in the risk of death or dependency at 6 months among patients treated with low-molecular-weight heparin. (From Ref. 22.)

danaparoid and 73.7% of patients assigned to placebo had favorable outcomes (P = .49). At 7 days, 59.2% of patients given danaparoid and 54.3% of patients receiving placebo had favorable outcomes (P = .07). Furthermore, for the same period, 33.9% of the former group and 27.8% of the latter group had "very favorable outcomes" (P = .01). Serious intracranial bleeding occurred within 10 days in 14 patients given danaparoid and in 4 patients receiving placebo (P = .05). It was concluded that despite an apparent positive response at 7 days, treatment with danaparoid is not associated with an improvement in favorable outcome at 3 months.

CONCLUSION

Low-molecular-weight heparin and heparinoid have emerged not only as a convenient alternative to standard unfractionated heparin, but have consistently been demonstrated in many clinical trials to be superior to heparin in terms of safety and efficacy. These clinical trials include the prevention and treatment of venous thromboembolism and the treatment of unstable angina. As such, LMWH and heparinoid may be considered as a new class of antithrombotic agent the clinical utility of which could be extended to other indications where heparin has been the traditional choice of treatment. Although controversial, many physicians still use heparin to treat acute ischemic stroke. Results of the FISS and TOAST trials suggest that there may be some justification for using LMWH or heparinoid in doses larger than those that are required for the prevention of DVT in patients presenting within the first 24 to 48 hours of stroke. However, at large doses, LMWH and heparinoid can cause increased bleeding, including intracranial hemorrhage, in acute stroke patients. Physicians should not regard LMWH or heparinoid as harmless, but should refine their skills in selecting the right patient for treatment.

REFERENCES

1. Barrowcliffe TW, Johnson EA, Thomas DP. Low Molecular Weight Heparin. Chichester: John Wiley & Sons, 1993.
2. Hirsh J. Low molecular weight heparin. Thromb Haemost 1993; 70:204–207.
3. Cade JF, Buchanan MR, Boneu B, et al. A comparison of the antithrombotic and haemorrhagic effects of low molecular weight heparin fractions: the influence of the method of preparation. Thromb Res 1984; 35:613–625.
4. Simonneau G, Charbonnier B, Decousus H, et al. Subcutaneous low-molecular-weight heparin compared with intravenous unfractionated heparin in the treatment of proximal deep vein thrombosis. Arch Intern Med 1993; 153:1541–1546.
5. Nurmohamed MT, Rosendaal FR, Büller HR, et al. Low-molecular-weight heparin versus standard heparin in general and orthopaedic surgery: a meta-analysis. Lancet 1992; 340:152–156.
6. Anderson DR, O'Brien BJ, Levin MN, Roberts R, Wells PS, Hirsh J. Efficacy and cost of low-molecular-weight heparin compared with standard heparin for the prevention of deep venous thrombosis after total hip arthroplasty. Ann Intern Med 1993; 119:1105–1112.
7. Bornstein NM, Norris JW. Deep vein thrombosis after ischemic stroke: rationale for a therapeutic trial. Arch Phys Med Rehabil 1988; 69:955–958.
8. Warlow C, Ogston D, Douglas AS. Venous thrombosis following strokes. Lancet 1972; 1:1305–1306.

9. McCarthy ST, Robertson D, Turner JJ, Hawkey CJ. Low dose heparin as a prophylaxis against deep-vein thrombosis after acute stroke. Lancet 1977; 2:800–801.
10. McCarthy ST, Turner J. Low-dose subcutaneous heparin in the prevention of deep-vein thrombosis and pulmonary emboli following acute stroke. Age Ageing 1986; 15:84–88.
11. Prins MH, Gelsema R, Sing AK, van Heerde LR, den Ottolander GJH. Prophylaxis of deep venous thrombosis with a low-molecular-weight heparin (Kabi 2165/Fragmin) in stroke patients. Haemostasis 1989; 19:245–250.
12. Sandset PM, Dahl T, Stiris M, Rostad B, Scheel B, Abildgaard U. A double-blind and randomized placebo-controlled trial of low molecular weight heparin once daily to prevent deep vein thrombosis in acute ischemic stroke. Semin Thromb Hemost 1990; 16(suppl):25–33.
13. Turpie AGG, Levin MN, Hirsh J, et al. Double-blind randomised trial of Org 10172 low-molecular-weight heparinoid in prevention of deep-vein thrombosis in thrombotic stroke. Lancet 1987; 1:523–525.
14. Turpie AGG, Gent M, Côté R, et al. A low-molecular-weight heparinoid compared with unfractionated heparin in the prevention of deep vein thrombosis in patients with acute ischemic stroke. Ann Intern Med 1992; 117:353–357.
15. Sandercock PAG, van den Belt AGM, Lindley RI, Slattery J. Antithrombotic therapy in acute ischaemic stroke: an overview of the completed randomised trials. J Neurol Neurosurg Psychiatry 1993; 56:17–25.
16. Lensing AWA, Prins MH, Davidson BL, Hirsh J. Treatment of deep vein thrombosis with low-molecular weight heparins: a meta-analysis. Arch Intern Med 1995; 155:601–607.
17. Théroux P, Waters D, Qiu S, McCans J, de Guise P, Juneau M. Aspirin versus heparin to prevent myocardial infarction during the acute phase of unstable angina. Circulation 1993; 88:2045–2048.
18. Cohen M, Adams PC, Parry G, et al. Combination antithrombotic therapy in unstable rest angina and non-Q-wave infarction in nonprior aspirin users: primary end points analysis from the ATACS trial. Circulation 1994; 89:81–88.
19. Gurfinkel EP, Manos EJ, Mejaíl RI, et al. Low molecular weight heparin versus regular heparin in the treatment of unstable angina and silent ischemia. J Am Coll Cardiol 1995; 26:313–318.
20. Fragmin During Instability in Coronary Artery Disease (FRISC) Study Group. Low-molecular-weight heparin during instability in coronary artery disease. Lancet 1996; 347:561–568.
21. Cohen M, Demers C, Gurfinkel E, et al. A comparison of low-molecular-weight heparin with unfractionated heparin for unstable coronary artery disease. N Engl J Med 1997; 337:447–452.
22. Kay R, Wong KS, Yu YL, et al. Low-molecular-weight heparin for the treatment of acute ischemic stroke. N Engl J Med 1995; 333:1588–1593.
23. Hommel M, for the FISS bis Investigators Group. Fraxiparine in Ischaemic Stroke Study (FISS bis). Cerebrovasc Dis 1998; 8(suppl 4):19.

24. Publications Committee for the Trial of ORG 10172 in Acute Stroke Treatment (TOAST) Investigators. Low molecular weight heparinoid, ORG 10192 (danaparoid), and outcome after acute ischemic stroke: a randomized controlled trial. JAMA 1998; 279:1265–1272.
25. Carter CJ, Kelton, JG, Hirsh J, Cerskus A, Santos AV, Gent M. The relationship between the hemorrhagic and antithrombotic properties of low molecular weight heparin in rabbits. Blood 1982; 59:1239–1245.

16

Thrombolytic Therapy for Acute Ischemic Stroke

Mark J. Alberts
Duke University Medical Center, Durham, North Carolina

INTRODUCTION AND HISTORY

In the past, much of stroke therapy has been centered around 4 major issues: (1) determining the territory and mechanism of the stroke; (2) preventing worsening and complications arising from the initial stroke; (3) taking steps to maximize rehabilitation and functional outcome; and (4) preventing a recurrent stroke. Yet the key issue of treatments designed to reverse or diminish the effects of an acute stroke has not been addressed in a comprehensive or aggressive manner until quite recently.

The delay in addressing the topic of acute stroke therapy may be partially due to the early experiences related to such treatments. As far back as 1958, there were trials evaluating the efficacy and safety of thrombolysis for acute ischemic stroke, with somewhat mixed results. Although some of these studies showed clinical efficacy, many were not randomized or blinded, and rates of symptomatic intracerebral hemorrhage (ICH) ranged from 3% to 8%.[1] In addition, many of these studies were done prior to the widespread use of head CT, making differentiation of an ICH from an ischemic stroke somewhat challenging. Clearly, treating a patient having an ICH with a thrombolytic agent is not optimal therapy!

After several trials of thrombolytics in the 1960s, relatively few large clinical studies were performed in the 1970s. However, the 1980s and 1990s saw a resurgence of interest in the use of thrombolytic agents for acute stroke. A recent literature review and meta-analysis identified at least 12 randomized trials of various thrombolytic agents for stroke.[2]

There are several factors responsible for the resurgent interest in this treatment modality. The widespread availability and use of head CT to assist in the diagnosis and management of stroke patients has certainly made the differentiation of ischemic stroke from other disorders relatively straightforward. The significant success of thrombolytic agents for acute myocardial infarction further heightened interest in this area.[3] A group of aggressive neurologists, neurosurgeons, and others interested in cerebrovascular disease has been a major factor in "pushing the envelope" for the development and testing of these and other new therapies for acute stroke patients.[4] Lastly, the availability of new agents (i.e., recombinant tissue plasminogen activator, rt-PA) and improved techniques of administration (i.e., microcatheters for intra-arterial use) have increased the safety and ease of administration for these therapies.

SCIENTIFIC BASIS

The concept underlying thrombolytic therapy for stroke is on one hand quite simple, but on the other hand rather profound. By lysing an occlusive clot in the cerebral circulation and reperfusing ischemic brain, one hopes to prevent cerebral infarction and improve the viability of ischemic brain by totally or partially reversing such ischemia. This should lead to improved functional outcomes for such patients.[5] These basic concepts raise other problematic issues: which patients have ischemic brain that is amenable to reperfusion; which clots are susceptible to lysis; could reperfusion lead to increased brain damage due to the production of toxic metabolites; can the ever-present risk of cerebral hemorrhage be limited?[1,6–9]

There are reasonable scientific (animal) and human clinical data demonstrating that in many cases of acute stroke there is a region of salvageable tissue (the so-called ischemic penumbra, IP) surrounding a core of infarcted tissue.[10,11] The presence and size of the IP appear to vary considerably from case to case, as does the survivability of this region. A combination of residual blood flow (denoting the severity of ischemia) and the duration of the insult appears to determine the size and life-span for the IP. Patients with good collateral flow can probably withstand vessel occlusions for longer periods of time with less permanent damage than patients with no or poor collaterals.

Based mostly on animal data, some researchers have suggested that the IP exists for about 3 to 4 hours.[12,13] Such statements belie the marked heterogeneity that is characteristic of strokes in humans. A myriad of factors can combine to either shorten or lengthen this time period. In addition, recent data using a combination of clinical and noninvasive tools to study brain metabolism (i.e., magnetic resonance spectroscopy, positron emission tomography) have demonstrated regions having characteristics consistent with an IP. Such regions have been observed to exist up to 12 to 17 hours after an ischemic stroke, with evidence of partial clinical recovery in some patients.[4,6,10,11,14,15] Other patients appear to have small or no IP regions even shortly after stroke onset.

Two general themes have emerged from these studies: (1) time cannot be the sole determinant of which patients have an IP, and therefore who will respond to lytic therapy, and (2) in general, the sooner patients are treated with lytic agents, the greater the chances of a good outcome.[5,6,16] Although it would seem that these two statements are contradictory, they are really complementary. In general, more rapid therapy should be the goal for all stroke patients. However, as more sophisticated means become available to define and measure the IP and cerebral viability, instead of using time as the key determinant, such tests may more precisely define which patients are candidates for treatment with lytic agents.[10] But until such tools are validated and become widely available, time will continue to be a key criterion for selecting patients.

It is well known that the types of lesions that occlude cerebral vessels differ depending on the location of the artery. Occlusions of the extracranial portion of the internal carotid artery (ICA) are often due to underlying atherosclerotic plaques with superimposed clot in some cases. The middle cerebral artery is often obstructed by a clot that has arisen from the heart or a proximal ICA lesion. Occlusion of small intracranial vessels leading to lacunar strokes can be due to either microatheromata or lipohyalinolysis.[17] While most lytic agents lyse acute clots quite well, their ability to rapidly lyse older clots that may cause cardioembolic strokes, as well as microatheromata that cause some lacunar strokes, is unclear. Results from some studies using IV TPA have produced conflicting data about the ability of this agent to reperfuse vessels with various occlusions.[18,19]

There is fairly convincing evidence from animal studies that acute reperfusion can lead to a dramatic increase in the levels of excitatory amino acids and other neurotransmitters, which by themselves can increase neuronal damage.[20,22] The extent to which these detrimental events can diminish the positive effects of reperfusion in humans with a stroke remains unclear. Another potentially important issue is one of reocclusion of a vessel following lysis. The extent to which this happens in stroke patients following treatment with lytics is unknown. My colleagues and I have certainly observed patients who improve rapidly during the administration of lytic agent, only to worsen minutes later (unrelated to an ICH). Whether this is due to reocclusion, toxic substances, or another process remains unclear.

The issue of lytic-induced cerebral hemorrhage is of grave concern, since any such events have the risk of making a stroke worse and leading to increased mortality.[23,24] Clearly, the reperfusion of dead brain is unlikely to improve clinical function, yet can lead to increased bleeding complications with potentially devastating clinical sequelae. This topic is discussed below in more detail.

PHARMACOLOGY

There are four major thrombolytic agents commonly used for cerebrovascular disease in the world as of 1998: streptokinase, tissue plasminogen activator, urokinase, and Ancrod. Several other agents, such as accelerated TPA and pro-urokinase, are under active development.

Streptokinase (SK) is a bacterial protein produced by group C hemolytic streptococci. In the body, SK combines with plasminogen to produce an activator complex, which then converts plasminogen to plasmin. Plasmin degrades fibrin clots as well as fibrinogen, and produces hypofibrinogenemia for about 24 to 36 hours following administration. This effect may be explained in part by the relatively long half-life of SK, along with the relative nonspecificity of the SK complex for clots (see Table 1). The SK activator complex is partially degraded by antistreptococcal antibodies. Hypotension and allergic reactions, as well as bleeding, are the most significant adverse reactions associated with SK administration. SK is typically administered by an intravenous (IV) infusion.[25]

Tissue plasminogen activator (TPA) used therapeutically is produced via recombinant DNA technology, and is therefore referred to as recombinant-TPA (rt-PA). It is a serine protease which preferentially binds to plasminogen in the presence of fibrin, making it more clot-specific. The effect is local fibrinolysis with fewer systemic effects, although there can be systemic effects in some patients. rt-PA has a shorter half-life than SK (see Table 1), and is metabolized in the liver. Commercially available rt-PA (Activase) is indicated for IV use only. Allergic reactions are extremely rare with rt-PA.[26]

Table 1 Pharmacology and Clinical Aspects of Thrombolytic Agents Used in Stroke Patients

Agent	Half-life	Typical route of administration	Clot selectivity[a]
Ancrod	3–5 hours	IV	+
Streptokinase	18–83 min[b]	IV	+
Tissue plasminogen activator	3–4 min	IV	+++
Urokinase	20 min	IA	+

[a]+, little or no clot selectivity; ++, moderate clot selectivity; +++, highly clot-selective.

[b]For streptokinase, the half-life is 18 minutes in patients with antistreptococcal antibodies, and 83 minutes in patients without such antibodies.

Urokinase (UK) is produced by kidney cells and excreted in the urine. Commercially available UK is prepared from cultured human kidney cells. It acts as a thrombolytic agent by converting plasminogen to plasmin, which then lyses fibrin and fibrinogen. It lacks the clot specificity of rt-PA. UK can be administered either IV or intra-arterially directly into an occluded artery.[27] In some cases it can be administered directly into the clot by using superselective catheters. Rare, mild allergic reactions have been reported when using UK.

Ancrod is a protein found in snake venom that acts as an anticoagulant and a thrombolytic agent. Its mechanism of action involves the cleavage of fibrinopeptide A from fibrinogen, which makes blood hypocoagulable. The removal of fibrinopeptide A from fibrinogen makes fibrin more soluble, since crosslinking is no longer possible. A circulating Ancrod-fibrin complex leads to further fibrinolysis. The half-life varies considerably, but can be up to 3 to 5 hours. Following prolonged Ancrod administration, fibrinogen levels often fall to zero.[28,29]

CLINICAL CONSIDERATIONS AND STUDIES

The clinical arena of thrombolytic therapy for acute ischemic stroke is complicated by several levels of heterogeneity. This includes variability in the stroke type and mechanism, the route of administration, variable treatment windows, and lastly the choice of lytic agent. There are a fair number of ischemic stroke subtypes and etiologies, ranging from small-vessel thrombotic to medium-vessel cardioembolic to large-vessel atherothrombotic, to name but a few.[17] It is perhaps unreasonable to expect any one therapy or agent to work equally well for all types of ischemic stroke, since clot location, size, age, etiology, and vessel wall pathology will vary. In addition, uncertainties with respect to patient selection (i.e., age, time window), concomitant diseases, and radiographic findings may further complicate such studies. Routes of administration for lytic agents currently consist of intravenous (IV), intra-arterial (IA), and selective IA (sIA) using microcatheters embedded within the clot. Also, the fact that many stroke patients recover spontaneously further complicates such studies.[15]

As with many areas of clinical uncertainty, it would be helpful to have large amounts of data upon which to base decisions. Cardiologists have been able to study such issues by using so-called megatrials of patients with myocardial infarction (MI). These trials typically enroll more than 10,000 patients, and in some cases study up to 40,000 patients.[3] Such trials are very unlikely to be done for lytic therapy of stroke patients for several reasons: (1) the number of available acute stroke patients is considerably smaller than for MI; (2) enrollment of stroke patients within a narrow time window is quite challenging; (3) smaller hospitals may not be able to participate in such large trials; and (4) the underlying heterogeneity of stroke may reduce the statistical power of even a modest-size trial to detect any meaningful differences.

Last are concerns about outcome measures. Some of the initial studies used angiographic criteria (i.e., reperfusion) as the primary outcome measure, while clinical changes were secondary endpoints.[1,18] At the time this seemed reasonable, since investigators were attempting to establish the biologic activity of thrombolytic agents in acute stroke patients. However, as indicated below, in some cases there was no clear correlation between angiographic and clinical outcomes. All of the recent, large, randomized studies have used clinical and functional outcome measures as their primary endpoints, which is in keeping with the FDA guidelines for such therapies.[1,2,18,19,23,30,31]

In the modern era (i.e., since head CT scans became widely available), there have been a number of fairly large, randomized trials of various lytic agents for stroke patients. Two of the large early studies using IV UK had very long enrollment windows (up to 30 days), did show evidence of efficacy, and had few bleeding complications.[32,33] In the late 1980s, a series of studies was begun using IV TPA in stroke patients. These studies included two large dose escalation studies performed in the mid to late 1980s. One study used IV TPA in stroke patients up to 8 hours after stroke onset.[18] This study used angiography pre- and post-TPA administration to evaluate vessel patency as the key endpoint. Only 34% of 93 treated patients demonstrated vessel patency immediately after TPA administration. There was no clear relationship between TPA dose and vessel patency, nor was there a correlation between dose and bleeding complications.[18] It is possible that insufficient numbers of patients were studied to identify an effective and safe dose in this study.

At the same time, the NIH was sponsoring a similar dose escalation study on patients within 3 hours of stroke onset. IV TPA was used, but without pretreatment or mandatory posttreatment angiography. These open studies found that up to 46% of stroke patients treated within 90 minutes of onset had significant early improvement in their neurologic status.[34,35] They also found that doses of TPA at or above 1.0 mg/kg resulted in higher rates of ICH.[24,34] Based on these results, a dose of 0.9 mg/kg was determined to offer a reasonable compromise between efficacy and minimal bleeding complications.

Several large, prospective studies of IV TPA and IV SK in stroke were then completed and reported (see Table 2). The first large randomized study of IV TPA for stroke in the modern era was the ECASS trial.[31] This study used a relatively high dose of TPA (1.1 mg/kg) with a 6-hour enrollment window. The choice of TPA dose is of significant interest. As stated above, the NINDS-TPA group found that TPA doses above 1.0 mg/kg were associated with a higher risk of ICH. However, the ECASS group chose to use an even higher dose, perhaps in an effort to attain improved efficacy.

Table 2 Recent Large Randomized Trials of Thrombolytic Agents in Stroke

Study name[a]	Age range	Drug/dose[b]	Patients	Outcome scales	Efficacy[c]	Sx ICH Rx/Pl[d]
ECASS	18–80	TPA 1.1 mg/kg	620	Barthel Rankin	NS	19.8%/6.5%
ECASS II	18–80	TPA 0.9 mg/kg	800	Rankin	NS	8.8%/3.4%
NINDS	18–85[e]	TPA 0.9 mg/kg	624	NIHSS[f] Barthel Rankin Glasgow Outcome	11%–13%	6.4%/0.6%
ATLANTIS	18–79	TPA 0.9 mg/kg	414	same as NINDS	NS	7.2%/0.7%
ASK	18–85	SK 1.5 M units + ASA 100 mg	340	Mortality Barthel	TW	12.6%/2.4%
MAST-E	22–94	SK 1.5 M units	310	Mortality Rankin	TW	21.2%/2.6%
MAST-I	none stated	SK 1.5 M units + ASA 300 mg	622	Mortality	TW[d]	10.0%/0.6%
PROACT II	18–85	9 mg pro-UK + IV heparin	180	Rankin	15%	10.2%/1.8%
STAT	≥18	Ancrod	500	Barthel	8%	5.2%/2%

[a]ECASS, European Cooperative Acute Stroke Study; NINDS, National Institute of Neurologic Disease and Stroke rt-PA Stroke Study; ATLANTIS, Alteplase Thrombolysis for Acute Non-Interventional Therapy in Ischemic Stroke; ASK, Australian Streptokinase Trial; MAST-E and MAST-I, Multicenter Acute Stroke Trial–(Europe or Italy). See text for details and references.

[b]TPA, recombinant tissue plasminogen activator (rt-PA); SK, streptokinase; ASA, aspirin; pro-UK, recombinant prourokinase.

[c]NS, no significant difference between treatment and placebo groups for the primary outcome measure; TW, treatment group did worse than placebo; specific numbers refer to absolute improvement in treatment groups vs. placebo.

[d]Sx ICH Rx/Pl, symptomatic intracerebral hemorrhage in treatment and placebo groups. Most studies reported intraparenchymal hematomas as those causing mass effect, and presumably neurologic worsening. These figures do not include cases of hemorrhagic transformation, which typically is not associated with clinical deterioration in most cases. The table reports the highest rate of ICH in the treatment group, if several rates are reported for different subgroups.

[e]An age exclusion was not formally included in the NINDS. However, due to ICH in several patients older than age 85 in that study, enrollment was informally limited to patients ≤ 85 years during the course of the study.

[f]NIHSS, National Institutes of Health Stroke Scale.

The results of ECASS were disappointing. There was no significant difference in the primary outcome measures (Barthel and Rankin) in the intention-to-treat analysis.[31] Of greater concern was the increased incidence of ICH, which approached 20% of the TPA group. Although a subgroup analysis identified patients (those without early CT scan changes) that did show some efficacy with TPA therapy, even this select group had an ICH rate of almost 20%.[31] Perhaps the higher TPA dose, combined with the prolonged enrollment window, may explain the poor efficacy and frequent bleeding complications seen in this study.

A second large trial was the NINDS rt-PA study.[19] This prospective study enrolled 624 patients in a double-blinded, placebo-controlled protocol. Half of the patients were treated within 90 minutes of stroke onset; the other half were treated from 91 to 180 minutes after stroke onset. Patients with early CT changes showing a large stroke were excluded, and the blood pressure had to be no greater than 185/110 before entry. The dose of rt-PA used was 0.9 mg/kg, with a maximum dose of 90 mg. This is considerably lower than the standard dose of 100 mg of IV rt-PA used for the treatment of acute MI, but stroke is clearly a different disease. Enrolled patients could not receive any antiplatelet agents or anticoagulants for 24 hours following TPA infusion. The endpoints consisted of neurologic and functional outcomes at 3 months after the stroke.[19]

This study found an 11% to 13% absolute increase in the number of rt-PA-treated patients vs. placebo having no or minimal neurologic disability 3 months after stroke onset. This positive effect was seen for patients in both time groups, and was present in patients with small-vessel, large-vessel, or embolic strokes.[19] As might be expected, the rt-PA group was more likely to have symptomatic intracerebral hemorrhage (ICH) than the placebo group (see Table 2). The incidence of symptomatic ICH was 6.4%, with half of those (2.9%) being fatal ICHs. There was no significant difference in mortality. Despite these bleeding complications, overall the rt-PA group had a significantly improved neurologic and functional outcome compared to the placebo group.

Some have criticized the NINDS rt-PA study as having enrolled patients with TIAs who would have improved even without lytic therapy. This issue could be raised with almost every acute stroke study, since such trials do not offer the luxury of waiting 24 hours to see if the symptoms resolve spontaneously. Patients who show early spontaneous improvement are typically excluded from all acute therapy trials, including the TPA studies. Even if there is a subpopulation of patients likely to improve without therapy, one would expect them to be equally distributed between the treatment and placebo groups.

Based on the results of the NINDS trial, in June 1996 the U.S. Food and Drug Administration approved IV TPA as the first agent for the acute treatment of stroke patients.[36] This approval carries many inclusion and exclusion criteria, the most important of which is a 3-hour time from stroke onset to the initiation of TPA therapy. Despite the excitement over this approval, there are several limitations to this study that deserve mention. All patients who improved did not do so equally across the various scales used in the assessments. The overall stroke severity in this study is somewhat less than in the ECASS and MAST-E studies (see below). Over 17,000 stroke patients had to be screened to ascertain the 624 who were treated. The main reason for exclusion was the time of presentation, which (as indicated below) will remain a challenge if this type of therapy is to be used in a widespread manner.

Questions and concerns have been raised about the longevity of the efficacy reported in the NINDS study. A follow-up study of the NINDS patients has shown persistent and statistically significant benefit in the rt-PA vs placebo treatment group up to 12 months after therapy.[37] There has also been concern about the relatively high cost of rt-PA therapy, which is approximately $2,000 per patient. A cost-benefit analysis of rt-PA in stroke patients has shown an overall cost saving in the range of $5 million per every 1,000 treated patients.[38]

Some physicians have questioned whether the results of the NINDS trial can be duplicated in routine clinical practice. Several follow-up studies of rt-PA usage postapproval have been published. In general, these studies have shown clinical efficacy consistent with the effects seen in the original NINDS study, with serious bleeding complications in the 5% to 6% range.[39] Certainly, when using rt-PA in stroke patients, it must be administered with close attention to the inclusion and exclusion criteria, as well as careful monitoring of the blood pressure and avoidance of concomitant medications that can precipitate bleeding postherapy.

Two large additional studies in rt-PA in acute stroke have recently announced results (although no formal publications were available at the time this chapter was written). The first was ECASS II, which is a European study that used rt-PA at a dose of 0.9 mg/kg, but with a 6-hour enrollment window. The other inclusion/exclusion criteria were similar (but not identical) to the NINDS study. In ECASS II, careful attention was given to excluding patients with early CT changes. The overall ECASS II results were negative, in that the treatment group did not show a statistically significant improvement, due in part to the very favorable outcomes seen in the placebo group. Bleeding complications appeared to be consistent with the NINDS rt-PA study. The other recent large study of rt-PA was ATLANTIS, which enrolled most patients within a 3- to 5-hour time window. This study was stopped early due to lack of efficacy, and also in light of the negative ECASS II study.

Streptokinase has been studied extensively in acute stroke. One large trial was the Multicenter Acute Stroke Trial–Italy (MAST-I), which randomized 622 patients into four treatment groups: placebo; IV SK (1.5 M units); SK plus 300 mg aspirin; and just aspirin.[30] All patients were treated within 6 hours of symptom onset. Other anticoagulants and antiplatelet agents were prohibited for 10 days following therapy, with the exception of subcutaneous heparin (maximum dose 15,000 U q.d.). An interesting aspect of this study was that informed consent was not routinely required from the enrolled patients. Patients in the SK group (with or without aspirin) had a 10-day fatality rate of 34% to 19%, compared to 10% for the aspirin group and 13% for the placebo group. For patients receiving SK and aspirin, the rate of symptomatic ICH was 10% vs. 0.6% for controls.[30] The majority of deaths in the SK group were related to cerebral causes (i.e., bleeding, edema, herniation). This study was discontinued early due to the high 10-day fatality rate.

The Australian Streptokinase Study (ASK) had a 4-hour treatment window, used 1.5 M units of SK (IV), and measured neurologic status 3 months after therapy.[40] All patients who were treated with SK also received 100 mg ASA within 4 hours of SK administration. A total of 340 patients were randomized in this double-blind, placebo-controlled protocol. The study was terminated early due to an increased risk of death and disability in the SK vs. placebo groups (48.3% vs. 44.6%, respectively). The rates of symptomatic ICH was 12.6% in the SK group and 2.4% in the placebo group. The outcomes were better for those patients treated within 3 hours of stroke onset, but even in this group there was not a statistically significant benefit in favor of SK compared to placebo.[40] Most of the poor outcomes were confined to the patients treated in the 3- to 4-hour time period. About one-third of patients receiving SK experienced significant hypotension, 2% had anaphylactic shock, and 6% experienced a rash.

The last reported large study is MAST-E, a study of IV SK with a 6-hour treatment window.[23] This study used 1.5 M units of SK, and allowed the use of IV heparin 12 hours after SK therapy. Most other studies of thrombolytic agents in stroke have prohibited the use of anticoagulants for 24 hours after the administration of the lytic agent. About one-third of the SK patients in MAST-E did receive heparin within 24 hours of SK therapy. The MAST-E study was stopped after 312 patients were enrolled due to an excessive 10-day mortality of 34% in the SK group compared to 18% for the placebo group.[23] The main cause for this excessive mortality was ICH. In this regard, the MAST-E mirrors the experience of MAST-I study (see above), each of which reported a high early mortality related to an increase in ICH and other cerebral causes.

There are several likely explanations for the high mortality and bleeding rates seen in the MAST and Australian studies. One explanation is that SK has a propensity to cause more brain bleeding than TPA. This may be due to the relative lack of clot selectivity of SK compared to TPA. Another factor may be the prolonged enrollment windows in these studies. Whereas the NINDS-TPA study had a 3-hour maximum treatment window, the other studies used 4- to 6-hour enrollment times. For reasons that are unclear, several of the European studies tended to enroll more severe stroke patients than the NINDS-TPA study. Larger strokes have a higher risk of hemorrhagic transformation compared to smaller strokes. Lastly, the early use of antiplatelet agents and anticoagulants in some of these studies may be a very significant factor in the increased rate of ICH. Based on these data, it seems reasonable to conclude that SK will not be a viable treatment for acute stroke in the foreseeable future.

In terms of the types of CNS hemorrhage following lytic therapy, the vast majority of such hemorrhages are asymptomatic hemorrhagic transformations of ischemic strokes. Such transformations occurs in 20% to 54% of stroke patients treated with lytics.[19,23,30,31,40] Of more concern are the symptomatic ICHs. In addition to the drug and time issues discussed above, several other clinical factors have been postulated to be important in causing such ICHs. Advanced age, hypertension, and stroke size appear to be among the most important factors.[24,31] Although it has been assumed that reperfusion is related to ICH, angiographic studies have not clearly shown that early reperfusion is associated with ICH.[18] Older patients are more likely to have underlying cerebral amyloid angiopathy (CAA), which is a common cause of ICH in the elderly.[41] Histologic studies have shown that approximately 40% of individuals above age 85 are likely to have evidence of CAA.[42] Studies of MI patients who receive TPA and develop an ICH have shown that CAA is found in about 60% of such patients.[43] Whether this is the explanation for some cases of ICH in stroke patients who receive lytics is unclear.

Patients with large or severe strokes and/or early CT changes appear to be more likely to experience CNS hemorrhage following lytic therapy.[19,23,31] This might reflect a larger mass of damaged brain tissue, which therefore is more likely to hemorrhage. Past studies have shown that stroke size is a key factor in predicting hemorrhagic transformation of embolic strokes.[44] On the other hand, patients with massive strokes are the ones who could potentially have the most to gain from reperfusion therapy, if done very soon after stroke onset. Subsequent analysis of the NINDS study showed that rt-PA-treated patients with early CT changes were more likely to have an ICH, with an odds ratio of 7.8. Patients with an NIHSS score >20 also had a higher risk of ICH, but this effect was not nearly as significant as the early CT changes. However, either group of patient still benefitted from rt-PA therapy, despite the increased risk of ICH.[45] As currently approved, the use of TPA in patients with early CT changes (mass effect, edema) or an NIH stroke scale score more than 20 is not a contraindication, but caution is advised. In general, early CT changes are very rare in stroke patients imaged within 3 hours of onset.[31] Therefore, if such changes are seen, it is important to requestion the patient and others to confirm the exact time of symptom onset and any other premonitory spells.

Intra-arterial UK or SK have been used fairly extensively at many medical centers for selected acute stroke patients. This may be partially based on the experiences of interventionalists using UK for peripheral occlusive disease, combined with the good efficacy and safety profile of UK for these indications. Hacke et al. reported one of the largest studies of UK in patients with posterior fossa strokes due to vertebrobasilar occlusive disease.[46] In this study of 65 patients, 43 were treated with UK or SK, and 22 were treated with standard therapy. Nineteen of the 43 patients treated with lytics had recanalization, and 14 of these patients survived. Only 3 of the 22 patients treated with conventional therapy survived. All of the patients without recanalization died. Since this study was neither randomized nor blinded, it is difficult to draw any definitive conclusions beyond saying that having normal blood flow to one's brainstem is a desirable state.

The PROACT study is investigating the use of sIA pro-urokinase (pro-UK) combined with heparin in patients with middle cerebral artery occlusions. All patients are treated within 6 hours of symptom onset. Preliminary results showed that sIA pro-UK was effective in producing clot lysis, with a recanalization rate of 58%, but a symptomatic hemorrhage rate of 15%. Reducing the dose of heparin appears to reduce the rate of ICH. However, there was no statistically significant correlation between recanalization and clinical improvement, although the number of treated patients was quite small.[47]

There have been several other series reporting the use of IA and sIA UK in acute stroke. The Oregon University team has treated 26 patients with IA UK for cerebral arterial occlusions.[48] They found complete or partial restoration of flow in 22 of 26 treated patients, and 14 patients had excellent clinical outcomes. Clinically significant cerebral hemorrhage developed in about 10% of treated patients. Another study treated 12 stroke patients with IA UK within 8 hours of stroke onset. Successful reperfusion using 160,000 to 500,000 IU was found in 75% of patients, with 50% of patients showing excellent clinical outcomes.[49] In most cases the UK was infused adjacent or into the clot. There were no hemorrhagic complications in this study.

In our experience, sIA UK is highly successful in lysing clots, with a recanalization rate of 85% to 90%. We typically use doses ranging from 200,000 to 750,000 IU, depending on the clot size and serial angiographic evaluation during the infusion. We have seen one case of clinically significant intracranial hemorrhage, and one case of a large groin hematoma using sIA UK. As with systemic TPA, we do not use systemic anticoagulants or antiplatelet agents for 24 hours following the administration of sIA-UK.

A significant challenge with using sIA UK is the need for an interventional team and angiography facilities, which are not available in many hospitals on a 24-hour/day basis. Such interventions obviously take time, which may further delay therapy. At this time it is unclear how useful sIA UK therapy will be or the number of patients that can be treated, even with a prolonged time window.

Ancrod has been evaluated in several large, prospective trials. One study enrolled and randomized 132 patients within 6 hours of stroke onset.[50] This is the largest prospective, randomized study of Ancrod in stroke reported to date. Patients received a 7-day IV infusion of placebo or Ancrod. Only 23% of the Ancrod group achieved the desirable fibrinogen reduction. There was no significant difference in neurologic outcome between the placebo and Ancrod groups, nor was there any evidence of excessive bleeding in the Ancrod group. Another large, randomized trial of Ancrod has been completed as this chapter is being written, but the results are not yet available.

In general, trials of lytic agents in acute stroke have reported very few significant systemic bleeding complications (typically < 1%). Perhaps the careful selection criteria of these trials serve to exclude patients at high risk for systemic bleeding events. For example, most studies exclude patients with recent surgery, biopsies, or systemic injuries. Hypotensive or allergic reactions have been seen most frequently with SK administration. The ASK trial reported a relatively high rate of complications, with 33% of patients having hypotension and 3.4% having peripheral bleeding related to SK administration.[40]

As of August 1998, the only approved therapy for acute ischemic stroke is rt-PA administered within 3 hours of stroke onset. Given all of the available data, one has to ask whether the NINDS rt-PA results are the exception that proves the rule, or simply the exception to the rule. Is the time window, choice of medication, and concomitant medications so narrow and specific that the other studies were seriously flawed and unlikely to show efficacy? Or might the NINDS rt-PA results be due to random chance? Do the benefits of TPA therapy clearly outweigh the risks? Opinions differ on this point.[51,52] If one examines the trial results for thrombolytic therapy in acute MI, one finds that a variety of agents are effective across a variety of treatment time windows (although earlier therapy is predictably more efficacious).[3] It would be comforting to have a similar range of positive results for the study of lytic agents in stroke patients. A recent meta-analysis of 12 randomized trials of various lytic agents in stroke patients did not reach any firm conclusions.[2] This analysis found that there was significant heterogeneity among the trials, which made comparisons difficult. Factors such as vessel size, clot type and age, collateral flow, type of drug, route of administration, time delays, and concomitant medications may all play significant roles in determining the efficacy and safety of lytic therapy.

There are several important issues related to thrombolytic therapy of stroke patients that were briefly noted above, and will now be discussed in more detail. One is early reocclusion. This is a common and important phenomenon in MI patients treated with lytics. The frequency of early reocclusion in stroke patients treated with lytics has not been well studied. I have seen this occur in at least one patient treated with IA UK for basilar artery thrombosis. This middle-aged woman had lysis of a distal basilar clot after 200,000 U of sIA-UK, then reoccluded the vessel in about 10 minutes. Infusion of another 500,000 U of sIA-

UK was required to lyse the second clot. The underlying vessel did not appear abnormal. In several cases patients receiving lytics show transient improvements, then return to baseline. This fluctuation may be due to reperfusion and reocclusion of a vessel, although proof is limited. There are reports that glycoprotein IIb/IIIa inhibitors can prevent this type of reocclusion.[53] Further studies are needed in this area to prove the safety and efficacy of these compounds in stroke patients treated with lytic agents.

Another issue is the occurrence of reperfusion injury following lysis. Acute reperfusion can lead to an increase in excitatory amino acid and free radical production. Animal models of stroke have shown that these events can considerably increase cerebral damage.[20,54,55] Whether similar events lead to clinical sequelae in human strokes following reperfusion is unclear, although preliminary studies suggest that similar events do occur.[56,57] There are a number of neuroprotective agents under development that could potentially be used to treat this complication.

TPA therapy for acute ischemic stroke remains grossly underutilized. Estimates indicate that about 1.5% of ischemic stroke patients in the United States are being treated with rt-PA. One major reason for this is the delayed time of presentation for most stroke patients. Studies suggest that only a small percentage of ischemic stroke patients present within 3 hours of symptom onset.[58] Physician concerns and a lack of hospital infrastructure may also contribute of the small number of stroke patients being treated with rt-PA.[59]

Much work needs to be done to improve stroke care and recognition. The cooperation and education of personnel involved in all phases of the acute stroke care are clearly necessary, ranging from EMS/EMT staffs to Emergency Department physicians and triage nurses, internists, family physicians, and others.[60] A multidisciplinary team approach is important for the safe and successful use of lytic agents in stroke patients.[4,61,62] In addition, the public requires significant education ranging from very basic information about stroke (i.e., what it is, symptoms of a stroke) to the emergency nature of this disease.[63] Recent studies have shown a paucity of knowledge in the general population about stroke.[64] Although educational efforts can be successful in some settings, it is likely that they will have to be repeated on a regular basis to have a consistent and persistent effect.[65] A "dual-track" approach is probably optimal, whereby educational effort aimed at health-care professionals is done in conjunction with public educational programs.

FUTURE STUDIES AND ISSUES

Several key issues are defining the direction of future studies of lytic agents in acute stroke: (1) Can different agents or modified administration techniques improve efficacy? (2) Is there a group of patients in which longer treatment time windows can be used safely? (3) Are there better methods to identify patients likely to benefit (or unlikely to benefit) from treatment with lytic agents?

The negative findings of studies of rt-PA with 6-hour treatment windows is a significant setback for expanding the number of treatable patients. Modified lytic agents that are more potent or more clot-selective are being studied in patients with acute MI. Whether these agents will also be studied in acute ischemic stroke is unclear. As stated above, there are ongoing studies using sIA UK in acute stroke. These studies in general use a 6-hour enrollment window, and require angiography and selective catheterization with infusion of the UK within the clot. Such studies have the advantage of determining the efficacy of UK in terms of clot lysis, as well as providing some correlation between reperfusion and clinical outcomes. They have the disadvantage of delaying therapy, since patients must undergo a cerebral angiogram prior to treatment.

There are two other promising areas. One is combination therapy using lytic agents and neuroprotective compounds. The theory is that combined therapy may enhance the effects of a single agent, and perhaps even extend the treatment time window. Since some neuroprotective agents can be given without a prior head CT scan, there is the potential for initiating therapy sooner, when the patient is still "in the field." Such combination therapy appears to be effective in animal stroke models.[66] However, there has yet to be a neuroprotective agent proven to be safe and effective in humans with stroke. Other challenges with combined therapy include a paucity of combined toxicology and pharmacokinetic data, along with dual exclusion criteria.

The other exciting area is the use of advanced neuroimaging techniques such as magnetic resonance spectroscopy (MRS), MR diffusion, and MR perfusion studies.[67] These modalities may be able to distinguish infarcted from ischemic brain, and could serve as a tool to identify patients likely to benefit from thrombolytic therapy. However, such technologies are not yet widely available, and performing additional studies may cause some delay in initiating therapy.

SUMMARY

We have entered into an era of active, as opposed to reactive, stroke therapy. The approval of IV rt-PA is the first step, although much work still needs to be done to improve the efficacy and safety of thrombolytic therapy and to make it available to more stroke patients. We are hopeful that rapid progress can be made in many of these areas, although if past experience is any guide, the challenges we face will be overcome "stroke-by-stroke."

Note added to proofs: Since this chapter was submitted, several important studies have been either published or presented in sufficient detail to justify this addendum. In ECASS II, the favorable outcome rate (defined as a amodified Rankin of 0 or 1) was 40.3% in the TPA group vs. 36.6% in the placebo group (p = 0.28). Symptomatic ICHs occurred in 8.8% of treated patients vs. 3.4% of controls.[68] Additional results for the ATLANTIS study have also been released. This study of IV TPA treated patients within a variety of time points, but most were treated within 3–5 hours of symptom onset. The rate of favorable outcomes was essentially identical between the TPA and placebo groups at 33%. Symptomatic ICHs occurred in 7.2% of TPA patients vs. 0.7% of controls.[69]

The results of PROACT II, which studied IA pro-urokinase plus IV heparin, were reported at a recent meeting. This study found a recanalization rate of 67% among patients receiving pro-UK vs. 18% in controls. The favorable outcome rate was 40% in the pro-UK group and 25% in controls, a significant difference (p = 0.043). Symptomatic ICHs occurred in 10.2% of treated patients and 1.8% of controls.[70]

The results of a large, prospective, placebo controlled trial of Ancrod were also announced. Treated patients received a 5 day intravenous infusion of Ancrod with adjustment of the dose to reduce serum fibrinogen to 40–69 mg/dl. This study found a favorable outcome in 42% of Ancrod patients compared to 34% of controls, which was a significant difference (p = 0.04). The rate of symptomatic ICHs was 5.2% in Ancrod patients vs. 2% in controls.[71]

Given this new data, acute stroke therapy with lytic agents may be changed. Treatment beyond 3 hours with TPA seems unlikely at this time. Intra-arterial pro-UK appears to be a reasonable option for patients treated up to 6 hours after stroke onset, provided they have an MCA occlusion. However, these results may encourage the treatment of patients with other large vessel occlusive lesions such as basilar and vertebral thrombosis. Ancrod may be an alternative to TPA within the 3 hour treatment window.

REFERENCES

1. Wardlaw J, Warlow C. Thrombolysis in acute ischemic stroke: does it work? Stroke 1992; 23:1826–1839.
2. Wardlaw J, Warlow C, Counsell C. Systematic review of evidence on thrombolytic therapy for acute ischaemic stroke. Lancet 1997; 350:607–614.
3. Van de Werf F, Califf RM, Armstrong PW, et al. Progress culminating from ten years of clinical trials on thrombolysis for acute myocardial infarction. GUSTO-I Steering Committee. Global utilization of streptokinase and tissue plasminogen activator for occluded coronary arteries. Eur Heart J 1995; 16:1024–1026.
4. Working Group on Emergency Brain Resuscitation. Emergency brain resuscitation. Ann Intern Med 1995; 122:622–627.

5. Levine SR, Brott TG. Thrombolytic therapy in cerebrovascular disorders. Prog Cardiovasc Dis 1992; 34:235–262.
6. Baron JC, von Kummer R, del Koppo GJ. Treatment of acute ischemic stroke. Challenging the concept of a rigid and universal time window [editorial]. Stroke 1995; 26:2219–2221.
7. Brott T, Haley EC, Levy DE, et al. The investigational use of tPA for stroke. Ann Emerg Med 1988; 17:1202–1205.
8. Pellegrini-Giampietro DE. Free radicals and the pathogenesis of neuronal death: cooperative role of excitatory amino acids. Adv Exp Med Biol 1994; 366:59–71.
9. Chan PH. Role of oxidants in ischemic brain damage. Stroke 1996; 27:1124–1129.
10. Fisher M, Takano K. The penumbra, therapeutic time window and acute ischaemic stroke. Baillieres Clin Neurol 1995; 4:279–295.
11. Heiss WD, Graf R. The ischemic penumbra. Curr Opin Neurol 1994; 7:11–19.
12. Hossmann KA. Viability thresholds and the penumbra of focal ischemia [see comments]. Ann Neurol 1994; 36:557–565.
13. Ginsberg M, Pulsinelli W. The ischemic penumbra, injury thresholds, and the therapeutic window for acute stroke. Ann Neurol 1994; 36:553–554.
14. Marchal G, Beaudouin V, Rioux P, et al. Prolonged persistence of substantial volumes of potentially viable brain tissue after stroke: a correlative PET-CT study with voxel-based data analysis. Stroke 1996; 27:599–606.
15. Furlan M, Marchal G, Viader F, et al. Spontaneous neurological recovery after stroke and the fate of the ischemic penumbra. Ann Neurol 1996; 40:216–226.
16. Camarata PJ, Heros RC, Latchaw RE. "Brain attack": the rationale for treating stroke as a medical emergency. Neurosurgery 1994; 34:144–157.
17. Caplan L. Diagnosis and treatment of ischemic stroke. JAMA 1991; 266:2413–2148.
18. del Zoppo GJ, Poeck K, Pessin MS, et al. Recombinant tissue plasminogen activator in acute thrombotic and embolic stroke. Ann Neurol 1992; 32:78–86.
19. National Institute of Neurologic Disorders and Stroke rt-PA Acute Stroke Study Group. Tissue plasminogen activator in acute ischemic stroke. N Engl J Med 1995; 333:1581–1587.
20. Obrenovitch TP, Richards DA. Extracellular neurotransmitter changes in cerebral ischaemia. Cerebrovasc Brain Metab Rev 1995; 7:1–54.
21. Siesjo BK, Katsura K, Zhao Q, et al. Mechanisms of secondary brain damage in global and focal ischemia: a speculative synthesis. J Neurotrauma 1995; 12:943–956.
22. Chan PH. Oxygen radicals in focal cerebral ischemia. Brain Pathol 1994; 4:59–65.
23. Multicenter Acute Stroke Trial–Europe Study Group. Thrombolytic therapy with streptokinase in acute ischemic stroke. N Engl J Med 1996; 35:145–150.
24. Levy DE, Brott TG, Haley EC Jr, et al. Factors related to intracranial hematoma formation in patients receiving tissue-type plasminogen activator for acute ischemic stroke. Stroke 1994; 25:291–297.
25. Anonymous. Streptase. In: Physicians' Desk Reference. Montvale, NJ: Medical Economics Data, 1998:578–580.
26. Anonymous. Activase. In: Physicians' Desk Reference. Montvale, NJ: Medical Economics Data, 1998:984–988.

27. Anonymous. Abbokinase. In: Physicians' Desk Reference. Montvale, NJ: Medical Economic Data, 1998:402–404.
28. Prentice CR, Hampton KK, Grant PJ, et al. The fibrinolytic response to Ancrod therapy: characterization of fibrinogen and fibrin degradation products. Br J Haematol 1993; 83:276–281.
29. Pollak VE, Glas-Greenwalt P, Olinger CP, et al. Ancrod causes rapid thrombolysis in patients with acute stroke. Am J Med Sci 1990; 299:319–325.
30. Multicentre Acute Stroke Trial–Italy (MAST-I) Group. Randomised controlled trial of streptokinase, aspirin, and combination of both in treatment of acute ischaemic stroke. Lancet 1995; 346:1509–1514.
31. Hacke W, Kaste M, Fieschi C, et al. Intravenous thrombolysis with recombinant tissue plasminogen activator for acute hemispheric stroke. European Cooperative Acute Stroke Study (ECASS). JAMA 1995; 274:1017–1025.
32. Abe T, Kazama M, Naito I, et al. Clinical evaluation for efficacy of tissue cultured urokinase (TCUK) on cerebral thrombosis by means of multi-center double-blind study. Blood Vessels 1981; 12:321-341.
33. Ohtomo E, Araki G, Itoh E, et al. Clinical efficacy of urokinase in the treatment of cerebral thrombosis. Clin Eval 1985; 13:711–751.
34. Brott TG, Haley EC Jr, Levy DE, et al. Urgent therapy for stroke. Part I. Pilot study of tissue plasminogen activator administered within 90 minutes. Stroke 1992; 23:632–640.
35. Haley EC Jr, Levy DE, Brott TG, et al. Urgent therapy for stroke. Part II. Pilot study of tissue plasminogen activator administered 91–180 minutes from onset. Stroke 1992; 23:641–645.
36. Activase, alteplase recombinant for acute ischemic stroke. Presented at the Peripheral and Centeral Nervous System Drug Advisory Committee Meeting, Bethesda, MD, June 6, 1996.
37. Kwiatkowski TG, Libman R, Frankel M, et al. The NINDS rt-PA stroke study. Sustained benefit at one year. Stroke 1998; 29:288.
38. Fagan SC, Morgenstern LB, Petitta A, et al. Cost-effectiveness of tissue plasminogen activator for acute ischemic stroke. Neurol 1998; 50:883–890.
39. Chiu D, Krieger D, Villar-Cordova C, et al. Intravenous tissue plasminogen activator for acute ischemic stroke: feasibility, safety, and efficacy in the first year of clinical practice. Stroke 1998; 29:18–22.
40. Donnan GA, Davis SM, Chamber BR, et al. Streptokinase for acute ischemic stroke with relationship to time of administration: Australian Streptokinase (ASK) Trial Study Group. JAMA 1996; 276:961–966.
41. Broderick J, Brott T, Tomsick T, et al. Lobar hemorrhage in the elderly. The undiminishing importance of hypertension. Stroke 1993; 24:49–51.
42. Masuda J, Tanaka K, Ueda K, et al Autopsy study of incidence and distribution of cerebral amyloid angiopathy in Hisayama, Japan. Stroke 1988; 19:205–210.
43. Sloan MA, Price TR, Petito CK, et al. Clinical features and pathogenesis of intracerebral hemorrhage after rt-PA and heparin therapy for acute myocardial infarction: Thrombolysis in Myocardial Infarction (TIMI) II Pilot and Randomized Clinical Trial combined experience. Neurology 1995; 45:649–658.

44. Okada Y, Yamaguchi T, Minematsu K, et al. Hemorrhagic transformation in cerebral embolism. Stroke 1989; 20:598–603.
45. NINDS rt-PA Stroke Study Group. Symptomatic intracerebral hemorrhage after t-PA for stroke. Stroke 1997; 28:2109–2118.
46. Hacke W, Zeumer H, Ferbert A, et al. Intra-arterial thrombolytic therapy improves outcome in patients with acute vertebrobasilar occlusive disease. Stroke 1988; 19:1216–1222.
47. del Zoppo G, Higashida R, Furlan A, et al. PROACT: a phase II randomized trial of recombinant pro-urokinase by direct arterial delivery in acute middle cerebral artery stroke. Stroke 1998; 29:4–11.
48. Barnwell SL, Nesbit GM, Clark WM. Local thrombolytic therapy for cerebrovascular disease: current Oregon Health Sciences University experience (July 1991 through April 1995). J Vasc Interv Radiol 1995; 6:78S–82S.
49. Barr JD, Mathis JM, Wildenhain SL, et al. Acute stroke intervention with intraarterial urokinase infusion. J Vasc Interv Radiol 1994; 5:705–713.
50. Ancrod Stroke Study Investigators. Ancrod for the treatment of acute ischemic brain infarction. Stroke 1994; 25:1755–1759.
51. Riggs J. Tissue-type plasminogen activator should not be used in acute ischemic stroke. Arch Neurol 1996; 53:1306–1308.
52. Brott T. Thrombolysis for stroke. Arch Neurol 1996; 53:1305–1306.
53. Wallace RC, Furlan AJ, Moliterno DJ, et al. Basilar artery rethrombosis: successful treatment with platelet glycoprotein IIB/IIIA receptor inhibitor. AJNR 1997; 18:1257–1260.
54. Siesjo BK, Zhao Q, Pahlmark K, et al. Glutamate, calcium, and free radicals as mediators of ischemic brain damage. Ann Thorac Surg 1995; 59:1316–1320.
55. Takagi K, Ginsberg MD, Globus MY, et al. Changes in amino acid neurotransmitters and cerebral blood flow in the ischemic penumbral region following middle cerebral artery occlusion in the rat: correlation with histopathology. J Cereb Blood Flow Metab 1993; 13:575–585.
56. Hegstad E, Berg-Johnsen J, Haugstad TS, et al. Amino-acid release from human cerebral cortex during simulated ischaemia in vitro. Acta Neurochir 1996; 138:234–241.
57. Castillo J, Davalos A, Naveiro J, et al. Neuroexcitatory amino acids and their relation to infarct size and neurological deficit in ischemic stroke. Stroke 1996; 27:1060–1065.
58. International Stroke Trial Collaborative Group. The International Stroke Trial: a randomized trial of aspirin, subcutaneous heparin, both, or neither among 19,435 patients with acute ischaemic stroke. Lancet 1997; 349:1569–1581.
59. Alberts MJ. Hyperacute stroke therapy with tissue plasminogen activator. Am J Cardiol 1997; 80:29D–34D.
60. Alberts M. Undergraduate and postgraduate medical education for cerebrovascular disease. Stroke 1995; 26:1849–1851.
61. Alberts M, Semantuverdi S, Graham G, et al. Acute stroke teams: results of a national survey. Stroke 1998; 29:2318–2320.
62. Gomez CR, Malkoff MD, Sauer CM, et al. Code stroke. An attempt to shorten inhospital therapeutic delays. Stroke 1994; 25:1920–1923.

63. Futrell N, Millikan CH. Stroke is an emergency. Dis Mon 1996; 42:199–264.
64. NSA/Gallup. National Stroke Awareness Survey. The Gallup Organization, 1991.
65. Alberts MJ, Perry A, Dawson DV, et al. Effects of public and professional education on reducing the delay in presentation and referral of stroke patients. Stroke 1992; 23:352–356.
66. Zivin J, Mazzarella V. Tissue plasminogen activator plus glutamate antagonist improves outcome after embolic stroke. Arch Neurol 1991; 48:1235–1238.
67. Fisher M, Prichard J, Warach S. New magnetic resonance techniques for acute ischemic stroke. JAMA 1995; 274:908–911.
68. Hacke W, Kaste M, Fieschi C, et al. Randomised double-blind placebo-controlled trial of thrombolytic therapy with intravenous alteplase in acute ischaemic stroke (ECASS II). Lancet 1998; 352:1245–1251.
69. Clark WM, Albers GW, for the ATLANTIS Stroke Study. The Atlantis rt-PA (Alteplase) Acute Stroke Trial: final results. Presented at the 24th American Heart Association International Conference on Stroke and Cerebral Circulation. Nashville, TN, 1999.
70. Furlan AJ, Higashida R, Wechsler L, et al. PROACT II: Recombinant prourokinase (r-ProUK) in acute cerebral thromboembolism: Initial trial results. Presented at the 24th American Heart Association International Conference on Stroke and Cerebral Circulation. Nashville, TN, 1999.
71. Sherman DG for the STAT Writers Group. Defibrinogenation with Viprinix (Ancrod) for the treatment of acute ischemic stroke. Presented at the 24th American Heart Association International Conference on Stroke and Cerebral Circulation. Nashville, TN, 1999.

17

Glutamate Receptor Antagonists for the Treatment of Acute Cerebral Ischemia

Daniel L. Small and Paul Morley
Institute for Biological Sciences, National Research Council of Canada, Ottawa, Ontario, Canada

Alastair M. Buchan
University of Calgary, Calgary, Alberta, Canada

INTRODUCTION

The glutamate hypothesis of neuronal cell death was derived from in vitro studies and then backed up by an array of in vivo studies of cerebral ischemia. This hypothesis causally associates the excitatory neurotransmitter glutamate in the ischemic neuron's inability to adequately buffer intracellular calcium which directly leads to the death of the cells (Fig. 1). Although glutamate is the principal excitatory amino acid neurotransmitter, there is a plethora of glutamate receptor subtypes and therefore pharmaceutical approaches. The receptors fall into three basic groups (Fig. 1): metabotropic receptors, which mediate second-messenger changes through G proteins; and two types of ionotropic receptors activated by N-methyl-D-aspartate (NMDA)- and α-amino-3-hydroxy-5-methyl-4-isoxazole propionic acid (AMPA)/kainate.

Experimentally, a series of glutamate receptor antagonists have been shown to be neuroprotective in both in vitro and in vivo models of ischemia. NMDA receptor antagonists will prevent the death of cultured neurons exposed to either brief periods of hypoxia or glutamate. In vivo, glutamate is released following ischemia (Fig. 1), and prior removal of glutamate afferents or pretreatment with either competitive or noncompetitive NMDA receptor antagonists, or competitive AMPA receptor antagonists, results in neuroprotection. The data demonstrating NMDA receptor antagonism–induced neuroprotection in global models of cerebral ischemia have been challenged since NMDA receptor antagonist neuroprotection likely results from drug-induced hypothermia rather than direct NMDA receptor blockade per se (Buchan and Pulsinelli, 1990). Both NMDA and AMPA receptor antagonists have, however, achieved more consistent neuroprotection in focal models of cerebral ischemia. Because of the direct clinical relevance of animal models of focal ischemia, a wave of clinical stroke trials with NMDA receptor antagonists have been undertaken (see Table 1).

These ongoing clinical trials with NMDA receptor antagonists have been plagued by problems of having to balance the risk of failure due to toxicity at too high a dose with the risk of failure due to a lack of efficacy at low doses. Simply stated, most NMDA receptor antagonists to date suffer from a low therapeutic index. Is this due to the fact that the animal models used to identify can-

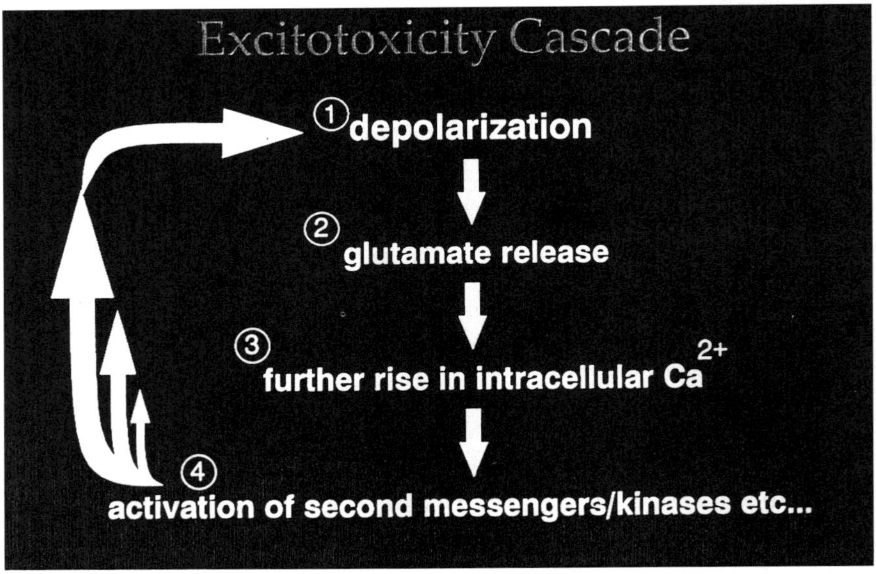

Figure 1 Cartoon depicting the proposed excitatory cascade following ischemia and potential sites of intervention ①-④. Initially there is a "presynaptic" depolarization ①, which results in an influx of calcium through N, P, and Q subtypes of voltage-gated calcium channels. This depolarization and calcium influx result in the release of glutamate ②, which activates postsynaptic NMDA, AMPA and metabotropic glutamate receptors for some of which various antagonists have been indicated in part 3 of this figure. This receptor activation results in a further increase in intracellular calcium ③ which in turn activates calcium-dependent downstream second messengers ④ such as kinases, lipases, proteases, and endonucleases. The whole cascade feeds forward upon itself, resulting in a pathological accumulation of intracellular calcium and the death of the cell.

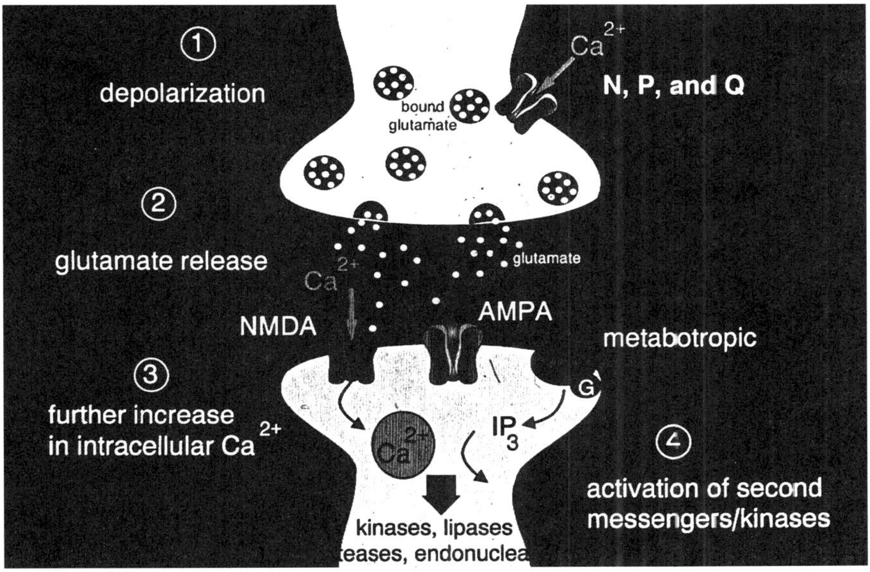

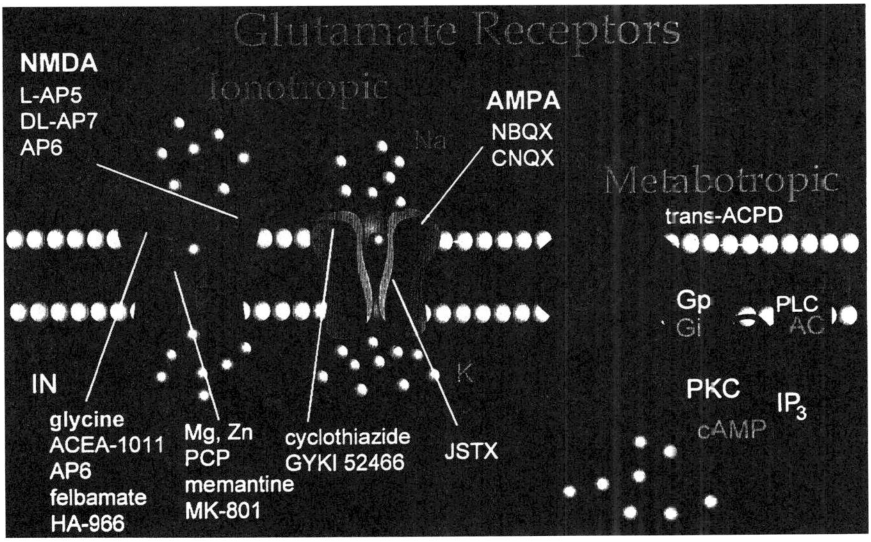

Figure 1 Continued

Table 1 NMDA and AMPA Receptor Antagonists Which Protect in Focal and Global Models of Ischemia

Target	Drug or drug class	Company (compound if applicable)	Protection in focal/global animal models		Clinical trial
NMDA receptors					
Competitive	Selfotel	Ciba/Novartis (CGS 19755)	Focal	Global	Phase II failed
	d-CPP	—	Focal	Global	?
Noncompetititve					
High affinity	Aptiganel (Cerestat)	Cambridge Neurosciences (CNS-1102)	Focal	?	Phase III discontinued
	Dizoclipine	Merck (MK-801)	Focal	Not global	Discontinued
Low affinity	Ketamine	—	Focal	Not global	—
	Dextromethorphan	Hoffman LaRoche	Focal	?	Discontinued
	Memantine	Merz/Neurobiological	Focal	Global	Phase II for AIDS dementia
	Remacemide	Astra Arcus	Focal	?	Phase II completed
	AR-R15896 AR	Astra Arcus	Focal	?	Phase II
	Magnesium	U.K. M.R.C.	?	?	Phase III started
Glycine site	Felbamate	Carter-Wallace (C-W 554)	?	?	?
	ACEA 1021 (Glystatin)	CoSensys	Focal	?	Phase II
	GV 150526	Glaxo Wellcome	Focal	Global	Phase III ongoing
	ACPC	Symphony (SYM-2030)	?	Global	Phase I

Polyamine site (NR2B selective)	Eliprodil	Syntholabo/Lorex (SL82.0715)	Focal	Global	Phase II discontinued
	CP-101,606	Pfizer	Focal	Global	Phase II
	Ro 25-6981	Hoffman LaRoche	?	?	?
Novel site	NPS 1506	NPS	Focal	?	Phase I
AMPA receptors					
Competitive	ZK-200775	Schering	?	?	Phase II
	YM872	Yamanouchi	Focal	?	Phase II
	YM90K	Yamanouchi	Focal	Global	Phase I
	S 17625-2	Servier	Focal	?	?
	PNQX	Parke-David (PD 15227)	Focal	?	?
	NBQX	NovoNordisk	Focal	Global	?
	LY 293558	Eli Lilly	Focal	?	?
Noncompetitive	GYKI 52466	Eli Lilly	Focal	Global	?
	JSTX	—	? Too toxic	Too toxic	—

didates for efficacy trials for stroke intervention do not appropriately represent the human pathophysiologic situation following a stroke? Or, alternatively, have clinical trials been prematurely initiated with inappropriate, perhaps toxic compounds?

The lack of success of clinical trials is not what was predicted by the postitive results in animal models. Doses that are effective in rodents are often far higher than that tested in the clinical protocols, and toxicity is not easily demonstrated in rats. Treatment in cerebral ischemia models is often initiated prior to the insult, yet treatment in the clinic is hampered by the fact that few patients present within a critical time period (<3 h; Adams et al., 1996) after the insult. In a study conducted at one U.S. center, only 42% of stroke patients presented within 24 h (Alberts et al., 1990). The best glutamate receptor antagonist for treatment in the clinic should be efficacious when administered several hours following the ischemic insult. The current studies using animal models also failed to address the question of the duration of treatment because the outcome measures in the models are usually taken following 1 to 2 days of reperfusion in focal ischemia and 3 to 7 days in global ischemia, whereas a patient's recovery must be measured in months and even years.

In this chapter we discuss the compounds in or about to enter clinical trials for acute stroke in a context of glutamate receptor biophysics and pharmacology, and propose a redressing of experimental studies to identify which subtypes of glutamate receptor subunits should be targeted. We predict that it should be possible to target a "subunit" of a glutamate receptor that will achieve neuroprotection with minimal toxicity.

GLUTAMATE RECEPTOR BIOPHYSICS AND PHARMACOLOGY

Ionotropic glutamate receptors NMDA, AMPA, and kainate are heteromeric tetramers which form cation permeable ion channels (Rosenmund et al., 1998). This allows for tremendous diversity in molecular structure and consequently will allow a new, much more selective approach to the pharmacology and behavior of glutamate receptor antagonists.

NMDA Receptors

Much of the diversity of NMDA receptors arises from the expression of the NR2 subunits, NR2A, NR2B, NR2C, and NR2D, each the product of a different gene with only 40% to 50% sequence homology (Conley, 1996). Expression of the NR1 subunit is ubiquitous throughout the brain as is NR2A, whereas NR2B is found in the cortex and hippocampus but not the cerebellum. NR2C and NR2D are found almost exclusively in the cerebellum and olfactory bulb, respectively. Developmentally, NR2B is expressed predominantly in the forebrain until P12, when NR2A and NR2C appear (Monyer et al., 1994). During development, NR2B and NR2C are transiently expressed in the cerebellum and in the hippocampus, respectively (Pollard et al., 1993). NR2C reappears in the hippocampus following a transient hypoxic-hypoglycemic insult (Perez-Velazquez and Zhang, 1994; Zhang et al., 1995; Small et al., 1997), suggesting a reemergence of a "developmental" NMDA receptor subunit following injury and hence possibly providing a selective therapeutic target.

Functionally, the Ca^{2+} permeability of NMDA receptors is about five times greater than that of other ionotropic glutamate receptors (Schneggenburger et al., 1993) due to an asparagine (N) residue in the TM2 region of the channel. Changing the N to glutamine (Q) or arginine (R) decreases the Ca^{2+} permeability, similar to manipulating the Q/R site of AMPA receptors (Burnashev et al., 1992). NR2C-containing receptors exhibit a smaller conductance (36 pS) than that for NR2A- or NR2B- containing receptors (50 pS) (Seeburg et al., 1995) but exhibit a weaker Mg^{2+} block.

Glycine is a coagonist which binds to an extracellular site(s) in the S1 and S2 regions of the NMDA receptor (O'Hara et al., 1993) with nM affinity (Ascher and Johnson, 1994). Since physiological concentrations of glycine are in the μM range (Curtis and Johnston, 1974), the NMDA receptor usually exists in the "glycine-primed" state. Glycine affinity also varies with subunit composition. The NR2A subunit confers a lower affinity for glycine than for the NR2B, NR2C, or NR2D subunits (Kutsuwada et al., 1992; Stern et al., 1992).

Polyamines, whose concentration transiently rises up to 14-fold following ischemia (Paschen et al., 1987), can either potentiate or block NMDA receptor responses, depending on their concentration (McGurk et al., 1990; Mayer and Westbrook, 1987). There may be at least three sites of polyamine interaction with NMDA receptors (Hollmann et al., 1993). The "flickery" block produced by high concentrations of polyamines is due to the molecule physically plugging the channel pore. At low μM concentrations, polyamines potentiate NMDA receptor responses. This effect is greatest in the N-terminal-containing NR1 subunit and is enhanced further when NR1 and NR2B subunits are combined (Williams et al., 1994).

Deactivation and desensitization of NMDA receptors occur more slowly than for AMPA receptors, and the affinity of NMDA receptors for glutamate is much greater than that for AMPA receptors (Sather et al., 1992). There are also subunit-specific differences in the affinities and deactivation rates; NMDA-mediated excitatory postsynaptic currents decay with time constants of 90, 400, 370, and 4,800 ms when NR1 subunits are coexpressed with NR2A, NR2B, NR2C, and NR2D subunits, respectively (Sucher et al., 1996).

AMPA Receptors

AMPA receptors are composed of the GluR1-GluR4 subunits which share about 70% sequence homology. GluR1-GluR3 subunits, unlike GluR4, are highly expressed in both the cerebral cortex and the hippocampus (Keinänen et al., 1990). There is abundant expression of GluR4 in CA1 and dentate gyrus, but levels are low in CA3 and CA4. Most subunits are expressed in the cerebellum but GluR2 is conspicuously absent from Bergmann glia. The flip splice variants of GluR subunits are more prominently and discretely expressed than the flop forms (Sommer et al., 1990). Developmentally, GluR1, GluR3, and GluR4 are expressed earlier than GluR2. Similarly, flip forms appear earlier during development than flop variants.

RNA editing of the AMPA receptors also increases with development (Bernard and Khrestchatisky, 1994; Standley et al., 1995). The major functional difference between the subunits is due to a single residue in the TM2 pore region where there is a glutamine (Q) residue in GluR1, GluR3, and GluR4 subunits and an arginine (R) in GluR2 subunits. Replacing the R with a Q confers an eightfold greater Ca^{2+} permeability, a double rectifying I-V relation (Boulter et al., 1990), and the channel is sensitive to block by intracellular polyamines (Bowie and Mayer, 1995; Seeburg, 1996). The R in GluR2 subunits is a product of posttranslational RNA editing of an adenosine to a guanosine by deamination (Yang et al., 1995). The efficiency of editing increases with age (Paschen and Djurcic, 1995; Bernard and Khrestchatisky, 1994; Standley et al., 1995). The conductance of AMPA receptors is relatively small (about 9 pS), (Conley, 1996). Expression of flip variants produces receptors with smaller current amplitudes and slower rates of desensitization than receptors possessing flop variants (Sommer et al., 1990).

Kainate Receptors

Kainate receptors are composed of KA1 and KA2 subunits, which share 70% homology, and GluR5, GluR6 and GluR7 subunits, which share 80% homology. There are no flip/flop variants for kainate receptors, but RNA editing of the TM2 (Q/R) site occurs in GluR5 and GluR6 subunits (Lomeli et al., 1994). Unlike in AMPA receptors where GluR2 editing occurs with 100% efficiency, GluR5 and GluR6 editing is 40% and 80% efficient, respectively (Paschen et al., 1995). Furthermore, there are two additional sites in GluR6, (I/V) and (Y/C), which effectively potentiate the functional consequences of Q/R site editing (Kohler et al., 1993). Kainate receptors are most abundantly expressed on the pyramidal cells of the CA3 region of the hippocampus and in cortical layers I, V, and VI (Gall et al., 1990). GluR5 is mainly present on cerebellar Purkinje cells. GluR6 and GluR7 are predominantly found in the dentate gyrus, CA3, and cerebellar granule cells. The conductance of kainate receptors (about 6 pS) is even smaller than that of AMPA or NMDA receptors (Conley, 1996).

GLUTAMATE RECEPTOR PHARMACOLOGY IN CEREBRAL ISCHEMIA

Although historically much of the pharmacology of NMDA receptors in cerebral ischemia has focused on the noncompetitive antagonist MK-801, the heterogeneity of the subunits that form the tetrameric ion channel has made for a diverse pharmacology in the past decade. Also, predictions of the therapeutic efficacy of NMDA receptor antagonists, based on preclinical studies, have been tested in clinical trials. The results of the trials that have tested clinical therapeutic efficacy of NMDA receptor antagonists so far have not borne out the optimism of preclinical predictions (see Table 1). Either the models used to predict clinical efficacy are inappropiate or the pharmacology of therapeutic intervention needs to be refined. Many of the problems associated with glutamate receptor antagonists in clinical trials are due to toxicity outweighing benefit. Agents with better therapeutic ratios are needed. This applies not only to NMDA receptor antagonists but also to the AMPA and kainate receptor antagonists which have just recently entered clinical trials. Perhaps agents with a better therapeutic ratio will be identified by redressing animal models with agents that exhibit greater subtype selectivity and/or more rapid kinetics. The remainder of this chapter will provide an overview of receptor pharmacology in experimental studies and clinical trials focusing on various pharmacological classes of compounds.

NMDA Receptor Antagonists

Competitive Antagonists

While there is some evidence that competitive NMDA receptor antagonists are neuroprotective in animal models (see Table 1), not all studies have reported significant neuroprotection with compounds of this class. They can be displaced by glutamate, necessitating very high antagonist concentrations to overcome the elevated cerebrospinal fluid levels of glutamate that occur during ischemia (Obrenovitch and Richards, 1995). The high levels of antagonist required to attenuate the pathological activation of the channel cause the adverse effects associated with many of the competitive NMDA receptor antagonists such as CGS 19755 (Selfotel), NPC 12626, and dCPP-ene (Muir and Lees, 1995). As a class, competitive NMDA receptor antagonists are well represented by Selfotel. The compound showed impressive preclinical data demonstrating dramatic neuroprotection in gerbil models of severe transient forebrain ischemia (Boast, 1988;

Boast et al., 1988) and the absence of psychotomimetic effects in monkeys at neuroprotective doses. However, in spite of an encouraging Phase II study, recruitment into Phase III clinical trials was halted early because in two Acute Stroke Studies Involving Selfotel Treatment (ASSIST) trials, as well as two concurrent traumatic brain injury trials, there was a higher cumulative, though not significant, increase in mortality in the combined Selfotel groups. The preclinical data suggesting Selfotel was neuroprotective were not supported by the clinical trials.

High-Affinity Noncompetitive NMDA Receptor Antagonists

Noncompetitive antagonists have the advantage that they should preferentially block pathological NMDA receptor activation when glutamate levels are high, while exhibiting minimal antagonistic behavior during normal receptor activation. Many of the noncompetitive receptor antagonists are use-dependent; i.e., since they bind within the channel pore, the channel must be open and therefore the receptor activated, for them to gain access to their binding sites (Rogawski, 1993). MK-801 is such an antagonist, producing a block of NMDA receptors by binding within the pore. It has received the most attention of all of the NMDA receptor antagonists and has been responsible for the immense efforts to develop glutamate antagonists for the treatment of stroke.

Examination of all studies investigating the neuroprotective efficacy of MK-801 in various global models of ischemia found that protection was observed only in studies that used a less severe insult, whereas no protection was seen in studies using more severe insults (Pulsinelli and Buchan, 1990). Furthermore, MK-801 is known to cause mild hypothermia, which itself is neuroprotective (Buchan and Pulsinelli, 1990; Corbett et al., 1990). Moreover, issues of neuroprotective efficacy aside, MK-801 produces adverse effects such as psychotomimetic effects, paranoid ideation, hallucinations, neuronal vacuolation, catatonia, and cardiovascular side effects, including peripheral vasoconstriction (Muir and Lees, 1995). These side effects are the reason for the failure of several noncompetitive NMDA receptor antagonists in clinical trials (see Table 1).

CNS-1102 (also called Aptiganel or Cerestat) is among the latest of many NMDA receptor antagonists which suffer from adverse CNS side effects and which has failed a Phase III safety and efficacy trial. Dextrorphan is a compound with an intermediate affinity, yet Phase II clinical trials were canceled due to some PCP-like effects and hypotension in patients receiving high doses. The clinical failure of intermediate noncompetitive receptor antagonists, like high-affinity antagonists, may result from their slow on rates and low therapeutic ratios relative to lower-affinity antagonists (Rogawski, 1993; Mealing et al., 1997).

Low-Affinity Noncompetitive NMDA Receptor Antagonists

Interest in noncompetitive antagonists which exhibit more rapid kinetics and lower affinity than the earlier compounds has recently increased (Jones and Rogawski, 1992; Parsons et al., 1995; Subramaniam et al., 1996; Mealing et al., 1997). Neuroprotection studies with these low-affinity, noncompetitive NMDA receptor antagonists, as with other NMDA receptor antagonists, are not without controversy. Although low-affinity, noncompetitive antagonists are generally associated with fewer adverse side effects and have better therapeutic ratios (Rogawski, 1993), there is evidence that their neuroprotective efficacy is not robust (Jensen and Auer, 1988; Germano et al., 1987; see Table 1). This may be due to the fact that many studies with these compounds were conducted with some of the earliest compounds which either exhibited minimal selectivity for individual NMDA receptor subunits or exhibited very slow kinetics and high affinity. Results with some newer compounds in this class which have faster kinetics and a lower affinity, e.g., memantine and AR-R15896AR, have been encouraging (Parsons et al., 1993; Black et al., 1995).

Clinically, in addition to the use of Mg^{2+} for the treatment of preeclampsia, a 3-year large-scale (2,700-patient) Phase III multicenter trial for the treatment of acute ischemic stroke began in October 1997. Patients, within 12 h of onset, are to receive placebo or IV magnesium (16 mmol over 15 min followed by 65 mmol over 24 h [Muir and Lees, 1997]). Given that Mg^{2+} may act as a neuroprotective agent through vascular and neuronal effects and that it is well tolerated, the results of these trials are anticipated with great enthusiasm. Phase II clinical trials for stroke with remacemide have been completed, and a Phase III trial for epilepsy is under way. Remacemide is very well tolerated, with dose-related dizziness and gastrointestinal upset being the most common adverse effects. Hopefully, the failure of high-affinity NMDA receptor antagonists in clinical trials will not adversely affect the future of low-affinity antagonists in clinical trials, should they prove effective in animal models of cerebral ischemia.

Glycine Site

There are fewer glycine site antagonists and they have received much less attention than the competitive and noncompetitive NMDA receptor antagonists. However, these agents have been gaining in popularity for stroke therapy because they have few adverse side effects (Muir and Lees, 1995; see Table 1). Agents like HA 966 and ACPC are partial agonists at the glycine site. As mentioned previously, physiological glycine levels saturate the glycine site of the NMDA receptors (Ascher and Johnson, 1994). A partial glycine site agonist with a very high affinity would be predicted to provide protection from pathological NMDA receptor activity while permitting physiological NMDA receptor activation. These agents provide neuroprotection in focal models of ischemia (Muir and Lees, 1995; Warner et al., 1995; Gill et al., 1995), while the ability of the glycine site antagonists to ameliorate damage in a global model of cerebral ischemia is less certain (Warner et al., 1995). Glycine site antagonists, as a class, is in its infancy in clinical trials, but a compound from Glaxo Wellcome, GV 150526, has progressed to Phase III trials for treatment of acute stroke (GAIN Americas) and will, upon completion, have enrolled 1,600 patients at 130 centers in the United States and Canada. This is in spite of earlier reports of elevated liver enzyme activities at high doses of the drug in safety trials (Haley, 1997). To date, doses of ACEA 1021 (Glystatin) higher than those demonstrated to be neuroprotective in animals have been infused in 53 stroke patients with no psychotomimetic effects or other safety concerns (Carter, 1996). ACEA is in Phase II clinical trials (see Table 1). It will be interesting to follow the development of this class of antagonists as more data are obtained.

Polyamine Site (NR2B Subunit Selective)

Of the few polyamine site NMDA receptor antagonists available, most, like eliprodil (Williams, 1993), ifenprodil (Williams, 1993), and CP-101,606 (White et al., 1995), have been reported to possess specificity for NR2B subunits of the NMDA receptor. These compounds are devoid of psychotomimetic effects and the vacuolation associated with other NMDA antagonists (Scatton et al., 1995; Pagnozzi et al., 1995). These compounds have proven neuroprotective in a number of models, particularly focal rather than global (Scatton et al., 1995; Toulmond et al., 1993; Menniti et al., 1995). Eliprodil progressed to Phase III clinical trials (Muir and Lees 1995) before being canceled due to a lack of efficacy. In addition to its action at NR2B receptor subunits, eliprodil also blocks Ca^{2+} and Na^{+} channels (Scatton et al., 1995). This lack of specificity could underlie the cardiovascular side effects seen in the eliprodil clinical trials, namely the dose-dependent prolongation of the corrected QT interval. Alternatively, the adverse cardiovascular effects could be due to the adrenergic activity shared by eliprodil and ifenprodil. It is unclear to what extent eliprodil's lack of specificity for NMDA receptors played in its failure in clinical trials. The lack of efficacy in trials might be attributed to the fact that it is a relatively low-affinity NMDA receptor antagonist.

To date, CP-101,606, a compound with a relatively high affinity for the NMDA receptor, like Ro 25-6981, has not been shown to have any adrenergic activity or any effects on Ca^{2+} or Na^{+} channels, but the development of this agent is in its infancy. CP-101,606 is currently in Phase II clinical trials. Like the noncompetitive PCP-site NMDA receptor antagonists, the polyamine site antagonists exhibit a use dependence and block better at higher concentrations of glutamate. Based on the argument made earlier for pore blockers, lower-affinity antagonists with rapid kinetics like isoxsuprine and eliprodil (Whittmore et al., 1996) should exhibit a better therapeutic ratio and therefore may prove to be more efficacious at lower doses (Rogawski, 1993). Either this argument does not hold true for this class of agents or the lack of efficacy of eliprodil was due to its lack of specificity at concentrations that were effective at the NMDA receptor. The results of trials with CP-101,606 and lower-affinity, more specific compounds are anxiously awaited.

NR2C Subunit-Selective Antagonists

Recently it was reported that there is an increased hippocampal expression of NR2C subunit mRNA following an in vitro hypoxic/hypoglycemic insult (Perez-Velazquez and Zhang, 1994; Small et al., 1998), suggesting the possible effectiveness of an NR2C-selective receptor antagonist. There are currently no known NR2C-selective antagonists. However, some compounds, such as phencyclidine (PCP), slightly prefer NR2C over NR2A and NR2B subunits, and agents like memantine which slightly prefer NR2A and NR2B over NR2C subunits (Monaghan and Larsen, 1997). Therefore, some crude pharmacological differentiation of the NR2 subunits is possible and these compounds will act as platforms for structure-activity relationship studies which should some day provide NR2 subunit-selective antagonists. There is also a recently described NMDA receptor antagonist, NPS 1506, which is reported to have a novel binding site and exhibit potentially advantageous pharmacological properties. Its subunit selectivity has not been reported but it is biologically active, has been demonstrated to be neuroprotective in a variety of animal models of stroke and is now in clinical trials, seemingly with none of the side effects associated with many other NMDA receptor antagonists. For now, a full characterization of postischemic changes in glutamate receptor subunit expression, at different times following the insult and in brain regions with different vulnerabilities to ischemic damage, would provide important insights into which compounds may show neuroprotective efficacy. Postischemic changes in NMDA receptor subunit expression may also explain why delayed treatment with NMDA receptor antagonists in global ischemia is not efficacious while treatment with AMPA receptor antagonists is (Li and Buchan, 1993).

AMPA and Kainate Receptor Antagonists

Competitive Antagonists

When all of the variables associated with the animal models of cerebral ischemia are considered, AMPA receptor antagonists are more effective than NMDA receptor antagonists (Xue et al., 1994). Although there are few AMPA receptor antagonists relative to the NMDA receptor antagonists, due in part to the high degree of sequence homology between AMPA receptor subunits (70%) as compared to NMDA receptor subunits (20% to 40%), the protection achieved with these agents is robust. In fact, the quinoxalinedione, NBQX, can be administered after a delay of as much as 12 hours and still provide significant protection against a global insult (Li and Buchan, 1993).

Antagonists that discriminate between AMPA and kainate receptors are rare. NS-102, SYM-2081, and phenobarbitone are reported to be selective for kainate receptors over AMPA receptors (Verdoorn et al., 1994), but further studies are required to verify this specificity. Among the competitive AMPA receptor antagonists are the quinoxalinediones, DNQX, CNQX, NBQX, PNQX, YM90K, and YM872. DNQX and CNQX exhibit little preference for AMPA receptors over kainate receptors whereas NBQX has demonstrated some selectivity for AMPA receptors over kainate receptors (Harris, 1995). AMOA, which has also demonstrated selectivity for AMPA receptors over kainate receptors, ameliorates damage due to transient forebrain ischemia (Frank et al., 1993). All quinoxalinediones, with the exception of YM872, are relatively insoluble in water. YM90K is in Phase I trials in Japan and PNQX is under development by Parke-Davis.

The insolubility of such compounds may result in similar nephrotoxicity associated with NBQX. Such toxicity would make it unlikely to successfully complete clinical trials. The highly soluble and neuroprotective YM872 (Small et al., 1998; Kawasaki-Yatsugi et al., 1998; Takahashi et al., 1998) is now in Phase II clinical trials and would seem more likely to succeed. A further complication of most quinoxalinediones is that they exhibit some activity at the NMDA receptor glycine site. In spite of these complications with competitive AMPA receptor antagonists, they have demonstrated the importance of AMPA receptors in animal models of cerebral ischemia. Therefore, development of more soluble and selective AMPA receptor antagonists is warranted. Given the problems associated with the use of competitive NMDA antagonists, namely competition with elevated glutamate concentrations in ischemic conditions, finding lower-affinity, use-dependent AMPA receptor antagonists could provide a safe, well-tolerated, neuroprotective therapy.

Noncompetitive Antagonists

Noncompetitive AMPA receptor antagonists primarily interact with the channel pore. The only other site at which channel activity has been reported to be antagonized is the GYKI site. GYKI 52466, borne out of efforts to develop 2,3-benzodiazepines as anxiolytics, acts like thiocyanate to antagonize AMPA receptor responses by accelerating desensitization rates (Kessler et al., 1996). Currently available AMPA receptor antagonists which interact with the channel pore are derived from spider and wasp toxins. One such toxin, JSTX, potently blocks only Ca^{2+}-permeable AMPA receptors (Blaschke et al., 1993). From site-directed mutagenesis studies, JSTX is thought to bind to the Q site in TM2. In spite of the tremendous neuroprotective potential of antagonists which selectively block Ca^{2+}-permeable AMPA receptors based on observations suggesting that there is a postischemic increase in the expression of the Ca^{2+}-permeable AMPA receptors (Pellegrini-Giampietro et al., 1992; Tsubokawa et al., 1995; Kawai et al., 1996), the toxic side effects of these compounds, ranging from nephrotoxicity to severe respiratory depression, have proven far too great to consider them as therapeutic agents. The development of compounds with similar selectivity, but less toxicity, perhaps a small, nonquinoxalinedionelike molecule, may result in an efficacious therapeutic intervention for cerebral ischemia.

CONCLUSION

Clinical success with glutamate receptor antagonists has been less than that predicted based on the explosion of experimental animal model studies initiated in the late 1980s. The results of these early experimental studies generated enthusiasm and hope for NMDA receptor antagonists and then subsequently for AMPA receptor antagonists. For the most part, many of the initial compounds demonstrating efficacy were severely hampered by toxicity problems upon further testing. It is the opinion of these authors that in the wake of the failure of several clinical trials, we should not abandon efforts with glutamate receptor antagonists, but rather we should redress these failures with a focus to identify the mechanism of toxicity and the mechanism of protection. Hopefully, these two drug mechanisms are separate and due to drug activity at different receptor subtypes. Given the heterologous behavior of glutamate receptors of different subtypes and subgroups, it is not unreasonable to anticipate identifying a unique pathological receptor subunit combination for which a drug may be selectively targeted. The continuing characterization of receptor structure-function relations combined with further analysis of postischemic receptors in resistant and vulnerable tissue promises to yield insight to whether more specific compounds will enjoy more success in clinical trials than their predecessors.

REFERENCES

Adams HP, Brott TG, Furlan AJ, Gomez CR, Grotta J, Helgason CM, Kwiatkowski T, Lyden PD, Marler JR, Torner J, Feinberg W, Mayberg M, Thies W (1996). Guidelines for thrombolytic therapy for acute stroke: a supplement to the guidelines for the management of patients with acute ischemic stroke: a statement for healthcare professionals from a special writing group of the stroke council, American Heart Association. Circulation 94:1167–1174.

Alberts M, Bertels C, Dawson D (1990). An analysis of time of presentation after stroke. JAMA 263:65–68.

Ascher P, Johnson JW (1994). The NMDA receptor, its channel, and its modulation by glycine. In Collingridge GL, Watkins JC, eds. The NMDA Receptor 2d ed. New York: Oxford University Press, pp. 177–205.

Bernard A, Khrestchatisky M (1994). Assessing the extent of RNA editing in the TMII regions of GluR5 and GluR6 kainate receptors during rat brain development. J Neurochem 62:2057–2060.

Black MA, Tremblay R, Mealing G, Ray R, Durkin JP, Whitfield JF, Blosser J, Morley P (1995). N-methyl-D-aspartate- or glutamate-mediated toxicity in cultured rat cortical neurons is antagonized by FPL 15896AR. J Neurochem 65:2170–2177.

Blaschke M, Keller BU, Rivossechi R, Hollmann M, Heinemann S, Konnerth A (1993). A single amino acid determines the subunit-specific spider toxin block of α-amino-3-hydroxy-5-methylisoxazole-4-propionate/kainate receptor channels. Proc Natl Acad Sci USA 90:6528–6532.

Boast CA (1988). Neuroprotection after brain ischemia: role of competitive N-methyl-D-aspartate antagonists. In: Liss AR, ed. Frontiers in Excitatory Amino Acid Research. New York: Alan R. Liss Inc., pp. 691–698.

Boast CA, Gerhardt SC, Pastor G, Lehmann J, Etienne PE, Liebman JM (1988). The N-methyl-D-aspartate antagonists CGS 19755 and CPP reduce ischemic brain damage in gerbils. Brain Res 442:345–348.

Boulter J, Hollmann M, O'Shea-Greenfield A, Hartley M, Deneris E, Maron C, Heinemann S (1990). Molecular cloning and functional expression of glutamate receptor subunit genes. Science 249:1033–1037.

Bowie D, Mayer ML (1995). Inward rectification of both AMPA and kainate subtype glutamate receptors generated by polyamine-mediated ion channel block. Neuron 15:453–462.

Buchan AM, Pulsinelli WA (1990). Hypothermia but not the N-methyl-D-aspartate antagonist, MK-801, attenuates neuronal damage in gerbils subjected to transient global ischemia. J Neurosci 10:311–316.

Burnashev N, Schoepfer R, Monyer H, Ruppersberg JP, Günther W, Seeburg P, Sakmann B (1992). Control by asparagine residues of calcium permeability and magnesium blockade in the NMDA receptor. Science 257:1415–1419.

Carter RB (1996). Anti-ischemic properties of ACEA 1021. CoCensys Symposium on Excitotoxicity and Apoptosis in Neurodegeneration and Cerebral Ischemia: Molecular Mechanisms and Therapeutic Implications. Nov. 15–16, Washington, D.C.

Conley EC (1996). The Ion Channel Facts Book: Extracellular Ligand-Gated Channels. London: Academic Press Limited.

Corbett D, Evans C, Thomas C, Wang D, Jonas RA (1990). MK-801 reduced cerebral ischemic injury by inducing hypothermia. Brain Res 514:300–304.

Curtis DR, Johnston GAR (1974). Amino acid transmitters in the mammalian CNS. Ergebnisse Physiol 69:97–188.

Frank I, Bruhn T, Diemer NH (1993). The effect of an AMPA antagonist (NBQX) on postischaemic neurone loss and protein synthesis in the rat brain. Exp Brain Res 95:70–76.

Gall C, Sumikawa K, Lynch G (1990). Regional distribution of mRNA for a putative kainate receptor in rat brain. Eur J Pharmacol 189:217–221.

Germano IM, Pitts LH, Meldrum BS, Bartkowski HM, Simon RP (1987). Kynurenate inhibition of cell excitation decreases stroke size. Ann Neurol 22:730–734.

Gill R, Hargreaves RJ, Kemp JA (1995). The neuroprotective effect of the glycine site antagonist 3R-(+)-cis-4-methyl-HA966 (L-687,414) in a rat model of focal ischaemia. J Cereb Blood Flow Metab 15:197–204.

Haley EC Jr (1997). Glycine antagonists in neuroprotection-I (GAIN-I). Stroke 28:232.

Harris EW (1995) Subtypes of glutamate receptors: pharmacological classification. In: Stone TW, ed. CNS Neurotransmitters and Neuromodulators: Glutamate. Boca Raton: CRC Press.

Hollmann M, Boulter J, Maron C, Beasley L, Sulivan J, Pecht G, Heinemann S (1993). Zinc potentiates agonist-induced currents at certain splice variants of the NMDA receptor. Neuron 10:943–954.

Jensen MI, Auer RN (1988). Ketamine fails to protect against ischaemic neuronal necrosis in the rat. Br J Anaesth 61:206–210.

Jones SM, Rogawski MA (1992). The anticonvulsant (±)-5-aminocarbonyl-10,11-dihydro-5H-dibenzo [a,d]cyclohepten-5,10-imine (ADCI) selectively blocks NMDA-activated current in cultured rat hippocampal neurons: kinetic analysis and comparison with dizocilpine. Mol Neuropharm 2:303–310.

Kawai N, Tsubokawa H, Oguro K, Masuzawa T (1996). Glutamate receptor subtype current in the postischemic hippocampal neurons. Int Acad Biomed Drug Res 11:89–96.

Kawasaki-Yatsugi S, Yatsugi S, Takahashi M, Toya T, Ichiki C, Shimizu-Sasamata M, Yamaguchi T, Minematsu K (1998). A novel AMPA receptor antagonist, YM872, reduces infarct size after middle cerebral artery occlusion in rats. Brain Res 793:39–46.

Keinänen K, Wisden W, Sommer B, Werner P, Herb A, Verdoorn TA, sakmann B, Seeburg PH (1990). A family of AMPA-selective glutamate receptors. Science 249:556–560.

Kessler M, Arai A, Quan A, Lynch G (1996). Effect of cyclothiazide on binding properties of AMPA-type glutamate receptors: lack of competition between cyclothiazide and GYKI 52466. Mol Pharmacol 49:123–131.

Kohler M, Burnashev N, Sakmann B, Seeburg PH (1993). Determinants of Ca^{2+} permeability in both TM1 and TM2 of high affinity kainate receptor channels: diversity by RNA editing. Neuron 10:491–500.

Kutsuwada T, Kashiwabuchi N, Mori H, Sakimura K, Kushiya E, Araki K, Meguro H, Masaki H, Kumanishi T, Arakawa M, Mishina M (1992). Molecular diversity of the NMDA receptor channel. Nature 358:36–41.

Li H, Buchan AM (1993). Treatment with an AMPA antagonist 12 hours following severe normothermic forebrain ischemia prevents CA1 neuronal injury. J Cereb Blood Flow Metab 13:933–939.

Lomeli H, Mosbacher J, Melcher T, Hoger T, Geiger JRP, Kuner T, Monyer H, Higuchi M, Bach A, Seeburg PH (1994). Control of kinetic properties of AMPA receptor channels by nuclear RNA editing. Science 266:1709–1712.

Mayer ML, Westbrook GL (1987). Permeation and block of N-methyl-D-aspartic acid receptor channels by divalent cations in mouse cultured central neurons. J Physiol 394:510–527.

McGurk JF, Bennett MVL, Zukin RS (1990). Polyamines potentiate responses of N-methyl-D-aspartate receptors expressed in *Xenopus* oocytes. Proc Natl Acad Sci USA 87:9971–9974.

Mealing GAR, Lanthorn TH, Small DL, Black MA, Laferriere NB, Morley P (1997). Antagonism of NMDA-evoked currents in rat cortical cultures by ARL 15896AR. J Pharmacol Exp Ther 281:376–383.

Menniti FS, Collins MA, Chenard BL, Shalaby IA, White WF (1995). CP-101,606, a potent and selective antagonist of forebrain NMDA receptors: in vitro neuroprotective activity. Soc Neurosci Abstr 21:37.1.

Monaghan DT, Larsen H (1997). NR1 and NR2 subunit contributions to N-methyl-D-aspartate receptor channel blocker pharmacology. J Pharmacol Exp Ther 280:614–620.

Monyer H, Brunashev N, Laurie DJ, Sakmann B, Seeburg PH (1994). Developmental and regional expression in the rat brain and functional properties of four NMDA receptors. Neuron 12:529–540.

Muir KW, Lees KR (1995). Clinical experience with excitatory amino acid antagonist drugs. Stroke 26:503–513.

Muir KW, Lees KR (1997). Intravenous Magnesium Efficacy in Stroke (IMAGES). Stroke 28:2105.

Obrenovitch TP, Richards DA (1995). Extracellular neurotransmitter changes in cerebral ischaemia. Cerebrovasc Brain Metab Rev 7:1–54.

O'Hara PJ, Sheppard PO, Thøgersen H, Venezia D, Haldemann BA, McGrane V, Houamed KM, Thomsen T, Gilbert CL, Mulvihill ER (1993). The ligand-binding domain in metabotropic glutamate receptors is related to bacterial periplasmic binding proteins. Neuron 11:41–52.

Pagnozzi MJ, Chambers LK, Menniti FS, Chenard BL, White WF (1995). CP-101,606, a potent and selective antagonist of forebrain NMDA receptors: in vivo activity. Soc Neurosci Abstr 21:439.9.

Parsons CG, Gruner J, Rozental J, Millar J, Lodge D (1993). Patch clamp studies on the kinetics and selectivity of N-methyl-D-aspartate receptor antagonism by memantine (1-amino-3,5-dimethyl-adamantan). Neuropharmacology 32:1337–1350.

Parsons CG, Quack G, Bresink I, Baran L, Przegalinski E, Kostowski W, Krzascik P, Hartmann S, Danysz W (1995). Comparison of the potency, kinetics and voltage-dependency of a series of uncompetitive NMDA receptor antagonists in vitro with anticonvulsant and motor impairment activity in vivo. Neuropharmacology 34:1239–1258.

Paschen W, Schmidt-Kastner R, Djuricic B, Messe C, Linn F, Hossmann KA (1987). Polyamine changes in reversible cerebral ischemia. J Neurochem 49:35–37.

Paschen W, Djuricic B (1995). Regional differences in the extent of RNA editing of the glutamate receptor subunits GluR2 and GluR6 in rat brain. J Neurosci Meth 56:21–29.

Paschen W, Schmitt J, Dux E, Djuricic B (1995). Temporal analysis of the upregulation of GluR5 mRNA editing with age: regional evaluation. Dev Brain Res 86:359–363.

Pellegrini-Giampietro DE, Zukin RS, Bennett MVL, Cho S, Pulsinelli WA (1992). Switch in glutamate receptor subunit gene expression in CA1 subfield of hippocampus following global ischemia in rats. Proc Natl Acad Sci USA 89:10499–10503.

Perez-Velazquez JL, Zhang L (1994). In vitro hypoxia induces expression of the NR2C subunit of the NMDA receptor in rat cortex and hippocampus. J Neurochem 63:1171–1173.

Pollard H, Khrestchatisky M, Moreau J, Ben-Ari Y (1993). Transient expression of the NR2C subunit of the NMDA receptor in developing brain. NeuroReport 4:411–414.

Pulsinelli WA, Buchan AM (1990). The NMDA receptor/ion channel: its importance to in vivo ischemic injury to selectively vulnerable neurons. In: Krieglstein J, Oberpichler H, eds. Pharmacology of Cerebral Ischemia. Stuttgart: Wissenschaftliche Verlagsgesellschaft, pp 169–175.

Rogawski MA (1993). Therapeutic potential of excitatory amino acid antagonists: channel blockers and 2,3-benzodiazepines. Trends Pharmacol Sci 14:325–331.

Rosenmund C, Stern-Bach Y, Stevens CF (1998). The tetrameric structure of a glutamate receptor channel. Science 280:1596–1599.

Sather W, Dieudonné S, MacDonald JF, Ascher P (1992). Activation and desensitization of N-methyl-D-aspartate receptors in nucleated outside-out patches from mouse neurons. J Physiol 450:643–672.

Scatton B, Avenet P, Benavides J, Besnard F, Carter C, Duverger D, Graham D, Langer AZ, Nowicki JP, Santamaria R, Schoemaker H (1995). Eliprodil, a neuroprotective agent which selectively blocks a subtype of NMDA receptor. In: Proceedings of the Symposium on Pre- and Post-Synaptic Modulation of the Glutamate Receptors: Molecular Pharmacology and Therapeutic Implications, Nov. 11, 1995; San Diego, CA.

Schneggenburger R, Zhou Z, Konnerth A, Neher E (1993). Fractional contribution of calcium to the cation current through glutamate receptor channels. Neuron 11:133–143.

Seeburg PH (1996). The role of RNA editing in controlling glutamate receptor channel properties. J Neurochem 66:1–5.

Seeburg PH, Burnashev N, Köhr G, Kuner T, Sprengel R, Monyer H (1995). The NMDA receptor channel: molecular design of a coincidence detector. Recent Prog Hormone Res 50:19–35.

Small DL, Murray CM, Monette R, Kawasaki-Yatsugi S, Morley P (1998). Neuroprotective effects of a novel AMPA receptor antagonist, YM872. NeuroReport 9:1287–1290.

Small DL, Poulter MO, Buchan AM, Morley P (1997). Alteration in NMDA receptor subunit mRNA expression in vulnerable and resistant regions of ischemia. Neurosci Lett 232:87–90.

Sommer B, Keinanen K, Verdoorn TA, Wisden W, Burnashev N, Herb A, Kohler M, Takagi T, Sakmann B, Seeburg PH (1990). Flip and flop: a cell specific functional switch in glutamate-operated channels of the CNS. Science 249:1580–1585.

Stand T, Wester PO (1993). A double blind randomized pilot trial of magnesium therapy in acute cerebral infarction. 7th Nordic Meeting on Cerebrovascular Diseases, 37. Copenhagen, July 15.

Standley S, Tocco G, Tourigny M-F, Massicotte G, Thompson RF, Baudry M (1995). Developmental changes in α-amino-3-hydroxy-5-methyl-4-isoxazole propionate receptor properties and expression in the rat hippocampal formation. Neuroscience 67:881–892.

Stern P, Béhé P, Schoepfer R, Colquhoun D (1992). Single channel conductances of NMDA receptor expressed from cloned cDNAs: comparison with native receptors. Proc R Soc (Lond) 250:271–277.

Subramaniam S, Donevan SD, Rogawski MA (1996). Block of the N-methyl-D-aspartate receptor by remacemide and its des-glycine metabolite. J Pharmacol Exp Ther 276:161–168.

Sucher NJ, Awobuluyi M, Choi Y-B, Lipton SA (1996). NMDA receptors: from genes to channels. Trends Pharmacol Sci 17:348–355.

Takahashi M, Ni JW, Kawasaki-Yatsugi S, Toya T, Yatsugi SI, Shimizu-Sasamata M, Koshiya K, Shishikura JI, Sakamoto S, Yamaguchi T (1998). YM872, a novel selective alpha-amino-3-hydroxy-5-methylisoxazole-4-propionic acid receptor antagonist, reduces brain damage after permanent focal cerebral ischemia in cats. J Pharmacol Exp Ther 284:467–473.

Takizawa S, Hogan M, Hakim AM (1991). The effects of a competitive NMDA receptor antagonist (CGS-19755) on cerebral blood flow and pH in focal ischemia. J Cereb Blood Flow Metab 11:786–793.

Toulmond S, Serrano A, Benavides J, Scatton B (1993). Prevention by eliprodil (SL 82.0715) of traumatic brain damage in the rat. Existence of a large (18 h) therapeutic window. Brain Res 620:32–41.

Tsubokawa H, Oguro K, Masuzawa T, Nakaima T, Kawai N (1995). Effects of a spider toxin and its analog on glutamate-activated currents in the hippocampal CA1 neurons after ischemia. J Neurophysiol 74:218–225.

Verdoorn TA, Johansen TH, Drejer J, Nielsen EO (1994). Selective block of recombinant GluR6 receptors by NS-102, a novel non-NMDA receptor antagonist. Eur J Pharmacol 269:43–49.

Warner DS, Martin H, Ludwig P, McAllister A, Keana JF, Weber E (1995). In vivo models of cerebral ischemia: effects of parenterally administered NMDA receptor glycine site antagonists. J Cereb Blood Flow Metab 15:188–196.

White WF, Ducat MF, Chenard BL, Butler TW, Ronau RT (1995). CP-101,606, a potent and selective antagonist of forebrain NMDA receptors: binding to a novel recognition site. Soc Neurosci Abstr 21:439.7.

Whittemore ER, Ilyin VI, Woodward RM (1996). Subtype-selective antagonism of NMDA receptors by nylidrin. Soc Neurosci Abstr 22:507.6.

Williams K (1993). Ifenprodil discriminates subtypes of the N-methyl-D-aspartate receptor: selectivity and mechanisms at recombinant heteromeric receptors. Mol Pharmacol 44:851–859.

Williams K, Zappia AM, Pritchett DB, Shen YM, Molinoff PB (1994). Sensitivity of the N-methyl-D-aspartate receptor to polyamines is controlled by NR2 subunits. Mol Pharmacol 45:803–809.

Xue D, Huang ZG, Barnes K, Lesiuk HJ, Smith KE, Buchan AM (1994). Delayed treatment with AMPA, but not NMDA antagonists reduces neocortical infarction. J Cereb Blood Flow Metab 14:251–261.

Yang J-H, Sklar P, Axel R, Maniatis T (1995). Editing of glutamate receptor subunit B pre-mRNA in vitro by site specific deamination of adenosine. Nature 374:77–81.

Zhang L, Miu P, Eubanks JH (1995). NMDA channel activities in rat CA1 hippocampal neurons following a brief hypoxic-hypoglycaemic challenge in brain slices. Soc Neurosci Abstr 21:392.1.

18

Drugs Enhancing or Slowing Recovery of Function

Larry B. Goldstein
Duke University Medical Center and Durham VA Medical Center, Durham, North Carolina

INTRODUCTION

Regardless of the initial severity of the neurological deficit, most stroke survivors exhibit some degree of recovery over time.[1–6] Along with the prevention of complications and secondary and tertiary prevention, optimization of the rate and degree of this "spontaneous" recovery is one of the primary goals of poststroke treatment. Whether intended to augment normal compensatory strategies for particular impairments[7] or to specifically improve lost functions,[8–11] the various techniques of physical, occupational, and speech therapy currently form the cornerstone for these interventions (see Chap. 12).

Based on the rapidly expanding knowledge of the fundamental neurobiology underlying normal recovery, a variety of innovative approaches for the management of stroke patients are currently being explored. For example "forced use",[12,13] sensory stimulation,[14] and suspended gait training in nonambulatory patients[15] represent some of these novel strategies. Offering the possibility of pharmacotherapy, laboratory studies have shown that drugs that influence the activity of specific central neurotransmitters can modulate the recovery process (Table 1). Although drug therapy to enhance recovery remains experimental, a knowledge of this emerging pharmacology is important for physicians caring for patients in the poststroke period, as several of the medications currently used to treat coincident medical problems may interfere with recovery.

IMPLICATIONS OF LABORATORY STUDIES

For the purposes of the present discussion, several general principles that arise from laboratory studies of the impact of drugs on recovery need to be reviewed (Table 1; see references 16, 17, and 18 for detailed reviews).

One important principle is that these drug effects are dose-dependent. For example, amphetamine is one of the most extensively studied drugs with the capacity to enhance recovery after focal brain injury. The dose-effect curve for amphetamine-promoted motor recovery in the rat forms an inverted "U" with the drug being ineffective at low and high doses.[19]

A second important principle is that the timing of drug administration may be critical. Some drugs may have opposite effects on an animal's ultimate behavioral deficit depending on when it is given in relationship to the injury.[19–21] For example, immediate postischemic administration of a benzodiazepine is neuroprotective after transient global ischemia models in the gerbil[22] and rat.[23,24] Other drugs, presumably acting through a GABA-ergic mechanism such as barbiturates,[25,26] phenytoin,[27] and muscimol[28–30] also have neuroprotective properties. In contrast, experimental studies show that benzodiazepines, barbiturates, phenytoin, and muscimol are harmful when given during the recovery period. Similarly, the anticholinergic scopolamine may be protective if given soon after a focal cortical lesion,[31–33] but harmful if given later.[34] Furthermore, the period of effectiveness of some drugs may be limited. Amphetamine results in the reinstatement of binocular depth perception in visually decorticated cats when the drug is given beginning 10 days after injury, but there is no behavioral improvement if administration is delayed for 3 months.[35] Thus, drugs may have their intended effects on recovery only if given during a specific "treatment window."

A third general principle is that the effects of certain drugs are dependent on the behavioral experience of the animal. Amphetamine's effect on motor recovery is blocked if rats are restrained rather than given motor practice after drug administration.[36] A smaller independent positive effect of the drug is found in rats that are allowed to freely ambulate but that are not given specific training.[37] The recovery of stereoscopic vision in visually decorticated cats also depends on visual experience after the drug is given.[35,38] The effects of drugs on recovery may also vary with the behavioral requirements of the task.[39]

CLINICAL STUDIES

Possible Detrimental Drug Effects in Humans

As can be appreciated by reviewing Table 2, several classes of drugs that laboratory studies suggest may affect recovery are used in the treatment of stroke patients. These drugs include certain antihypertensive agents, certain anti-

Table 1 Selected Laboratory Studies of Drug Effects on Recovery After Focal Brain Injury

Transmitter/drug/class	Action	Effect on recovery
Norepinephrine		+
Amphetamine	Sympathomimetic	+
Phentermine	Sympathomimetic	+
Phenylpropanolamine	Sympathomimetic	+
Methylphenidate	Sympathomimetic	+
Yahimbine	α_2-AR antagonist	+
Idazoxan	α_2-AR antagonist	+
Clonidine	α_2-AR agonist	–
Haloperidol	α_1-AR antagonist	–
Prazosin	α_1-AR antagonist	–
Propranolol	β-AR antagonist	Neutral
GABA		–
Diazepam	GABA Agonist	–
Muscimol	GABA Agonist	–
Anticonvulsants		
Phenytoin		–
Phenobarbital		–
MK-801		–/Neutral
Carbamazepine		Neutral
Antidepressants		
Trazodone	5HT reuptake blocker	–
Fluoxetine	5HT reuptake blocker	Neutral
Despiramine	NE reuptake blocker	+
Amitriptyline	Mixed 5HT & NE reuptake blocker	–/Neutral
Dopamine		
Haloperidol	Butyrophenone	–
Fluanisone	Butyrophenone	–
Droperidol	Butyrophenone	–
Spiroperidol	Antagonist	–
Apomorphine	Agonist	+

A "–" indicates a detrimental effect, a "+" indicates a beneficial effect; NE, norepinephrine; 5HT, serotonin; AR, adrenergic receptor.

convulsants, anxiolytics, and major tranquilizers. We carried out a retrospective study of physician prescribing patterns to determine how frequently these and other medicines were being prescribed for patients recovering from stroke (Fig. 1).[40] Over 80% of individuals were taking at least one drug at the time of the stroke. Sixty-five percent of patients were receiving multiple drugs. Anti-

Table 2 Principles from Laboratory Studies

1. The effects of drugs on recovery are dose-dependent.
2. There may be a "treatment window."
3. Drug therapy may need to be combined with training.
4. The effects of drugs on recovery may vary with the behavioral requirements of the task.

hypertensives such as clonidine and prazosin and sedative hypnotics including benzodiazepines were among the most commonly prescribed agents. The number of stroke patients prescribed sedative-hypnotic agents more than doubled over the first 2 days of hospitalization (17% to 44%), including a doubling of the number receiving benzodiazepines (10% to 20%). Thus, several of the drugs that have deleterious effects on recovery of function in laboratory animals were commonly prescribed for stroke patients for the treatment of coincident medical conditions. Subsequent studies carried out in different populations of stroke patients have had similar results.[41,42]

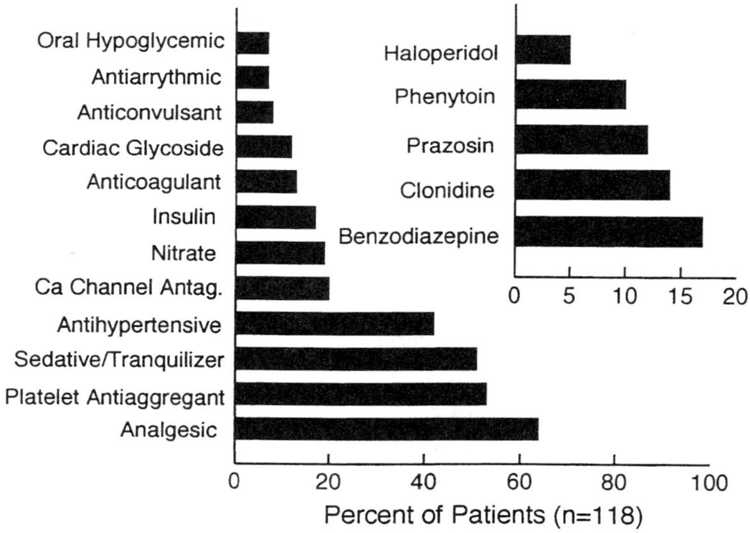

Figure 1 Drugs prescribed following stroke. The drugs prescribed for patients admitted to the hospital within 48 hours of a carotid distribution ischemic stroke were recorded[40]. The percentage of patients prescribed the indicated drugs are shown. This study indicates that several of the drugs that have deleterious effects on recovery of function in laboratory animals are commonly prescribed for stroke patients for the treatment of coincident medical conditions (inset). Revised from Goldstein.[67]

Determining whether the detrimental effects of drugs anticipated from laboratory studies also occur in humans recovering from stroke is difficult. Largely anecdotal reports indicate that treatment with haloperidol[16,43] and certain antihypertensives[44] may interfere with language recovery in aphasic stroke. We performed a retrospective study that tested the hypothesis that selected drugs that are harmful in recovering laboratory animals would also interfere with motor recovery in human stroke patients.[41] These potentially deleterious drugs included the antihypertensives clonidine and prazosin, neuroleptics, benzodiazepines, and phenytoin. The motor recoveries of stroke patients who received one or a combination of these drugs were compared to the recoveries of a similar group of patients who were not given any of these agents (Fig. 2). The two groups were similar in with respect to a variety of characteristics including age, blood pressure, gender, and medical comorbidity. Motor function was measured prospec-

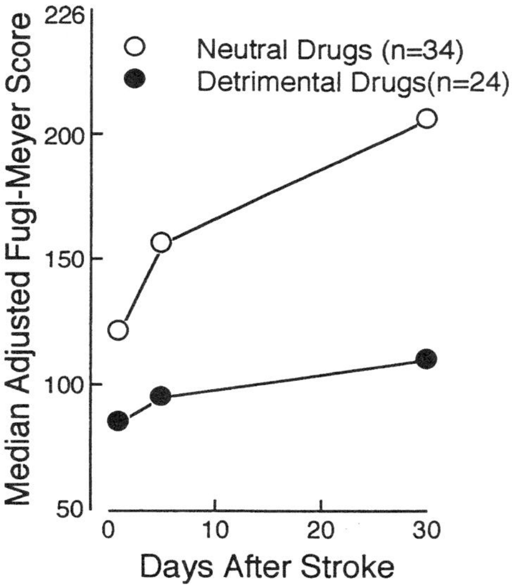

Figure 2 Effect of “detrimental drugs” on short-term motor recovery. Motor function was measured prospectively with the Fugl-Meyer Assessment[47] in a cohort of patients with ischemic stroke.[41] The medications taken by these patients at the time of stroke or during the subsequent hospitalization were determine by review of their medical records. The patients were then divided into two groups. One group (“detrimental” drug group) had received one or a combination of the drugs hypothesized to be harmful based on laboratory animal experiments. The remaining patients, all of whom had received at least one drug, were included in the “neutral” drug group. Patients in the “detrimental” drug group had greater initial deficits and recovered motor function slower than patients in the “neutral” drug group. (From Ref. 18.)

tively with the Fugl-Meyer Assessment by observers who were blind to the study hypothesis. As a group, those who received one or a combination of the hypothesized "detrimental" drugs had significantly slower motor recoveries than a comparable group of patients who did not receive one of these drugs. A multivariate analysis indicated a significant effect of "drug group" after correcting for the contributions of other variables including the initial severity of the deficit.

Supporting the findings of the previous study, the deleterious effect of certain drugs on recovery was also found in a separate cohort of patients with anterior circulation ischemic stroke.[42] These patients were control subjects in a prospective acute stroke interventional trial.[45] Nearly 40% of the control patients enrolled in this study received one or a combination of the antihypertensives clonidine and prazosin, neuroleptics, benzodiazepines, phenytoin, or phenobarbital. The most commonly prescribed of the potentially detrimental medications were benzodiazepines, and the most commonly given of these was triazolam. Although the reason a medication was given was not recorded, triazolam was likely prescribed for its soporific effect. Although the groups of patients who did or did not receive one of the "detrimental" drugs were not prospectively randomized, they were quite similar with respect to the presence of a variety of comorbid conditions and patient characteristics that could impact on the recovery process. As with the previous study, stepwise regression models indicate that drug group had a detrimental effect on motor recovery independent of the degree of the initial motor impairment, comorbid conditions, and other patient characteristics. This harmful effect was also found when independence in activities of daily living was measured serially with the Barthel Index (Fig. 3).

Because both of these studies involved retrospective analyses, it cannot be certain that the reason for the administration of a given drug rather than the drug itself influenced recovery. Another limitation is that these studies did not permit an analysis of the impact of specific "detrimental" drugs, nor did they permit analyses of dose or timing effects.

Pharmacological Enhancement of Recovery

Based on laboratory studies, variables such as drug dose, treatment window, and the use of concomitant training would be expected to be critical factors in studies of the effects of drugs on recovery in human stroke patients. Most of these variables have not been rigorously studied through clinical trials; however, several small trials have been completed.

Motor Impairments

Amphetamine. Motivation in elderly patients refractory to rehabilitation procedures improves with amphetamine treatment.[46] The first study of am-

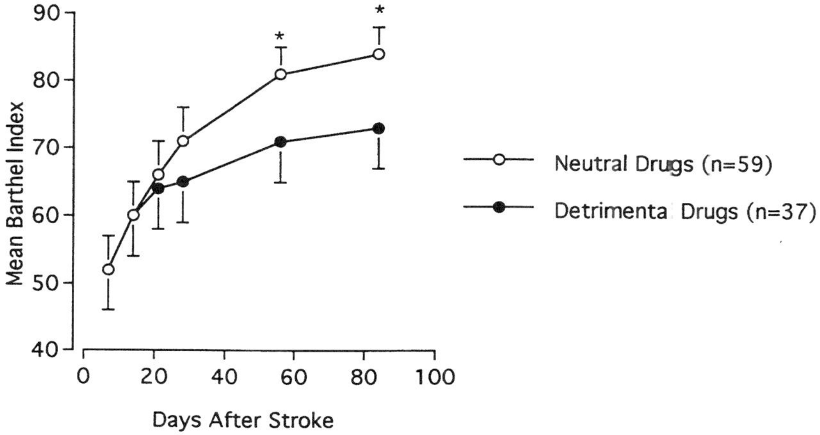

Figure 3 Effect of "detrimental drugs" on recovery of activities of daily living. The drugs prescribed to placebo control stroke patients enrolled in a prospective randomized clinical trial[45] were recorded prospectively. The patients were then divided into two groups. One group ("detrimental" drug group) had received one or a combination of the drugs hypothesized to be harmful based on laboratory animal experiments. The remaining patients, all of whom had received at least one drug, were included in the "neutral" drug group. The graph gives the mean Barthel Index for patients in each group. Patients in the "detrimental" drug group had similar initial deficits but had poorer recoveries than patients in the "neutral" drug group. (From Ref. 42.)

phetamine's effects on recovery after stroke was carefully designed to simulate the paradigm used in the laboratory experimental studies (Fig. 4) Eight patients with stable motor deficits were randomized to receive either a single dose of amphetamine or placebo within 10 days of carotid distribution ischemic stroke. Motor function was measured with a reliable and validated scale, the Fugl-Meyer Assessment.[47] Within 3 hours of drug administration, all of the patients underwent intensive physical therapy (e.g., drug administration was coupled with task-specific experience). The following day, the patients' abilities to use their affected limbs were reassessed. Overall, the amphetamine-treated group had a significant improvement in motor performance while there was little change in the placebo-treated group. This study was important in that it suggested that the drug effect observed in the laboratory might occur in humans, but had significant limitations. The study involved only a small group of highly selected patients and the results might not be generalizable. Only two of the four patients receiving amphetamine had a "dramatic" motor improvement (the intervention had a variable effect even in this highly selected group). Because only very short-term motor recovery was

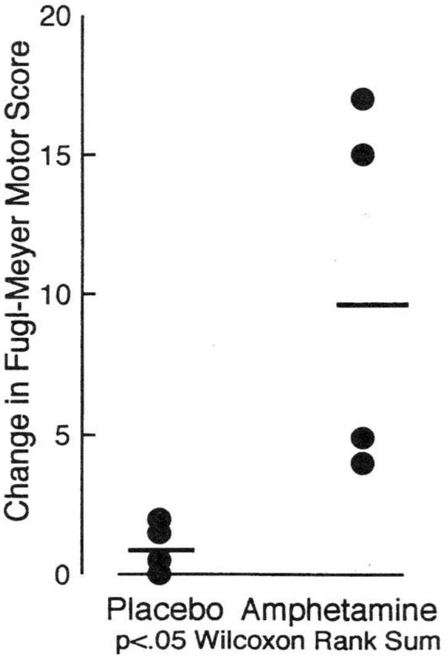

Figure 4 Effect of amphetamine on short-term motor recovery after stroke. In a double-blind trial, eight patients with stable motor deficits were randomized to receive a single dose of 10 mg d-amphetamine or placebo followed by physical therapy within 10 days of ischemic stroke.[68] The differences in Fugl-Meyer scores between baseline and 24 hours after treatment for the amphetamine-treated stroke patients and controls are shown. (From Ref. 18.)

measured, the longer-term efficacy of amphetamine administration remained uncertain, and there were no data from the study with regard to the longer-term efficacy of amphetamine administration. Due to concern about the potential harmful effects of sympathomimetic agents in patients immediately following stroke, studies reproducing and extending this finding have been lacking. Until recently, this study provided some of the only controlled data of a beneficial effect of amphetamine treatment on motor recovery in humans.

A second double-blind, placebo-controlled trial, reported in abstract form, was negative.[48] In this study, 12 patients were given 10 mg amphetamine daily for 14 days followed by 5 mg for 3 days. Twelve patients receiving placebo. Interventions began more than 1 month after the stroke, and the administration of the drug/placebo was not tightly linked with physical therapy sessions. Thus, this study varied in several significant ways from the previous trial. These differences include a different dosing regimen, a longer delay between stroke and treatment, and a lack of a tightly coupled drug–physical therapy regimen.

A third double-blind, placebo-controlled trial of the effects of amphetamine on motor recovery in rehabilitation patients was subsequently performed (Fig.

5).[49] This study included five amphetamine-treated and five placebo-treated patients. Drug or placebo was given once every 4 days for 10 sessions beginning 15 to 30 days after stroke. Each dose was given in tight conjunction with a session of intensive physical therapy. Motor function was again measured with the Fugl-Meyer Assessment, with the final evaluation being performed 1 week after the last dose. Patients treated with amphetamine had significantly greater improvements in motor scores than placebo-treated patients. Although preliminary, these results suggest that amphetamine administration combined with physical therapy may enhance motor recovery in humans stroke patients, that the effect is still present at least 1 year after drug treatment is halted, and that the effect is present even when the intervention is delayed for up to 1 month after stroke. In combination with the principles learned from the laboratory, these three clinical studies suggest that drug dose, timing, and the tight coupling of drug was physical therapy may be critical determinants of whether the treatment is efficacious.

Methylphenidate. Nonspecific stimulant medications including methylphenidate have been used in cognitively impaired brain-injured patients for many years. The drug has also been used in the treatment of poststroke depres-

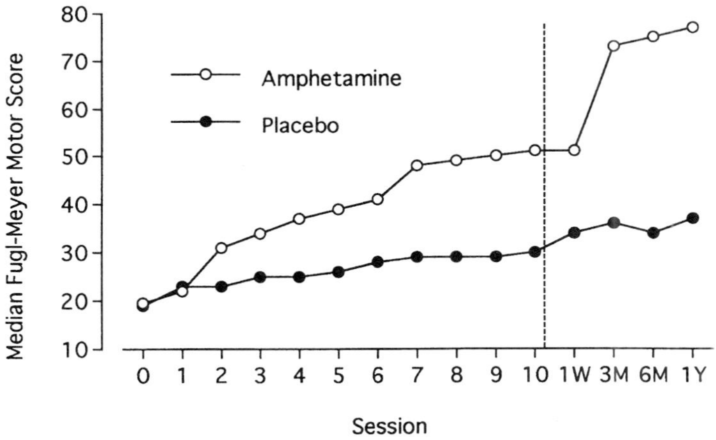

Figure 5 Effect of amphetamine on motor recovery in stroke rehabilitation patients. Beginning 16 to 30 day after stroke, 10 hemiplegic patients were randomly assigned to receive either 10 mg d-amphetamine or placebo combined with physical therapy every fourth day for 10 sessions. Motor function was measured prospectively with the Fugl-Meyer Assessment.[47] Off-drug follow-up assessments (to the right of the vertical dotted line) were performed after 1 week (1W), 3 months (3M), 6 months (6M) and 1 year (1Y). Patients who received d-amphetamine coupled with physical therapy had significantly improved motor function compared to placebo treated patients even as long as 1 year later. (From Ref. 49.)

sion in patients undergoing rehabilitative therapy.[50–52] Only limited data are available concerning the drug's impact on neurological impairments.[53] This study did not find any effect of the drug on physical performance despite significant effects on cardiovascular function. However, variables shown to be important from laboratory studies and suggested from the clinical amphetamine trials previously reviewed (e.g., timing in relationship to brain injury, tight conjunction of drug administration, and physical therapy) were not considered in the design of this early study.

Tricyclic Antidepressants. Clinical depression is associated with impaired recovery after stroke in humans.[54] Tricyclic antidepressants are commonly used to treat mood disorders in stroke patients. Trazodone, a drug that impairs recovery from hemiplegia in the rat (see Table 1), was found to improve outcome as measured with the Barthel index in depressed stroke patients.[55] However, trazodone was given in only a single dose in the animal study, and repeated dosing likely has a different effect on neurotransmitter levels. Other clinical studies have found a beneficial effect of the serotonin reuptake blocker fluoxetine[56] and no significant effect of the norepinephrine reuptake blockers maprotiline[56] and nortriptyline.[57]

Other Catecholaminergic Drugs. Phenoxybenzamine caused slight transient worsening of the neurologic deficit in several stroke patients, but this might have been due to the hemodynamic effects rather than a specific effect on the recovery process.[58]

Aphasia

Amphetamine. Speech pathologists have begun to study the effects of amphetamine on language recovery after stroke.[59,60] In one study,[60] six aphasic patients had language function rated with the Porch Index of Communicative Ability[61] 10 to 30 days after stroke. Based on this initial evaluation, 6-month language scores were predicted for each patient. All patients were then given 10 mg d-amphetamine followed by speech therapy every fourth day for 10 sessions. The patients' actual scores after 3 months were then compared with their 6-month predicted scores. Most patients achieved or exceeded their 6-month predicted scores by the time of the 3-month evaluation. Although promising, this study needs to be interpreted cautiously as it was a feasibility trial that lacked control subjects.

Bromocriptine. Preliminary uncontrolled studies suggested that the administration of bromocriptine, a dopamine agonist, improved fluency in certain aphasics.[62–64] However, two small controlled studies were negative.[65,66] These disappointing results may have been due to a variety of factors. Both controlled trials included patients long after stroke, and one included several patients with traumatic brain injury. Both studies titrated patients to a maximally tolerated dose (e.g., because of inverted U-shaped dose response curve, a lower dose may have been efficacious). It is unclear whether drug administration was tightly coupled with active speech therapy.

Other Drugs. One retrospective study found that both thiazide diuretics and a mixed group of antihypertensives were associated with impaired language recovery in aphasic stroke patients.[44] Propranolol, a drug that had no effect on motor recovery in experimental studies, also had no effect on language recovery in these patients.

RECOMMENDATIONS

It is clear that certain drugs influence behavioral recovery in laboratory animals with focal brain injury. These drug effects can be either beneficial or harmful to the recovery process. Importantly, similar drug effects may occur in humans. In choosing drugs to treat coincident medical problems in stroke patients, although overriding concerns often dictate that a specific drug be used, this emerging pharmacology should be kept in mind. Given the available data, the use of a β-adrenergic receptor antagonist is preferable to either an α_1-adrenergic receptor antagonist or an α_2-adrenergic receptor agonist in the treatment of hypertension following stroke. Thiazide diuretics should be used cautiously. Haloperidol and other neuroleptics are potentially harmful, and until the pharmacology of the effects of major tranquilizers are better understood, they should be withheld whenever possible in patients recovering from stroke. Recommendations concerning the choice of specific tricyclic antidepressants in stroke patients must await further laboratory and clinical studies. However, the preliminary data currently available suggest that if the choice of antidepressants is not dictated by other concerns, a serotonin reuptake blocker such as fluoxetine may be preferable. Benzodiazpines, especially when used only as sleep aides, should generally be avoided. Of the anticonvulsants experimentally tested during the recovery period, the only drug not found to be harmful is carbamazepine. This drug should be considered when nonemergent treatment of seizure disorders are necessary in stroke patients. The use of specific drugs to enhance recovery should still be viewed as experimental. However, pharmacotherapy capable of improving recovery after stroke may be possible in the future.

REFERENCES

1. Duncan PW, Goldstein LB, Matchar D, Divine GW, Feussner J. Measurement of motor recovery after stroke. Outcome assessment and sample size requirements. Stroke 1992; 23:1084–1089.
2. Newman M. The process of recovery after stroke. Stroke 1972; 3:702–710.
3. Wade DT, Langton HR, Wood VA, Skilbeck CE, Ilsmail HM. The hemiplegic arm after stroke: measurement and recovery. J Neurol Neurosurg Psychiatry 1983; 46:521–524.
4. Loewen SC, Anderson BA. Predictors of stroke outcome using objective measurement scales. Stroke 1990; 21:78–81.
5. Wade DT, Wood VA, Hewer RL. Recovery after stroke—the first three months. J Neurol Neurosurg Psychiatry 1985; 48:7–13.
6. Kinsella G, Ford B. Acute recovery patterns in stroke patients. Med J Aust 1980; 2:662–666.
7. Wescott EJ. Traditional exercise regimens for the hemiplegic patient. Am J Phys Med 1967; 46:1012–1023.
8. Bobath B. Adult Hemiplegia: Evaluation and Treatment. London: William Heinemann Medical Books, 1984.
9. Brunnstrom S. Movement Therapy in Hemiplegia. A Neurophysiological Approach. New York: Harper & Row Publishers, 1970.
10. Wolf SL, Binder-Macleod SA. Electromyographic biofeedback applications to the hemiplegic patient. Phys Ther 1983; 63:1393–1403.
11. Basmajian JV, Gowland CA, Finlayson AJ, et al. Stroke treatment: comparison of integrated behavioral–physical therapy vs traditional physical therapy programs. Arch Phys Med Rehabil 1987; 68:267–272.
12. Wolf SL, Lecraw DE, Barton LA, Jann BB. Forced use of hemiplegic upper extremities to reverse the effect of learned nonuse among chronic stroke and head-injured patients. Exp Neurol 1989; 104:125–132.
13. Tabu E, Crago JE, Burgio LD, et al. An operant approach to rehabilitation medicine: overcoming learned nonuse by shaping. J Exp Anal Behav 1994; 61:281–293.
14. Johansson K, Lindgren I, Widner H, Wiklund I, Johansson BB. Can sensory stimulation improve the functional outcome in stroke patients? Neurology 1993; 43:2189–2192.
15. Hesse S, Bertelt C, Jahnke MT, et al. Treadmill training with partial body weight support compared with physiotherapy in nonambulatory hemiparetic patients. Stroke 1995; 26:976–981.
16. Feeney DM, Sutton RL. Pharmacotherapy for recovery of function after brain injury. CRC Crit Rev Neurobiol 1987; 3:135–197.
17. Feeney DM, Sutton RL. Catecholamines and recovery of function after brain damage. In: Stein DG, Sabel BA, eds. Pharmacological Approaches to the Treatment of Brain and Spinal Cord Injury. New York: Plenum Publishing Corporation, 1988: 121–142.
18. Goldstein LB. Basic and clinical studies of pharmacologic effects on recovery from brain injury. J Neural Transplant Plast 1993; 4:175–192.

19. Goldstein LB. Pharmacology of recovery after stroke. Stroke 1990; 21(suppl III):139–142.
20. Goldstein LB. Pharmacologic modulation of recovery after stroke: clinical data. J Neuro Rehab 1991; 5:129–140.
21. Goldstein LB. Drugs and stroke recovery. Neurology 1996; 46:1187–1188.
22. Schwartz RD, Huff RA, Yu X, Carter ML, Bishop M. Postischemic diazepam is neuroprotective in the gerbil hippocampus. Brain Res 1994; 647:153–160.
23. Johansen FF, Diemer NH. Enhancement of GABA neurotransmission after cerebral ischemia in the rat reduces loss of hippocampal CA1 pyramidal cells. Acta Neurol Scand 1991; 84:1–6.
24. Schwartz RD, Yu X, Katzman MR, Hayden-Hixson DM, Perry JM. Diazepam, given postischemia, protects selectively vulnerable neurons in the rat hippocampus and striatum. J Neurosci 1995; 15:529–539.
25. Sternau LL, Lust WD, Ricci AJ, Ratcheson R. Role for g-aminobutyric acid in selective vulnerability in gerbils. Stroke 1989; 20:281–287.
26. Smith AL, Hoff JT, Nielsen LS, Larson CP. Barbiturate protection in acute focal cerebral ischemia. Stroke 1974; 5:1–7.
27. Boxer PA, Cordon JJ, Mann ME, et al. Comparison of phenytoin with noncompetitive N-methyl-D-aspartate antagonists in a model of focal brain ischemia in the rat. Stroke 1990; 21(suppl III):47–51.
28. Lyden PD, Lonzo L. Combination therapy protects ischemic brain in rats. A glutamate antagonist plus a g-aminobutyric acid agonist. Stroke 1994; 25:189–196.
29. Lyden PD, Hedges B. Protective effect of synaptic inhibition during cerebral ischemia in rats and rabbits. Stroke 1992; 23:1463–1470.
30. Lyden P, Lonzo L, Nunez S. Combination chemotherapy extends the therapeutic window to 60 minutes after stroke. J Neurotrauma 1995; 12:223–230.
31. Hayes RL, Lyeth BG, Dixon CE, Stonnington HH, Becker DP. Cholinergic antagonist reduces neurologic deficits following cerebral concussion in the rat. J Cereb Blood Flow Metab 1985; 5(suppl 1):S395–S396.
32. Lyeth BG, Ray M, Hamm RJ, et al. Postinjury scopolamine administration in experimental traumatic brain injury. Brain Res 1992; 569:281–286.
33. Saponjic RM, Hoane MR, Barbay S, Barth TM. Scopolamine facilitates recovery of function following unilateral electrolytic sensorimotor cortex lesions in the rat. Restor Neurol Neurosci 1995; 8:205–212.
34. De Ryck M, Duytschaever H, Janssen PAJ. Ionic channels, cholinergic mechanisms, and recovery of sensorimotor function after neocortical infarcts in rats. Stroke 1990; 21(suppl III):158–163.
35. Feeney DM, Hovda DA. Reinstatement of binocular depth perception by amphetamine and visual experience after visual cortex ablation. Brain Res 1985; 342:352–356.
36. Feeney DM, Gonzalez A, Law WA. Amphetamine, haloperidol, and experience interact to affect the rate of recovery after motor cortex injury. Science 1982; 217:855–857.
37. Goldstein LB, Davis JN. Post-lesion practice and amphetamine-facilitated recovery of beam-walking in the rat. Restor Neurol Neurosci 1990; 1:311–314.

38. Hovda DA, Sutton RL, Feeney DM. Amphetamine-induced recovery of visual cliff performance after bilateral visual cortex ablation in cats: measurements of depth perception thresholds. Behav Neurosci 1989; 103:574–584.
39. Schmanke TD, Avery RA, Barth TM. The effects of amphetamine on recovery of function after cortical damage in the rat depend on the behavioral requirements of the task. J Neurotrauma 1996; 13:293–307.
40. Goldstein LB, Davis JN. Physician prescribing patterns after ischemic stroke. Neurology 1988; 38:1806–1809.
41. Goldstein LB, Matchar DB, Morgenlander JC, Davis JN. The influence of drugs on the recovery of sensorimotor function after stroke. J Neuro Rehab 1990; 4:137–144.
42. Goldstein LB. Sygenin Acute Stroke Study Investigators. Common drugs may influence motor recovery after stroke. Neurology 1995; 45:865–871.
43. Porch B, Wyckes J, Feeney DM. Haloperidol, thiazides, and some antihypertensives slow recovery from aphasia. Soc Neurosci Abstr 1985; 11:52.
44. Proch BE, Feeney DM. Effects of antihypertensive drugs on recovery from aphasia. Clin Aphasiol 1986; 16:309–314.
45. SASS Investigators. Ganglioside GM1 in acute ischemic stroke: the SASS trial. Stroke 1994; 25:1141–1148.
46. Clark ANG, Mankikar GD. d-Amphetamine in elderly patients refractory to rehabilitation procedures. J Am Geriatr Soc 1979; 27:174–177.
47. Fugl-Meyer AR, Jaasko L, Leyman I, Olsson S, Steglind S. The post-stroke hemiplegic patient. I. A method for evaluation of physician performance. Scand J Rehab Med 1975; 7:13–31.
48. Reding MJ, Solomon B, Borucki SJ. Effect of dextroamphetamine on motor recovery after stroke. Neurology 1995; 45(suppl 4):A222.
49. Walker-Batson D, Smith P, Curtis S, Unwin H, Greenlee R. Amphetamine paired with physical therapy accelerates motor recovery after stroke—further evidence. Stroke 1995; 26:2254–2259.
50. Johnson ML, Roberts MD, Ross AR, Witten CM. Methylphenidate in stroke patients with depression. Am J Phys Med Rehabil 1992; 71:239–241.
51. Lazarus LW, Moberg PJ, Langlsey PR, Lingam VR. Methylpenidate and nortriptyline in the treatment of poststroke depression: a retrospective comparison. Arch Phys Med Rehabil 1994; 75:403–406.
52. Lazarus LW, Winemiller DR, Lingam VR, et al. Efficacy and side effects of methylphenidate for poststroke depression. J Clin Psychiatry 1992; 53:447–449.
53. Larsson M, Ervik M, Lundborg P, Sundh V, Svanborg A. Comparison between methylphenidate and placebo as adjuvant in care and rehabilitation of geriatric patients. Comp Gerontol 1988; 2:53–59.
54. Morris PLP, Raphael B, Robinson RG. Clinical depression is associated with impaired recovery from stroke. Med J Aust 1992; 157:239–242.
55. Reding MJ, Orto LA, Winter SW, Fortuna IM, Di Ponte P, McDowell FH. Antidepressant therapy after stroke. A double-blind trial. Arch Neurol 1986; 43:763–765.
56. Dam M, Tonin P, De Boni A, et al. Effects of fluoxetine and maprotiline on functional recovery in poststroke hemiplegic patients undergoing rehabilitation therapy. Stroke 1996; 27:1211–1214.

57. Lipsey JR, Pearlson GD, Robinson RG, Rao K, Price TR. Nortriptyline treatment of post-stroke depression: a double-blind study. Lancet 1984; 1:297–300.
58. Meyer JS, Miyakawa Y, Welch KMA, et al. Influence of adrenergic receptor blockade on circulatory and metaboloic effects of disordered neurotransmitter function in stroke patients. Stroke 1976; 7:158–167.
59. Homan R, Panksepp J, Mcsweeny J, et al. d-Amphetamine effects on language and motor behaviors in a chronic stroke patient. Soc Neurosci Abstr 1990; 16:439.
60. Walker-Batson D, Unwin H, Curtis S, et al. Use of amphetamine in the treatment of aphasia. Restor Neurol Neurosci 1992; 4:47–50.
61. Porch B. The Porch Index of Communicative Ability. Administration, Scoring, and Interpretation. 3d ed. Palo Alto: Consulting Psychologists Press, 1981.
62. Albert ML, Bachman DL, Morgan A, Helm-Estabrooks N. Pharmacotherapy for aphasia. Neurology 1988; 38:877–879.
63. Bachman DL, Morgan A. The role of pharmacotherapy in the treatment of aphasia. Aphasiology 1988; 3–4:225–228.
64. Sabe L, Leiguarda R, Starkstein SE. An open-label trial of bromocriptine in nonfluent aphasia. Neurology 1992; 42:1637–1638.
65. Gupta SR, Mlcoch AG, Scolaro C, Moritz T. Bromocriptine treatment of nonfluent aphasia. Neurology 1995; 45:2170–2173.
66. Sabe L, Salvarezza F, Cuerva AG, Leiguarda R, Starkstein S. A randomized, double-blind, placebo-controlled study of bromocriptine in nonfluent aphasia. Neurology 1995; 45:2272–2274.
67. Goldstein LB. Restorative neurology. In: Wilkins RH, Rengachary SS, eds. Neurosurgery. 2d ed. New York: McGraw-Hill Book Company, 1996:459–470.
68. Crisostomo EA, Duncan PW, Propst MA, Dawson DB, Davis JN. Evidence that amphetamine with physical therapy promotes recovery of motor function in stroke patients. Ann Neurol 1988; 23:94–97.

19
Subarachnoid Hemorrhage

E. Clarke Haley, Jr.
University of Virginia Health System, Charlottesville, Virginia

INTRODUCTION

Subarachnoid hemorrhage (SAH) is a frequently devastating neurological illness that has been the beneficiary of a resurgence in interest in recent decades. Hippocrates described clinical scenarios compatible with subarachnoid hemorrhage, and Morgagni suspected intracranial arterial aneurysms as the cause of "meningeal apoplexy" in the mid-1700s.[1] The first published neuropathological demonstration of a ruptured intracranial aneurysm was by Cheyne in 1812. Surgical attempts to prevent rebleeding began with proximal ligation of parent arteries in the early 1900s. Dr. Walter Dandy performed the first direct surgical clipping of an intracranial aneurysm in 1937. The mid-20th century was a time of controversy in the treatment of SAH. Clinicians argued first over the benefits of surgery versus conservative treatment for ruptured aneurysms,[2] then over the timing of surgery.[3] When Ecker described the phenomenon of delayed cerebral vasospasm in 1951, he was greeted with great skepticism. In 1990, Dr. Charles Drake lamented that despite recent advances in medical and surgical treatment, the outcome from treatment of SAH had not changed in 30 years.[4] Recent clinical and epidemiological evidence suggests that with modern multitargeted therapy, improvements in outcome from SAH can now be demonstrated.[5]

SAH affects approximately 30,000 patients annually in North America, and in contrast to trends for ischemic stroke and intraparenchymal hemorrhage, the incidence of SAH is not decreasing.[5] About 80% of spontaneous SAH is caused by ruptured saccular arterial aneurysms; the remaining 20% is associated with ruptured fusiform or mycotic aneurysms, spontaneous intracranial arterial dissections, ruptured arteriovenous malformations, subarachnoid extension of intraparenchymal hematomas, or unknown causes.

Table 1 lists the distribution and frequency of ruptured saccular intracranial aneurysms. The pathogenesis of these lesions is not clearly understood. Attention has focused on defects in the internal elastic lamina and media at branch points of intracranial arteries, yet it is unclear whether these defects are congenital, acquired, or whether there is an interaction of both.[6] The incidence of aneurysms found at autopsy in patients under 10 years of age approaches zero.[7] Serial angiograms performed on unoperated aneurysms have shown that about 50% will increase in size over time[8]; also, as angiography may not accurately delineate the true diameter of aneurysms, since part of the wall may be occupied by layered thrombus, this may be an underestimate of the growth potential for saccular aneurysms. Other systemic arteriopathies have been associated with intracranial aneurysm formation, such as that associated with polycystic kidney disease, fibromuscular dysplasia, Ehlers-Danlos syndrome, neurofibromatosis, and others.[9] Intracranial atherosclerosis may predispose to fusiform intracranial aneurysms. A familial clustering of ruptured aneurysms is well described, and more of these patients have multiple aneurysms.[10] A genetic defect in connective tissue formation in these cases is highly suspected.

CLINICAL PRESENTATION AND NATURAL HISTORY

The Ictus

The clinical history of a patient with a ruptured intracranial aneurysm is one of the most distinctive in medicine, yet the diagnosis is frequently missed initially.[11] The abrupt onset of a severe, atypical headache, frequently described as "the worst headache of my life," is characteristic of this disorder. The onset of the headache may or may not be associated with a brief loss of consciousness, nausea and/or vomiting, focal neurological deficits (including cranial nerve palsies), or

Table 1 Location and Frequency of Ruptured Saccular Aneurysms

Aneurysm site	Proportion
Internal carotid artery	29.8%
Middle cerebral artery	22.3%
Anterior communicating/ anterior cerebral artery	39.0%
Vertebrobasilar arteries	7.6%
Other	2.5%

Source: Ref. 3.

stiff neck. Remarkably, of patients surviving to reach the hospital for evaluation and treatment, 70% will be fully alert or only drowsy and will have no motor or speech deficit.[12] A high index of suspicion must be maintained, as identification of the "warning leak" may be life-saving.[13]

Admission Neurological Grade

The most powerful predictor of outcome following an initial SAH is the neurological status on admission to the hospital. Table 2 outlines two commonly used grading scales, the Hunt and Hess scale devised in the 1960s,[14] and the World Federation of Neurological Surgeons scale developed in the 1980s.[15] Both scales have valuable prognostic capability in terms of predicting mortality, as well as favorable outcome (see below), regardless of management strategy.

The pathophysiology of altered levels of consciousness in the first 24 hours following the ictus is easily understood in some patients, yet obscure in others. Acute elevations in intracranial pressure with aneurysm rupture (or rebleeding) have been recorded in experimental models[16] as well as humans.[17] Accompanying reductions in global cerebral blood flow may account for alterations in consciousness in some patients. Most patients who survive the ictus have compensatory mechanisms that are quickly recruited to lower intracranial pressure into normal ranges. These compensatory mechanisms may be confounded, however, by acute obstruction of cerebrospinal fluid drainage by the subarachnoid (or, in

Table 2 Grading Scales and Outcome

Grade	Neurological status	Mortality	Favorable outcome[a]
Hunt and Hess Scale			
1	Asymptomatic	11%	
2	Severe headache or meningismus; no neurological deficit (except cranial nerve palsy)	26%	
3	Drowsy; minimal neurological deficit	33%	
4	Stuporous; moderate to severe neurological deficit	71%	
5	Comatose; decerebrate posturing	100%	
WFNS Scale			
1	GCS = 15; no motor deficit	7%	85%
2	GCS = 12–14; no motor deficit	11%	79%
3	GCS = 13–14; major motor deficit	19%	68%
4	GCS = 7–12; deficit present or absent	30%	46%
5	GCS = 3–6; deficit present or absent	44%	35%

[a]Favorable Outcome is either good recovery or moderate disability on the Glasgow Outcome Scale.
Source: Refs. 3, 15.

some cases, intraventricular) blood clot. Obstructive hydrocephalus may result, with frequently profound effects on level of consciousness. In other patients, aneurysms may rupture into the substance (parenchyma) of the brain itself, producing an intracerebral hematoma which may exert detrimental mass effects on adjacent and remote structures. Finally, in patients who cannot be demonstrated to have either raised intracranial pressure, hydrocephalus, or mass effects, some have proposed that the acute explosion of blood at arterial pressure inside the closed skull exposes the brain to an injury resulting in generalized brain swelling.[18]

Rebleeding

Defining the natural history of untreated ruptured intracranial aneurysms is more difficult than might be appreciated, since there has been a tendency for surgical harvesting of the most favorable cases since the 1950s. Moreover, studies prior to the widespread availability of computerized tomography (CT) scanning probably confused rebleeding with both hydrocephalus and delayed cerebral vasospasm. Data from the Cooperative Aneurysm Study on the Timing of Aneurysm Surgery, which was a prospective epidemiological survey in > 3,500 patients admitted within 3 days of the ictus,[3] documented that the incidence of rebleeding was about 4% on the calendar day of the ictus and then was constant at 1% to 2% per day for the next 4 weeks. Then there was a gradual fall to approximately 3% per year at 6 months. A long-term cohort study showed that this 3% per-year rate of rebleeding remains constant for up to 20 years of follow-up.

Clinically, rebleeding is frequently a catastrophic event if it occurs in the first month; about 70% of patients who rebleed will die within 6 months.[3] Abrupt changes in neurological status or abrupt increases in headache should prompt emergency head CT scanning to rule out an increase in acute intracranial blood. Lumbar puncture is not required or recommended to make the diagnosis of rebleeding. In fact, some evidence suggests that lumbar puncture actually increases the incidence of rebleeding,[19] presumably by lowering CSF pressure and thereby increasing the transmural bursting pressure of the aneurysm.

Hydrocephalus

Varying degrees of ventriculomegaly are common on admission CT scans in patients admitted within 3 days of SAH. Retrospective series report an incidence of acute hydrocephalus of 20% to 27%[20,21]; the prospective Cooperative Aneurysm Study reported 15%.[22] While many patients with hydrocephalus on admission CT scan may not have altered levels of consciousness, a higher incidence of acute hydrocephalus has been observed in patients admitted with poor neurological grades and those with large amounts of subarachnoid and/or intraventricular blood.[3] Patients with hydrocephalus following SAH have a worse prognosis.

Hydrocephalus may also develop either subacutely, during the first 2 weeks, or late, following discharge from the hospital. In the subacute cases, increasing headache or changes in level of consciousness may be confused with either rebleeding or vasospasm. In the chronic phase, patients may present with behavior or memory and gait disturbances characteristic of bifrontal lobe dysfunction. Many patients with chronic hydrocephalus are apparently asymptomatic, however.[23]

Vasospasm

Following aneurysmal SAH, approximately 70% to 80% of patients will have some degree of narrowing of one or more cerebral arteries visible on cerebral angiography.[24] The narrowing may begin within 2 days of the SAH and may persist for weeks, but usually subsides by 21 days if the patient survives. The peak incidence and severity of this delayed narrowing of cerebral vessels, termed angiographic vasospasm, is 9 ± 2 days. In approximately half of patients with angiographic vasospasm (or 30% to 40% of the total), the arterial narrowing is either so severe or so widespread that symptomatic cerebral ischemia develops, so-called symptomatic vasospasm or delayed ischemic neurological deficit. Clinically, the most common presentation is a decline in the level of consciousness, but disorientation, agitation, or focal or multifocal neurological deficits (e.g., aphasia, hemiparesis) may develop over just a few minutes to a few hours. Fever and increased headache may further confound the clinical picture. Symptomatic vasospasm commonly develops between days 4 and 14 following the hemorrhage.

If left untreated, about half of patients with symptomatic vasospasm (or 15% of the total) will either die or have a permanent neurological deficit attributable to brain infarction. In the Cooperative Study on the Timing of Aneurysm Surgery, conducted before the widespread use of hypertensive/hypervolemic therapy or calcium antagonists, symptomatic vasospasm was the leading cause of combined death and disability in patients with aneurysmal SAH.[3]

The precise pathophysiology of cerebral vasospasm remains unclear, although increasing evidence points to oxyhemoglobin released from degenerating red cells in the subarachnoid clot as the major mediator.[25] The amount (thickness) and distribution of subarachnoid blood clot visible on admission CT scan obtained within the first 3 days after the hemorrhage are correlated with the incidence and distribution of arterial narrowing on subsequent cerebral angiograms,[26] and are also prognostic for development of delayed ischemic deficits.[27]

Seizures

Loss of consciousness with tonic posturing of the extremities is a frequent occurrence at the hemorrhage ictus, being reported in about 25% of patients.[28] Whether this represents true electrical and clinical seizure activity or merely decerebrate posturing or other "release phenomena" related to the acute, massive increase in intracranial pressure, is unknown.[29] Similar behaviors may be seen with rebleeding, so the incidence figures for seizures occurring prior to operative clipping of the aneurysm may be confounded. In postoperative patients, seizures occur in 3% to 5% during the acute hospitalization.[30] The long-term incidence of recurrent seizures, or epilepsy, following discharge is difficult to determine, but may be estimated at about 5%.[31]

Medical Complications

Patients with acute SAH are frequently critically ill. In addition to the neurological complications described above, patients with SAH are at risk for serious, nonneurological medical complications related not only to their immobility and neurological deficits but also to the profound autonomic and endocrinologic changes that occur with acute extravasation of blood at arterial pressure into the subarachnoid space, as well as complications from medical and surgical interventions (e.g., fluid overload). Recently, Solenski and colleagues focused attention on nonneurological medical complications in a large, prospective series of North American SAH patients.[32] In that series, medical complications accounted for nearly a fourth of overall mortality, equaling the mortality from rebleeding and vasospasm, and exceeding that from direct effects of the hemorrhage.

Cardiac complications were the most frequent, with 35% of patients reported to have a variety of arrhythmias; 5% of arrhythmias were reported to be severe or life-threatening. Pulmonary complications, on the other hand, were more likely to be severe and result in mortality. Pulmonary edema, both neurogenic and from fluid overload, was reported in 23% of patients. Adult respiratory distress syndrome (ARDS) was reported in 4% of patients, but accounted for 28% of mortality attributed to medical complications. The onset of either cardiac or pulmonary complications was frequently associated with either the day of, or the day following aneurysm surgery.

Electrolyte disturbances, particularly hyponatremia, are common in the first 2 weeks following SAH. Recent studies suggest a relationship of hyponatremia to excessive natriuresis and volume contraction, rather than excessive antidiuretic hormone (ADH) secretion.[33] The mechanism of the natriuresis is unclear. In the chronic stages following SAH, hyponatremia may occur in association with increased extracellular fluid volume, a picture more consistent with the syndrome of inappropriate ADH.

Outcome

Estimates of overall outcome from the modern management of North American patients with aneurysmal SAH come from two sources: large, prospective cohort studies such as the North American experience in the International Cooperative Study on Timing of Aneurysm Surgery conducted from 1980 to 1983,[12] and prospective population-based studies such as the King County Survey conducted from 1987 to 1989.[34] The population-based studies provide a truer picture of overall management, as they include patients who die prior to admission to a hospital and include patients who are not referred to major neurosurgical referral centers. On the other hand, the number of patients examined is necessarily smaller, so confidence intervals around outcome proportions are broader, making the estimates less precise. Extrapolation of results from large, randomized clinical trials is even more hazardous because of the introduction of selection bias in addition to referral bias.

Figure 1 illustrates the outcomes from both studies. The Glasgow Outcome Scale,[35] although developed for use in patients with head trauma, has been adopted for use in SAH outcome studies because of its ease of administration and excellent reliability (low interobserver variability). In the King County study, 28% of patients had died, while 58% had favorable outcomes (either Good Re-

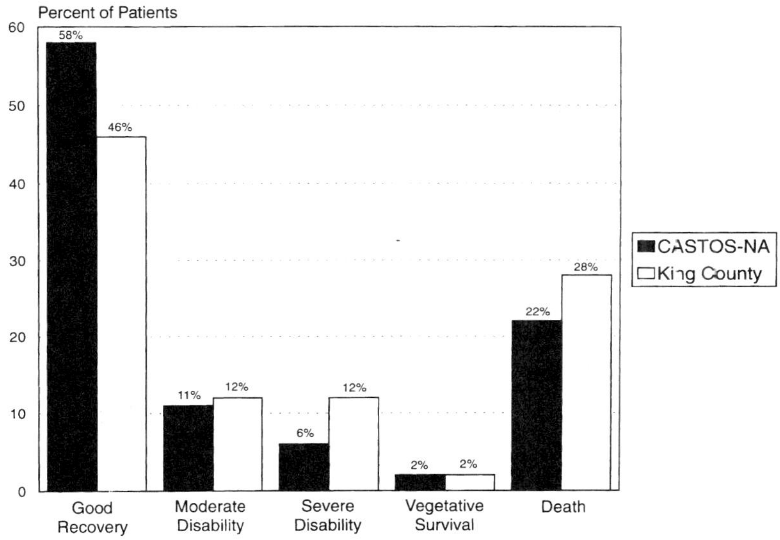

Figure 1 Bar graph depicting the overall outcome by the Glasgow Outcome Scale in the North American experience in the Cooperative Aneurysm Timing of Surgery Study (CASTOS-NA) and the King County survey of subarachnoid hemorrhage. Data from CASTOS-NA are at 6 months; King County follow-up was at 1 year.

covery or Moderate Disability, but able to live independently with minimal assistance in activities of daily living) at 1 year after the hemorrhage. Outcomes reported in the Cooperative Study were somewhat better, with 22% dead and 70% with favorable outcome, but this may merely be a reflection of the referral bias cited above.

Figure 2 illustrates the primary causes of death and disability in the Randomized Trial of Nicardipine in the Subarachnoid Hemorrhage conducted in North American centers.[36] Clearly, prevention and improved management of vasospasm, rebleeding, surgical complications, and medical complications represent opportunities for improving the outcome from SAH, as these complications occur in the hospital under direct medical supervision. Perhaps with urgent intervention, as in trauma and acute ischemic stroke, even the direct effects of the initial hemorrhage might be ameliorated.

DIAGNOSIS AND EVALUATION

History, CT Scanning, Lumbar Puncture

The diagnosis of SAH must be suspected on the basis of the history of the onset of the headache. While focal neurological deficits (e.g., third nerve palsy) may

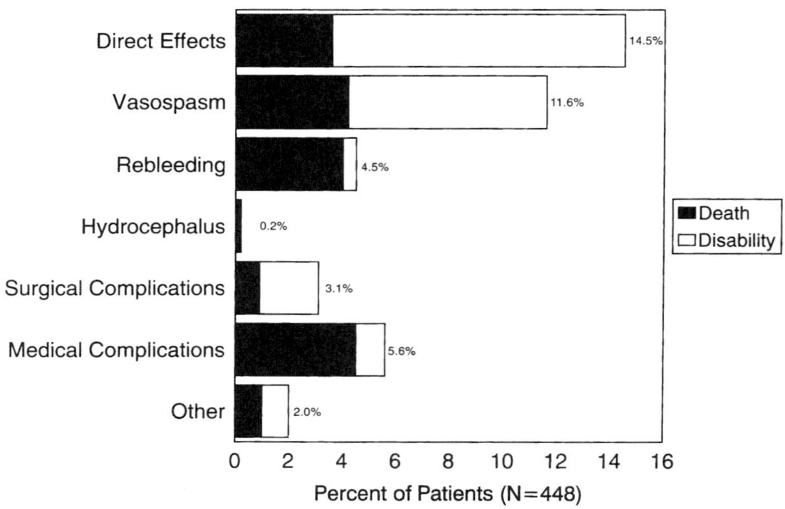

Figure 2 Bar graphs illustrating the rates of death and disability (any outcome on the Glasgow Outcome Scale other than Good Recovery or Death) by primary cause as reported by the treating investigators in the Randomized Trial of Nicardipine in Subarachnoid Hemorrhage.

be clues, these are most frequently absent in patients surviving to reach the hospital. Patients with a history of the abrupt onset of a severe, atypical headache should undergo emergency noncontrasted head CT scanning.[38] If this study is performed on the calendar day of the ictus with modern-generation equipment, the diagnostic yield of visible subarachnoid blood clot is > 90%. If the CT scan is positive for blood, then diagnostic lumbar puncture is unnecessary and may be dangerous. However, a negative CT scan, even on the day of the ictus, does not completely exclude SAH; patients with appropriate histories and negative CT scans should undergo diagnostic lumbar puncture by an experienced clinician. This is even more important if the initial CT scan is not performed until after the first day, as the yield of CT scanning progressively declines with time. Magnetic resonance imaging (MRI) is not recommended to establish the diagnosis of acute SAH.[37]

The amount and distribution of blood clot observed on the initial CT scan constitute a strong prognostic factor for outcome and are predictive of symptomatic vasospasm. Table 3 shows the relationship of CT blood clot to outcome and ischemic deficits from vasospasm from the Cooperative Study. The distribution of blood on initial CT scan may also be a clue to the source of bleeding in patients found to have multiple aneurysms. Head CT scanning is also useful in patients with neurological worsening after admission. Neurological worsening after admission is frequently multifactorial, so noninvasive measures to detect cerebral vasospasm may not exclude concomitant hydrocephalus, brain edema, or rebleeding.

Cerebral Angiography

Patients with SAH diagnosed by CT scan or lumbar puncture should undergo diagnostic cerebral angiography to detect the source of bleeding, usually an aneurysm.[37] In approximately 20% to 25% of patients, no source of bleeding will be identified. However, a repeat angiogram after approximately 1 week may yield an aneurysm that was not visible on the initial angiogram in an additional 1% to 2% of cases. Magnetic resonance angiography (MRA) and spiral CT angiogra-

Table 3 Relationship of CT Subarachnoid Blood to Incidence of Ischemic Deficits

Amount of CT blood	% Focal ischemic deficits
None	12.2%
Focal thin	29.0%
Diffuse	37.5%
Focal thick	44.0%

phy may be used in selected emergency situations when patients may be too ill to undergo selective catheterization, but still do not have the sensitivity necessary to be recommended for routine use.

Postoperative angiography is frequently used to check clip placement; in some centers, intraoperative angiography is used for this purpose. Incompletely clipped aneurysms represent a recurrent hemorrhage risk.[38] Selective catheter angiography also remains the gold standard for detection of cerebral vasospasm.

Transcranial Doppler

The ability to detect Doppler signals from intracranial arteries was immediately recognized to have potential applicability in the detection of cerebral vasospasm following subarachnoid hemorrhage.[39] Subsequent experience has shown that this technique may have significant limitations, including lack of sensitivity, operator variability, and inability to obtain signals from up to 10% of patients. Nevertheless, in experienced hands, the detection of markedly elevated blood flow velocities[40] or rapidly rising velocities[41] in the middle cerebral arteries has sufficient specificity to make the test clinically useful for detecting arterial narrowing, either asymptomatic or symptomatic.

Insufficient data exist to recommend cerebral blood flow measurement by a variety of techniques, transcranial cerebral oxygen saturation, or electrical brain mapping as an adjunct to the management of patients with SAH.[37]

MANAGEMENT

Preoperative Care

The goals of the preoperative management of patients with aneurysmal SAH are to prevent rebleeding and brain ischemia, reduce pain, and prevent or manage neurological or medical complications. Specific measures to prevent rebleeding are discussed below. In experienced neurosurgical referral centers, patients are usually admitted to either an intensive care unit or an acute stroke care and monitoring unit where trained personnel can perform frequent clinical assessments of neurological function. Strict bedrest in a darkened room with restricted visitation is frequently prescribed. Pneumatic compression boots are used to prevent deep-vein thrombosis. Stool softeners are prescribed to prevent straining at bowel movements.

Rigorous attention must be paid to patient fluid and electrolyte balance. Fluid restriction and induced hypotension have been shown not to reduce rebleeding, and outcomes were worse than with no treatment, probably because of exacerbation of brain ischemia from vasospasm.[42,43] Recall that patients receiving routine maintenance fluids alone may still become volume-contracted and hyponatremic.[33] Gentle hypervolemia with isotonic fluids is therefore recommended. Hyponatremia should not be treated with fluid restriction, but rather with volume and sodium replacement.[37]

Hypertension (systolic blood pressure > 160 mm Hg) is treated with caution, particularly during the period of risk for vasospasm. Slower-acting agents such as labetalol or hydralazine are preferred. Frequently, relief of pain or emptying of a full bladder will have dramatic salutary effects.

Studies on the utility of anticonvulsant drug therapy in either the acute or chronic stage following SAH have been conflicting. While administration of anticonvulsants in the acute period does not appear to prevent the subsequent development of a seizure disorder,[31] most North American experts use prophylactic anticonvulsant drugs (usually phenytoin) to prevent seizures during the perioperative period when the results of a seizure could be catastrophic. Routine long-term anticonvulsant use following SAH is not recommended.[37]

The use of large doses of corticosteroids continues to be prevalent among North American neurosurgeons despite lack of evidence that they provide a benefit. The presumed benefit of steroids in the acute period following SAH is that they may reduce brain edema and perivascular inflammation that may promote vasospasm. Potential side effects include steroid psychosis, gastrointestinal bleeding, pancreatitis, increased susceptibility to infection including sepsis, masking of the clinical signs of infection, and poor wound healing. The American Heart Association did not address the use of corticosteroids in their Guidelines statement.[37]

Surgery

Craniotomy with direct surgical clipping of the ruptured aneurysm continues to be strongly recommended for most patients as the procedure of choice to prevent rebleeding.[37] The timing of aneurysm surgery continues to be a matter of clinical judgment, though a preponderance of North American neurosurgeons have adopted a preference for early surgery, especially in patients admitted in good neurological grades (Hunt and Hess grades I–III). The North American experience in the Timing of Surgery study suggested that overall mortality was not increased by planned early surgery, and that the proportion of patients who ultimately achieved a good recovery was significantly higher in the group planned for early surgery.[12] As in the overall study, patients planned for surgery during days 7 to 10 following the hemorrhage had significantly worse outcomes, probably reflecting the concomitant influence of delayed cerebral vasospasm during that time interval.

Surgical alternatives to direct clipping of the neck of the aneurysm, such as coating or wrapping of the aneurysm, or proximal carotid ligation, have generally been unsuccessful. Incompletely clipped aneurysms also continue to confer risk of both rupture and regrowth. Use of temporary clips on the parent artery intraoperatively may assist in the dissection and clipping of difficult aneurysms; induced intraoperative hypotension is now no longer recommended.[37]

Prevention and Treatment of Vasospasm

There have been a number of important developments in the treatment of delayed cerebral vasospasm following aneurysmal SAH during the last 15 years. While a specific antagonist to the primary spasmogen has not yet been developed, several other strategies appear to be effective, though none is 100%.

In 1989, the U.S. Food and Drug Administration approved oral nimodipine, a dihydropyridine calcium antagonist, for use in patients with SAH admitted in good neurological grade (Hunt and Hess grades I–III). Table 4 summarizes the results of the five studies upon which the recommendation was based.[44] In each study, poor outcome was reduced, though only in the British Aneurysm Trial was the difference statistically significant for overall outcome at 3 months. Angiograms performed in the course of these studies did not show a reduction of the incidence or severity of the arterial narrowing by nimodipine. The beneficial effects are therefore surmised to be on the basis of improved collateral blood flow or possibly a neuroprotectant effect from reduced intracellular calcium accumulation in the ischemic tissue.

The North American participants in the Cooperative Aneurysm Study tested high doses of the dihydropyridine calcium antagonist nicardipine given intravenously for up to 14 days following aneurysmal SAH.[24,36] The incidence and severity of both angiographic and clinically symptomatic vasospasm were reduced by nicardipine, but overall outcome was no different from that with standard management which, in these participating centers, included intentional hypervolemia and induced hypertension. Fewer patients treated with nicardipine required hypervolemic/hypertensive therapy in this study.

Hypervolemic/hypertensive therapy has never been subjected to testing in a randomized, controlled clinical trial, but the anecdotal evidence that it is effective is so strong that many experts believe that such a trial would be unethical. The extensive anecdotal experience has been painstakingly compiled by Dorsch.[45,46] His analysis suggests that prophylactic hypervolemic therapy may reduce the incidence of symptomatic vasospasm by about one-third, and that combined hypervolemic/hypertensive therapy in patients with clinically symptomatic vasospasm may reduce mortality by about one-third and improve good recovery by about one-third.

Hypervolemic/hypertensive therapy is aggressive medical treatment that should be administered by experienced clinicians in an intensive care unit setting. Complications such as fluid overload and pulmonary edema are common.[47] If treatment is begun after brain infarction is already well established, fatal brain

Table 4 Prospective, Randomized Clinical Trials of Oral Nimodipine After Aneurysmal Subarachnoid Hemorrhage

	Allen (1983)	Philippon (1986)	Neil-Dwyer (1987)	Petruk (1988)	BRANT (1989)
Nimodipine treatment	0.35 mg/kg q4h × 21 days	60 mg q 4 h × 21 days	60 mg q4h × 21 days	90 mg q4h × 21 days	60 mg q4h × 21 days
Total patients	125	170	75	188	1,115
Exclusions	9	100	25	34	561
Placebo	60	39	25	82	276
Nimodipine	56	31	25	72	278
Admit neurologic grade	I-II	I-III	I-V	III-V	I-V
Interval to treatment after SAH	≤96 h	≤72 h	≤96 h	≤96 h	≤96 h
Follow-up period	21 days	21 days	3 mo	21 days, 3 mo	21 days, 3 mo
Assessment scale	5-step	GOS	GOS	GOS	GOS
Results					
Favorable outcome	NR	NR P13	(GOS 1–2) N19 (76%) (52%)	(GOS 1–2) N28 (39%) P28 (34%)	(GOS 1–2) N223 (80%) P185 (67%)
Poor outcome	(GOS 3–5) N1 (2%)[a] P8 (13%)[a]	(GOS 3–5) N3 (10%)[a] P13 (33%)[a]	(GOS 3–5) N6 (24%) P12 (48%)	(GOS 3–5) N44 (61%) P54 (66%)	(GOS 3–5) N55 (20%) P91 (33%)
Death	N1 (2%)[a] P3 (5%)[a]	N3 (10%)[a] P7 (18%)[a]	N1 (4%) P6 (24%)	N34 (47%) P32 (39%)	N43 (15%) P60 (22%)
Relative risk reduction in poor outcome	(86%)[a,b]	(71%)[a,b]	50%	7%	40%†

BRANT, British Aneurysm Nimodipine Trial; GOS, Glasgow Outcome Scale; NR, not reported; N, nimodipine; P, placebo.
[a]Patients with vasospasm only.
[b]Statistically significant $P<.05$.

edema may be induced. The therapy is not recommended for patients with unsecured aneurysms because of the risk of inducing rebleeding.

In several specialized centers, angioplasty of narrowed cerebral vessels with microcatheter-directed balloons[48] or with superselective injections of the vasodilator papaverine[49] has been used successfully in selected patients. The efficacy of the routine use of this treatment for patients with symptomatic vasospasm has not been established. The treatment is therefore reserved for those patients who have failed other measures. Again, however, prompt intervention must be used before infarction is well established.

Several other potential therapies have been reported to have promising results, but definitive proof of efficacy awaits further study. Cisternal irrigation with the thrombolytic agent tissue plasminogen activator at the time of early surgical clipping of the aneurysm is a theoretically attractive approach that showed promise in experimental animal studies[50] and in small, uncontrolled series of patients.[51,52] A small, randomized, controlled trial suggested that the incidence and severity of angiographic vasospasm were reduced by the treatment, and there were suggestions of benefit on overall outcome in patients fully complying with the protocol.[53] However, the intent-to-treat results were disappointing with regard to overall outcome.

Therapeutic trials with drugs that have putative neuroprotectant effects, such as the 21-aminosteroid, tirilazad mesylate, have also had mixed results. In a randomized trial of over 1,000 patients in Europe and Australasia, treatment with tirilazad, 6 mg/kg/day, begun within 48 hours of the SAH and continued through day 10 following the hemorrhage, was associated with a nearly 50% relative reduction in mortality compared to patients treated with either placebo or lower doses of tirilazad.[54] The incidence of symptomatic vasospasm was also reduced, but the difference was not statistically significant. In a similar trial conducted in North America, no significant improvement in either mortality or vasospasm could be demonstrated.[55] One hypothesis for the discrepant findings is that patients in North America were more likely to receive concomitant anticonvulsant medication, which has the effect of lowering blood levels of tirilazad. Further studies of tirilazad in patients with SAH are ongoing.

Treatment of Hydrocephalus

Management of acute hydrocephalus following SAH is problematic. Ventriculostomy and cerebrospinal fluid drainage can lower intracranial pressure and result in prompt neurological improvement in some patients admitted in poor neurological grades.[23] However, the procedure may result in an increased incidence of rebleeding and may be associated with infectious complications including ventriculitis and meningitis. Many neurosurgeons take the approach of operating urgently on the aneurysm and placing the ventriculostomy at the time of surgery, but after the aneurysm has been secured. As the blood in the subarachnoid space is resorbed postoperatively, the ventriculostomy can be clamped and removed in most instances. Permanent shunting is avoided, if possible, because of the tendency for these devices to malfunction over time.

Hydrocephalus evolving during the second week is frequently communicating hydrocephalus and may be treated with serial lumbar puncture or a lumbar drain for several days.[37] If the hydrocephalus persists, permanent cerebrospinal fluid diversion may be necessary. Patients with chronic hydrocephalus may be managed in a similar fashion.

Antifibrinolytic Therapy

Administration of preoperative antifibrinolytic drugs was investigated in several controlled studies conducted in the 1980s. A consistent pattern emerged suggesting that while antifibrinolytic drugs did appear to reduce the incidence of rebleeding, any benefit was obviated by an increased incidence of death and disability from symptomatic vasospasm.[56] For this reason, most North American neurosurgeons have largely abandoned the use of these drugs, opting instead for early aneurysm surgery.

Detachable Coils/Balloon Trapping

Since 1990, interventional neuroradiological techniques have been used to treat aneurysms. Most studies have enrolled patients who were felt to be poor surgical risks because of either the nature of the aneurysm (size or location) or poor medical condition. Use of detachable platinum coils that promote luminal thrombosis of the aneurysm has been reported to result in complete occlusion of 81% of small-necked aneurysms, but only 19% of wide-necked aneurysms.[57] The use of detachable balloons placed inside the aneurysm has been less successful. Detachable balloons to occlude the parent artery both proximal and distal to large carotid aneurysms may be a reasonble treatment in some cases.

FUTURE DIRECTIONS

Prevention

Clearly, rupture of an unsuspected cerebral aneurysm can be a catastrophic event, and while medical and surgical treatment may have improved recently, a far more effective approach to reducing the toll of morbidity and mortality from SAH is prevention. Epidemiological studies have identified hypertension, smoking, and binge alcohol drinking as potentially modifiable risk factors for SAH.[37] However, the benefit of either hypertension treatment, or smoking and drinking cessation on subsequent risk for SAH has not been definitively shown, and the magnitude of any benefit from these interventions is likely to be small. There are also other compelling health reasons for modifying these factors, so definitive studies to prove a benefit for SAH reduction are unlikely to be performed.

A far more fruitful avenue for consideration is the identification and potential treatment of unruptured aneurysms. Much additional work needs to be done in this regard, however. To date, the natural history (i.e., rupture rate) of unruptured aneurysms is unknown. This question is currently being investigated in a large retrospective and prospective cohort study, the International Study of Unruptured Intracranial Aneurysms. Moreover, the optimal management of these aneurysms continues to be a matter of controversy. Many surgical series cite very low rates of morbidity and mortality for clipping of unruptured aneurysms,[58] but these studies were retrospective and potentially biased. Moreover, what role, if any, do the newer interventional radiological techniques (e.g., coiling) play in the management of unruptured aneurysms? If screening for unruptured aneurysms is to be done, who should be screened, and how should it be done? Is MRA adequate, or will selective contrast angiography be required in high-risk individuals? These are all important issues for future research.

Direct Effects

The results of several recent clinical trials now suggest that direct effects of the initial hemorrhage may be the leading cause of death and disability following SAH, replacing vasospasm, which has seen improvements in management over the last decade. While treatment of the direct effects of the initial hemorrhage may seem to be a dauntless task, combination of treatments designed for traumatic head injury or acute ischemic stroke (e.g., neuroprotectant drugs[59]) with ultra-early intervention protocols may potentially be a fruitful avenue for investigation. As with acute ischemic stroke, it may be that the speed with which treatment is delivered may be more important than precisely which treatment is used.

Improved Diagnosis

Finally, it may be argued that with improvements in management of rebleeding and vasospasm, it becomes more important to make an early diagnosis and rapid referral to experienced neurological and neurosurgical centers in cases of SAH. Patient and physician recognition of the clinical symptoms, followed by appropriate diagnostic studies, are the key to improved outcomes from this disease in the future.

Note added in proof: Unruptured Aneurysms. Since submission of this manuscript, important observations regarding the natural history and surgical treatment of unruptured intracranial aneurysms have been published.[60] A Guidelines Statement by the Stroke Council of the American Heart Association on the management of these lesions is in preparation.

ACKNOWLEDGMENTS

The author is grateful to Dr. William Longstreth for providing supplemental data from the King County Survey, and Dr. James Torner for providing additional information from the Cooperative Aneurysm Timing of Surgery Study for this manuscript.

REFERENCES

1. McHenry LC. Garrison's History of Neurology. Springfield, IL: C.C. Thomas, 1969.
2. Graf CJ, Nibbelink DW. Cooperative aneurysm study of intracranial aneurysms and subarachnoid hemorrhage: report on a randomized treatment study III. Intracranial surgery. Stroke 1974; 5:559–601.
3. Kassell NF, Torner JC, Haley EC, Jane JA, Adams HP, Kongable GL. The international cooperative study on the timing of aneurysm surgery. Part 1. Overall management results. J Neurosurg 1990; 73:18–36.
4. Drake CG. Management of cerebral aneurysm. Stroke 1981; 12:273–283.
5. Ingall TJ, Whisnant JP, Wiebers DO, O'Fallon WM. Has there been a decline in subarachnoid hemorrhage mortality? Stroke 1989; 20:718–724.
6. Weir BKA. Pathology. In: Aneurysms Affecting the Nervous System. Baltimore: Williams and Wilkins, 1987:209–261.
7. Riggs H, Rupp C. Miliary aneurysms: relation of anomalies of the circle of Willis to formation of aneurysms. Arch Neurol Psychiatry 1943; 49:615–616.
8. Bjorkesten G, Troupp H. Changes in the size of intracranial arterial aneurysms. J Neurosurg 1962; 19:583–588.
9. Weir BKA. Medical, Neurologic, and Ophthalmologic Aspects of Aneurysms. In: Aneurysms Affecting the Nervous System Baltimore; Williams and Wilkins, 1987. pp. 54–133.
10. Rankainen A, Hernesniemi J, Tromp G. Special features of familial intracranial aneurysms: Report of 215 familial aneurysms. Neurosurgery 1995; 37:43–47.
11. Kassell NF, Kongable GL, Torner JC, Adams HP Jr, Mazuz H Delay in referral of patients with ruptured aneurysms to neurosurgical attention. Stroke 1985; 16:587–590.
12. Haley EC, Kassell NF, Torner JC and the Participants. The international cooperative study on the timing of aneurysm surgery: the North American experience. Stroke 1992; 23:205–214.

13. Leblanc R. The minor leak preceding subarachnoid hemorrhage. J Neurosurg 1987; 66:35–39.
14. Hunt WE, Hess RM. Surgical risk as related to the time of intervention in the repair of intracranial aneurysms. J Neurosurg 1968; 28:14–20.
15. Drake CG. Report of World Federation of Neurological Surgeons Committee on a Universal Subarachnoid Hemorrhage Grading Scale. J Neurosurg 1988; 68:985–986.
16. Jakubowski J, Bell BA, Symon L, Zawirske MB, Francis DM. A primate model of subarachnoid hemorrhage: change in regional cerebral blood flow, autoregulation carbon dioxide reactivity, and central conduction time. Stroke 1982; 13:601–611.
17. Hayashi M, Kobayshi H, Munemoto S, Yamamoto S. Changes in intracranial pressure during the rupture of an intracranial aneurysm and the prognosis in regard to life. Brain Nerve 1982; 34:187–193.
18. Fisher CM. Clinical syndromes in cerebral thrombosis, hypotensive hemorrhage and ruptured saccular aneurysm. Clin Neurosurg 1975; 22:117–174.
19. Duffy GP. Lumbar puncture in spontaneous subarachnoid haemorrhage. Br Med J 1982; 285:1163–1164.
20. Milhorat TH. Acute hydrocephalus after aneurysmal subarachnoid hemorrhage. Neurosurgery 1987; 20:747–753.
21. van Gijn J, Hijdra A, Wijdicks EF, Vermeulen M, van Crevel H. Acute hydrocephalus after aneurysmal subarachnoid hemorrhage. J Neurosurg 1985; 63:355–362.
22. Graff-Radford NR, Torner J, Adams HP Jr, Kassell NF. Factors associated with hydrocephalus after subarachnoid hemorrhage: a report of the Cooperative Aneurysm Study. Arch Neurol 1989; 46:744–752.
23. Hasan D, Vermeulen M, Wijdicks EF, Hijdra A, van Gijn J. Management problems in acute hydrocephalus after subarachnoid hemorrhage. Stroke 1989; 20:747–753.
24. Haley EC, Kassell NF, Torner JC and the Particpants. A randomized trial of nicardipine in subarachnoid hemorrhage: angiographic and transcranial Doppler ultrasound results. A report of the Cooperative Aneurysm Study. J Neurosurg 1993; 78:548–553.
25. MacDonald RL, Weir BKA, Runzer TD, Grace MGA, Findlay JM, Saito K, Cook DA, Mielke BW, Kanamaru K. Etiology of cerebral vasospasm in primates. J Neurosurg 1991; 75:415–424.
26. Fisher CM, Kistler JP, Davis JM. Relation of cerebral vasospasm to subarachnoid hemorrhage visualized by computerized tomographic scanning. Neurosurgery 1980; 6:1–9.
27. Adams HP Jr, Kassell NF, Torner JC, Haley EC. Predicting cerebral ischemia after aneurysmal subarachnoid hemorrhage: influences of clinical condition, CT results, and antifibrinolytic therapy. A report of the Cooperative Aneurysm Study. Neurology 1987; 37:1586–1591.
28. Sundaraam MB, Chow F. Seizures associated with spontaneous subarachnoid hemorrhage. Can J Neurol Sci 1986; 13:229–231.
29. Hart RG, Byer JA, Slaughter JR, Hewlett JE, Easton JD. Occurrence and implications of seizures in subarachnoid hemorrhage due to ruptured intracranial aneurysms. Neurosurgery 1981; 8:417–421.
30. Kassell NF, Boarini DJ. Perioperative care of the aneurysm patient. Contemp Neurosurg 1984; 6:1–6.

31. Notani M, Kawamura H, Amano K, Tanikawa T, Kawabatake H, Iseke H, Shiwaku T, Nagao T, Kakinoki Y, Kitamura K. The incidence of postoperative epilepsy and prophylactic anticonvulsants in patients with intracranial aneurysm. Neurol Surg 1984; 12:269–274.
32. Solenski NJ, Haley EC, Kassell NF, Kongable G, Germanson T, Truskowski L, Torner JC and the Participants. Medical complications of aneurysmal subarachnoid hemorrhage: a report of the multicenter, cooperative aneurysm study. Crit Care Med 1995; 23:1007–1017.
33. Wijdicks EF, Vermeurlen M, ten Haaf JA, Hijdra A, Bakker WH, van Gijn J. Volume depletion and natriuresis in patients with a ruptured intracranial aneurysm. Ann Neurol 1985; 18:211–216.
34. Longstreth WT, Nelson LM, Koepsell TD, van Belle G. Clinical course of spontaneous subarachnoid hemorrhage: a population-based study in King County, Washington. Neurology 1993; 43:712–718.
35. Jennett B, Bond M. Assessment of outcome after severe brain damage: a practical scale. Lancet 1975; 1:480–484.
36. Haley EC, Kassell NF, Torner JC and the Participants. A randomized controlled trial of high-dose intravenous nicardipine in aneurysmal subarachnoid hemorrhage. A report of the Cooperative Aneurysm Study. J Neurosurg 1993; 78:537–547.
37. Mayberg MR, Batjer HH, Dacey R, Diringer M, Haley EC, Heros RC, Sternau LL, Torner J. Guidelines for the management of aneurysmal subarachnoid hemorrhage. A statement for healthcare professionals from a special writing group of the Stroke Council, American Heart Association. Circulation 1994; 90 2592–2605.
38. Lin T, Fox AJ, Drake CG. Regrowth of aneurysm sacs from residual neck following aneurysm clipping. J Neurosurg 1989; 70:556–560.
39. Aaslid R, Huber P, Nornes H. Evaluation of cerebrovascular spasm with transcranial Doppler ultrasound. J Neurosurg 1984; 60:37–41.
40. Sloan MK, Haley EC, Kassell NF, Henry ML, Stewart SR, Beskin RR, Sevilla EA, Torner JC. Sensitivity and specificity of transcranial Doppler ultrasonography in the diagnosis of vasospasm following subarachnoid hemorrhage. Neurology 1989; 39:1514–1518.
41. Harders AG, Gilsbach JM. Time course of blood velocity changes related to vasospasm in the circle of Willis measured by transcranial Doppler ultrasound. J Neurosurg 1987; 66:718–728.
42. Wijdicks EF, Vermeurlen M, Hijdra A, van Gijn J. Hyponatremia and cerebral infarction in patients with ruptured intracranial aneurysms: is fluid restriction harmful? Ann Neurol 1985; 17:137–140.
43. Torner JC, Nibbelink DW, Burmeister LF. Statistical comparisons of end results of a randomized treatment study. In: Sahs AL, Nibbelink DW, Torner JC, eds. Aneurysmal Subarachnoid Hemorrhage: Report of the Cooperative Study. Baltimore, MD: Urban & Schwarzenberg, 1981:249–276.
44. Wong MCW, Haley EC. Calcium antagonists: stroke therapy coming of age. Stroke 1990; 21:494–501.
45. Dorsch NWC, King MT. A review of cerebral vasospasm in aneurysmal subarachnoid haemorrhage. Part I. Incidence and effects. J Clin Neurosci 1994; 1:19–26.

46. Dorsch NWC. A review of cerebral vasospasm in aneurysmal subarachnoid haemorrhage. Part II. Management. J Clin Neurosci 1994; 1:78–92.
47. Levy M, Giannotta S. Cardiac performance indices during hypervolemic therapy for cerebral vasospasm. J Neurosurg 1991; 75:27–31.
48. Newell DW, Eskridge JM, Mayberg MR, Grady MS, Winn HR. Angioplasty for the treatment of symptomatic vasospasm following subarachnoid hemorrhage. J Neurosurg 1989; 71:654–660.
49. Kassell NF, Helm G, Simmons N, Phillips CD, Cail WS. Treatment of cerebral vasospasm with intra-arterial papaverine. J Neurosurg 1992; 77:848–852.
50. Findlay JM, Weir BKA, Gordon P, Grace M, Baughman R. Safety and efficacy of intrathecal thrombolytic therapy in a primate model of cerebral vasospasm. Neurosurgery 1989; 24:491–498.
51. Findlay JM, Weir BKA, Kassell NF, Disney LB, Grace MGA. Intracisternal recombinant tissue plasminogen activator after aneurysmal subarachnoid hemorrhage. J Neurosurg 1991; 75:181–188.
52. Ohman J, Servo A, Heiskanen O. Effect of intrathecal fibrinolytic therapy on clot lysis and vasospasm in patients with aneurysmal subarachnoid hemorrhage. J Neurosurg 1991; 75:197–201.
53. Findlay JM, Kassell NF, Weir BKA, Haley EC, Kongable GL, Germanson T, Truskowski L, Alves WM, Holness RO, Knuckey NW, Yonas H, Steinberg GK, West M, Winn HR, Ferguson G. A randomized trial of intraoperative, intracisternal tissue plasminogen activator for the prevention of vasospasm. Neurosurgery 1995; 37:168–178.
54. Kassell NF, Haley EC, Apperson-Hansen C, Alves WM and the Participants. Randomized, double-blind, vehicle-controlled trial of tirilazad mesylate in patients with aneurysmal subarachnoid hemorrhage: a cooperative study in Europe, Australia, and New Zealand. J Neurosurg 1996; 84:221–228.
55. Haley EC, Kassell NF, Apperson-Hansen C, Maile MH, Alves WM and the Participants. A randomized, double-blind, vehicle-controlled trial of tirilazad mesylate in patients with aneurysmal subarachnoid hemorrhage: a cooperative study in North America. J Neurosurg. 1997; 86:467–474.
56. Haley EC, Torner JC, Kassell NF. Antifibrinolytic therapy and cerebral vasospasm. Neurosurg Clin North Am 1990; 1:349–356.
57. Guglielmi G, Vinuela F, Duchwiler G, Dion J, Lylyk P, Berenstein A, Strother C, Graves V, Halbach V, Nichols D. Endovascular treatment of posterior circulation aneurysms by electrothrombosis using electrically detachable coils. J Neurosurg 1992; 77:515–524.
58. Nakagawa T, Haski K. The incidence and treatment of asymptomatic, unruptured cerebral aneurysms. J Neurosurg 1994; 80:217–223.
59. Fisher M. An overview of cytoprotective therapy for acute ischemic stroke. In: Moskowitz MA, Caplan LR, eds. Cerebrovascular Diseases, Nineteenth Princeton Stroke Conference, Boston: Butterworth-Heinemann, 1995:391–401.
60. The International Study of Unruptured Intracranial Aneurysms Investigators: Unruptured intracranial aneurysms—risk of rupture and risks of surgical intervention. N Engl J Med 1998; 339:1725–1733.

20

Medical Management of Intracerebral Hemorrhage

Lewis B. Morgenstern
University of Texas, Houston, Texas

Derk W. Krieger
The Cleveland Clinic Foundation, Cleveland, Ohio

Intracerebral hemorrhage (ICH) is perhaps the most frustrating type of stroke. While mortality and morbidity are particularly high, specific therapy remains largely an enigma. In this chapter we review the current care of patients with ICH, describe new trends in therapy, and speculate on future avenues of research.

EPIDEMIOLOGY AND RISK FACTORS OF PRIMARY ICH

ICH accounts for 10% to 15% of all stroke.[1] Mortality from ICH approaches 50% in most series.[2] African-Americans (AAs) are at greatest risk from mortality secondary to ICH, particularly at younger ages. With advancing ages, as ICH mortality increases, the relative gap between AAs and non-Hispanic whites (NHWs) closes. In those over 75, AAs and NHWs have similar ICH mortality. Hispanic-Americans (HAs) have a large burden of ICH at younger ages relative to NHWs, but are relatively protected at older ages.[3]

Hypertension remains the single most important risk factor for ICH with a relative risk of approximately 4-5.[1] Still, hypertension is found in only about 50% of patients with spontaneous ICH.[4] Although the pathophysiology of ICH seems to emphasize weakening of small arteries by chronic blood pressure elevation, the precise mechanism is unknown. The classic teaching of so-called Charcot-Bouchard microaneurysm formation and rupture has become lore, but certainly does not explain spontaneous ICH in nonhypertensives and probably many hypertensives. Acute space-occupying lesions such as ICH have been shown in animal models to cause acute hypertension. Therefore, a patient with ICH with acute hypertension, but without a clear history of chronic hypertension, cannot be considered to have a "hypertensive hemorrhage." In these patients other risk factors and causes of secondary hypertension should be rigorously sought after.

Tobacco use, while clearly a risk factor for subarachnoid hemorrhage and ischemic stroke, has not convincingly been linked to the etiology of ICH.[1] Ethanol use seems protective at low levels and very detrimental at higher consumption rates.[5] Diabetes mellitus and anticoagulant use also contribute to ICH risk.[6] The presence of apolipoprotein E e4 has recently been shown to increase the risk of amyloid-angiopathy-related ICH.[7]

SECONDARY CAUSES OF ICH

Table 1 reviews the differential diagnosis of ICH. Amyloid angiopathy is important in the etiology of ICH in the elderly population, causing ICH in about 50% of cases in the over-80 group.[4] Diagnosis can only be made by biopsy, an unappealing option since there is no specific treatment. Coagulopathy, either pharmacologic, genetic, or acquired, is a rare cause of ICH. Hemorrhagic transformation of ischemic stroke or venous infarction must always be considered. Hemorrhage into a tumor, particularly metastatic melanoma, renal cell carcinoma, and choriocarcinoma[1] must be considered. Since lung tumors are so much more common, although less likely to bleed, they still account for a large portion of tumor hemorrhage. Primary brain tumors including gliomas and hemangioblastoma can mimic primary ICH. Arteriovenous malformations (AVMs) and aneu-

Table 1 Differential Diagnosis of the Etiology of ICH

Hypertension and idiopathic (primary)
Traumatic contusion
Amyloid angiopathy
Anteriovenous malformation
Cerebral congenital aneurysm rupture
Cerebral mycotic aneurysm rupture and infective endocarditis
Hemorrhagic conversion of ischemic stroke
Cerebral venous infarction
Cerebral vasculitis and collagen vascular disorders
Coagulopathy
Cocaine
Stimulant drugs
Thrombolytic therapy
Hemorrhage into primary or secondary brain tumor

rysms should always be in the differential, but are usually easily discriminated from primary ICH (see Diagnosis below).

Drug use, particularly cocaine, has been implicated as an etiology of secondary ICH.[8,9] Sympathomimetic agents such as phenylpropanolamine have been implicated by anecdotal reports,[4] but well-controlled studies have not been reported to date. Thrombolytic therapy with recombinant tissue plasminogen activator (rt-PA) for acute ischemic stroke is associated with a 6.4% risk of symptomatic ICH.[10] Rt-PA for acute myocardial infarction carries a <1% risk of ICH. Traumatic brain injury causing cerebral contusion can mimic ICH,[1] and frequently is accompanied by other intracranial bleeding including subdural and epidural hemorrhage.

DIAGNOSIS

Although some of us hold fast to the belief that we can distinguish ischemic from hemorrhagic stroke at the bedside, the reality is that only a noncontrast CT scan is so talented. Although headache is two to three times as common in ICH as ischemic stroke,[11,12] it is still prevalent in a quarter of patients with acute ischemic stroke. Symptoms of increased intracranial pressure (ICP) including decreased level of consciousness can occur in both disorders and are unreliable as discriminating tools.

Our diagnostic evaluation (see Fig. 1) begins with a careful history and physical examination. Our goal is to exclude secondary causes of ICH. A noncontrast CT scan is performed urgently. The most common locations for spontaneous ICH are:[4] lobar (40% to 50%), putamen (40%), cerebellum (5% to 10%), thalamus (5%), and pons (5%). Clues to the presence of a cerebral AVM or aneurysm are the presence of subarachnoid blood and location close to the circle of Willis, where aneurysm formation is most common. A clearly defined putamenal ICH without subarachnoid blood by CT in a hypertensive patient is almost certainly primary in nature and a cerebral angiogram is unwarranted. In contrast, a lobar hematoma close to the Sylvian fissure with surrounding subarachnoid blood should raise prompt suspicion of a middle cerebral artery aneurysm and lead to an urgent cerebral angiogram. Angiography is an invasive procedure which keeps a critically ill patient away from the ICU and perhaps definitive therapy until completion. It should be performed only when the history and CT findings support the possibility of vascular anomaly.

As discussed below, hematoma volume is the best predictor of outcome from ICH. As Figure 2 demonstrates, volume is estimated from CT by measuring the greatest diameter (A) of the hematoma and multiplying that by the perpendicular diameter at that location (B) and multiplying that product by the "thickness." The thickness based on the number of CT sections the hematoma is

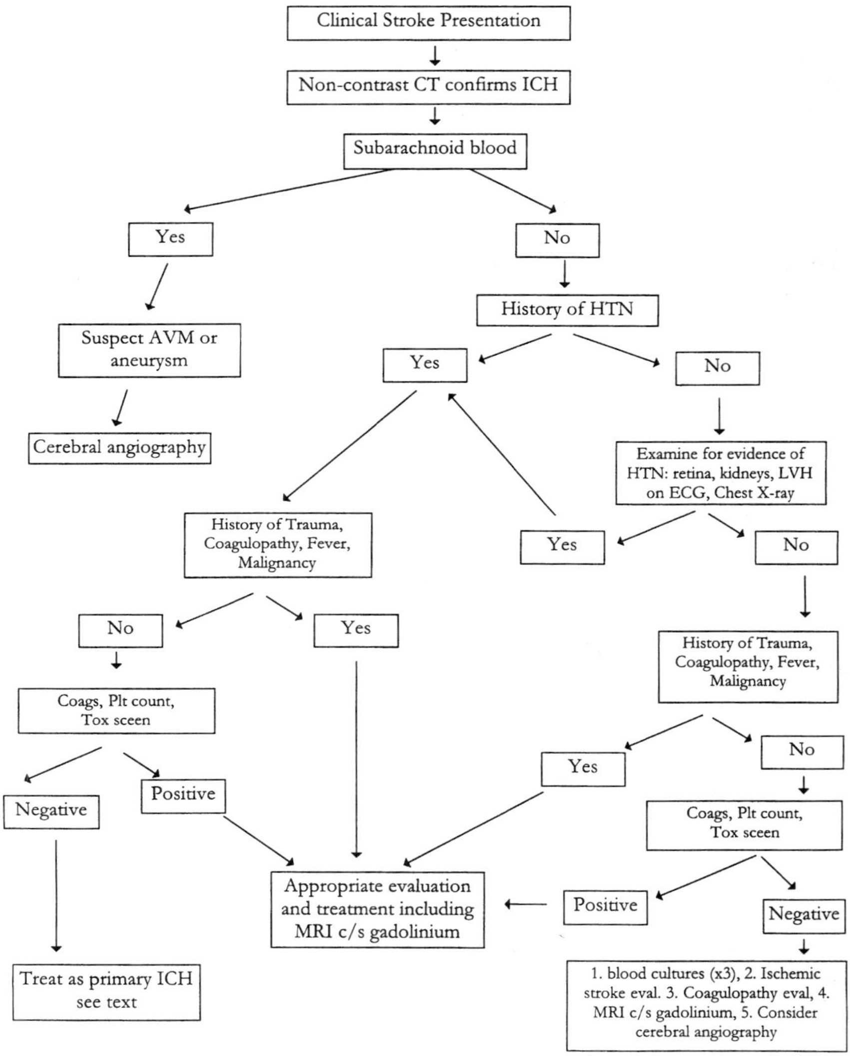

Figure 1 Diagnostic evaluation of patients with ICH.

clearly visualized and whether the slices are 5 mm or 1 cm cuts (C). This product (A × B × C) is then divided by 2 to yield the approximate volume of the hematoma, (A × B × C)/2. This method is simple, quick, and well validated.[13]

Particularly when a clear history is not found, but in all patients, we search hard for other secondary etiologies. All patients should have a complete blood count, platelets, protime, and partial thromboplastin time. History of coagulopathy or bleeding diathesis should prompt hematology consultation. We perform a toxicology screen in all patients and have been surprised by some of the results.

Frequently an MRI scan is performed in patients with ICH to search for underlying etiologies. This is frequently of little use. Blood obscures visualization of underlying structures during the first 3 to 6 weeks following hemorrhage. An AVM or tumor may be overlooked if an MRI is done too early. We review CT scans of "suspicious" ICHs with our neuroradiology colleagues and together decide if and when an MRI is indicated. Often delay saves money and yields a more accurate diagnosis. Of course, the diagnosis of vascular malformation or tumor should be made as promptly as possible. A cerebral angiogram may be most helpful in certain situations.

EMERGENCY DEPARTMENT MANAGEMENT

Symptoms and signs depend on the extent and localization of the ICH. Within the first few hours, ICHs often bring about a progressive deteriorating clinical course. There is a narrow time window of opportunity for treatments aimed at attenuation or reversal of brain injury.

Initial medical management of stroke patients at the scene begins with protection of the airway. The initial response in the treatment of an acute stroke must focus upon an approach similar to that advocated in *advanced cardiac and trauma life support* courses. The importance of controlling and securing the airways in patients with neurological emergencies cannot be overemphasized. The decision to intubate frequently seems more complex than it ought to be.[14]

Since the brain tolerates anoxia for only a short period, ventilation and oxygenation are the initial treatment goals. Control of the airway does not necessarily require endotracheal intubation, and physicians should be familiar with the various methods available to assure a patent, secured airway. In stroke patients it is usually not the difficulty breathing but the reduced ability to clear the airway, either due to impaired consciousness or brainstem dysfunction, that prompts endotracheal intubation. For many stroke patients, oropharyngeal and nasopharyngeal airways are most appropriate. The choice of either one depends on the presence of an intact gag reflex. The insertion technique for an oropharyngeal airway (size 3–5 for adults) involves opening the mouth and insertion of the airway approximately one-fourth of the way in a reverse position, then rotating it as further insertion takes place. Since this maneuver often induces the patient's gag reflex, a nasopharyngeal airway (size 7–8 for adults) may be better tolerated by a patient with intact gag reflex. Before inserting an oropharyngeal airway, the mouth and pharynx should be cleared of secretions using a rigid pharyngeal suction tip.

The advantages of endotracheal airways over oro- or nasopharyngeal airways include limiting aspiration, allowing for efficient ventilation and oxygenation, allowing for suctioning of trachea and bronchi, and providing a route of administration of some drugs. In conclusion, alert patients with intact gag reflex may be provided with supplementary oxygen via nasal cannula or face mask; with decreasing consciousness a naso- or oropharyngeal tube should be inserted, and with inability to protect the airway, endotracheal intubation is recommended.

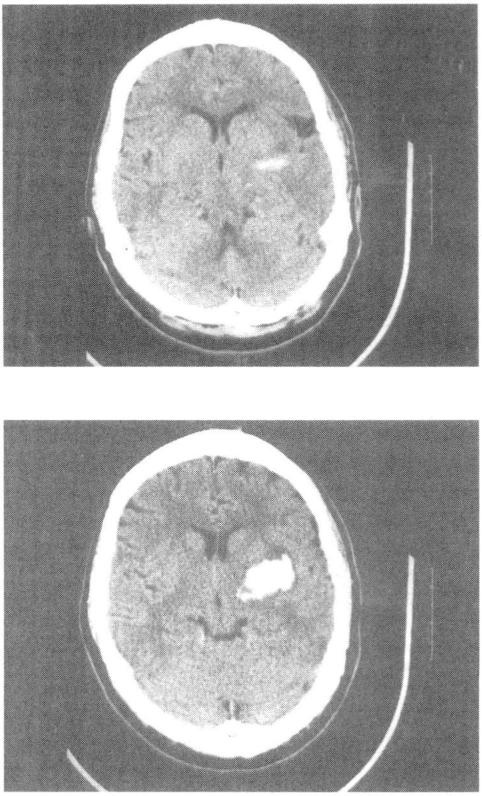

(a)

(b)

Figure 2 Noncontrast CT scan of a spontaneous hypertensive left putamenal ICH. Each hash mark on the scale to the right of each image is 1 cm. The volume of the hematoma is estimated by the (A × B × C)/ 2 method, where A = the greatest diameter (Fig. 2b), B = the diameter perpendicular to A, and C = the thickness measured as the number of CT slices where the hematoma is visualized (a-e) multiplied by slice thickness. CT slices are 1 cm on this scan. A = 4 cm , B = 2 cm, C = 5 cm; therefore hematoma volume is approximately 20 mL.

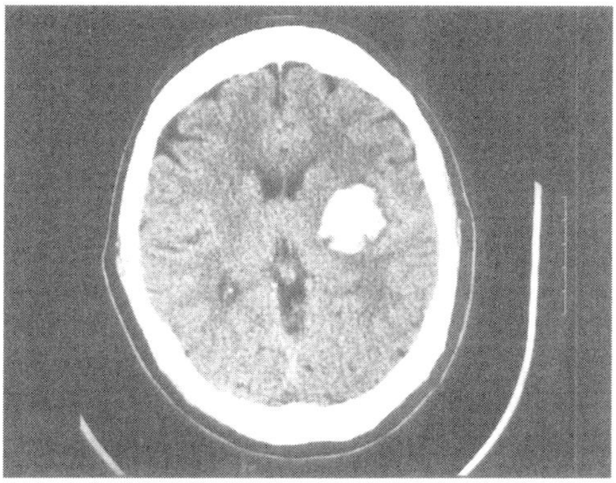

(c)

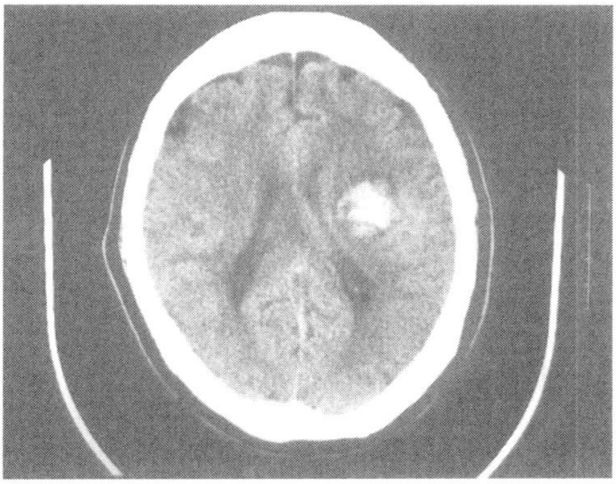

(d)

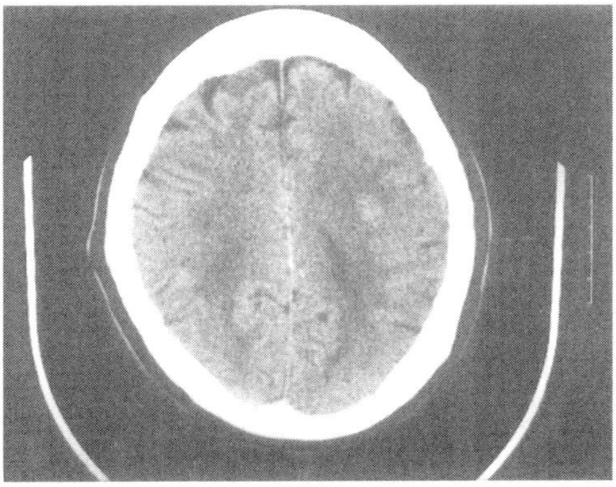

(e)

Medications used during endotracheal intubation vary somewhat depending upon the condition of the patient, familiarity of the physician, and availability. For acute stroke patients with presumably elevated ICP, a relatively rapid induction, using approximately 0.02 mg/kg pancuronium, followed by 100 mg succinylcholine, 2 to 3 mg/kg thiopental, and 75 mg lidocaine is recommended.[15,16] This combination of medication will blunt the rise of ICP and autonomic responses associated with intubation. If elevated ICP is not an issue, a combination of a short-acting benzodiazepine and fentanyl is usually sufficient. For stroke patients the decision whether to perform an orotracheal or nasotracheal intubation depends on the acuity of the neurological decline. Nasotracheal tubes are better tolerated in conscious patients; however, they require that the patient ventilate spontaneously during the procedure.

All patients should receive supplemental oxygen when first seen. Its prolonged use is guided by the degree of hypoxemia as indicated by blood gas analysis or pulse oximetry. In patients who require intubation the initial ventilator settings should be: intermittent mandatory ventilation (IMV) at 10 breaths/min; tidal volume (V_t) 10 cc/kg; fraction of oxygen (FiO_2) 1.0 (=100%); and pressure support of 7 to 10 cm H_2O. The IMV mode of ventilation will provide the patient with the minimal respiratory rate set, but the patient will be able to breathe additionally as necessary. The respiratory rate suggested for initial ventilator setting is a reasonable number to remember if the goal is to maintain normal CO_2.

Along with airway protection and oxygenation, circulation and cerebral perfusion support become necessary. Continued cerebral perfusion is vital due to the poor tolerance of neural tissue to ischemia. Cardiac output and blood pressure must be maintained using fluid resuscitation and pressor drugs. For the immediate situation until arrival in the emergency room, fluid replenishment with intravenous crystalloids in the range of 10 to 15 cc/kg normal saline is recommended.[17,18] In patients with a history of severe cardiomyopathy or congestive heart failure, and in those who display obvious rales upon chest auscultation, fluid replenishment should be withheld until arrival and assessment in the emergency room.

In the emergency room the diagnosis of ICH needs to be established by noncontrast brain CT. Concomitantly, serum chemistry, coagulation studies, urine analysis, EKG, and chest x-ray should be obtained emergently. Monitoring of fluid management includes possible placement of a central venous line to guide fluid replenishment and insertion of a Foley catheter to record urine output. A continuous blood pressure recording using an arterial line is indicated in all patients with abnormal blood pressure readings in the field. Approximately 10% to 20% of ICHs are reported to develop seizures.[19–21] Currently, some advocate treating patients with antiepileptics preventively, using fosphenytoin, loading dose 20 mg/kg and continuation according to serum levels.

The emergency management of patients with ICH depends largely on their clinical status; thus, neurological examination must be carried out expeditiously to establish the level of function. The neurological exam should be practically focused to determine the level of consciousness as well as motor and language performance. This is also the time to interview members of the family, inquiring about specific pieces of information necessary to decide on the further management of the patient. According to current practice and knowledge, we recommend consideration of the following guidelines on specific management in patients with ICH. (1) Patients need to be admitted to a critical care unit for close observation and immediate repeat CT if the patient's neurologic status declines; (2) if present, coagulation abnormalities need to be corrected; (3) in the event of occlusive hydrocephalus and depressed level of consciousness, a ventriculostomy should be performed; and (4) urgent surgical evacuation is indicated individually on the basis of size, location, and etiology of hemorrhage, neurological status, and comorbidity (see surgical section).

BLOOD PRESSURE MANAGEMENT AND RECURRENCE

A controversial point regards the management of blood pressure in patients with acute ICH in the emergency department and intensive care unit. While it is now accepted that blood pressure control in patients with subarachnoid hemorrhage and an unclipped aneurysm is critical to prevent rebleeding, no such consensus exists for ICH. Theoretically, since the mechanism of ICH is thought to be rupture of a microaneursym or rupture of a weakened vessel, continued hypertension may increase the chance of recurrent hemorrhage. Indeed, studies have demonstrated that 14% to 33% of ICHs expand if measured within the first 6 hours after symptom onset.[22,23] The problem is that the data to support an etiologic role of hypertension in early hematoma extension is lacking. In fact, Mayer et al.[24] demonstrated that level of blood pressure in the emergency department did not predict which patients with ICH worsen. Blood pressure also did not correlate with hematoma expansion or clinical deterioration in recent studies.[23,25,26] One study did find that presenting blood pressure and poor early control correlated with worse outcome.[27] This study selected 87 of the 378 patients with ICH at a large urban hospital and performed a retrospective analysis. This study has been criticized[28] for methodologic reasons; its conclusions, while hypothesis generating, are dubious at best.

Opponents to lowering blood pressure in acute ICH point to ischemic stroke as a model for the hazards of decreasing blood pressure in the acute stroke patient.[29] Since patients with chronic hypertension autoregulate so that higher blood pressures are necessary to drive cerebral blood flow, precipitously lowering blood pressure to a "normal range" in acute stroke may decrease cerebral blood flow to a critical level in patients with ICH. Researchers are becoming increasingly aware that part of the pathophysiology of cerebral injury in ICH is regional brain ischemia caused by the hematoma, which compresses surrounding vascular structures, and vasoconstrictive properties inherent in hematoma fluid.[30] These areas, which already receive only borderline perfusion, may become necrotic if cerebral blood flow is further compromised by acutely lowering blood pressure.

While the debate rages, these theoretical concepts drive our therapy at the bedside. We treat the patient rather than the numbers. Patients with chronic hypertension and acute ICH do well with modest blood pressure control (10% to 15% over 12 to 24 hours) with a mean arterial pressure goal of 110 to 130 depending on initial blood pressure readings. We use agents such as intravenous labetalol, enalapril, and nicardipine which have smooth onset and easy titration. We avoid nifedipine, because it can lower blood pressure too quickly. We also avoid sodium nitroprusside and other nitrates due to their theoretical ability to increase cerebral edema.

DEFINITIVE THERAPY

Therapy for ICH is largely supportive. Efforts to rigorously test specific therapies for clot removal and pharmacotherapy have only recently come to the forefront of stroke research. We will consider both surgical and nonsurgical approaches. As we comment at the end of this section, the possibility of combining these approaches is likely to hold the greatest hope for ICH treatment.

Surgery

In a population-based study in Cincinnati, Broderick et al. reported that only 34 of the 188 ICH patients underwent surgical treatment.[31] Only 15 of the 34 had surgery within 12 hours of symptom onset. In Houston,[32] we have reported the results of a prospective study of 58 patients who received either early clot evacuation or best medical therapy. The last 26 of these patients were randomized in a single-site clinical trial of early surgery versus best medical therapy. We defined "early surgery" by evacuation within 12 hours of symptom onset. Open craniotomy was used in all surgical cases.

Our preliminary results suggested that early surgery decreased mortality by 18% (27% vs. 9%) in our randomized group at 1 month, but that functional outcome was unchanged by surgery in survivors at 1 month. We have continued to add to these small numbers and will soon reexamine our data with our larger sample size.

Other studies generally support such conclusions. Volpin[33] in a retrospective study found that surgery on comatose patients with ICH volumes between 26 and 85 ml improved survival. The timing of surgery was not reported. In a prospective study, Juvela[34] found no surgical benefit with late surgery (within 48 hours) except in severely impaired patients who had better survival with surgery but no functional improvement. Batjer[35] performed a clinical trial on putamenal ICH including patients presenting to the emergency department within 24 hours of symptom onset. After 21 patients the study was stopped without any surgical benefit shown.

Timing may be the key. As we discussed previously, investigators have recently turned their attention to regional ischemia in the area around an ICH. We know from animal models and human studies on acute ischemic stroke that the therapeutic time window to salvage ischemic neurons is on the order of 6 hours. Perhaps early clot evacuation may reduce regional ischemia. In a retrospective review of 100 patients treated with open craniotomy within 7 hours of symptom onset, Kaneko et al.[36]report an impressive 7% mortality rate and good outcome in 35%.

Newer surgical techniques including stereotactic and endoscopic surgery are receiving increasing attention.[37] The instillation of thrombolytic material directly into the hematoma, while counterintuitive on initial glance, may lead to clot lysis and decompression.[38]

A recommendation for surgical referral is therefore based on small trials. Before the results of a multicenter clinical trial are obtained, discussions with patients and families cannot be dogmatic. We feel the evidence reviewed above suggests that if clot evacuation is offered it should be done early, certainly within 12 hours of onset, but "the earlier the better." We explain to families that while this procedure may be life saving, the quality of life in the survivor may be extremely poor. We restrict recommending surgery to patients who have a 30-cc or larger hematoma and significant dysfunction: either motor, speech, or level of consciousness.

Experimental Therapy

If surgery alone is not the entire answer, perhaps other therapies may add promise. One strategy now being considered is combining surgery with anti-ischemic therapy. We will need to await the results of neuroprotective trials in ischemic stroke to see the first agent proven effective. Kanno et al [39] have used hyperbaric oxygen and early surgery in combination to treat patients with ICH. There is a great potential to combine a variety of agents and surgical procedures, intravenous and locally, both before, during and after surgery.

CRITICAL CARE MANAGEMENT OF THE ICH PATIENT

The critical care management of patients with ICH aims at cerebral perfusion support, fine-tuning of fluid replacement, and management of increased ICP (see Table 2). Neurocritical care management in patients with ICH also includes the perioperative management, control of complications, and selection of patients for specific strategies. Since none of the various approaches has been sufficiently tested for efficacy in prospective trials, currently, firm recommendations for specific strategies cannot be made.

Hemostatic Agents

If the patient has a coagulopathy, it must be reversed as soon as possible. In many instances, coagulopathic states in patients with ICH can be inferred from the CT, demonstrating a blood level within the hematoma usually not seen with primary ICH. Blood should be drawn to measure hematocrit, hemoglobin, partial thromboplastin time, prothrombin time/INR, platelet count, and fibrinogen. Fresh-frozen plasma and vitamin K should be used for patients on coumadin therapy. Effects of heparin can be neutralized by an infusion of protamine. Four to six units of cryoprecipitate or fresh-frozen plasma, and 1 U of single donor platelets are recommended for ICH patients on thrombolytic agents.[40] Patients with known factor deficiencies, such as hemophilia, must receive their deficient factor or fresh-frozen plasma. Patients with known platelet disorders such as leukemia should receive platelet transfusions. Patients on aspirin or other antiplatelet agents should discontinue taking them but do not need platelet transfusion. It is thought that further increase of hematoma volume and recurrence of ICH may be prevented by these measures.[41]

Cerebral Perfusion Support and Fluid Resuscitation

Under normal conditions, most of the blood constituents do not affect the cerebral vessels owing to the presence of the blood-brain barrier, which limits their

Table 2 Therapeutic Management of Intracranial Hypertension with ICH[a]

1. Osmotherapy
2. Hyperventilation
3. Surgical treatment
   a. evacuation of ICH with impending transtentorial herniation
   b. ventriculostomy for hydrocephalus occlusus accompanying ICH
   c. early evacuation of ICH with size >30 cc (?)

[a]For details see text.

access to the vascular smooth muscle. In contrast, oxygen and CO_2 diffuse freely across this barrier. Arterial hypercapnia and hypoxia will result in arterial dilatation, hypocapnia, and vasoconstriction. It has been demonstrated experimentally that the blood-brain barrier is defective in the vicinity of the ICH, thus allowing for transfer of various blood constituents that may alter regional blood flow regulation.[42] Cerebral blood flow studies in human traumatic and nontraumatic ICH indicate an altered blood flow surrounding the hematoma.[43,44]

In general, cerebral perfusion pressure (CPP) is maintained within a range of 60 to 160 torr. Below 60 torr, vasodilatation of the cerebral arterioles is maximal and cerebral blood flow becomes linearly and directly dependent upon CPP. Above 160 torr, the microvasculature is maximally constricted, and sustained hypertension will lead to fragmentation of the endothelial surfaces with a rise in arterial resistance and decline in cerebral blood flow. The CPP is determined by the difference between mean arterial blood pressure (MAP) and the sum of the cerebral venous pressure (CVP) plus the intracranial pressure (ICP). Under normal conditions the CVP (5 torr supine) and the ICP (10 to 15 torr supine) are negligible and the MAP is the major determinant of the CPP. Arteriolar MAP minus ICP represents the perfusion pressure at the capillary bed. Therefore, in brain tissue surrounding ICH with already altered regional blood flow, small changes in systemic blood pressure may be precarious and put this tissue at further risk for demise.

Currently, the principal variable subjective to manipulation is the MAP. Crystalloids and colloids can be used to increase the intravascular volume . Crystalloids are solutions that contain sodium as their major osmotically active agent (normal saline or Ringer's lactate). In healthy adults approximately a quarter of the volume of isotonic crystalloids administered as a bolus will remain in the intravascular space within 30 minutes. In patients with either increased capillary permeability or hypoalbuminemia the portion that remains intravascularly may be much less. Colloids, on the other hand, due to their high osmotic activity, are fluids with a greater tendency to remain confined to the intravascular space (albumin 5% and 25%, dextran 40 and 70, hydroxyethyl starch). In order to manage the intravascular volume to enhance cerebral blood flow a number of hemodynamic variables need to be considered.

State of hydration and adequacy of cardiac function can be roughly inferred from either the central venous pressure, pulmonary wedge pressure, or right ventricular end-diastolic volume. In patients with ICH on the critical care unit we prefer the use of colloids in combination with furosemide as a first line of defense to treat mass effect. The main advantage of colloids plus furosemide over mannitol is that the latter dehydrates the intravascular space to a greater degree, whereas colloids have a tendency to conserve intravascular volume. In patients with significant ICH the target minimum of CPP is >70 torr. If volume expansion (pulmonary wedge pressure of 14 to 16 torr) is insufficient to maintain CPP, vasopressors are added. A combination of dopamine (at 2 μg/kg/min) and phenylephrine is best suited to promote MAP.

Management of Intracranial Hypertension

Brain edema begins to develop in the vicinity of the hematoma within the first several hours after onset. Mass effect from the hematoma with adjacent edema may have deleterious effects including transtentorial herniation, the most serious consequence after ICH. The majority of acute deaths within the first few days after ICH result from these processes. The requirement of a constant monitoring device is controversial.[45,46] Currently, we suggest utilization of either a fiber optic intraparenchymal pressure device or a frontal ventriculostomy in patients with clinical deterioration to a GCS <9 secondary to presumed elevated ICP.

To facilitate clinical management, patients with significant intracranial hypertension are best intubated. Depending on the evolution of the underlying mass effect, sedation (the use of propofol is recommended) and additional paralysis (the use of intermittent or continuous vecuronium is recommended) may be required. The ventilator is generally set at tidal volumes of 8 to 10 cc/kg (ideal weight) at rates of 10 to 12 breaths per minute. A minimum of 5 cm H_2O of PEEP and the minimum FiO_2 to maintain SaO_2>90% is advocated. Minute ventilation is adjusted to maintain $PaCO_2$ between 35 to 40 torr. The use of hyperventilation is not recommended unless intracranial hypertension cannot be controlled with osmotherapy alone and the patient is considered a candidate for surgery.[47,48] The same applies for the use of barbiturates that may be helpful to prevent progression in those patients awaiting emergency hematoma evacuation. If hyperventilation is intended, respiratory rate may have to be increased to rates between 14 and 18 breaths per minute and titrated to results of arterial blood gases. Prolonged periods of hyperventilation should be avoided since cerebral vasoconstriction aggravates ischemic brain injury.

Steroids, widely used for reducing brain edema in patients with brain tumors, have failed to show benefit with strokes.[49,50] There is no improvement in 21-day mortality with steroids; additionally, the rate of complications, mostly infection and deterioration of diabetes mellitus, are significantly increased with steroids.

Another controversial issue regarding treatment of patients with intracranial hypertension is the position of the head. Although traditionally elevated 30°, it can be argued that the reduction in venous pressure induced by head elevation at the level of the superior sagittal sinus may be counteracted by the concomitant reduction in hydrostatic carotid artery pressure.[51]

Hyperosmolar agents such as mannitol and glycerol are reported to be potential agents for reducing brain edema. The intravenous infusion of 200 mL 10%

glycerol over 30 minutes significantly increases cerebral blood flow in the affected hemisphere in patients with acute ICH.[52] Glycerol doses of 0.2 to 1.0 g/kg/h leading to plasma concentrations of 10 to 30 mOsm/L are necessary to control ICP in patients with cerebral edema.[53] A 20% mannitol solution administered intravenously (5 to 15 mL/kg) induces a rapid but transient decrease in elevated ICP. The agent causes initial systemic hypervolemia followed by extensive diuresis. The onset of action is only minutes for mannitol but may be up to 3 hours for glycerol; the duration of action lasts up to 6 to 9 hours for mannitol, and 10 hours for glycerol. A 10% solution of glycerol in saline (200 mL in 2 h q6–12 h) acts more slowly and mildly than mannitol does. With hyperosmolar agents attention should be paid to acute pulmonary edema, dehydration, and electrolyte imbalance. In addition, rebound ICP increases may occur hours after administration (less likely with glycerol).

Control of Complications

ICH is often complicated by respiratory and urinary tract infection. Body postures should be changed at appropriate intervals, and patients with ICP crises requiring paralysis should be rested at a Rotorest bed. An indwelling urinary catheter is necessary in all patients with ICH subject to manipulation of the intravascular volume. When infections are suspected, empiric antibiotic coverage is implemented while cultures are pending.

Although no specific risk factor can be identified, gastrointestinal complications are a prevalent complication in acutely brain-injured patients. In a consecutive series of 19 patients with severe head injury, 15 patients had some and 7 cases had marked incidence of gastrointestinal hemorrhage.[54] We suggest H_2-channel blocker, or proton-pump inhibitors, for all patients treated on a critical care unit for serious ICH.

The syndrome of inappropriate secretion of antidiuretic hormone is fairly common in patients with acute ICH. It is characterized by an excess of sodium excretion into the urine associated with a low plasma concentration. Although hyponatremia may exacerbate brain edema, correction should be made gradually by restricting the water intake and, only if unsuccessful, loading salt, or with furosemide administration.

Epilepsy complicates ICH. Development of persistent seizures appears to correlate with the extent of brain injury. Although early reports suggested that prophylactic administration of antiepileptic drugs would prevent epileptogenesis, controlled studies have failed to corroborate this assumption. In patients with severe head injury, the presence of an intracranial hematoma has a robust association with the development of posttraumatic epilepsy.[55] Treatment strategies for prevention or prophylaxis of symptomatic epilepsy after ICH must await absolute knowledge of mechanisms. As already discussed in the emergency treatment section, currently, some recommend preventive antiepileptic therapy for a period of 4 weeks after onset. Antiepileptic therapy is then continued after this period in the presence of EEG evidence for seizure activity or if clinically warranted.

PROGNOSIS

Outcome from spontaneous supratentorial ICH has received some attention. These predictors are basically natural history studies since early surgery was utilized in only a trivial number of patients. Tuhrim et al.[56] have validated two models of predicting mortality from ICH based on clinical presentation. The simpler, which involves hematoma volume, Glascow Coma Scale (GCS), and pulse pressure, has a good sensitivity and specificity. This and other models require calculation from a predictive equation.[57,58] Broderick et al.[59] found that only 1 of 71 patients with hematoma volume >30 cc recovered to functional independence. Hematoma volume and ventricular extension are recognized as the best overall predictors of outcome.[26,60]

REFERENCES

1. Thrift AG, Donnan GA, McNeil JJ. Epidemiology of intracerebral hemorrhage. Epidemiol Rev 1995; 17:361–381.
2. Juvela S. Risk factors for spontaneous intracerebral hemorrhage. Stroke. 1995; 26:1558–1564.
3. Morgenstern LB, Spears WD. A triethnic comparison of intracerebral hemorrhage mortality in Texas. Ann Neurol 1997; 42:919–923.
4. Wityk RJ, Caplan LR. Hypertensive intracerebral hemorrhage. Epidemiology and clinical pathology. Neurosurg Clin North Am 1992; 3:521–532.
5. Juvela S. Risk factors for impaired outcome after spontaneous intracerebral hemorrhage. Arch Neurol. 1995; 52:1193–1200.
6. Juvela S. Prevalence of risk factors in spontaneous intracerebral hemorrhage and aneurysmal subarachnoid hemorrhage. Arch Neurol. 1996; 53:734–740.
7. Greenberg SM, Briggs ME, Hyman BT, et al. Apolipoprotein E e4 is associated with the presence and earlier onset of hemorrhage in cerebral amyloid angiopathy. Stroke 1996; 27:1333–1337.
8. Levine SR, Brust JCM, Futrell N, et al. A comparative study of the cerebrovascular complications of cocaine: alkaloidal versus hydrochloride—a review. Neurology 1991; 41:1173–1177.
9. Kibayashi K, Mastri AR, Hirsch CS. Cocaine induced intracerebral hemorrhage: analysis of predisposing factors and mechanisms causing hemorrhagic strokes. Hum Pathol 1995; 26:659–663.

10. The National Institute of Neurological Disorders and Stroke rt-PA Stroke Study Group. Tissue plasminogen activator for acute ischemic stroke. N Engl J Med 1995; 333:1581–1587.
11. Vastergaard K, Andersen G, Nielsen MI, Jensen TS. Headache in stroke. Stroke. 1993; 24:1621–1624.
12. Jorgensen HS, Jespersen HF, Nakayama H, et al. Headache in stroke: the Copenhagen stroke study. Neurology 1994; 44:1793–1797.
13. Kothari RU, Brott T, Broderick JP, et al. The ABCs of measuring intracerebral hemorrhage volumes. Stroke. 1996; 27:1304–1305.
14. Marino PL. Tubes, blowouts, and the occult. In: Marino PL, ed. The ICU Book. Philadelphia: Lea and Febiger, 1991:383–390.
15. Van Aken H, Van Hemelrijck J. An overview of the influence of anesthesia on cerebral blood flow and cerebral metabolism. Minerva Anestesiol 1993; 59:615–20.
16. Hacke W, Stingele R, Steiner T, Schuchardt V, Schwab S. Critical care of acute ischemic stroke. Intens Care Med 1995; 21(10):856–862.
17. Frank JI. Management of intracranial hypertension. Med Clin North Am 1993; 77(1):61–76.
18. Andrews BT. Fluid and electrolyte disorders in neurosurgical intensive care. Neurosurg Clin North Am 1994; 5:707–23.
19. Ropper AH, Davis KR. Lobar cerebral hemorrhages: acute clinical syndromes in 26 cases. Ann Neurol 1980; 8:141–147.
20. Kase CS, Williams JP, Wyatt DA, Mohr JP. Lobar intracerebral hematomas. Clinical and CT analysis of 22 cases. Neurology 1982; 32:1146–1150.
21. Faught E, Peters D, Bartolucci A, Moore L, Miller PC. Seizures after primary intracerebral hemorrhage. Neurology 1989; 39:1089–1090.
22. Brott T, Brodrick J, Kothari R, et al. Early hemorrhage growth in patients with intracerebral hemorrhage. Stroke 1997; 28:1–5.
23. Fujii Y, Tanaka R, Takeuchi S, et al. Hematoma enlargement in spontaneous intracerebral hemorrhage. J Neurosurg. 1994; 80:51–57.
24. Mayer SA, Sacco RL, Shi T, Mohr JP. Neurologic deterioration in noncomatose patients with supratentorial intracerebral hemorrhage. Neurology. 1994; 44:1379–1384.
25. Mayer SA. Hematoma enlargement in intracerebral hemorrhage. J Neurosurg 1994; 81:333 (letter).
26. Qureshi AI, Safdar K, Weil EJ, et al. Predictors of early deterioration and mortality in black americans with spontaneous intracerebral hemorrhage. Stroke 1995; 26:1764–1767.
27. Dandapani B, Suzuki S, Kelley RE, et al. Relation between blood pressure and outcome in intracerebral hemorrhage. Stroke 1995; 26:21–24.
28. Leys D, Mounier-Vehier F, Mounier-Vehier C, Carre A. Relationship between blood pressure and outcome in intracerebral hemorrhage. Stroke 1995; 26:1126–1127 (letter).
29. Powers WJ. Acute hypertension after stroke: the scientific basis for treatment decisions. Neurology. 1993; 43:461–467.
30. Mendelow AD. Mechanisms of ischemic brain damage with intracerebral hemorrhage. Stroke 1993; 24(suppl I):115–117.

31. Broderick J, Brott T, Tomsick T, et al. Management of intracerebral hemorrhage in a large metropolitan population. Neurosurgery 1994; 34:882–887.
32. Morgenstern LB, Pasteur W, Grotta JC. Randomized trial of early surgery for hemispheric intracerebral hemorrhage. Stroke. 1996; 27:195 (abstract).
33. Volpin L, Cervellini P, Colombo F, et al. Spontaneous intracerebral hematomas: a new proposal about the usefulness and limits of surgical treatment. Neurosurgery 1984; 15:663– 666.
34. Juvela S, Heiskanen O, Poranen A, et al. The treatment of spontaneous intracerebral hemorrhage. A prospective randomized trial of surgical and conservative treatment. J Neurosurg 1989; 70:755–758.
35. Batjer HH, Reisch JS, Allen BC, et al. Failure of surgery to improve outcome in hypertensive putaminal hemorrhage. Arch Neurol 1990; 47:1103–1106.
36. Kaneko M, Tanaka K, Shimada T, et al. Long-term evaluation of ultra-early operation for hypertensive intracerebral hemorrhage in 100 cases. J Neurosurg 1983; 58:838–842.
37. Auer LM, Deinsberger W, Niederkorn K, et al. Endoscopic surgery versus medical treatment for spontaneous intracerebral hematoma: a randomized study. J Neurosurg 1989; 70:530–535.
38. Schaller C, Rohde V, Meyer B, Hassler W. Stereotactic puncture and lysis of spontaneous intracerebral hemorrhage using recombinant tissue-plasminogen activator. Neurosurgery 1995; 36:328–335.
39. Kanno T, Nagata J, Nonomura K, et al. New approaches in the treatment of hypertensive intracerebral hemorrhage. Stroke 1993; 24(suppl I):96–100.
40. Adams HP, Brott TG, Furlan AJ et al. Guidelines for thrombolytic therapy for acute stroke: a supplement to the guidelines for the management of patients with acute ischemic stroke. Circulation 1996; 94:1167–1174.
41. Feldmann E. Intracerebral hemorrhage. Curr Concepts Cerebrovasc Dis Stroke 1991; 26:1–6.
42. Jenkins A, Mendelow D, Graham D, Nath F, Teasdale G. Experimental intracerebral haematoma: the role of blood constituents in early ischemia. Br J Neurosurg 1990; 4:45– 51.
43. Sills C, Villar-Cordova C, Pasteur W, et al. Demonstration of hypoperfusion surrounding intracerebral hematoma in humans. J Stroke Cerebrovasc Dis 1996; 1:17–24.
44. McLaughlin MR, Marion DW. Cerebral blood flow and vasoresponsivity within and around cerebral contusions. J Neurosurg 1996; 85:871–876.
45. Frank J. Large hemispheric infarction, deterioration, and intracranial pressure. Neurology 1995; 45:1286–1290.
46. Schwab S, Aschoff A, Spranger M, Albert F, Hacke W. The value of ICP monitoring in acute hemispheric stroke. Neurology 1996; 47:393–398.
47. Fortune JB, Feustel PJ, Graca L, Hasselbarth J, Kuehler DH. Effect of hyperventilation, mannitol, and ventriculostomy drainage on cerebral blood flow after head injury. J Trauma 1995; 39:1091–1097.
48. Van Santbrink H, Maas AJR, Avezaat CJJ. Continuous monitoring of partial pressure of brain tissue oxygen in patients with severe head injury. Neurosurgery 1996; 38:21–31.

49. Norris JW, Hachinski VC. High dose steroid treatment in cerebral infarction. Br Med J 1986; 292:21–23.
50. Poungvarin N, Bhoopat W, Viriyavejakul A, et al. Effects of dexamethasone in primary supratentorial intracerebral hemorrhage. N Engl J Med 1987; 316:1229–1233.
51. Feldman Z, Kanter MJ, Robertson CS, Contant CF, Hayes C, Sheinberg MA, Villareal CA, Narayan RK, Grossman RG. Effect of head elevation on intracranial pressure, cerebral perfusion pressure, and cerebral blood flow in head injured patients. J Neurosurg 1992; 77:651–652.
52. Sasaki T, Matsuzaki T, Nakagawa J, et al. Improvement of CBF by glycerol administration in hypertensive intracerebral hemorrhage. Brain Nerve (Tokyo) 1983; 35:505–510.
53. Pitlick WH, Pirikitakuhlr P, Painter MJ, Wessel HB. Effect of glycerol and hyperosmolality on intracranial pressure. Clin PharmTher 1982; 31:466–471.
54. Gudeman SK, Wheeler CB, Miller JD, Halloran LG, Becker DP. Gastric secretory and mucosal injury response to severe head trauma. Neurosurgery 1983; 12:175–179.
55. Willmore LJ. Post-traumatic epilepsy: cellular mechanisms and implications for treatment. Epilepsia 1990; 31(suppl 3):67–73.
56. Tuhrim S, Horowitz DR, Sacher M, Godbold JH. Validation and comparison of models predicting survival following intracerebral hemorrhage. Crit Care Med 1995; 23:950–954.
57. Mase G, Zorzon M, Biasutti E, et al. Immediate prognosis of primary intracerebral hemorrhage using an easy model for the prediction of survival. Acta Neurol Scand 1995; 91:306–309.
58. Lisk DR, Pasteur W, Rhoades H, et al. Early presentation of hemispheric intracerbral hemorrhage: prediction of outcome and guidelines for treatment allocation. Neurology 1994; 44:133–139.
59. Broderick JP, Brott TG, Duldner JE, et al. Volume of intracerebral hemorrhage. A powerful and easy-to-use predictor of 30-day mortality. Stroke 1993; 24:987–993.
60. Radberg JA, Olsson JE, Radberg CT. Prognostic parameters in spontaneous intracerebral hematomas with special reference to anticoagulant treatment. Stroke 1991; 22:571–576.

21

Misrepresentations, Extrapolations, and Problems in the Use of Aspirin in Stroke Prevention

Henry J. M. Barnett
The John P. Roberts Research Institute, London, Ontario, Canada

An extraordinarily powerful medication, as readily available as chewing gum, frequently goes on sale in supermarkets for less than 1¢ per pill. Aspirin is inexpensive, ubiquitous, and in most countries is the staple remedy for the relief of pain. Its popularity has persisted over the past 100 years. Now, for 25 years it has been recognized as an antithrombotic drug because of its antiplatelet properties. The little headache pill has come to play an important role in preventing or at least delaying two of our commonest causes of death: heart attack and ischemic stroke.

Misrepresentations and extrapolations have confused the progress of our understanding of the role of aspirin in stroke prevention. At first there was an understandable skepticism that an over-the-counter drug had sufficient potency to reduce substantially major morbidity and mortality from the commonest vascular diseases. A former Canadian provincial deputy minister of health was heard in the early 1980s to interrupt a conversation relating to aspirin in this new role by remarking: "But isn't this use of aspirin little more than a joke?" Most recently a 1997 article by a science writer in The Economist has epitomized this tendency to misstatement.[1] The expressions of uncritical and poorly informed opinions have probably helped to perpetuate, at least with the public, the continuing confusion. In the aforementioned article, the importance of aspirin's antithrombotic role was not minimized, but the facts were jumbled and the writer perpetuated some misleading statements. He attributed the interest in aspirin's antithrombotic usefulness to three sequential events:

1. The report began by stating that the interest in the antithrombotic usefulness of aspirin dated back to 1971, when Sir John Vane determined that aspirin "blocked the production of postglandins from platelets and endothelial cells." He went on to say that this led to the Physicians Health Study.

2. The Economist story stated that in the Physicians Health Study of 22,000 male U.S. doctors, one tablet of aspirin daily had been shown to cut the incidence of heart attacks by half, and established that "the drug can also prevent thrombosis and strokes."

3. The article stated that based on these observations, "Peto and Collins in 1988 and 1994 confirmed the benefit of aspirin by meta-analyses."

The first of these statements suggests that pathophysiological and clinical observations were in an orderly sequence to the biochemical and physiological studies which established the inhibition by aspirin of prostaglandin production in the platelet and of the production in the endothelial cell of prostacyclin. The facts of this interesting saga are quite different and are sketched out herewith.

Fisher noted in 1959 that recurrent amaurosis fugax was due to platelet-fibrin embolism.[2] Mustard and his colleagues in 1965 discovered that sulfinpyrazone altered platelet survival.[3] In the same year the platelet-inhibiting properties of dipyridamole were reported.[4] Mustard and colleagues in Toronto in 1967 and Weiss in New York in the same year noted that platelet aggregation in the presence of collagen was inhibited by aspirin.[5,6]

Despite the inference in the Economist article, clinical studies did not wait for the biochemical and physiological determination of the mode of action of the platelet-inhibiting drugs. In 1969 Acheson and Hutchinson reported on the negative effect of dipyridamole in reducing stroke.[7] Harrison and Marshall in 1971 published intriguing observations based on the treatment of two patients with amaurosis fugax whose events were remarkably reduced during aspirin administration[8] (Fig. 1) Their two-case publication stands as a remarkable example of the occasional penetrating insight which may ensue from the lowly case report. These observations and the report by Mundall et al. in 1972 of aspirin benefit in a single patient with recurrent amaurosis fugax in association with thrombocytosis constituted the pilot studies to form the basis for large clinical trials.[9] Even before the publication of these case reports Mustard urged the author of this article to launch a randomized trial of aspirin in patients with TIA and minor stroke, including those with amaurosis and hemisphere events. The planning began in 1970, the first patient entered in 1971, and the results were published in 1978.[10] Randomization involved 585 patients in a study of factorial design. In the patients in the aspirin-containing arms of the trial, 1,300 mg aspirin daily was shown to reduce the relative risk of stroke and death by 31%. In the subgroup of men alone, for stroke and death this reduction was 51%, and no benefit was detected for women (Fig. 2). This gender difference appears now to be related to the rela-

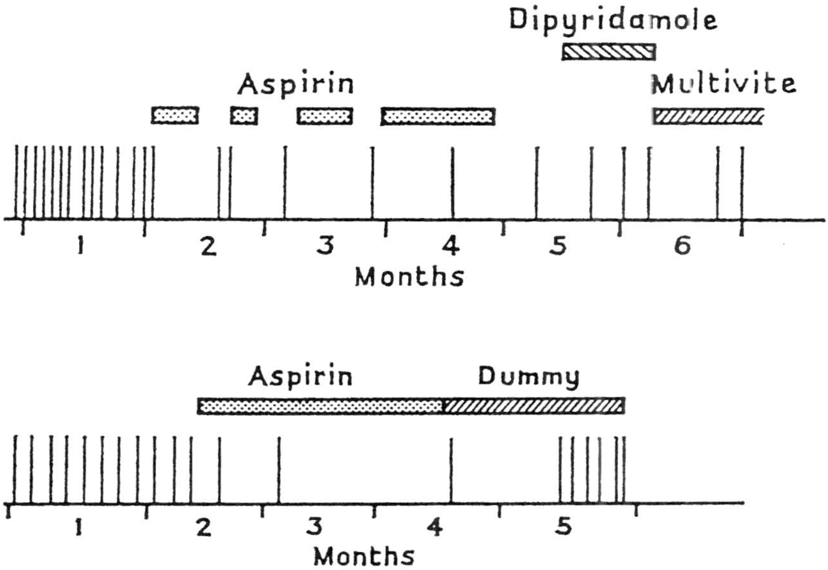

Figure 1 Two patients with multiple recurrent attacks of amaurosis fugax experienced a decreased number of events with the administration of 600 mg aspirin, not with dipyridamole (150 mg), multivitamins, or placebo. The earliest "pilot study" in 1971 of aspirin therapy. (From Ref. 8.)

tively better prognosis enjoyed by women after TIA or minor stroke.[11] The Canadian study had too few female subjects and it is likely that a type II error ensued. Subsequent trials have detected benefit for women at a rate below that for men. Nevertheless, aspirin is effective in both sexes.

The Harrison and Marshall "pilot study" and the Canadian Cooperative Study began at about the same time as the very preliminary experimental observations on the inhibition of prostaglandins by aspirin were being made and published.[12] The first human observation evaluating the effect of aspirin upon prostaglandin levels involved three patient volunteers who were each given 600 mg of aspirin. The later discovery of prostacyclin was based on observations published by Moncado, Vane, and associates just about the time that the Canadian trial was concluding.[13]

The next statement from The Economist, that one aspirin a day prevents heart attack and stroke, is distorted. The Physicians Health Study in fact did not administer one tablet of aspirin per day. Instead all subjects in the trial were randomized to receive 325 mg aspirin or placebo every other day.[4] There was a

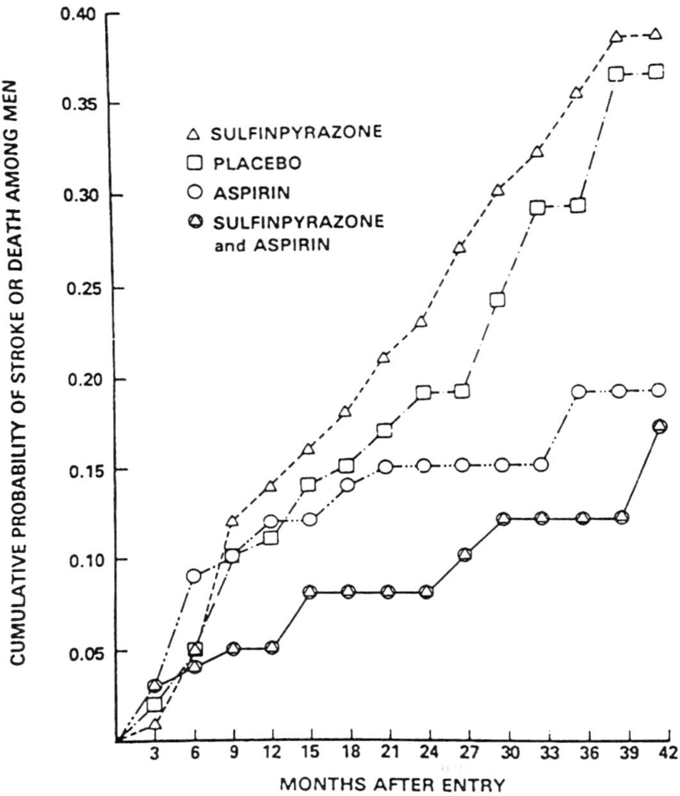

Figure 2 Cumulative probability of stroke or death among men in the Canadian Cooperative Study. The placebo and sulfinpyrazone groups had similar survival curves; the aspirin-containing groups fared significantly better. (From Ref. 10.)

substantial reduction in fatal and nonfatal myocardial infarction (44%), but it is inaccurate to claim that stroke reduction was observed (Table 1). Some, including the author of this chapter, believe that because of this failure and for a number of other reasons, the correct dose of aspirin to be utilized in stroke prevention is unknown and the question of proper dose remains unsettled. It is speculation only that the dose to prevent heart attacks is the same as that to prevent stroke. Van Gijn, although a strong proponent of low-dose aspirin for all vascular territories threatened with thrombosis, paradoxically expresses the opinion that these differing vascular disease territories may respond differentially to different antithrombotics including antiplatelet drugs.[15] The same differential for

Table 1 Physicians' Health Study[a]

Outcome	ASA	Placebo	P value
MI	139	239	<.00001
Stroke	119	98	NSD

[a]Male doctors—22,071, ages 40–48.
Aspirin—325 mg, alternate days vs. placebo.
Follow-up—60.2 months.
Compliance—87%.
In the study there was a 44% relative risk reduction in myocardial infarction, but no benefit in terms of stroke reduction or of total mortality.[14]

aspirin dose may apply to different vascular territories, threatening ischemia due to thrombosis.

The meta-analyses combining all drugs employed and all types of patients threatened with thrombosis find a 22% to 23% risk reduction of stroke, myocardial infarction, or vascular death.[16] The assumption is accepted in these meta-analyses that a dose ideal for myocardial infarction will be ideal for stroke. Without equivocation, unstable angina and patients with acute myocardial infarction are treated beneficially with doses ranging from 50 mg to 1300 mg.[17–19] In patients afflicted with unstable angina, postmortem studies have revealed that most victims of this disorder have platelets clumped in the intramyocardial arterioles downstream from irregular plaques in the large coronary arteries.[20] There is a 60% to 75% reduction of fatal myocardial infarction in these subjects when they receive a dose of aspirin varying from 325 to 1,300 mg a day.[17,18] Reductions of outcome events of this magnitude have not been encountered in any of the series of stroke-threatened patients. It may be that this difference in benefit is due to the importance of other causative mechanisms of TIA and stroke—for example, cholesterol or atheromatous debris emboli. These types of emboli are not seen in coronary artery disease because the vessels involved are of a different caliber and the atheromatous lesions are correspondingly smaller.

The Anti-Platelet Collaborators in their 1994 publication identified 14,000 patients treated for TIA or stroke with an odds reduction of 23% for nonfatal strokes.[16] A subsequent meta-analysis confirms benefit in stroke reduction alone but not at a statistically significant level.[21] It may be that the dose best for one vascular system is not necessarily the best for other vascular systems. The present author, as well as Dyken, has addressed this problem in detail.[22,23] No randomized trial of patients with TIA or minor stroke utilizing < 650 mg has reported > 18% relative risk reduction, the range being from 7% to 18%.[24,25] The trials utilizing larger doses have indicated a benefit ranging from 24% to 37% relative risk reduction.[10,26–30] These comparisons cannot be taken as proof of difference but they constitute a source of major concern that the matter of dose is unsettled. The meta-analyses may be giving a figure for benefit diluted by the low-dose studies.

In the surgical arm of the North American Symptomatic Carotid Endarterectomy Trial (NASCET), patients receiving aspirin in the perioperative period in larger dose (650 to 1,300 mg) experienced a 1.1% to 2.7% stroke rate, compared with 6.5% to 7.5% for those taking 325 mg or less. These data-generated observations have led to the hypothesis that larger doses of aspirin are required when the carotid artery is denuded of its endothelium, exposing excessive amounts of collagen. Experimentally, excess amounts of collagen have been shown to increase the amount of aspirin required to inhibit platelet function.[31] The hypothesis generated from NASCET is now being evaluated with 2,800 patients randomized in the Aspirin in Carotid Endarterectomy Trial (ACE), which will conclude in August 1998.[32] The patients in this trial about to undergo endarterectomy for any reason are receiving by random assignment either 80, 325, 975, or 1,300 mg for 2 days prior to and for 3 months after endarterectomy. Ipsilateral stroke is the primary outcome event to be evaluated.

A survey of 120 world stroke leaders reports that a mean dose of 325 mg aspirin has been selected as the common choice among the "experts."[33] This judgment is based on personal preference, reading of the existing incomplete data, faith in the ability of meta-analyses to substitute for direct-comparison clinical trials, faith in the concept that thrombosis in any arterial vascular system is identical to the process in all arterial vascular systems, and not based on appropriately designed comparable studies. Scientific truth is rarely achieved by a majority vote, and the plural of anecdote is not data.

Three compelling reasons have made it important to examine the appropriateness of the dose and to ensure that the minimal required dose is known:

1. The higher therapeutic dosage of aspirin, specifically the 1,300 mg used in the Canadian Cooperative Study, was later hypothesized to be conducive to increased thrombosis. Blocking the cyclo-oxygenase enzyme in the endothelial cell and thereby inhibiting the production of the antiaggregant prostacyclin was though to be undesirably antagonistic to the desirable effect of blocking the platelet-produced aggregant thromboxane B_2.

2. More aspirin was hypothesized to make many patients more prone to hemorrhage, including intracerebral bleeding.[14]

3. The gold standard, aspirin, against which to test new drugs must be used in its optimal dose or the comparisons of any new drug with it can be misleading.

It is time to look back upon the evidence supporting or denying these two hypotheses and evaluate the impact of the uncertainty regarding the optimal dose in the trials of drugs putatively superior to aspirin.

For the hypothesized increase in the tendency of stroke or vascular death from the higher doses, no trials have produced any data suggesting that less is better, or that the higher therapeutic doses (975 to 1,300 mg per day) are liable to increased thrombogenesis and thus increased numbers of outcome events.[16,34] The single stroke prevention trial which tested lower dose (300 mg) against higher dose (1,200 mg) reported an equal and low benefit in both arms, with a nonsignificant trend favoring the higher dose.[24] Experimentally, thrombosis will occur if massive doses of aspirin are used, but such doses are well beyond the range utilized in the clinical trials of stroke prevention.

Regarding the tendency of larger doses to result in more hemorrhagic complications, the concern may have been overstated. NASCET has had scrupulous follow-up on 2,534 patients who have completed 11,000 patient-years of the daily use of the enteric-coated aspirin supplied to all patients in the trial. Intracranial hematomas, hemorrhagic transformation of cerebral infarction, and wound hematomas occurred at all therapeutic dose levels ranging from 325 mg to 1300 mg per day.[35] No dose level exhibited a difference in these complications. Because there was no placebo arm in this trial, these total numbers of intracranial hemorrhage and of wound-site bleeding cannot be causally assigned with certainty to aspirin.

Serious gastrointestinal hemorrhage was slightly but not significantly more common in those receiving higher dose. In the considerable experience provided by 11,000 patient-years of enteric-coated aspirin use, a total of only 33 major gastrointestinal bleeding episodes was reported. These are undesirable but rare, occurring in 1.1% of patients who had taken daily aspirin for an average of 5 years and in whom the average daily dose was approximately 650 mg. Only one fatal upper gastrointestinal hemorrhage occurred. This patient was not taking a large daily dose of aspirin but was receiving 650 mg daily. A second patient died of a myocardial infarction possibly influenced by the presence of an anemia associated with chronic melena due to upper gastrointestinal bleeding. The hemoglobin was reduced to 85 g/L (normal 140 to 180 g/L). The dose being taken was 325 mg daily. Two conclusions arise from these observations on gastrointestinal bleeding. First, it is a very uncommon phenomenon. Second, it occurs with nearly equal frequency at all therapeutic dose levels. These conclusions have two caveats. First, patients were not given aspirin if they had a recent (2-year) history of serious upper gastrointestinal discomfort or bleeding. Second, the observations apply only to enteric-coated aspirin. There is no doubt that the tolerability of aspirin decreases with higher dosage of regular aspirin. Because compliance to therapy is an important consideration, a drug that produces a predictably high number of patients with epigastric discomfort is not desirable. Much of the distress found with regular (plain or buffered) aspirin appears to be avoided with enteric coating. Observations in NASCET suggest that the enteric-coated variety leads to less upper abdominal distress. Admittedly, this matter requires more careful scrutiny than the design of NASCET permitted.

At times the medical journals and the public press have combined to present strong opinions on the subject of the risk of hemorrhage with aspirin. The editor-in-chief of the New England Journal of Medicine, basing his comments upon the preliminary report of the Physicians Health Study, cautioned that aspirin might be a cause of hemorrhagic stroke.[36] Of a total of 150 strokes in this preliminary report of this study, 13 of the strokes in the aspirin group and 6 in the placebo group were said to have been "hemorrhagic."[37] Splitting these down into those with moderate, severe, or fatal hemorrhagic strokes, there were 12 in total, of which 10 were in the aspirin arm of the trial. This difference was reported as significant. After 1 year of further follow-up of the original two cohorts, there were a total of 217 strokes of which 19 were moderate, severe, or fatal—13 in the aspirin group and 6 in the placebo group. Three strokes said to be hemorrhagic had been added to the aspirin and four to the placebo treatment arms. Significance was gone. The previous "significance" attributed to a subgroup of a subgroup was in all probability due to the spin of chance. The editorial, frequently quoted, was not followed by subsequent explanation when the subject had come into clearer perspective with the continuation of the follow-up period of the trial. No definition of hemorrhagic stroke was given, and no description was given of what imaging evaluations were used to prove the hemorrhagic nature of the stroke. Modern studies have shown the serious imperfections in making a diagnosis of hemorrhagic stroke when CT or MR images are replaced by clinical judgment alone.

In late 1996, the Lancet report on a retrospective study of 550 patients presenting to many participating institutions in a trial evaluating the cause of melena and hematemesis.[38] The patients who presented with these signs of upper gastrointestinal bleeding and 1,202 control subjects from the Framingham community census role were interviewed to inquire of their aspirin usage, as to both dose and type of formulation. The total study involved only 19 patients who had been regularly taking enteric-coated aspirin, as compared to a total of 154 patients regularly taking plain or buffered aspirin. By comparison with the control group they stated that the 17 patients with melena or hematemesis who took enteric-coated aspirin in a dose of 325 mg daily or less had a multivariate relative risk of 2.7 (Cl 1.4 to 5.3), not different from that seen with the use of plain or buffered aspirin. Because there were only two patients and 10 control subjects who took >325 mg per day, the report conceded that there were insufficient data to evaluate enteric-coated aspirin "at this level" (*sic*). The report went on to concede that their findings regarding enteric-coated aspirin (19 patients altogether) were inconsistent with findings from endoscopic studies. Nevertheless, they drew conclusions equating the risk of enteric-coated and plain aspirin despite the very few patients taking the enteric variety. Time, the news magazine, picked up on this report and in a prominent box under the "Health Report" section made the following remarks:

> Here's a warning to those who figure that coated or buffered aspirin protects the stomach from bleeding. The chance of that side effect is related to the amount—not the type—of aspirin used. Recommendation: take the smallest effective dose.[39]

No one should deny that aspirin causes gastrointestinal bleeding. It is difficult, however, to accept the data upon which the conclusions are reached that therapeutic coating confers no protection nor that the dose of enteric-coated aspirin is a major factor in hemorrhage. Further controlled observations are needed and should be conducted.

The third concern relates to the proper dose of ASA to use as the benchmark for new drugs. The first putative successor to aspirin, ticlopidine, was tested against 1,300 mg aspirin.[40] A modest difference in stroke prevention was noted, favoring ticlopidine over aspirin. No explanation has been forthcoming to account for the fact that the difference between the two drugs was all realized in the first 6 months of the trial (Fig. 3). Was it just by chance? If that is the case, the two drugs are of equal value, one not better than the other. Ticlopidine was shown

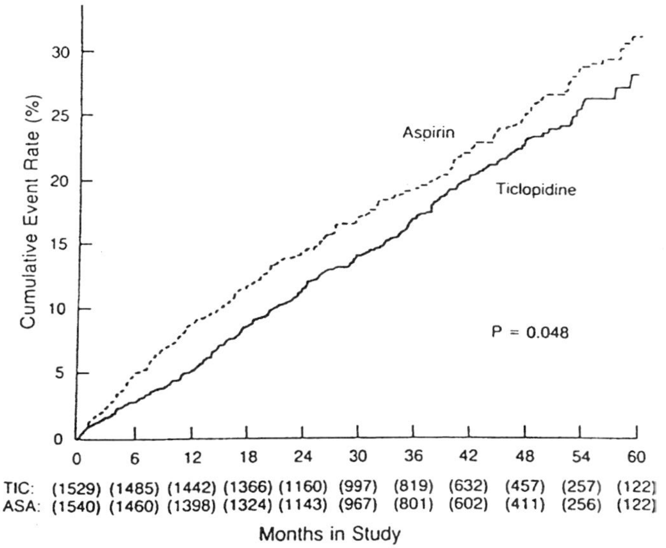

Figure 3 Cumulative event rate survival curves for nonfatal stroke or death from any cause in the TASS trial. The modest differences between ticlopidine and aspirin were all achieved within the first 6 months of therapy. (From Ref. 40.)

to be beneficial against placebo in the only other stroke prevention trial that evaluated this drug in patients who had experienced a completed stroke[41] (Fig. 4). Despite extensive promotion, ticlopidine remains the second choice of platelet inhibitor for stroke-threatened patients and stroke victims to reduce the chance of recurrence.[33] The modest difference between aspirin and ticlopidine is not impressive; diarrhea is a common complication, and 16% of instances of bone marrow suppression known to the manufacturers have proved fatal.[42] It is good, though, to have an alternative platelet inhibitor to utilize when patients cannot tolerate aspirin or when symptoms continue despite its use in adequate dosage.

No data exist which establish the efficacy for the strategy of replacing aspirin with ticlopidine in the presence of recurring symptoms. Patients who continue to have TIA despite aspirin have been dubbed "aspirin failures." No one knows, of course, whether or not the continuing TIAs are evidence that the aspirin therapy possibly has not "failed" but may in fact successfully have prevented TIAs from proceeding on to stroke. Nor is it known that patients who "fail" are likely to respond to a change in platelet inhibitor. The fact has long been recognized that untreated TIAs go in flurries. In the absence of a disciplined trial their cessation erroneously may be attributed to a shift from aspirin to another plate-

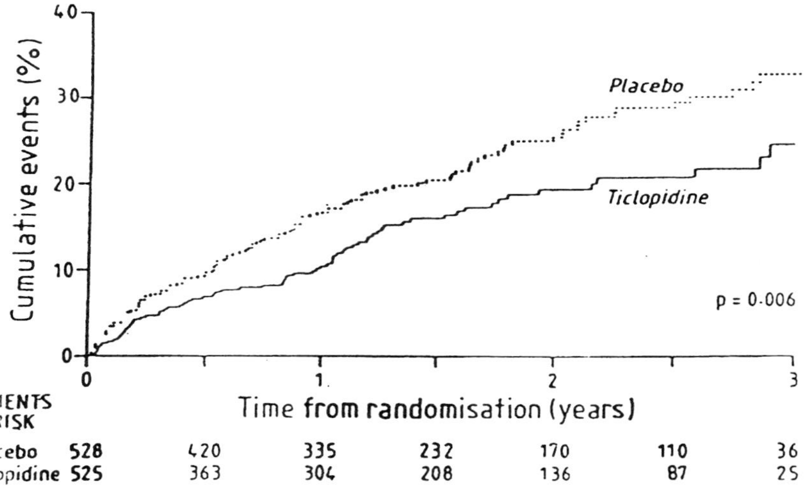

Figure 4 Survival curves for the occurrence of stroke, myocardial infarction, or vascular death in the placebo and ticlopidine groups in the CATS trial of patients with completed stroke. The combined rates for the three outcomes were 15% in the placebo and 11% in the ticlopidine group, a relative risk reduction favoring ticlopidine of 30% and an absolute reduction of 4%. (From Ref. 41.)

let inhibitor. Before making this change, three steps are recommended. First, if the patient is on low aspirin dose, an increase to no less than three 325 mg enteric-coated aspirin daily is recommended. Second, a search should be made for the possibility that the TIAs are not of platelet-fibrin origin. Possibilities to be considered are that they may be coming from atheromatous and cholesterol debris arising from the aorta, or that they are of hemodynamic origin.[43] Third, inquiry should be made if they are induced by exercise or postural change or even from exposure to bright light if they are manifest by amaurosis fugax.[44] A case report here is instructive.

An 81-year old retired cardiologist began to experience episodes of amaurosis fugax on a twice-weekly basis. These followed cessation of coumadin therapy given for 3 months after a valve replacement. Each lasted 2 to 3 minutes. Anticoagulants were reinstated and later were combined with aspirin therapy, 325 mg daily. When the combination failed to reduce the number of recurrent events, he was regarded as a "failed therapy" patient and given a prescription for ticlopidine. Prior to its use he sought a second opinion. His arteriogram was reviewed. The bifurcation had been declared the site of moderate stenosis but there were no oblique views, and the intracranial images evidenced collateral filling of the middle cerebral artery from the side opposite to the ocular symptoms. Thus, the available pictures suggested a near-occlusion despite the lack of convincingly severe stenosis visible at the carotid bifurcation. The patient was taken into a windowless room and the lights were extinguished. A bright light overhead was turned on and he looked directly at it for 2 minutes. The light then was switched off. Covering the involved eye and then the good eye, alternately, revealed that the corridor light coming through from beneath the door of the darkened room was almost indiscernible for 2 minutes in the eye afflicted with recurrent amaurosis but was readily discernible at once with the uninvolved eye. These observations justified repeat angiography which identified, in oblique views, a nearly complete stenosing occlusion of the ipsilateral internal carotid artery. A carotid endarterectomy was performed and his amaurosis events have not recurred for 2 years of follow-up. It was clearly demonstrated that his "aspirin failure" status was due to the fact that he was not afflicted with amaurosis of thromboembolic, but of hemodynamic nature.

The newest platelet-inhibiting drug to have gone beyond the trial stage is clopidogrel. For reasons not stipulated in the report, the investigators tested it against only 325 mg aspirin while the related compound ticlopidine produced by the same pharmaceutical company had been tested against 1300 mg.[45] Patients did not require stroke-threatening symptoms for entry into the study but could have experienced either TIA, stroke, intermittent claudication, or myocardial infarction. Stroke, as an outcome event, was not by itself significantly reduced. Benefit was found in the combined outcome events (Figs. 5,6) it has been calculated from the publication of results from the clopidogrel trial that 222 patients

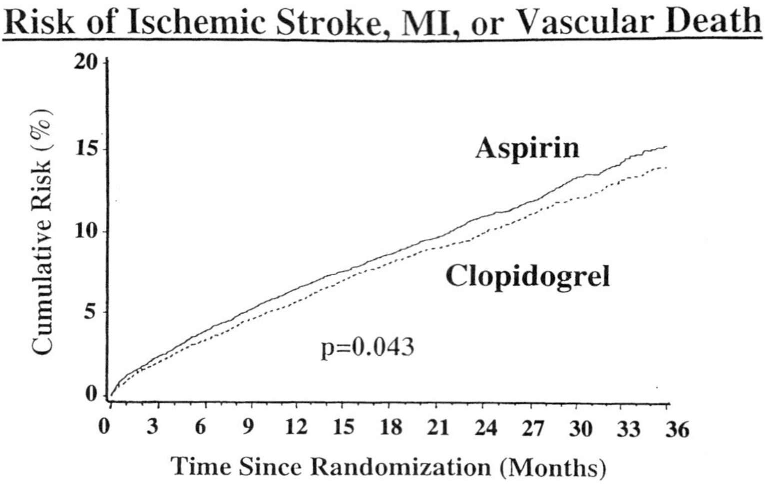

Patients	A:	9586	9190	8087	6139	3979	2143	542
at Risk	C:	9599	9247	8191	6160	4053	2170	539

Figure 5 Cumulative risk of any of the three outcome events in the trial of aspirin vs. clopidogrel. Although the differences were statistically significant, the benefit of clopidogrel over aspirin was a disappointing 0.5% absolute risk reduction favoring clopidogrel. (From Ref. 45.)

are required to be changed from aspirin to clopidogrel therapy for 1 year to prevent one stroke (M. Eliasziw, personal communication, 1997). Once again, no more than a marginal difference between aspirin and clopidogrel was observed. Nobody knows how the results would have emerged had the same dose of aspirin been utilized as in the ticlopidine studies.

Attempts are being made to rehabilitate an older platelet inhibitor—dipyridamole. It is troublesome that the investigators of the latest trial chose to test this drug in a factorial design with one arm of the trial containing only a placebo.[46] This was done despite the fact that in their own earlier study they had established a 38% stroke reduction with aspirin plus dipyridamole, and many other trials and meta-analyses had proven already very convincingly that aspirin alone was efficacious.[47] Not only were patients denied a proven therapy in favor of placebo, but the investigators dropped the aspirin dose to 25 mg b.i.d., a dose never tested, let alone proven efficacious in stroke prevention. The combination of aspirin (50 mg) and dipyridamole (400 mg) yielded a benefit in stroke and death which was just below the level found in the Canadian Cooperative Study or the AICLA trial, both of which utilized 10 times the ASA dose.[10,28]

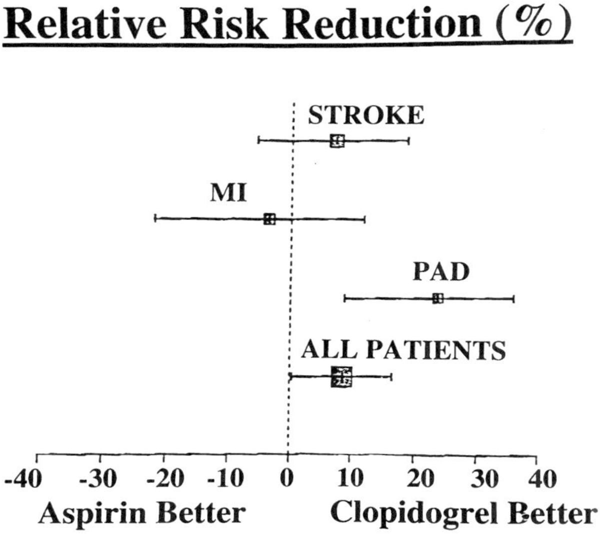

Figure 6 Relative risk reduction and 95% Cl by disease subgroup in the CAPRIE trial. The overall benefit was statistically significant combining stroke, myocardial infarction, and peripheral vascular disease. The stroke reduction was moderate but not significant. (From Ref. 45.)

Despite strong argument to the contrary, pharmacological benefit still does not equate with clinical benefit.[48] This very low dose of aspirin cannot be justified on the basis of any clinical studies against another dose or placebo in stroke-threatened patients. In the case of dipyridamole it is important to recall that in three previous trials combining aspirin in higher dose (900 to 1,300 mg daily) with dipyridamole in a total of 1,575 patients, the combined therapy was no better than aspirin alone.[27,28,49] A trial utilizing other dose(s) of aspirin with and without dipyridamole is essential before this drug is considered of proven benefit. When and if repeated, this trial must be monitored more scrupulously than this latest study appears to have been.[50] It will be unethical for anyone to repeat a trial utilizing a placebo. This ethical requirement was breached in the ESPS2 trial. Until information about the correct dose of aspirin is finalized, this drug cannot be recommended.

In conclusion, some final comments deserve consideration about the best platelet-inhibiting drug and best dose of aspirin if it is to remain the first choice and the standard for other trials: the only totally acceptable way in which the enigma of choice and dose can be resolved is by continuing careful comparative clinical trials. Until these trials are conducted the uncertainties defined in this essay will persist. Pharmacologists produce no more than surrogate evidence of clinical applicability no matter how impressive the in vitro evidence which is amassed, either for a low aspirin dose or for therapy combined with another platelet inhibitor. An early pathophysiological study in patients who had suffered cerebral thrombosis, involving bleeding time, platelet adhesion, and platelet aggregation, and involving the testing of 11 consecutive therapeutic sequences in 17 patients, convinced the investigators that the optimum aspirin dose was 500 to 1,000 mg daily.[51] Disturbing to those who are complacent about the in vitro evidence that low dose is adequate are studies showing that cell-cell interactions between platelets and erythrocytes promote platelet reactivity.[52] Prior platelet tests have not been conducted in the presence of red cells. The investigators in this trial concluded by recommending a loading dose of 500 mg aspirin. Studies comparing the comparative effect of very low dose (81 mg) and low dose (325 mg) after exercise in human subjects found that the collagen-induced aggregation was greater with 325 mg than with 81 mg.[53] Because of the possibility of plaque rupture, with its extensive collagen exposure and platelet activation, they recommended the higher dose in post–myocardial infarction patients. A dose > 325 mg was not studied. Another group reported that platelet inhibition was optimized by a loading dose of 300 mg but were of the opinion that maintenance dose need only be 40 mg per day.[54] All of these observations were related to platelet function and not to outcome results in clinical trials. The best ongoing dose is left unsettled. The bedside, not the test tube, is the required laboratory for finalizing this matter.

SUMMARY

1. It can be stated without equivocation that the risk of stroke can be reduced by the use of platelet inhibitors.

2. It is the opinion of the writer that aspirin is the first choice for stroke-threatening subjects but that the best dose is not known. The writer recommends between 650 and 975 mg per day. Very definite opinions to the contrary have been expressed, many by those who favor a low dose (325 mg) or a very low dose (81 mg).[55,56]

3. The rationale for the insistence upon low dose no longer exists.[22] There is no evidence that a high dose, up to 1,300 mg per day, increases the chance of stroke or myocardial infarction. There is good evidence emerging that the intracranial, the endarterectomy wound site, and serious gastrointestinal bleeding complications are decidedly uncommon and are either related or are questionably related at best to higher than to lower dose.

4. The dose to be used in stroke prevention should be based on good comparative clinical trials instead of pharmacological in vitro studies and statistical manipulation.

What will happen in the future? The dose question may be settled, or a better drug than anything available to date may emerge. Mark Twain noted that predictions were difficult to make, especially into the future! This applies to the future of aspirin, the dose of aspirin, and the place of other platelet inhibitors in stroke prevention.

ACKNOWLEDGMENTS

The author wishes to acknowledge the assistance in crafting this manuscript of Ms. Heather Meldrum and Dr. Michael Eliasziw. Grateful thanks go to SmithKline Beecham who provided the Ecotrin for 11 years to all patients in the NASCET trial. Mrs. Cathy Wild was very helpful with the production of this paper.

REFERENCES

1. Anonymous. An aspirin a day keeps the doctor at bay. The Economist August 9, 1997:69–70.
2. Fisher CM. Observations of the fundus oculi in transient monocular blindness. Neurology 1959; 9:333.
3. Smythe HA, Ogryzlo MA, Murphy EA, et al. The effect of sulfinpyrazone (Anturan) on platelet economy and blood coagulation in man. Can Med Assoc J 1965; 92:818–821.
4. Emmons PR, Harrison MJ, Honour AJ, Mitchell JR. Affect of a pyrimido pyrimidine derivative on thrombus formation in the rabbit. Nature 1965; 208:255–257.
5. Evans G, Nishizawa EF, Packham MA, Mustard JF. The effect of acetylsalicylic acid (aspirin) on platelet function. Blood J Hematol 1967; 30:550.
6. Weiss HJ, Aledort LM. Impaired platelet/connective-tissue reaction in man after aspirin ingestion. Lancet 1967; 2:495–497.
7. Acheson J, Danta G, Hutchinson EC. Controlled trial of dipyridamole in cerebral vascular disease. BMJ 1969; 1:614–15.
8. Harrison MJG, Marshall J, Meadows JC, Russell RWR. Effect of aspirin in amaurosis fugax. Lancet 1971; 743–744.
9. Mundall J, Quintero P, von Kaulla KN, Harmon R, Austin J. Transient monocular blindness and increased platelet aggregability treated with aspirin. Neurology 1972; 22(3):280–285.
10. Canadian Cooperative Study Group. A randomized trial of aspirin and sulfinpyrazone in threatened stroke. N Engl J Med 1978; 299:53–59.
11. Dyken ML. Antiplatelet aggregating agents in transient ischemic attacks and the relationship of risk factors. In: Breddin K, Loew D, Uberla K, et al., eds. Prophylaxis of Venous, Peripheral, Cardiac and Cerebral Vascular Diseases with Acetylsalicylic Acid. Stuattgart, Germany: Schattauer Verlag, 1981:141–148.

12. Smith JB, Willis AL. Aspirin selectively inhibits prostaglandin production in human platelets. Nature New Biol 1971; 231:235–237.
13. Moncada S, Gryglewski RJ, Bunting S, Vane JR. An enzyme isolated from arteries transforms prostaglandin endoperoxides to an unstable substance that inhibits platelet aggregation. Nature 1976; 263:663–665.
14. Steering Committee of the Physicians' Health Study Research Group. Final report on the aspirin component of the ongoing Physicians' Health Study. N Engl J Med 1989; 321:129–135.
15. van Gijn J, Algra A. Secondary stroke prevention with antithrombotic drugs: what to do next? Cerebrovasc Dis 1997; 7(suppl 6):30–32.
16. Antiplatelet Trialists Collaboration. Collaborative overview of randomised trials of antiplatelet therapy. Prevention of death, myocardial infarction, and stroke by prolonged antiplatelet therapy in various categories of patients. BJM 1994; 308:81–106.
17. Lewis HD, Davis JW, Archibald DG, et al. Protective effects of aspirin against acute myocardial infarction and death in men with unstable angina: results of veterans administration cooperative study. N Engl J Med 1983; 309:396–403.
18. Cairns J, Gent M, Singer J, et al. A study of aspirin (ASA) and/or sulfinpyrazone in unstable angina. Circulation 1984; 70(suppl II):415.
19. De Caterina R, Giannessi D, Boem A, Bernini W, Battaglia D, Michelassi C, Dell'Amico F, L' Abbate A, Patrignani P, Patrono C. Equal antiplatelet effects of aspirin 50 or 324 mg/day in patients after acute myocardial infraction. Thromb Haemost 1985; 54(2):528–532.
20. Davies MJ, Thomas AC, Knapman PA, Hangartner JE. Intramyocardial platelet aggregation in patients with unstable angina suffering sudden ischemic cardiac death. Circulation 1986; 73(3):418–427.
21. Barnett HJM, Eliasziw M, Meldrum HE. Drugs and surgery in the prevention of ischemic stroke. N Engl J Med 1995; 332:238–248.
22. Barnett HJM, Kaste M, Meldrum HE, Eliasziw M. Aspirin dose in stroke prevention: beautiful hypotheses slain by ugly facts. Stroke 1996; 27:588–592.
23. Dyken ML. Controversies in stroke: past and present: the Willis Lecture. Stroke 1993; 24:1251–1258.
24. UK-TIA Study Group. The United Kingdom transient ischemic attack (UK-TIA) aspirin trial: final results. J Neurol Neurosurg Psychiatry 1991; 54:1044–1054.
25. SALT Collaborative Group. Swedish Aspirin Low-dose Trial (SALT) of 75 mg aspirin as secondary prophylaxis after cerebrovascular ischaemic events. Lancet 1991; 338:1345–9.
26. Fields WS, Lemak NA, Frankowski RF, Hardy RJ. Controlled trial of aspirin in cerebral ischemia. Stroke 1977; 8:301–316.
27. Guiraud-Chaumeil B, Rascol A, David JL, Boneu B, Clanet M, Bierme R. Prévention des récidives des accidents vasculaires cérébraux ischémiques par les anti-agrégants plaquettaires: résultats d'un essai thérapeutique contrôlé de 3 ans. Rev Neurol (Paris) 1982; 138:367–385.
28. Bousser MG, Eschwege E, Haguenau M, et al. "AICLA" controlled trial of aspirin and dipyridamole in the secondary prevention of athero-thrombotic cerebral ischemia. Stroke 1983; 14:5–14.

29. Sorensen PS, Pedersen H, Marquardsen J, et al. Acetylsalicylic acid in the prevention of stroke in patients with reversible cerebral ischemic attacks: a Danish cooperative study. Stroke 1983; 14:15–22.
30. Swedish Cooperative Study. High-dose acetylsalicylic acid after cerebral infarction. Stroke 1987; 18:325–334.
31. O'Brien JR, Etheringon MD. How much aspirin? Thromb Haemost 1990; 64(3):486.
32. Thorpe KE, Taylor DW, for the North American Symptomatic Carotid Endarterectomy Trial Collaborators: ASA and Carotid Endarterectomy. Abstract presented at the 22nd International Joint Conference on Stroke and Cerebral Circulation, Anaheim, CA, Feb. 6–8, 1997.
33. Busch M, Masuhr F, Einhaupl, KM. Medical and surgical prevention of stroke: experiences around the world. Cerebrovasc Dis 1997; 7(suppl):22–28.
34. Matchar DB, McCrory DC, Barnett HJM, Reussner JR. Medical treatment for stroke prevention. Ann Intern Med 1994; 121(1):41–53.
35. Munson RJ, Sharpe BL, Finan JW, Eliasziw M, Hachinski VC, Barnett HJM for the North American Symptomatic Carotid Endarterectomy Trial (NASCET) Group. The NASCET Experience of Bleeding Complications of Patients on Aspirin. Abstract presented at the 22nd International Joint Conference on Stroke and Cerebral Circulation, Anaheim, CA Feb. 6–8, 1997.
36. Relman AS. Aspirin for the primary prevention of myocardial infarction. N Engl J Med 1988; 318(4):245–246.
37. Steering Committee of the Physicians' Health Study Research Group. Preliminary report: findings from the aspirin component of the ongoing Physicians' Health Study. N Engl J Med 1986; 318(4):262–264.
38. Kelly JP, Kaufman DW, Jurgelon JM, Sheehan J, Koff RS, Shapiro S. Risk of aspirin-associated major upper-gastrointestinal bleeding with enteric-coated or buffered product. Lancet 1996; 348:1413–1416.
39. Croning B. Health report. Time Dec. 30, 1996–Jan. 6, 1997:12.
40. Hass WK, Easton JD, Adams HP Jr, Pryse-Phillips W, Molony BA, Anderson S, Kamm B, for the Ticlopidine Aspirin Stroke Study Group. A randomized trial comparing ticlopidine hydrochloride with aspirin for the prevention of stroke in high-risk patients. N Engl J Med 1989; 321:501–507.
41. Gent M, Blakely JA, Easton JD, Ellis DJ, Hachinski VC, Harbison JW, Panak E, Roberts RS, Sicurella J, Turpie AGG, CATS Group. The Canadian American Ticlopidine Study (CATS) in thromboembolic stroke. Lancet 1989; June 3:1215–1220.
42. Barentt HJM, Eliasziw M, Meldrum HE. Prevention of ischemic stroke (reply). N Engl J Med 1995; 333:460.
43. Amarenco P, Cohen A, Tzourio C, Bertrand B, Hommel M, et al. Atherosclerotic disease of the aortic arch and the risk of ischemic stroke. N Engl J Med 1994; 331:1474–1479.
44. Furlan AJ, Whisnant JP, Kearns TP. Unilateral visual loss in bright light. An unusual symptom of carotid artery occlusive disease. Arch Neurol 1979; 36(11):675–676.
45. CAPRIE Steering Committee. A randomised, blinded, trial of clopidogrel versus

aspirin in patients at risk of ischaemic events (CAPRIE). Lancet 1996; 348:1329–1339.
46. Diener HC, Cunha L, Forbes C, Sivenius J, Smets P, Lowenthal A. European Stroke Study 2. Dipyridamole and acetylsalicylic acid in the secondary prevention of stroke. J Neurol Sci 1996; 143:1–13.
47. ESPS Group. The European Stroke Prevention Study (ESPS) principal endpoints. Lancet 1987; Dec. 12:1351–1354.
48. Vane JR, Meade TW. Second European Stroke Prevention Study (ESPS 2): clinical and pharmacological implications. J Neurol Sci 1997; 145(2):123–125.
49. American-Canadian Co-operative Study Group. Persantine. Aspirin trial in cerebral ischemia: endpoint results. Stroke 1985; 16:406–415.
50. Enserink M. Fraud and ethics charges hit stroke drug trial. Science 1996; 274:2004–2005.
51. Lejeune A, Fattet M, Degos JD. Aspirin dose, bleeding time, platelet adhesion and aggregation in cerebral thrombosis. Int J Clin Pharmacol Ther Toxicol 1988; 26(5):237–242.
52. Santos MT, Valles J, Aznar J, Marcus AJ, Broekman MJ, Saifer LB. Prothrombotic effects of erythrocytes on platelet reactivity. Reduction by aspirin. Circulation 1997; 95:63–68.
53. Feng D, McKenna C, Murillo J, Mittleman MA, Gebara OC, Lipinska I, Muller JE, Tofler GH. Effect of aspirin dosage and enteric coating on platelet reactivity. Am J Cardiol 1997; 80:189–193.
54. Buerke M, Pittroff W, Meyer J, Darius H. Aspirin therapy: optimized platelet inhibition with different loading and maintenance doses. Am Heart J 1995; 130:465–472.
55. Hart RG, Harrison MJG. Aspirin wars: the optimal dose of aspirin to prevent stroke. Stroke 1996; 27:585–587.
56. Patrono C, Roth GJ. Aspirin in ischemic cerebrovascular disease: how strong is the case for a different dosing regimen? Stroke 1996; 27:756–760.

22

Alternatives to Aspirin: Advantages and Disadvantages

Tom Jeerakathil and Ashfaq Shuaib
University of Alberta Hospital, Edmonton, Alberta, Canada

INTRODUCTION

The previous chapter discussed in detail the rationale for the use of aspirin in the prevention of stroke in patients with a TIA or completed stroke. Despite a number of advances in the understanding of antiplatelet mechanisms and the introduction of many new medications, aspirin remains the first-line therapy in stroke prevention in most patients. According to the Antiplatelet Trialists Collaboration meta-analyses, from 1988 and 1994 there is an approximately 22% odds reduction in the risk of stroke recurrence with the use of antiplatelet therapy as a whole as compared to placebo.[1,2] Approximately half of the patients included in the meta-analysis were on aspirin monotherapy; the others were on either aspirin plus another antiplatelet agent, or on another agent alone. The dose of aspirin most commonly used to prevent stroke varies between 30 mg and 1,300 mg/day. Dr. H.J.M. Barnett discusses details concerning the appropriate dose of aspirin and the evidence supporting the use of aspirin in the previous chapter.

There are several situations where alternatives to aspirin may be considered. Alternative therapy should obviously be tried in patients who cannot tolerate aspirin. Many patients who have a TIA or stroke may already be on aspirin for other indications, including preexisting cardiac disease or a prior cerebral ischemic event. These patients have been referred to as aspirin failures, and a trial of another antiplatelet agent may be warranted. In studies where aspirin has been compared to other antiplatelet medications, some studies have shown the alternative therapies to be marginally superior to aspirin.[3,4] A rationale for the first-line use of the alternative medications based on their superior prevention profile has thus been offered for primary use. It has also been suggested that prior to changing the antiplatelet agent, one should consider increasing the dose of aspirin in patients who are on lower doses (especially if the dose is < 300 mg).[5] This chapter reviews the published literature on additional antiplatelet agents that have been used in the prevention of noncardioembolic stroke. Antiplatelet therapy for the prevention of cardioembolic stroke will be discussed in another chapter.

ANTIPLATELET AGENTS TESTED IN CONTROLLED PROSPECTIVE TRIALS

Ticlopidine

Ticlopidine is the first of a new generation of antiplatelet agents, called thienopyridines, that selectively and irreversibly inhibit the ADP-related activation of platelet aggregation.[6–10] These compounds have a different mechanism of action than aspirin, which acts by preventing the formation of thromboxane A_2 by irreversibly inhibiting platelet cyclo-oxygenase. Ticlopidine was synthesized in 1972. Clopidogrel was synthesized 13 years later and is several times more potent. Ticlopidine and clopidogrel inhibit platelet adhesion to the vascular subendothelium and intimal proliferation in animal models.[11,12] Both drugs inhibit the ADP-induced exposure of the GPIIb/IIIa receptor complex but do not directly interfere with the receptor (see Figs. 1,2).[9,10] Both drugs have been compared to aspirin in large prospective trials.[3,4,13]

There are two large clinical trials that tested the efficacy of ticlopidine in patients with transient ischemic attacks (TIA) and stroke.[3,14] One study compared the efficacy against aspirin in patients with TIAs or minor stroke (Ticlopidine Aspirin Stroke Study, TASS) while the second study was a placebo-controlled study in patients with completed stroke (Canadian American Ticlopidine Study, CATS). The TASS study recruited 3,069 subjects with a TIA or mild stroke within the previous 3 months. Patients treated with aspirin were given a dose of 1,300 mg/day and ticlopidine was offered in a dose of 500 mg/day. In the TASS study,

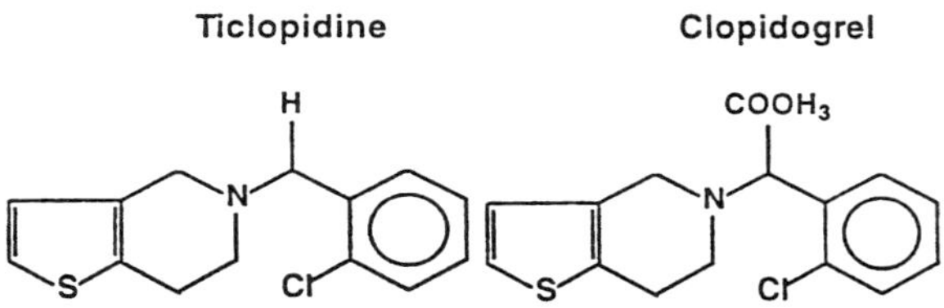

Figure 1 Thienopyridines (From Ref. 9.)

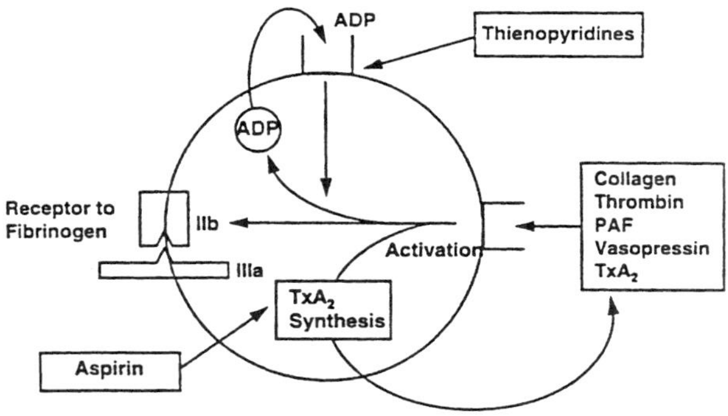

Figure 2 Mechanism of action of thienopyridines. TxA_2 = Thromboxane A_2; PAF = platelet-activating factor. (From Ref. 9.)

the average yearly risk for the primary composite outcome of stroke or death from any cause was significantly less in the ticlopidine group (6.6%) than the aspirin group (7.6%). Overall there was a 14% relative risk reduction in ticlopidine-treated patients compared to aspirin-treated patients. Significantly better protection was sustained through the entire duration of the trial in the ticlopidine-treated group. There was also a significant reduction in the risk of stroke (fatal and non-fatal) in the ticlopidine-treated group (20% relative risk reduction; annual event rate 3.7% in the ticlopidine group and 4.6% in the aspirin group). The relative risk reduction of the composite outcome of stroke, MI, or vascular death was 6% in favor of ticlopidine but did not reach significance.[3]

In the second large trial, CATS, the efficacy of ticlopidine was compared to placebo in 1,072 patients with a completed stroke. Patients with a cardio-embolic stroke were excluded. Atherothrombotic stroke was the most frequent stroke type, comprising 74% of patients in the study. For the primary outcome of stroke, myocardial infarction, or vascular death, there was a significant relative reduction in on-treatment (30%) and intention-to-treat (23%) analysis. Other outcome events including stroke, MI, and all deaths or all strokes were reduced but reached statistical significance only in the on-treatment analysis.[14]

Serious side effects can develop in a significant number of patients treated with ticlopidine. Neutropenia was seen in 2.4% of patients and was severe in 0.8% of patients in the TASS study. It is therefore strongly recommended that the white cell count (specifically neutrophil count) be evaluated every 2 weeks for the first 3 months on therapy. The risk of developing neutropenia after the initial 3 months is very small. Treatment requires discontinuation of the medication. Other hematological complications noted with patients on ticlopidine include thrombocytopenia, thrombotic thrombocytopenic purpura (TTP), and aplastic anemia.[15,16] Diarrhea may be seen in up to 20% of patients and may be the reason for discontinuing therapy in approximately 5% to 6% of patients.[3,14] In most cases, the diarrhea will respond to a temporary reduction in dosage. Some clinicians have reported the occurrence of lymphocytic colitis in patients on ticlopidine therapy.[17–19] This condition may manifest as severe and chronic diarrhea. Whether this condition is an adverse effect of ticlopidine therapy or an unrelated occurrence remains to be seen. Skin rash (12% to 15%) and hepatic dysfunction (4%) are other complications that may require discontinuation of the drug.[20]

Ticlopidine has been used extensively in the treatment of patients with TIA and stroke. Most current recommendations would suggest that the drug be used as a second-line therapy in patients who either cannot tolerate aspirin or continue to have symptoms on aspirin.[1,21] Ticlopidine is occasionally used in combination with aspirin or warfarin in patients who continue to have symptoms while on monotherapy with one or the other agent. While we have used the combination in an occasional patient, it must be emphasized that the combination therapy has not been evaluated in prospective studies.

Clopidogrel

Clopidogrel is a second-generation thienopyridine compound synthesized in 1985. Its mechanism of action is similar to ticlopidine but is many times more potent and may have significantly fewer serious side effects. Clopidogrel is inactive in vitro and its activity depends on hepatic biotransformation. By blocking the platelet ADP receptor, clopidogrel indirectly inhibits the binding of fibrinogen to its platelet receptor, the glycoprotein GP IIb–IIIa. The platelet inhibition induced by clopidogrel persists for several days after the medication is stopped and slowly diminishes as new platelets are formed and join into the circulation (see Fig. 3).[22,23]

The efficacy of clopidogrel was compared to aspirin in a large prospective randomized, double-blinded study in patients presenting with stroke, myocardial infarction, or peripheral vascular disease. The Clopidogrel versus Aspirin in Patients at Risk of Ischemic Events (CAPRIE) trial enrolled 19,195 patients (> 6,300 patients in each clinical subgroup) to aspirin 325 mg or clopidogrel 75 mg/day. The incidence of the composite outcome of stroke, myocardial infarction, or vascular death was 5.32% in the clopidogrel group and 5.83% in the aspirin group. This reflects a significant 8.7% relative risk reduction (intention to treat) in favor of clopidogrel. Based on these data, clopidogrel would be expected to prevent 24 major events per 1,000 patients per year. This compares to a prevention of 19 events per 1,000 patients in the aspirin-treated group.[4] This would equate

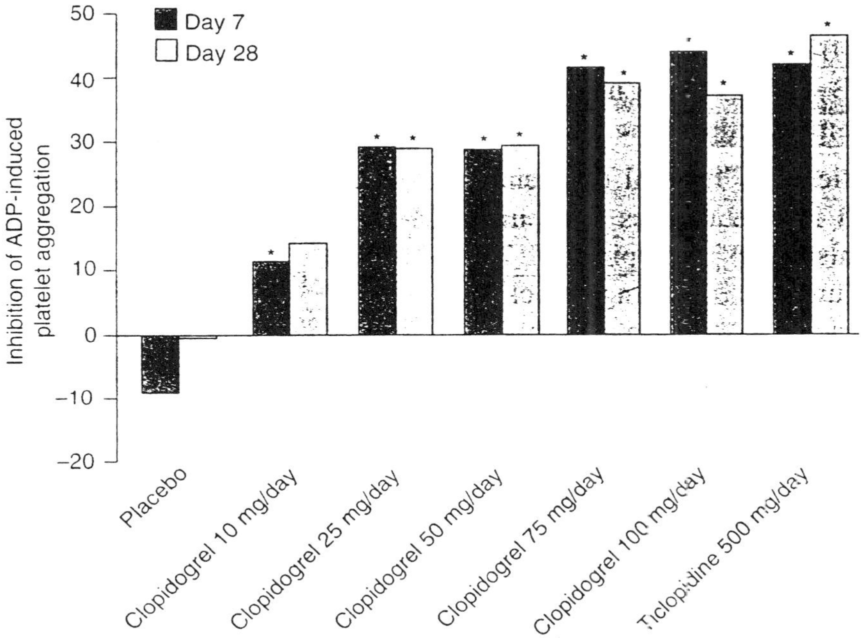

Figure 3 Inhibition of platelet aggregation by clopidogrel 10 to 100 mg/day, ticlopidine 500 mg/day, and placebo. Percentage of ADP (5 μmoles/L)-induced inhibition on days 7 and 28 vs. day 0. $^*P<.05$ vs. placebo (TT). (From Ref. 22.)

to a 26% increase in the number of events prevented during clopidogrel versus aspirin treatment.

The study was powered to detect a realistic treatment effect in the overall cohort but not in each of the three clinical subgroups. Despite this, a subgroup analysis was carried out looking at the composite endpoint in each of the clinical subgroups. The relative risk reductions, 95% confidence intervals, and *P* values are as follows: stroke group 7.3% (–5.7 to 18.7; *P* = .26); MI group –3.7% (–22.1 to 12.0; *P* = .66); peripheral vascular disease group 23.8% (8.9 to 36.2; *P* = .0028). A test for heterogeneity was positive (*P* = .042), suggesting that the benefit of clopidogrel may not be identical across all three groups. Clopidogrel may be more effective in patients with peripheral vascular disease, but no comment can be made on how it compares to aspirin in patients with prior stroke or MI, as the subgroup analyses were not significant and the trial was not adequately powered to rule out a difference.

As shown above, the relative risk reduction in the subgroup of patients who had MI as a qualifying event was negative (–3.7). This suggests that patients on clopidogrel do worse than those on aspirin, although the result did not reach significance. For this reason, an additional analysis was carried out combining patients in the peripheral vascular disease and stroke subgroups with remote history of MI (n = 2,144), and the patients in the MI subgroup, examining a total of 8,446 patients. The overall relative risk reduction in favor of clopidogrel was 7.4% (95% CI –5.2 to 18.6). This result did not reach significance and does not confirm that clopidogrel is superior to aspirin in the subset of patients with previous MI. It was, however, in keeping with the overall findings of the study.[4]

In the clinical subgroup of patients with previous stroke, the clopidogrel-treated patients had a lower absolute number of recurrent nonfatal strokes (298 vs. 322) and a very slightly higher number of fatal strokes (17 vs. 16) than the aspirin group. This difference was not subject to analysis, so it is not known how clopidogrel compares to aspirin in the secondary prevention of stroke alone. Ticlopidine, on the other hand, has been shown to provide a significantly greater relative risk reduction of fatal or nonfatal stroke than aspirin (RRR 20%).[3] Concerning the composite outcome of stroke, MI, or vascular death, the two drugs show a similar relative risk reduction above aspirin (6% for ticlopidine, 7% for clopidogrel), but the difference was significant only for clopidogrel.[3,4] It is difficult to make accurate comparisons between the two trials because of differences in the baseline characteristics of the study populations, the size of the trials, and differences in some of the endpoints. A reasonable conclusion is that ticlopidine is marginally superior to aspirin in the prevention of stroke and also death from any cause, and that clopidogrel is marginally superior to aspirin in the prevention of the composite of stroke, MI, or vascular death.

An important advantage of clopidogrel was the significantly lower rate of complications. The most frequent adverse events in the CAPRIE trial were indigestion/nausea/vomiting, occurring significantly more in the aspirin group (17.59%) than in the clopidogrel group (15.01%) (see Fig. 4). Bleeding disorders occurred in about 9.3% of patients for both treatments. Rash was more common in the clopidogrel group, and 0.9% of clopidogrel patients had to discontinue therapy because of rash compared to 0.41% of aspirin patients. Diarrhea occurred in 4.46% of clopidogrel patients compared to 4.61% of aspirin patients, but no therapy was discontinued as a result of it.[4] Clopidogrel has a better safety profile than ticlopidine. It has been extensively tested in patients with cerebrovascular, cardiovascular, and peripheral vascular diseases. The 75-mg once-a-day treatment, combined with a significantly smaller risk of hematological, hepatic, gastrointestinal, and other systemic complications compared to ticlopidine, makes it an attractive alternative. The medication has, however, only recent been intro-

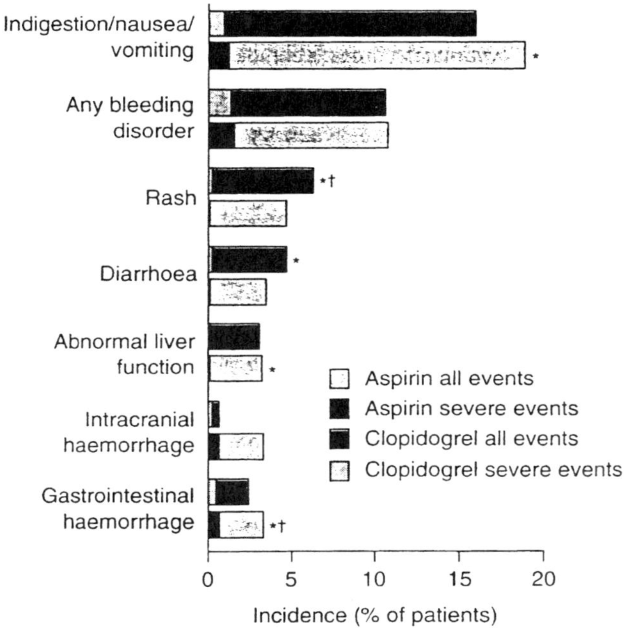

Figure 4 Adverse events reported in patients who received clopidogrel 75 mg/day (n = 9,599) or aspirin 325 mg/day (n = 9,586) in the CAPRIE (G) trial. $*P<.05$ for all events; †$p<0.05$ for severe events. (From Ref. 22.)

duced on the market, and definitive judgments regarding its safety require further information.

Dipyridamole

Dipyridamole has been available as an antiplatelet agent for cardiac disease for a number of years. One small study evaluated the efficacy of dipyridamole alone in stroke prevention with negative results.[24] Dipyridamole inhibits platelet cAMP phosphodiesterase and therefore prevents the degradation of cAMP to AMP. Elevated platelet cAMP levels reduce platelet reactivity.[10] Dipyridamole also enhances the synthesis and release of prostacyclin and inhibits its degradation.[25] Given their differing mechanisms of action, it was thought that combining dipyridamole with aspirin may have additive effects. Three studies examined the combination of aspirin and dipyridamole versus placebo for secondary stroke prevention.[26–28] The AICLA controlled trial of aspirin and dipyridamole in the secondary prevention of atherothrombotic cerebral ischemia (AICLA)[26] found no significant difference between the combination and placebo, nor did the French study (Toulouse-TIA),[28] but both were small trials. The larger European Stroke Prevention Study (ESPS) showed an impressive 38% relative risk reduction over placebo for the combination of 225 mg dipyridamole and 990 mg aspirin daily.[27] AICLA and the French study as well as a third study, called the American-Canadian Co-Operative Study,[29] also compared the combination of aspirin and dipyridamole with aspirin alone. None found any significant difference between the combination of both drugs and aspirin alone.

The effects of aspirin alone, dipyridamole alone, or a combination of the two medications versus placebo were studied in the second European Stroke Prevention Trial (ESPS-II).[30] In 1996, ESPS-II published its results. The dose of aspirin was only 50 mg/day. Dipyridamole was used in a dose of 200 mg twice a day in specially designed sustained-release capsules. The study involved 6,602 patients who were followed for 2 years. The primary endpoints included stroke, sudden death, and death from any cause. The low dose of aspirin (18% relative risk reduction; $P = .013$; odds ratio 0.79; 95% CI 0.65–0.97) and dipyridamole (16% relative risk reduction; $P = .039$; odds ratio 0.81; 95% CI 0.67–0.99) were both significantly better than placebo in stroke prevention. The combination of the two medications was significantly better than either medication alone (37% risk reduction; $P < .001$; odds ratio 0.59; 95% CI 0.48–0.73).

Hemorrhagic complications were seen more frequently in the low-dose aspirin or combination group than dipyridamole alone. Patients on a dipyridamole regimen reported more frequent diarrhea and headaches. Gastrointestinal events and headaches were major reasons for discontinuation of a dipyridamole regimen. There were a number of controversial aspects to the study; it has been criticized for including a placebo arm and for irregularities in the conduct of the trial. These and other details are discussed in the preceding chapter. We would recommend that dipyridamole be used in combination with aspirin in patients who cannot tolerate the higher dose of aspirin (> 325 mg/day) and who continue to have events. It is important that the drug be used only in combination with low-dose aspirin. It is only the combination that appears to be better than aspirin alone. It is also important to remember that the medication used in the ESPS-II trial was the higher-dose, sustained-release preparation that has not become available on the market at the time of publication.

Sulfinpyrazone

Sulfinpyrazone is another antiplatelet drug that has been evaluated in the secondary prevention of stroke. The Canadian Cooperative Study of aspirin, sulfinpyrazone, and placebo in secondary stroke prevention showed no benefit for sulfinpyrazone alone. The combination of sulfinpyrazone plus aspirin was no more effective than aspirin alone.[31] Sulfinpyrazone is not currently recommended in the secondary prevention of stroke, given the existing evidence and the availability of more proven medications.

Glycoprotein IIb–IIIa Antagonists

When platelets adhere to the vessel wall, they require activation of the glycoprotein IIb–IIIa receptor (GPIIb–IIIa) as the final step for platelet aggregation.[32–34] A number of peptides that block the GPIIb–IIIa receptor have been synthesized and are undergoing clinical trials in patients with TIA and stroke. Some such agents have already been successfully tested in patients with unstable angina or myocardial infarction.

The chimeric recombinant antibody abciximab (ReoPro) was shown in the EPIC trial to reduce the incidence of death, myocardial infarction, or the need for urgent intervention by up to 35% compared to placebo in high-risk patients undergoing coronary artery angioplasty or atherectomy.[35] The EPILOG and RAPPORT trials showed similar benefits.[36,37] The synthetic cyclic heptapeptide eptifibatide was shown in the IMPACT II trial to reduce the occurrence of myocardial infarction and other negative outcomes in patients undergoing unplanned or emergency coronary stenting.[38] Another IIb-IIIa inhibitor, tirofiban, reduced negative ischemic outcomes in similar patients in the RESTORE and PRISM-PLUS trials.[39,40]

Some trials of GPIIb-IIIa antagonists have demonstrated an increase in major bleeding in the treatment arms; whether this is an unavoidable adverse effect of certain of these compounds remains to be seen. A Phase II study of a new oral medication, SB 214857, has been performed in patients with recent myocardial infarction, unstable angina, stroke, or TIA; the results are pending. A number of other trials are also in preparation. If Phase III clinical trials show benefits and the medications are tolerable, they would add a new dimension to the prevention of stroke and other vascular diseases in stroke patients.

NONRESPONSE TO ASPIRIN

The response to treatment with aspirin is not the same in all patients. Some stroke patients have elevated levels of platelet reactivity. When aspirin treatment is initiated, platelet activity falls toward normal within hours in > 90% of patients. While the activity remains normal in the majority of subjects, platelet reactivity returns to an enhanced level in approximately 33% of patients. These patients have been called secondary nonresponders. In one study where 1,500 mg/day aspirin was used in 180 patients, the risk of stroke, myocardial infarction, or sudden death was significantly higher in the nonresponders than the responders over a 2-year follow-up. Vascular complications were seen in 5 of 114 patients (4.4%) who responded to aspirin, compared to 24 of 60 patients (40%) in nonresponders.[41]

Other studies have also demonstrated that there is variability in individual response to aspirin therapy in terms of the degree of prolongation of bleeding time and the effect on platelet adhesiveness.[42–44] In other words, aspirin may not have the same antiplatelet effect in all individuals. The results of these studies are very dramatic, but it remains to be confirmed that nonresponse in the laboratory corresponds with a higher rate of clinical events.

Identification of nonresponders may be difficult at present, as some of the laboratory tests used to distinguish responders from nonresponders are not widely available and may not be easily reproducible. The bleeding time may be a better test to identify patients who would be most likely to benefit from ASA therapy.[42] Until further advances are made in this area, patients who continue to have symptoms on high-dose aspirin may be considered clinical nonresponders and may be treated with alternative medications.

SUMMARY

For a number of years aspirin was the only antiplatelet agent available for stroke prophylaxis. During the last two decades ticlopidine and clopidogrel have been tested as two alternative medications to aspirin (see Table 1). While the two medications have shown significant superiority over aspirin in prospective and double-blind studies, the success has not been sufficient to justify a switch to the newer medications. The possibility of more severe side effects, especially with ticlopidine, and the additional cost are in part responsible for the reluctance. We recommend the use of ticlopidine or clopidogrel in patients who either cannot tolerate aspirin or who have strokes or TIAs despite being on at least 325 mg aspirin per day. There is a good theoretical reason to combine ticlopidine or clopidogrel with aspirin in the secondary prevention of stroke or other vascular disease. The combination of these two classes of medications with different mechanisms of antiplatelet action may be more efficacious than one class alone, and this may be a direction for future trials. Currently there are no data supporting the combination of aspirin and a thienopyridine derivative.

Dipyridamole has been shown in recent studies to work well in combination with low-dose aspirin as an antiplatelet agent. Again there is controversy surrounding the large ESPS-II trial. Despite such reservations, the combination of small-dose aspirin and dipyridamole may have a place in the management of patients who cannot tolerate aspirin or continue to have symptoms while on as-

Table 1 Doses, Mechanisms of Action, and Side Effects of Some Alternative Antiplatelet Agents

Drug	Dose	Mechanism	Side effects
Ticlopidine	250 mg twice daily	Blocks the platelet ADP receptor; inhibits GPIIb-IIIa mediated platelet adhesion	Diarrhea 20%, rash 12–15%, bleeding 9%, neutropenia 2.4%, hepatic dysfunction 4%, GI bleeding 0.5%, aplastic anemia, TTP
Clopidogrel	75 mg daily	Blocks the platelet ADP receptor; inhibits GPIIb-IIIa mediated platelet adhesion	Diarrhea 4.6%, indigestion/nausea/vomiting 15%, rash 6%, bleeding 9.3%, GI bleeding 2%
Dipyridamole	200 mg sustained release, twice daily alone or in combination with ASA 25 mg bid	Blocks platelet phosphodiesterase and elevates platelet cAMP; enhances prostacyclin	(For dipyridamole alone): bleeding 4.7%, headache 37.2%, nausea 14.8%, diarrhea 15.4%[a]

[a]Note: a high rate of minor adverse events occurred in the placebo group (nausea 13.7%, diarrhea 9.3%, headache 32.4%) as well in the in the dypyridamole regimens in the ESPS-II.
Sources: Refs. 3, 4, 14, 30.

pirin. Other medications, such as the GPIIb–IIIa antagonists, may be on the horizon as new agents for use in the secondary prevention of stroke.

Finally, the identification of ASA nonresponders may help clinicians to determine those individuals who may benefit from first-line therapy with alternative antiplatelet agents. This is a promising area of research, but more information is required before the phenomenon of ASA nonresponse will influence clinical decisions.

REFERENCES

1. Antiplatelet Trialists' Collaboration. Collaborative overview of randomized trials of antiplatelet therapy. 1. Prevention of death, myocardial infarction, and stroke by prolonged antiplatelet therapy in various categories of patients. BMJ 1994; 308:81–106.
2. Antiplatelet Trialists' Collaboration. Secondary prevention of vascular disease by prolonged antiplatelet treatment. BMJ 1988; 296:320–331.
3. Hass WK, Easton DJ, Adams HP Jr, Pryse-Phillips W, Molony BA, Anderson S, Kamm B. A randomized trial comparing ticlopidine hydrochloride with aspirin for the prevention of stroke in high risk patients. N Engl J Med 1989; 321:501–507.
4. CAPRIE Steering Committee. A randomized blinded trial of clopidogrel versus aspirin in patients at risk of ischaemic events (CAPRIE). Lancet 1996; 348:1329–1339.
5. Dyken ML, Barnett HJM, Easton JD, Field WS, Fuster V, Hachinski V, Norris JW, Sherman DG. Low-dose aspirin and stroke: "It ain't necessarily so." Stroke 1992; 23(10):1395–1399.
6. Dyken ML. Aspirin with and without dipyridamole. Cerebrovasc Dis 1997; 7(suppl 6):10–16.
7. Panak E, Maffrand JP, Picard-Fraire C, Vallee E, Blanchard J, Roncucci R. Ticlopidine: a promise for the prevention and treatment of thrombosis and its complocations. Haemostasis 1983; 13(suppl 1):1–54.
8. McTavish D, Faulds D, Goa KL. Ticlopidine. An updated review of its pharmacology and therapeutic use in platelet-dependent disorders. Drugs 1990; 40:238–259.
9. Bousser MG, Roberts RS, Gent M. Ticlopidine and clopidogrel in secondary stroke prevention. Cerebrovasc Dis 1997; 7(suppl 6):17–23.
10. Schror K. Antiplatelet drugs: a comparative review. Drugs 1995; 50(1):7–28.
11. Reece AH, Walton PL. Inhibition of intimal proliferation of rabbit aorta by ticlopidine. Thromb Haemost 1979; 42:367.
12. Herbert J, Tissinier A, Defreyn G, et al. Inhibitory effect of clopidogrel on platelet adhesion and intimal proliferation after arterial injury in rabbits. Arterioscler Thromb 1993; 13:1171–1179.
13. Bellavance A. Efficacy of ticlopidine and aspirin for prevention of reversible cerebrovascular ischemic events: the ticlopidine aspirin stroke study. Stroke 1993; 24:1452–1457.

14. Gent M, Blakely JA, Easton JD, Ellis DJ, Hachinski VC, Harbison JW, Panak E, Roberts RS, Sicurella J, Alexander GG, Turpie AGG, CATS Group. The Canadian American Ticlopidine Study (CATS) in thromboembolic stroke. Lancet 1989; I:1215–1220.
15. Kovacs MJ, Soong PY, Chin-Yee IH. Thrombotic thrombocytopenic purpora associated with ticlopidine. Ann Pharmacother 1993; 27:1060–1061.
16. Yeh SP, Hsueh EJ, Wu H, Wang YC. Ticlopidine-associated aplastic anemia. A case report and review of the literature. Ann Hematol 1998; 76:87–90.
17. Schmeck-Lindenau HJ, Kurtz W, Heine M. Lymphocytic colitis during ticlopidine therapy (letter). [German.] Dtsch Med Wochenschr 1998; 123(15):479.
18. Aviles P, Gisbert MC, Berbegal SJ, Lopez BI. Ticlopidine-induced lymphocytic colitis (letter). [Spanish.]. Med Clin (Barc) 1996; 106(8):317.
19. Personal communications with Dr. Dan Sadowski and Dr. Nancy I.A. Byles. Division of Gastroenterology, Department of Medicine, University of Alberta, 1998.
20. Murray JC, Kelly MA, Gorelick PB. Ticlopidine: a new antiplatelet agent for the secondary prevention of stroke. Clin Neuropharmacol 1994; 17:23–31.
21. Barnett HJ, Eliasziw M, Meldrum HE. Drugs and Surgery in the prevention of ischemic stroke. N Engl J Med 1995; 332(4):238–248.
22. Coukell AJ, Markham A. Clopidogrel. Drugs 1997; 54(5):745–750.
23. Boneu B, Destelle G. Platelet anti-aggregating activity and tolerance of clopidogrel in atherosclerotic patients. Thromb Haemost 1996; 76:939–943.
24. Acheson J, Danta G, Hutchinson EC. Controlled trial of dipyridamole in cerebral vascular disease. BMJ 1969; i:614–615.
25. Moncada S, Korbut R. Dipyridamole and other phosphodiesterase inhibitors act as antithrombotic agents by potentiating endogenous prostacyclin. Lancet 1978; i:1286–1289.
26. Bousser MG, Eshwege E, Haguenau M, Lefauconnier JM, Thibult N, Touboul D, et al. "AICLA" controlled trial of aspirin and dipyridamole in the secondary prevention of atherothrombotic cerebral ischemia. Stroke 1983; 14:5–14.
27. European Stroke Prevention Study Group. ESPS: principal end points. Lancet 1987; ii:1351–1355.
28. Guiraud-Chaumeil B, Rascol A, David J, Boneu B, Clanet M, Bierme R. Prevention des recidives des accidents vasculaires cerebraux ischemiques par les anti-aggregants plaquettaires. Rev Neurol (Paris) 1982; 138:367–385.
29. American-Canadian Co-operative Study Group. Persantine aspirin trial in cerebral ischemia. 2. Endpoint results. Stroke 1985; 16:406–415.
30. Diener HC, Cunha C, Forbes J, Sivenius P, Smets P, Lowenthal A. European Stroke Prevention Study 2. Dipyridamole and ascetylsalicylic acid in the secondary prevention of stroke. J Neurol Sci 1996; 143:1–13.
31. Canadian Cooperative Study Group. A randomized trial of aspirin and sulfinpyrazone in threatened stroke. N Engl J Med 1978; 299:53–9.
32. Kieffer N, Phillips DR. Platelet membrane glycoproteins: functions in cellular interactions. Annu Rev Cell Biol 1990; 6:329–357.
33. George JN, Caen JP, Nurden AT. Glanzmann's thromboasthenia: the spectrum of clinical disease and molecular abnormalities in 64 patients. Blood 1990; 75:1383–1395.

34. Nurden AT, Duperat VG, Nurden P. Platelet function and pharmacology of antiplatelet drugs. Cerebrovasc Dis 1997; 7(suppl 6):2–9.
35. EPIC Investigators. Use of monoclonal antibody directed against the platelet glycoprotein IIb–IIIa receptor in high-risk coronary angioplasty. N Engl J Med 1994; 330:956–961.
36. EPILOG Investigators. Platelet glycoprotein IIb–IIIa receptor blockade and low dose heparin during percutaneous coronary revascularization. N Engl J Med 1997; 336:1689–1696.
37. Brener SJ, Barr LA, Burchenal J, Katz S, George BS, Jones AA, Moliterno DJ, Topol EJ. A randomized, placebo controlled trial of abciximab with primary angioplasty for acute MI: the RAPPORT Trial. Circulation 1997; 96(suppl I):I–473. Abstract.
38. IMPACT-II Investigators. Randomized placebo-controlled trial of effect of eptifibatide on complications of percutaneous coronary intervention: IMPACT-II. Lancet 1997; 349:1422–1428.
39. RESTORE Investigators. Effects of platelet glycoprotein IIb/IIIa blockade with Tirofiban on adverse cardiac events in patients with unstable angina or acute myocardial infarction undergoing coronary angioplasty. Circulation 1997; 96:1445–1453.
40. Ferguson JJ. Meeting highlights, 46th Annual Scientific Sessions of the American College of Cardiology—antiplatelet therapy in acute coronary syndromes. Circulation 1997; 96:367–368.
41. Grotemeyer KH, Scharafinski HW, Hussedt IW. Two-year follow-up of aspirin responder and aspirin non-responder. A pilot study including 180 post-stroke patients. Thromb Res 1993; 71:397–403.
42. Buchanan MR, Brister SJ. Individual variation in the effects of ASA on platelet function: implications for the use of ASA clinically. Can J Cardiol 1995 ;11(3):221–227.
43. Cortelazzo S, Marchetti M, Orlando E, Falanga A, Barbui T, Buchanan MR. Aspirin increases the bleeding side effects in essential thrombocythemia independent of the cyclooxygenase pathway: role of the lipoxygenase pathway. Am J Hematol 1998; 57:277–282.
44. Mueller MR, Salat A, Stangl P, Murabito M, Pulaki S, Boehm D, Koppensteiner R, Ergun E, Mittlboeck M, Schreiner W, Losert U, Wolner E. Variable platelet response to low-dose ASA and the risk of limb deterioration in patients submitted to peripheral arterial angioplasty. Thromb Haemost 1997; 78:1003–1007.

23

Anticoagulation for Prevention of Cardioembolic Stroke

Oscar Benavente and Robert G. Hart
University of Texas Health Science Center, San Antonio, Texas

CARDIOEMBOLIC STROKE

Emboli arising from the heart account for approximately 20% of all ischemic strokes.[1] Advances in imaging techniques have lead to recognition of new cardiac disorders potentially responsible for embolic stroke. Because the underlying cardiac condition is often evident before stroke occurs and antithrombotic therapies are notably effective, cardiogenic emboli to the brain are among the most preventable causes of stroke.

With a thorough cardiac workup, a potential source of cardiogenic emboli can be identified in at least 30% of all patients with ischemic stroke. However, potential cardioembolic sources often coexist with other risk factors for cardiovascular disease.[2–4] Thus, the identification of a potential cardioembolic source is not usually sufficient for diagnosis.

Cardioembolic stroke is caused by several very different cardiac disorders, each with a unique natural history and a variable response to antithrombotic therapy (Fig. 1).

The embolic material originating from the heart and proximal aorta can be quite diverse. The thrombi may be formed by different proportions of platelets and fibrin, cholesterol fragments, tumor particles, or bacterial clusters. The natural history and response to antithrombotic therapy of each of these conditions are unique, and consequently, each source of cardioembolic strokes should be considered separately.

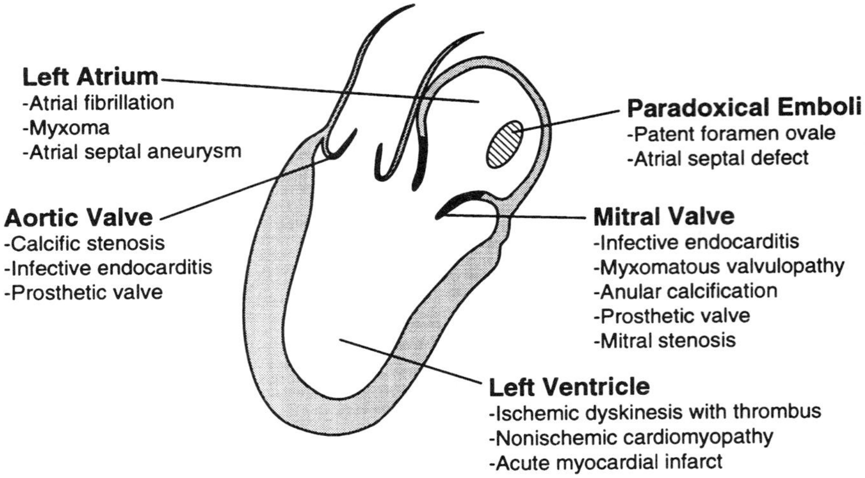

Figure 1 Common sources of cardiogenic emboli.

The incidence of ischemic stroke associated with cardioembolic sources has a wide variation. Cardioembolic sources of stroke can be divided according to the stroke risk into "major risk," where the risk for stroke is well established, and "minor risk," where the risk for stroke has been incompletely established. The former carries a substantial annual risk of emboli and usually antithrombotic therapy is warranted for primary prevention. On the contrary, the so-called minor sources of emboli have a low or uncertain risk of embolism, and antithrombotic therapy is usually reserved for secondary prevention (Table 1). [5]

ATRIAL FIBRILLATION

Atrial fibrillation (AF) is the most common cardiac arrhythmia, affecting 0.7% of the general population of the United States (1.8 million people). Its prevalence increases with age—about 5% at age 65 years and approximately 10% at the age of 80 years. AF is equally distributed in the two sexes. The mean age of individuals affected is about 75 years.[6]

Nonvalvular AF is responsible for about 16% (range 11% to 29%) of all ischemic strokes. [2,3,7–11] In patients >70 years of age with ischemic stroke, AF is present in more than one-third.[12] AF-associated stroke is a common cause of disabling stroke in the elderly, particularly in elderly women.[12] Nonvalvular AF is a recognized independent risk factor for ischemic stroke.[13] The risk of ischemic

Table 1 Potential Cardioembolic Sources

Major risk
Atrial fibrillation
Mitral stenosis
Prosthetic cardiac valves
Recent myocardial infarction (especially large anterior wall)
Left ventricular thrombus (more if mobile and protruding)
Atrial myxoma
Infective endocarditis
Marantic endocarditis
Dilating cardiomyopathies (nonischemic)
Minor risk
Mitral valve prolapse
Patent foramen ovale
Atrial septal aneurysm
Aortic arch atheromatous plaques
Left ventricular regional wall motion abnormalities
Mitral annular calcification
Calcified aortic stenosis

stroke increases fivefold (from 1% to 5%/year) in elderly patients (mean age 70 years) with nonvalvular AF, and about 18-fold in patients with AF and rheumatic mitral stenosis.[14] AF accounts for about half of the cardioembolic strokes (Fig. 2).

Most embolic strokes in patients with AF are caused by the embolism of thrombi forming in the appendage of the left atrium (Fig. 3).[15,16] About 70% of ischemic strokes in AF patients are embolic[14–17,19]; however, approximatly 30% of AF-associated strokes are secondary to intrinsic cerebrovascular disease, atheroma of the proximal aorta, or other cardioembolic sources.[15,16] The formation of thrombi in the left atrium appendage in AF patients is precipitated by the sluggish flow from ineffective atrial contraction. However, AF alone may not be enough to promote thrombi formation; other factors must also contribute. Associated cardiovascular disease and age appear to influence the stroke rate in AF, and hence also influence the formation of atrial appendage thrombi. Embolic events are intermittent in AF, sometimes separated by years. A balance between clot formation and inhibition is possibly present in the atrial appendage of these patients. The balance is influenced by atrial size, appendage flow velocities, and coagulation factors. Therefore, the type and intensity of antithrombotic therapy to inhibit appendage thrombi may differ between AF patients and over time for individual patients.

The overall incidence of ischemic stroke among people with AF is about 5%/year, however, the rate of stroke varies widely, depending on coexisting car-

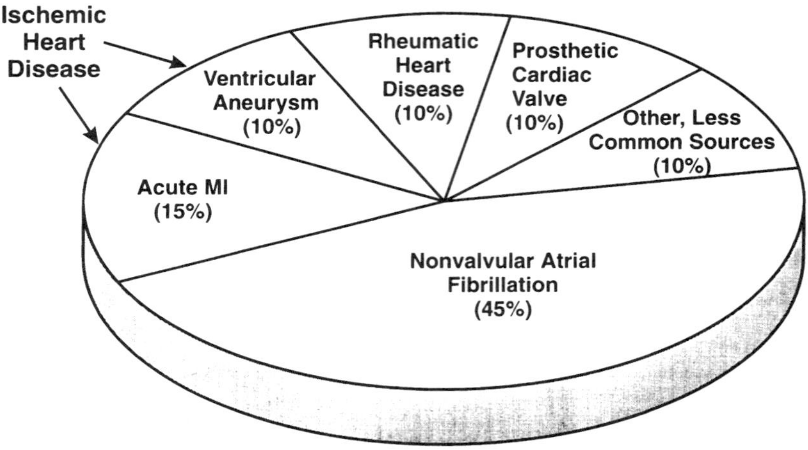

Figure 2 Etiology of cardioembolic stroke.

diovascular disorders.[18–21] Identification of subgroups of AF patients with relatively high vs. low absolute rates of stroke is important for selecting prophylactic antithrombotic therapy.[17,19–24] Prospective studies have shown that hypertension, prior TIA/stroke, and left ventricular systolic dysfunction are indepenently

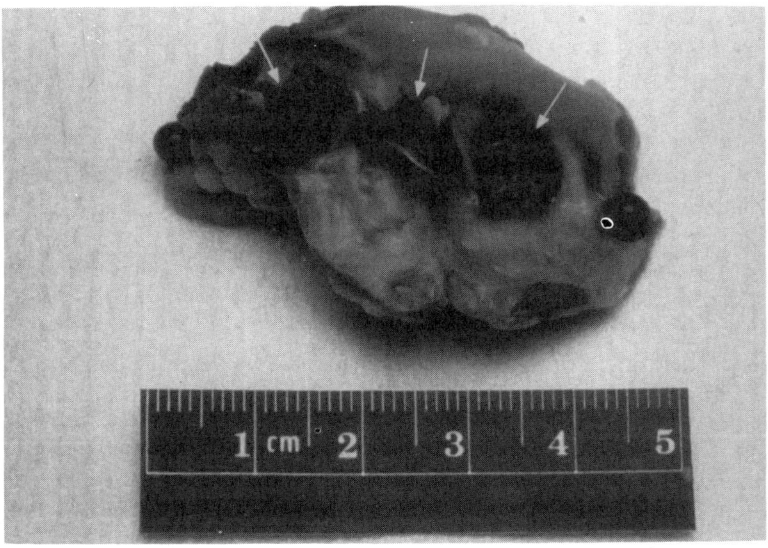

Figure 3 Thrombi in the appendage of the left atrium in a patient with chronic AF.

Table 2 Risk Stratification in Atrial Fibrillation Patients High-Risk Variables

History of hypertension (includes systolic blood pressure >160)
Prior TIA or stroke
Diabetes
Recent heart failure
Age >65 years

Table 3 Stroke Rates in Atrial Fibrillation Patients

Unselected AF patient	5%/year
Low-risk AF patient	2%/year
High-risk AF patient	8%/year

predictive of stroke in AF patients.[18,21,24–26] Echocardiographic studies identified left ventricular systolic dysfunction to be strongly, consistently and independently associated with subsequent stroke in patients with AF[25,27] (Tables 2, 3)

Stroke Prevention in AF

The efficacy of antithrombotic therapies to prevent stroke in nonvalvular AF has been well established by recent randomized clinical trials.[1,23–34] An aggregate analysis of six clinical trials showed that anticoagulation with warfarin reduces ischemic stroke by nearly 70% compared to the rate in untreated patients,[18,29] and an efficacy analysis indicated an even greater benefit (Fig. 4). In addition, the increase in major bleeding among elderly anticoagulated AF patients in these trials was only 0.3% to 2.0%/year with a target INR 1.5 to 4.0.[18,29,35] Participants in these trials were carefully selected to minimize bleeding risks and were followed closely on clinical trial protocols.

The risk of major hemorrhage in elderly AF patients on oral anticoagulants seems to be related to the intensity of anticoagulation, patient age, and fluctuation in INR.[36–38] The optimal intensity of anticoagulation to prevent ischemic stroke and minimize the risk of bleeding probably varies according to the individual stroke risk. Low-intensity anticoagulation (INR target range 2.0 to 3.0) is effective in primary stroke prevention for AF patients. However, warfarin proved to be more effective in high-risk patients with prior TIAs or strokes when a higher INR target (2.5 to 4.2) was used.[38]

The efficacy of aspirin for stroke prevention in AF patients has been tested in three randomized clinical trials. Pooled analysis showed a risk reduction of 21% (range 15% to 44%, $P = 0.05$), compared to placebo,[28–30] however, aspirin

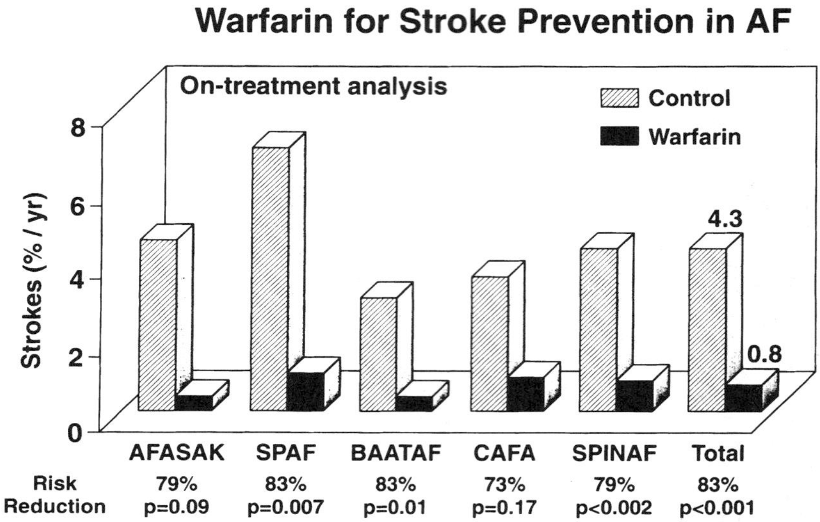

Figure 4 Warfarin for stroke prevention. AFASAK: Atrial fibrillation, Aspirin, Anticoagulation study from Copenhagen, Denmark; SPAF: Stroke Prevention in Atrial Fibrillation; BAATAF: Boston Area Anticoagulation Trial in Atrial Fibrillation; CAFA: Canadian Atrial Fibrillation Anticoagulation; SPINAF: Veterans Affairs Stroke Prevention in Nonrheumatic Atrial Fibrillation.

was significantly less effective than warfarin in these trials (Fig. 5).[29,31,35] Overall, warfarin reduces the risk of stroke by 50% compared to aspirin in AF patients. Aspirin may be more efficacious in preventing noncardioembolic strokes in AF-patients.[16,39]

Unquestionably, warfarin is highly efficacious for preventing stroke in AF patients and relatively safe for selected patients. Aspirin offers less benefit, possibly by decreasing noncardioembolic strokes in these patients. The choice of antithrombotic prophylaxis should be based upon the risk stratification. Long-term anticoagulation cannot be recommended for all unselected patients with AF since most of them will not experience strokes, even if untreated. Low-risk AF patients with a relatively small stroke rate would not significantly benefit by the use of warfarin, since the absolute risk reduction will be small (~1%/year). In these patients anticoagulation may not be warranted.[38a] On the contrary, AF patients who have a high risk for ischemic stroke (>7%) because of a history of hypertension, prior TIA or stroke, diabetes, or ventricular dysfunction would have a significantly lower stroke rate if anticoagulated (Table 4).

High-risk patients suitable for anticoagulation benefit extensively from warfarin. For high-risk patients aged 75 years or younger, an intensity INR of

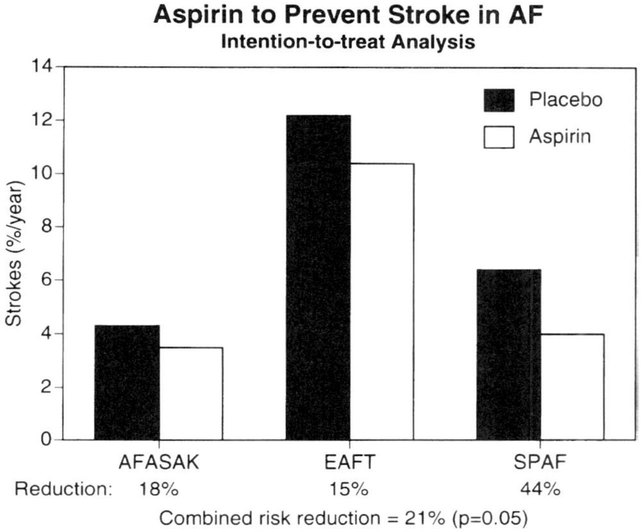

Figure 5 Aspirin to prevent stroke in AF. Intention-to-treat analysis. AFASAK: Atrial fibrillation, Aspirin, Anticoagulation study from Copenhagen, Denmark; EAFT: European Atrial Fibrillation Trial; SPAF: Stroke Prevention Atrial Fibrillation Trial.

2.0 to 3.0 is effective and safe; for those older than 75 years, a slightly lower target (INR 2.0) appears appropriate in order to minimize bleeding complications.[35–37] For secondary prevention, a range closer to an INR of 3.0 may be optimal.[38] Patients <60 years with "lone" AF may not require antithrombotic therapy, considering that the intrinsic risk for stroke is small.[19] The efficacy of aspirin in low-risk AF patients is still unproven, and its use is empirical.[40]

Several issues concerning stroke prevention in AF patients are still unsettled. There is not sufficient clinical evidence that cardioversion followed by prolonged maintenance of sinus rhythm will reduce embolism.[41,42] The choice of intensity of anticoagulation and risk/benefit of combining antiaggregant agents

Table 4 Anticoagulation in Atrial Fibrillation: Effect of Risk Stratification

		Number needed to treat with warfarin to prevent 1 stroke/year	
	Stroke rates	Any stroke	Disabling stroke
Unselected AF patient	5%/year	33	70
Low-risk AF patient	2%/year	83	160
High-risk AF patient	8%/year	16	25

with anticoagulants for the prevention of ischemic stroke and vascular death in elderly AF patients are equally unresolved issues. This is especially important for AF patients >75 years, who often are at a higher risk for warfarin-related hemorrhage.[30,37] Higher intensities of anticoagulation may be required to prevent ischemic stroke when multiple risk factors are present. A validated risk stratification scheme to stratify AF patients who would most benefit from antithrombotic therapy is needed.

MYOCARDIAL INFARCTION

The stroke rate in survivors of myocardial infarction (MI) is about 1% to 2%/year.[43–45] Since coronary artery atherosclerosis often coexists with primary cerebrovascular disease, not all the strokes in these individuals are cardioembolic.[46,47] The risk of stroke is particularly high during the first 3 months after the MI.[40,43,48]

The use of long-term anticoagulants post-MI is associated with a 75% risk reduction in the incidence of stroke; however, this represents only an absolute risk reduction of 1%/year. At the same, time anticoagulation (INR 2.5 to 4.5) has an associated excess incidence of intracerebral hemorrhage (ICH) of 10-fold, or 0.4%/year. In addition, ICHs have a higher mortality and are more disabling than ischemic strokes.[49] In summary, we would need to treat 1000 unselected MI survivors to prevent approximately 10 strokesper year, and for every 1,000 patients treated, four would suffer a disabling or fatal ICH. Therefore, the net benefit is minimal. The risk vs. benefit of a lower-intensity anticoagulation (INR 1.6 to 2.5) has not been tested in this setting.[50,51] Aspirin reduces the incidence of stroke in patients with prior MI, with a relative risk reduction of 30%, but with a very small absolute risk reduction (<0.5%). Because of such small net benefit, oral anticoagulation cannot be routinely recommended in an *unselected* group of post-MI patients to prevent stroke.

There are, however, specific subsets of patients with prior MI that are at higher risk of ischemic stroke and benefit from anticoagulation. Patients who suffered an anterior wall MI have a higher risk for stroke than patients with MI in other locations.[43,44,46] The presence of left ventricular thrombi post-MI is associated with a much higher incidence of embolic stroke (approximatley 5% to 10% over the following 6 to 12 months).[1,52] In this setting, anticoagulants reduce the stroke risk by 60%,[1] so its use is indicated for 3 to 6 months after the thrombi is diagnosed. There is some evidence indicating that chronic thrombus (>6 months) have less emboliogenic potential; thus anticoagulation after this period would be reasonable only if the thrombus is mobile and/or protruding.[53]

The presence of AF in MI survivors markedly increases the risk for embolic stroke,[18,43,54,55] and anticoagulation is routinely recommended in this situation. The presence of congestive heart failure in patients with prior MI also seems to increase the risk of ischemic stroke.[43,44,56,57] The risk of stroke increases by 1% to 2%/year when CHF is present in MI survivors. Despite doubling the incidence when compared with patients without CHF, the stroke risk is still relatively low, and anticoagulation may not substantially benefit these patients.

In summary, oral anticoagulation (INR 2.5 to 4.8) to prevent stroke does not substantially benefit unselected patients following acute MI. The value of lower-intensity anticoagulation (INR 1.6 to 2.5) and antiplatelet agents for stroke prevention in this setting is still unproven. On the other hand, patients with prior MI and AF or acute left ventricular thrombi are at higher risk of embolic stroke, and anticoagulation (INR 2.0 to 3.0) is routinely recommended for stroke prevention.

PROSTHETIC CARDIAC VALVES

Despite progress in valve design and effective anticoagulant therapy, systemic embolism remains a serious threat in patients following heart valve replacement. The rate of embolism is high in patients with mechanical prosthetic cardiac valves, and even in properly anticoagulated patients the rate of embolism is 2% to 4%/year.[59–63] Embolism is more frequent with valves in mitral position, multiple valves and cage-ball valves. The presence of atrial stasis is a risk factor for thrombogenicity; atrial stasis is influenced by valve type and position, atrial fibrillation, and ventricular pacemakers.

Permanent anticoagulation is generally recommended to prevent embolic stroke and valve thrombosis for all mechanical prosthetic valves. It is also recommended for bioprosthetic valves in mitral position if associated with AF, enlarged left atria, or ventricular pacemakers and if there is evidence of atrial thrombi or prior thromboembolism.[59]

Long-term anticoagulation is warranted for patients with bioprosthetic valves in the mitral position plus atrial fibrillation. Also, anticoagulation is recommended when the prosthetic valve is associated with an enlarged (>5.5 cm) left atrium, atrial thrombi, prior embolism, or a ventricular pacemaker.[59] Bioprosthetic valves in the aortic position in patients with sinus rhythm may not require chronic anticoagulation since the stroke rate is relatively low. Warfarin is recommended for a period of 3 months after valve implant.[59]

Thrombogenicity of specific valves varies, as do factors influencing thromboembolic risk; thus, multiple factors should be considered before selecting prophylactic antithrombotic therapy. In the past, the intensity of use of anticoagulation for mechanical valves was between INR 3.0 and 4.5. Now it is believed that a lower intensity (INR 2.5 to 3.5) would be as effective as a higher intensity[59]; however, this issue is still controversial. Adding antiplatelet agents, such as aspirin or dipyridamol, to warfarin further reduces embolism; however, this therapeutic strategy may increase the risk of bleeding (mostly minor bleeds when aspirin is added).[60]

The success of antithrombotic therapy in primary stroke prevention in patients with prosthetic valves is influenced by several factors: type of prosthesis; factors associated with left atrial stasis; underlying cardiovascular disease; and tolerability of antithrombotic therapies. The optimal or appropiate intensity of anticoagulation and the decision to use additional antiplatelet agents in individual patients depends upon of the presence of the above-mentioned risk factors and the valve type.

In fully anticoagulated patients, the incidence of stroke is about 1%/year and most of the emboli are minor, leaving mild residual deficits.[63,64] When stroke occurs in anticoagulated patients, transesophageal echocardiography (TEE) should usually be performed to search for infective valve vegetations, thrombi, spontaneous echodensities, or atrial thrombi.[65] Anticoagulation may be increased if embolism from the left atrium is suspected, while adding an antiplatelet agent might be useful if stroke is attributed to associated cerebrovascular disease or to valve-related thrombi.

PATENT FORAMEN OVALE

Patent foramen ovale (PFO) has been associated with stroke in several case-controll studies, particularly in young individuals without other recognized cause for stroke. This is due to its potential role as a conduit for paradoxical embolism.[66–69] Precordial contrast echocardiography detects some degree of interatrial shunting in about 18% of normal controls,[66,68,70–72] especially during early systole or Valsalva-provoking activities such as coughing.[73,74] The fossa ovalis and the size of PFO can be directly visualized by TEE.[72,75,76] Transcranial Doppler (TCD) can detect injected microbubbles that bypass the pulmonary capillaries to enter the cerebral circulation, and correlates well with the TEE evidence of PFO in the majority of patients.[77–82] The size of the PFO patency varies from 1 to 9 mm at autopsy.[82] The volume of shunting depends on both the size of the PFO and the difference in atrial pressures.

The prevalence of PFO in young adults with TIA or ischemic stroke is increased (about 40%, range 32% to 48%),[66–69,78] especially among those with cryptogenic ischemic stroke, where its prevalence in some series is >50%.[66,72,78,82] Hence, the frequency of PFO is increased two to three times among young adults with cerebral ischemia, and PFO is clearly associated with cryptogenic stroke in young adults.[68] In older stroke patients, the presence of PFO is lower, probably because its importance as an independent risk factor is offset by the higher prevalence of other stroke mechanisms.[72,83–85]

The mechanism of PFO-associated stroke is thought to be due to paradoxical embolism in many patients. Paradoxical embolism is when the embolic material originating in the venous system or right chambers migrates into the systemic circulation, through vascular shunts that bypass the pulmonary vasculature. Emboli can arise from thrombi in the crural pelvic veins or in the right chamber of the heart; however, the source of embolism is often not found.

Several lines of evidence challenge the concept that paradoxical embolism is the most common underlying mechanism of stroke in patients with PFO. First, in patients with isolated PFOs the shunting during Valsalva maneuver involves only a small fraction of cardiac output, and the chance that this degree of shunting will result in recurrent emboli is remote.[86] Second, deep-venous thrombosis is identified in only about 10% of PFO-associated stroke. Further, PFOs are associated with mitral valve prolapse and atrial septal aneurysms; both are independent potential cardioembolic sources.[68,87,88] Atrial septal aneurysms are present in about 25% of young patients with PFO-associated stroke.[68,88] and their presence alone has been associated with a high risk of embolic stroke (see below).[68] It is possible that in as many as half of the stroke patients with PFO-associated stroke , PFO and stroke coexist by chance.

The management of patients with PFO-associated stroke is controversial since the recurrence rate of stroke is relatively low (1%/year), even when patients are treated with aspirin or short-term anticoagulation.[89] The use of antiplatelet agents seems to be a valid alternative in patients who suffer a stroke when deep venous thrombosis is not present. The use of long-term anticoagulation seems appropiate when a venous source of emboli is present. Surgical closure of PFOs is a relatively safe procedure, but its value is unclear, given the uncertainties in pathogenesis, recurrence rate of stroke, and comparative efficacy of antithrombotic agents.[88,90–92]

ATRIAL SEPTAL ANEURYSMS

Atrial septal aneurysms are bulging areas in the interatrial septum identified by TEE in about 1% of normal hearts and in approximately 10% of patients with ischemic stroke.[76,88,93–102] Atrial septal aneurysms are often fenestrated and are associated with PFO, atrial septal defects, and mitral valve prolapse.[68,97,100,102–104] The possible mechanisms for cardioembolic stroke in patients with atrial septal aneurysms include paradoxical embolism,[68,104] intra-anerysm thrombus formation,[100,101,105] and associated mitral valve prolapse.[68,105,106]

The risk for initial stroke and the natural history of recurrent stroke in patients with atrial septal aneurysm are unknown. The presence of coexistent PFO or mitral valve prolapse appears to influence the stroke risk.[68] Optimal antithrombotic therapy for these patients is unclear.[107]

ANTICOAGULATION IN ACUTE CARDIEMBOLIC STROKE

Cardioembolic strokes have a higher incidence of secondary hemorrhagic transformation than other types of ischemic stroke; therefore, this makes early anticoagulation potentially risky. The available data do not allow accurate, evidence-based estimates of the risk vs. benefit of early anticoagulation for patients with cardioembolic stroke.

The risk of early recurrent stroke or systemic embolism following a recent cardioembolic stroke in untreated patients is estimated to be about 10% during the first week,[1] and is especially high during the first 5 or 6 days after an acute cardioembolic stroke.[108,109] The overall risk of early recurrent stroke is strongly influenced by the specific cardioembolic source (i.e. ,lower for nonvalvular atrial fibrillation).

Pooled data from case series and one small controlled trial [110–112] suggest that heparin reduces early stroke recurrence by about 70% in patients with cardioembolic stroke. However, the increased risk of symptomatic intracranial hemorrhage (ICH) in early-anticoagulated patients could offset the benefit obtained by early anticoagulation.

Even in patients who are not on anticoagulants, cardioembolic strokes frequently undergo spontaneous hemorrhagic transformations.[113–116] The mechanism of delayed hemorrhagic transformation in embolic stroke in most patients appears to be the reperfusion of infarcted or ischemic brain tissue following distal migration or dissolution of the embolus. Serial CT scans disclose up to 40% frequency of delayed hemorrhagic transformation in nonanticoagulated patients.[117,118] Autopsy series showed hemorrhagic transformation even in a higher percentage (50% to 70%) of nonanticoagulated patients.[116] A prospective MRI study that imaged patients 3 weeks following cardioembolic stroke reported a 70% incidence of hemorrhagic transformation.[115] The great majority of hemorrhagic transformations are asymptomatic in patients not receiving anticoagulants.

The relationship between anticoagulants and clinically significant delayed hemorrhage is controversial. The incidence and time course of asymptomatic hemorrhagic transformation do not seem to be affected by anticoagulation[119]; however, the degree and likelihood of associated clinical deterioration are augmented.[114,119,120] The incidence of symptomatic hemorrhagic transformation in acutely anticoagulated patients varies widely (from 1% to 25%).[109,113,114,121,122]

Patients with a large infarct, excessive anticoagulation, and hemorrhagic infarction on initial CT scan are at higher risk for symptomatic hemorrhagic transformation. Small case series have advocated the use of anticoagulants in patients with early hemorrhagic infarction on CT scan.[109,110,123,124] It appears that hemorrhagic infarction may not be an absolute contraindication to anticoagulation, especially in individual patients who are at high risk of recurrent embolism. But, given the lack of prospective studies and the relatively small number of patients in these anecdoctal case series, early anticoagulation in hemorrhagic infarction cannot be routinely recommended due to safety concerns. Delaying anticoagulation for 1 to 2 weeks following detection of hemorrhagic infarction may be prudent.

At the present time it is impossible to make firm guidelines regarding anticoagulation in acute cardioembolic stroke because of the paucity of adequate data. Two large clinical trials (TOAST and IST) should shed light on critical issues soon. The risk vs. benefit of early anticoagulation is influenced by the specific cardioembolic source and the size of the infarct. For patients at relatively low risk for early stroke recurrence, including those with nonvalvular atrial fibrillation or recent myocardial infarction without associated ventricular thrombi, deferring anticoagulation for several weeks may reduce the risk of hemorrhagic deterioration, particularly for patients with moderate to large infarct size or uncontrolled hypertension. Initiation of anticoagulation with oral warfarin (without the use of heparin) is an adequate alternative for these patients.

For patients at high risk for recurrent embolization (i.e., mechanical prosthetic valve, intracardiac thrombus, AF with valvular disease or congestive heart failure), early anticoagulation is tentatively recommended, particularly if there are no associated risk factors for brain hemorrhage. Intravenous boluses of heparin and excessive anticoagulation should be avoided.

The value of antiplatelet agents and low-dose subcutaneous heparin in this setting has not been systematically assessed. Both could be alternatives to intravenous heparin, particularly in patients at low risk of early recurrent stroke (i.e., nonvalvular AF).[15]

Patients with prosthetic valves who are fully anticoagulated at the time of the stroke represent a management challenge, and reversing anticoagulation in patients with large infarcts or with infarcts already visible on early CT scan (<6 to 12 hours) should be considered. Anticoagulation is not indicated for embolic stroke secondary to native-valve infective endocarditis.[125]

REFERENCES

1. Cerebral Embolism Task Force. Cardiogenic brain embolism: the second report of Cerebral Embolism Task Force. Arch Neurol 1989; 46:727–741.
2. Bogusslavsky J, Cachin C, Regli F, Despland PA, Van Melle G, Kappenberger L. Cardiac sources of embolism and cerebral infarction—clinical consequences and vascular concomitants. Neurology 1991; 41:855–859.
3. Horning CR, Brainin M, Mast H. Cardioembolic stroke: results from three current stroke data banks. Neuroepidemiolgy 1994; 13:318–323.
4. Ramirez-Lassepas M, Cipolle RJ, Bjork RJ. Can embolic stroke be diagnosed on the basis of neurological clinical criteria? Arch Neurol 1987; 44:87–89.

5. Sherman DG, Dyken ML, Gent M, Harrison MJG, Hart RG. Antithrombotic therapy for cerebrovascular disorders: an update. Chest 1995; 108:444S–456S.
6. Feinberg WM, Blackshear JL, Laupacis A, Kronmal R, Hart RG. Prevalence, age distribution, and gender of patients with atrial fibrillation. Arch Intern Med 1995; 155:469–473.
7. van Merwijk G, Lodder J, Bamford J, Kester ADM. How often is nonvalvular atrial fibrillation the cause of brain infarction. J Neurol 1990; 237:205–207.
8. Broderick JP, Philips SJ, O'Fallon WM, Frye RL, Whisnant JP. Relationship of cardiac disease to stroke ocurrence, recurrence and mortality. Stroke 1992; 23:1250–1256.
9. Mohr JP, Caplan LR, Melski JW, et al. The Harvard Cooperative Stroke Registry: A prospective registry. Neurology 1978; 28:754–762.
10. Britton M, Gustafsson C. Nonrheumatic atrial fibrillation as a risk factor for stroke. Stroke 1985; 16:182–88.
11. Sandercock P, Bamford J, Dennis M, Burn J, Slattery J, Jones L, et al. Atrial fibrillation and stroke: prevalence in different types of stroke and influence on early and longterm prognosis. (Oxfordshire community stroke project). Br Med J 1992; 305:1460–1465.
12. Asplund K, Carlberg B, Sundstrom G. Stroke in the elderly. Cerebrovasc Dis 1992; 2:152–157.
13. Wolf PA, Abbot RD, Kammel WB. Atrial fibrillation as an independent risk factor for stroke: The Framinghan Study. Stroke 1991; 22:983–988.
14. Wolf PA, Dawber TR, Thomas HE, Kannel WB. Epidemiologic assessment of chronic atrial fibrillation and risk of stroke: The Framinghan Study. Neurology 1978; 28:973–977.
15. Bogousslavsky J, Van Melle G, Regli F, et al. Pathogenesis of anterior circulation stroke in patients with atrial fibrillation: The Lausanne Stroke Registry. Neurology 1990; 40:1046–1050.
16. Miller VT, Rothrock JF, Pearce LA, Feinberg WM, Hart RG, Anderson DC. Ischemic stroke in patients with atrial fibrillation: effect of aspirin according to stroke mechanism. Neurology 1993; 43:32–36.
17. Moulton AW, Singer DE, Haas JS. Risk factors for stroke in patients with nonrheumatic atrial fibrillation: a case-control study. Am J Med 1991; 91:156–161.
18. Atrial Fibrillation Investigators. Risk factors for stroke and efficacy of antithrombotic therapy in atrial fibrillation: analysis of pooled data from five randomized clinical trials. Arch Intern Med 1994; 154:1949–957.
19. Kopecky SL, Gersh BJ, McGoon MD, et al. The natural history of lone atrial fibrillation: a population-based study over three decades. N Engl J Med 1987; 317:669–674.
20. Stroke Prevention in Atrial Fibrillation Investigators. Predictors of thromboembolism in atrial fibrillation. II. Echocardiographic features in patients at risk. Ann Intern Med 1991; 1:6–12.
21. Stroke Prevention in Atrial Fibrillation Investigators. Predictors of thromboembolism in atrial fibrillation. I. Clinical features in patients at risk. Ann Intern Med 1992; 116:1–5.

22. Cabin HS, Clubb KS, et al. Risk for systemic embolization of atrial fibrillation without mitral stenosis. Am J Cardiol 1990; 65:1112–1116.
23. Peterson P, Kastrup J, et al. Risk factors for thromboembolic complications in chronic atrial fibrillation. Arch Intern Med 1990; 150:819–821.
24. van Latum JC, Koudstaal PJ, Venables GS, et al. Predictors of major vascular events in patients with a transient ischemic attack or minor ischemic stroke and with nonrheumatic atrial fibrillation. Stroke 1995; 16:801–806.
26. Stroke Prevention in Atrial Fibrillation Investigators. Risk factors for thromboembolism during aspirin therapy in atrial fibrillation. J Stroke Cerebrovasc Dis 1995; 5:147–157.
27. Leung DYC, Black IW, Cranney GB, Hopkins AP, Walsh WF. Prognostic implications of left atrial spontaneous echo contrast in nonvalvular atrial fibrillation. J Am Coll Cardiol 1994; 24:255–262.
28. Stroke Prevention in Atrial Fibrillation Investigators. Stroke prevention in atrial fibrillation: final results. Circulation 1991; 84:527–539.
29. European Atrial Fibrillation Trial Study Group. Secondary prevention of vascular events in patients with nonrheumatic atrial fibrillation and recent transient ischemic attack or minor ischemic stroke. Lancet 1993; 342:1255–1262.
30. Peterson P, Boysen G, Godtfredson J, Andersen ED, Andersen B. Placebo-controlled, randomized trial of warfarin and aspirin for prevention of thromboembolic complications in chronic atrial fibrillation. the Copenhagen AFASAK study. Lancet 1989; 1:175–179.
31. Peterson P, Boysen G. Prevention of stroke in atrial fibrillation. N Engl J Med 1990; 323:482.
32. Boston Area Anticoagulation Trial for Atrial Fibrillation Investigators. The effect of low-dose warfarin on the risk of stroke in nonrheumatic atrial fibrillation. N Engl J Med 1990; 323:1505–1511.
33. Connolly SJ, Laupacis A, Gent M, Roberts RS, Cairns JA, Joyner C, CAFA Study Coinvestigators. Canadian Atrial Fibrillation Anticoagulation (CAFA) Study. J Am Coll Cardiol 1991; 18:349–355.
34. Harenberg J, Weuster B, Pfitzei M, Dempfle C-E, Stehle G, Kubler W, Schlierf G. Prophylaxis of embolic events in patients with atrial fibrillation using low molecular weight heparin. Semin Thromb Hemost 1993; 19(suppl):116–121.
35. Stroke Prevention in Atrial Fibrillation Investigators. Warfarin versus aspirin for prevention of thromboembolism in atrial fibrillation. Stroke Prevention in Atrial Fibrillation II Study. Lancet 1994; 343:687–691.
36. Hart RG, Boop B, Anderson DC. Oral anticoagulants and intracranial hemorrhage: facts and hypotheses. Stroke 1995; 26:1471–1477.
37. Stroke Prevention in Atrial Fibrillation Investigators. Bleeding during antithrombotic therapy for atrial fibrillation. Arch Intern Med 1996; 156:409–416.
38. European Atrial Fibrillation Trial Study Group. Optimal oral anticoagulant therapy in patients with nonrheumatic atrial fibrillation and recent cerebral ischemia. N Engl J Med 1995; 333:5–10.
38a. Stroke Prevention in Atrial Fibrillation Investigators. Patients with nonvalvular atrial fibrillation at low risk of stroke during treatment with aspirin. JAMA 1998; 279(16):1273–1277.

39. Miller VT, Pearce LA, Feinberg WM, Rothrock JF, Anderson DC, Hart RG. Differential effect of aspirin versus warfarin on clinical stroke types in patients with atrial fibrillation. Neurology 1996; 46:238–240.
40. Antiplatelet Trialists Collaboration. Collaborative overview of randomized trials of antiplatelet therapy (Part I). Br Med J 1994; 308:81–106.
41. Dish DL, Greenberg ML, Holzberg PT, Malenka DJ, Birkmeyer JD. Managing chronic atrial fibrillation: a Markov decision analysis comparing warfarin, quinidine and low-dose amiodarone. Ann Intern Med 1994; 120:449–457.
42. Middlekauff HR, Stevenson WG, Gornbein JA. Antiarrhythmic prophylaxis vs. warfarin anticoagulation to prevent thromboembolic events among patients with atrial fibrillation: a decision analysis. Arch Intern Med 1995; 155:913–920.
43. Tanne D, Goldbourt U, Zion M, Reicher-Reiss H, Kaplinsky E, et al. Frequency and prognosis of stroke/TIA among 4808 survivors of acute myocardial infarction. Stroke 1993; 24:1490–1495.
44. Bodenheimer MM, Sauer D, Shareef B, Brown MW, Fleiss JL, Moss AJ. Relation between myocardial infarction location and stroke. J Am Coll Cardiol 1994; 24:61–66.
45. McAllen PM, Marshall J. Cerebrovascular incidents after myocardial infarction. J Neurol Neurosurg Psychiatry 1977; 40:951–955.
46. Martin R, Bogousslavsky J for the Lausanne Stroke Registry Group. Mechanisms of late stroke after myocardial infarction. J Neurol Neurosurg Psychiatry 1993; 56:760–764.
47. Stratton JR, Nemanich JW, Johannessen KA, Resnick AD. Fate of left ventricular thrombi in patients with remote myocardial infarction or idopathic cardiomyopathy. Circulation 1988; 78:1388–1393.
48. Dexter DD, Whisnant JP, Connolly DC, O'Fallon WM. The association of stroke and coronary heart disease: a population study. Mayo Clin Proc 1987; 62:1077–1083.
49. Stroke Prevention in Atrial Fibrillation Investigators. Bleeding during antithrombotic therapy in patients with atrial fibrillation. Arch Intern Med 1996; 156:409–416.
50. Second Report of the Working Party on Anticoagulant Therapy in Coronary Thrombosis to the Medical Research Council. An assessment of long-term anticoagulant administration after cardiac infarction. BMJ 1964; ii:837–844.
51. United States Veterans Administration. Long-term anticoagulant therapy after myocardial infarction. JAMA 1980; 243:661–669.
52. Keren A, Goldberg S, Gottlieb S, et al. Natural history of left ventricular thrombi: their appearance and resolution in the posthospitalization period of acute myocardial infarction. Am Heart J 1990; 119:73–78.
53. Cairns JA, Hirsch J, Lewis HD, Resnekov L, Theroux P. Antithrombotic agents in coronary artery disease. Chest 1992; 102(suppl):456–481.
54. Behar S, Tanne D, Zion M, et al. Incidence and prognostic significance of chronic atrial fibrillation among 5,839 consecutive patients with acute myocardial infarction. Am J Cardiol 1992; 70:816–818.
55. Komrad MS, Coffey CE, Coffey KS, McKinns R, Massey EW, Califf RM. Myocardial infarction and stroke. Neurology 1984; 34:1403–409.

56. Katz SD, Marantz PR, Biasucci L, et al. Low incidence of stroke in ambulatory patients with heart failure. Am Heart J 1993; 126:141–146.
57. Dunkman WD, Johnson GR, Carson PE, Bhat G, Farrel L, Cohn JN. Incidence of thromboembolic events in congestive heart failure. Circulation 1993; 87(suppl VI):94–101.
58. Acute Infarction Ramipril Efficacy (AIRE) Study Investigators. The effect of ramipril on mortality and morbidity of survivors of acute myocardial infarction with clinical evidence of heart failure. Lancet 1993; 392:821–828.
59. Stein PD, Alpert JS, Copeland J, Dalen JE, Goldman S, Turpie AGC. Antithrombotic therapy in patients with mechanical and biological prosthetic heart valves. Chest 1995; 108(suppl):371.S–379.S.
60. Turpie AGC, Gent M, Laupacis A, et al. Comparison of aspirin with placebo in patients treated with warfarin after heart-valve replacement. N Engl J Med 1993; 329:524–529.
61. Butchart EG, Lewis PA, Grunkemeier GL, Kulatilake N, et al. Low risk of thrombosis and serious embolic events despite low-intensity anticoagulation: experience with 1,004 Medtronic Hall valves. Circulation 1988; 78(suppl I):66–77.
62. Saour JN, Sieck JO, Mamo LAR, Gallus AS. Trial of different intensities of anticoagulation in patients with prosthetic heart valves. N Engl J Med 1990; 322:428–430.
63. Kuntze CE, Ebels T, Eijgelaar A, van der Heide JNH. Rates of thromboembolism with three different mechanical heart valve prostheses: Randomized study. Lancet 1989; 1:514–517.
64. Altman R, Rouvier J, Gurfinkel E, D'Ortencio O, Manzanel R, LaFuente L, Favaloro RG. Comparison of two levels of anticoagulant therapy in patients with substitute heart valves. J Thorc Cardiovasc Surg 1991; 101:427–431.
65. Scott PJ, Essop R, Wharton GA, Williams GJ. Left atrial clot in patients with mitral prostheses: increased rate of detection after recent systemic embolism. Int J Cardiol 1991; 33:141–148.
66. Lechat P, Mas JL, Lascault G, et al. Prevalence of patent foramen ovale in patients with stroke. N Engl J Med 1988; 319:1148–1152.
67. Webster MWI, Smith HJ, Sharp DN, et al. Patent foram ovale in young stroke patients. Lancet 1988; 2:11–12.
68. Cabanes L, Mas JL, Cohen A, Amrenco P, Cabanes PA, et al. Atrial septal aneurysm and patent foramen ovale as risk factors for cryptogenic stroke in patients less than 55 years of age. A study using transesophageal echocardiography. Stroke 1993; 24:1865–1873.
69. DiTullio M, Sacco RL, Gopal A, Mohr JP, Homma S. Patent foramen ovale as a risk factor for cryptogenic stroke. Ann Intern Med 1992; 117:461–465.
70. Dubourg O, Bourdaris JP, Farcot JC, Gueret P, Terdjman M, Ferrier A, Rigaud M, et al. Contrast echocardiographic visualization of cough-induced right to left shunt through a patent foramen ovale. J Am Coll Cardiol 1984; 4:587–594.
71. Louie EK, Konstadt SN, Rao TL, Scanlon PJ. Transesophageal echocardiographic diagnosis of right to left shunting across the foramen ovale in adults without prior stroke. J Am Coll Cardiol 1993; 21:1231–1237.
72. Hausmann D, Mugge A, Becht I, Daniel WG. Diagnosis of patent foramen ovale

by transesophageal echocardiography and association with cerebral and peripheral events. Am J Cardiol 1992; 70:1668–672.
73. Lynch JJ, Schuchard GH, Gross CM, Wann LS. Prevalence of right-to-left atrial shunting in a healthy population: detection by Valsalva maneuver contrast echocardiography. Am J Cardiol 1984; 68:1478–1480.
74. Strunk BL, Cheitlin MD, Stulburg MS, Schiller NB. Right-to-left interarterial shunting through a patent foramen ovale despite normal intracardiac pressures. Am J Cardiol 1987; 60:413–415.
75. Chenzbraun A, Pinto FJ, Schnittger I. Biplane transesophageal echocardiography in the diagnosis of patent foramen ovale. J Am Soc Echocardiogr 1993; 6:417–421.
76. Albers GW, Comess KA, DeRook FA, Bracci P, Atwood JE, Bolger A, et al. Transesophageal echocardiographic findings in stroke subtypes. Stroke 1994; 25:23–28.
77. Kamik R, Stollberger C, Valentin A, Winkler WB, Slany J. Detection of patent foramen ovale by transcranial Doppler ultrasound. Am J Cardiol 1992; 69:560–562.
78. Schminke U, Ries S, Daffertshafer M, Staedt U, Hennerici M. Patent foramen ovale: a potential source of cerebral embolism? Cerebrovasc Dis 1995; 5:133–138.
79. Jauss M, Kaps M, Keberle M, Haberbosch W, Dorndorf W. A comparison of transesophageal echocardiography and transcranial Doppler sonography with contrast medium for detection of patent foramen ovale. Stroke 1994; 25:1265–1267.
80. Klotzsch C, Janssen G, Berlit P. Transesophageal echocardiography and contrast TCD in the detection of a patent foramen ovale: experience with 111 patients. Neurology 1994; 44:1603–1606.
81. Teague SM, Sharma MK. Detection of paradoxical cerebral echo contrast embolization by transcranial Doppler ultrasound study. Stroke 1991; 22:740–745.
82. Hagen PT, Scholz DG, Edwards WD. Incidence and size of patent foramen ovale during the first 10 decades of life: an autopsy study of 965 normal hearts. Mayo Clin Proc 1984; 59:17–20.
83. DeBelder MA, Tourikis L, Leech G, Camm AJ. Risk of patent foramen ovale for thromboembolic events in all age groups. Am J Cardiol 1992; 69:1316–320.
84. Stollberger C, Slany J, Schuster I, Leitner H, Winkler WB, Karnik R. The prevalence of deep venous thrombosis in patients with suspected paradoxical embolism. Ann Intern Med 1993; 119:461–465.
85. Jones EF, Calafiore P, Donnan GA, Tonkin AM. Evidence that patent foramen ovale is not a risk factor for cerebral ischemic in the elderly. Am J Cardiol 1994; 74:596–599.
86. Falk RH. PFO or UFO? The role of a patent foramen ovale in cryptogenic stroke. Am Heart J 1991; 121:124–126.
87. Beeson G, Bogousslavsky J, Hommel M, Stauffer JC, Biche JP. Patent foramen ovale in young stroke patients with mitral valve prolapse. Acta Neurol Scand 1994; 89:23–26.
88. Hanna S, Sun JP, Furlan AJ, Stewart WJ, Sila CA, Tan M. Patent foramen ovale and brain infarct. Stroke 1994; 25:782–786.

89. Bogousslavsky J, Garazi S, Jeanrenaud X, Aebisher M, Van Melle G for the Laussane Stroke with Paradoxal Embolism Study Group. Stroke recurrence in patients with patent foramen ovale: the Laussane Study. Neurology 1996; 46:1301–13005.
90. Bridges ND, Hellenbrand W, Latson L, Fifiano J, Newburger JW, Lock JE. Transcatheter closure of patent foramen ovale after presumed paradoxical embolism. Circulation 1982; 56:1902–1908.
91. Devuyst G, Jeanrenaud X, Guffi M, Aerischer N, Hurni M, et al. Surgical closure of patent foramen ovale with stroke: a pilot study. Cerebrovasc Dis 1995; 5:239 (abstract).
92. Ende DJ, Rao S. Transcatheter occlusion of patent foramen ovale with Sideris' buttoned device to prevent recurrence of paradoxical embolism. Circulation 1994; 90(suppl):I-387 (abstract).
93. Hofmann T, Kasper W, Meirnertz T, Geibel A, Just H. Echocardiographic evaluation of patients with clinically suspected arterial emboli. Lancet 1990; 336:1421–1424.
94. Cujec B, Polasek P, Voll C, Shuaib A. Transesophageal echocardiography in the detection of potential cardiac source of embolism in stroke patients. Stroke 1991; 22:727–733.
95. Leung DY, Black IW, Cranney CB, Walsh WF, Grimm RA, Stewart WJ, Thomas JD. Selection of patients for transesophageal echocardiography after stroke and systemic embolic events. Role of transthoracic echocardiography. Stroke 1995; 26:1820–1824.
96. Labovitz AJ, Camp A, Castello R, Martin TJ, et al. Usefulness of transesopahgeal echocardiography in unexplained cerebral ischemia. Am J Cardiol 1993; 72:1448–1452.
97. Homma S, Di Tullio MR, Sacco RL, Mihalatos D, Li Mandri G, Mohr JP. Characteristics of patent foramen ovale associated with cryptogenic stroke. A biplane transesophageal echocardiographic study. Stroke 1994; 25:582–586.
98. Belkin RN, Kisslo J. Atrial septal aneurysm: recognition and clinical relevance. Am Heart J. 1990; 120:948–857.
99. Shenoy MM, Vijaykumar PM, Friedman SA, Greif E. Atrial septal aneurysm associated with systemic embolism and interatrial right-to-left shunt. Arch Intern Med 1987; 147:605–606.
100. Belkin RN, Hurwitz BJ, Kisslo KB. Atrial septal aneurysm: association with cerebrovascular and peripheral embolic events. Stroke 1987; 18:856–862.
101. Di Pasquale G, Andreoli A, Grazi P, Dominici P, Pinelli G. Cardioembolic stroke from atrial septal aneurysm. Stroke 1988; 19:640–623.
102. Lucas C, Goullard L, Marchau M, Godefroy O, Rondepierre P, et al. Higher prevalence of atrial septal aneurysms in patients with ischemic stroke of unknown cause. Acta Neurol Scand 1994; 89:210–213.
103. Mugge A, Daniel WG, Angermann C, Spes C, et al. Atrial septal aneurysm in adult patients: A multicenter study using transthoracic and transesophageal echocardiography. Circulation 1995; 91:2785–2792.

104. Zabaigoitia-Reyes M, Herrera C, Gandhi DK, Mehlman DJ, McPherson DD, Talano JV. A possible mechanism for neurologic ischemic events in patients with atrial septal aneurysm. Am J Cardiol 1990; 66:761–764.
105. Belkin RN, Welish SJ, Figueroa R, Marks SJ, Alas L, Singh BM, et al. Atrial septal aneurysm associated thrombus and stroke: demonstration with transesophageal echocardiography. J Stroke Cerebrovasc Dis 1991; 1:142–145.
106. Schneider B, Hanrath P, Vogel P, Meinertz T. Improved morphologic characterization of atrial septal aneurysm by transesophageal echocardiography: Relation to cerebrovascular events. J Am Coll Cardiol 1990; 16:1000–1009.
107. Garazi S, Bogousslavsky J, Moncayo J, Jeanrenaud X, et al. Stroke recurrence with atrial septal aneurysm. Cerebrovasc Dis 1995; 5:231 (abstract).
108. Yasaka M, Yamaguchi T, Oita J, Sawada T, Schichiri M, Omae T. Clinical features of recurrent embolization in acute cardioembolic stroke. Stroke 1993; 24:1681–1685.
109. Cerebral Embolism Study Group. Immediate anticoagulation of embolic stroke: Brain hemorrhage and management options. Stroke 1984; 15:779–789.
110. Lodder J, Vanderlugt PJ. Evaluation of the risk of immediate anticoagulation treatment in patients with embolic stroke of cardiac origin. Stroke 1983; 14:42–46.
111. Koller RL. Recurrent embolic cerebral infarction and anticagulation. Neurology 1982; 32:283–285.
112. Cerebral Embolism Study Group. Immediate anticoagulation of embolic stroke: A randomized trial. Stroke 1983; 14:668–676.
113. Lodder J. CT-detected hemorrhagic infarction: relation with the size of the infarct, and the presence of midline shift. Acta Neurol Scand 1984; 70:329–335.
114. Hart RG, Easton JD. Hemorrhagic infarcts. Stroke 1986; 17:586–589.
115. Hornig CR, Bauer T, Simon C, Trittmacher S, Dorndorf W. Hemorrhagic transformation in cardioembolic cerebral infarction. Stroke 1993; 24:465–468.
116. Lodder J, Krune-Kubat B, Broekman J. Cerebral hemorrhage infarction at autopsy: cardiac embolic cause and the relationship to the cause of death. Stroke 1986; 17:626–629.
117. Okada Y, Yamaguchi T, Minematsu K, et al. Hemorrhagic transformation in cerebral embolism. Stroke 1989; 20:598–603.
118. Hornig CR, Dorndorf W, Agnoli AL. Hemorrhagic cerebral infarction: A prospective study. Stroke 1986; 17:179–185.
119. Cerebral Embolism Study Group. Cardioembolic stroke, immediate anticoagulation and brain hemorrhage. Arch Intern Med 1987; 147:636–6340.
120. Calandre L, Ortega J, Bermejo F. Anticoagulation and hemorrhagic infarction in cerebral embolism secondary to rheumatic heart disease. Arch Neurol 1984; 41:1152–1154.
121. Shields RW, Laureno R, Lachman T, Victor M. Anticoagulant related hemorrhage in acute cerebral embolism. Stroke 1984; 15:426–437.
122. Chamarro A, Vila N, Saiz A, Alday M, Tolosa E. Early anticoagulation after large cerebral embolic infarction: a safety study. Neurology 1995; 45:861–865.

123. Rothrock JF, Dittrich HC, McAllen S, Taft BJ, Lyden PD. Acute anticoagulation following cardioembolic stroke. Stroke 1989; 20:730–734.
124. Pessin MS, Estol CJ, Lafranchise F, Caplan LR. Safety of anticoagulation after hemorrhagic infarction. Neurology 1993; 43:1298–1303.
125. Hart RG, Foster JW, Luther MF, Kanter MC. Stroke in infective endocarditis. Stroke 1990; 21:695–700.

24
Atherosclerotic Intracranial Arterial Stenosis

Marc I. Chimowitz
Emory University, Atlanta, Georgia

INTRODUCTION

Atherosclerotic stenosis of the major intracranial arteries (carotid siphon, middle cerebral artery, vertebral artery, basilar artery) is an important cause of ischemic stroke, especially in blacks, Asians, and Hispanics.[1–8] In the United States, intracranial stenosis causes approximately 40,000 ischemic strokes annually. This chapter will focus on the epidemiology, prognosis, diagnosis, and treatment of intracranial arterial stenosis.

EPIDEMIOLOGY OF INTRACRANIAL OCCLUSIVE DISEASE: IMPACT OF RACE

Studies performed in the 1960s established the importance of atherosclerotic intracranial large-artery occlusive disease as a cause of stroke.[1–3,5,9] In the Joint Study of Extracranial Arterial Occlusion, in which 3,788 patients with signs and symptoms of ischemic cerebrovascular disease underwent four-vessel angiography, stenotic lesions were identified in 7.7% of basilar arteries, 4.4% of intracranial verterbral arteries, 6.7% of intracranial carotid arteries, 3.8% of middle cerebral arteries (MCA), 3.2% of anterior cerebral arteries (ACA), and 2.6% of posterior cerebral arteries (PCA). Overall, 6.1% of patients in the study (84% of whom were white) had isolated intracranial occlusive disease.[1] Subsequent studies have confirmed that approximately 5% to 10% of ischemic strokes in whites are caused by intracranial stenosis.[6,10–13] These studies probably underestimate the true frequency of intracranial stenosis as a cause of stroke because angiography, the most reliable method for establishing this diagnosis, was only performed in 38% to 75% of patients.

Several studies have also suggested that blacks are more likely to develop intracranial large artery atherosclerosis than whites.[2,3,6–9,14,15] In a study of patients with anterior circulation ischemia, the rates of MCA occlusion were 90% in black males and 12% in white males.[16] In another study of patients with posterior circulation ischemia, distal basilar artery and intracranial branch lesions were significantly more frequent in blacks, whereas severe extracranial vertebral artery disease was five times more common in whites.[17] Several recent studies have shown that 15% to 29% of TIAs or strokes in blacks are caused by stenosis of a major intracranial artery.[6–8] In one study in which angiography was performed in 45 consecutive blacks with carotid distribution TIA, 13 patients (29%) had isolated stenosis of the ipsilateral carotid siphon (6 patients), MCA stem (4 patients), or an MCA branch (3 patients). In comparison, only 12 patients (24%) had extracranial internal carotid artery stenosis.[8]

Studies of Japanese, Chinese, and Hispanic patients have shown that these racial groups are also at high risk of developing intracranial atherosclerosis.[4,6,18,19] One study of patients with symptomatic anterior circulation ischemia showed that 83% of severely stenotic lesions in Japanese Asians involved the intracranial arteries, whereas 85% of severe lesions in American whites involved the extracranial internal carotid artery.[18] In another study comparing Chinese living in the United States with American whites, the Chinese patients had significantly higher rates of intracranial carotid artery and MCA stenoses.[19] The explanation for the variance in the distribution of cerebral atherosclerosis in different races is uncertain. Some studies have suggested that genetic susceptibility to intracranial large artery disease in blacks, Hispanics, and Asians plays a major role 19,20; other studies suggest that the influence of lifestyle and risk factor profiles on the distribution of atherosclerosis may be most important.[6,21]

Of the 550,000 patients suffering a stroke annually in the United States, approximately 467,500 (85%) patients suffer an ischemic stroke.[22,23] Given that the ratio of whites to blacks in the United States population is 6.6 and that blacks have twice the incidence of stroke, approximately 358,000 whites and 109,000 blacks suffer an ischemic stroke annually in the United States. Since approximately 6% of ischemic strokes in whites and at least 15% of ischemic strokes in blacks are caused by intracranial large-artery atherosclerosis, approximately 40,000 patients (21,480 whites, 16,350 blacks) suffer a stroke each year in the United States as a result of intracranial atherosclerosis. The importance of intracranial atherosclerosis as a cause of stroke is underscored when one considers that two other common causes of stroke, nonvalvular atrial fibrillation and extracranial carotid stenosis, account for approximately 70,000 and 85,000 strokes, respectively, in the United States each year.[24,25]

PROGNOSIS OF PATIENTS WITH SYMPTOMATIC INTRACRANIAL STENOSIS

The long-term prognosis of carotid siphon stenosis has mostly been studied retrospectively. Two studies of patients with symptomatic or asymptomatic siphon stenosis showed that the rates of ipsilateral stroke from carotid siphon disease was low, but the rates of stroke from other causes (e.g., coexistent extracranial carotid stenosis) and death from CAD were high.[26,27] In one of these studies, 66 patients with carotid siphon stenosis > 50% were followed for an average of 3.9 years. Ten patients (15%) had a stroke and 33 patients (50%) died. Eight of the 10 patients with stroke had ipsilateral siphon stenosis, and in six of these there was tandem extracranial carotid stenosis. Therefore, only two of the strokes could be attributed solely to carotid siphon stenosis. Fifty five percent of the deaths were caused by CAD.[26] In another study of 15 patients with carotid siphon stenosis > 50% followed for a mean of 51 months, only one patient (7%) had a stroke that could be attributed to the siphon stenosis, and five patients (33%) died (3 from CAD, 1 cerebellar hemorrhage, 1 basilar thrombosis).[27]

Another retrospective study of 58 patients found a much higher rate of stroke caused by carotid siphon stenosis.[28] Patients in this study had symptomatic or asymptomatic carotid siphon stenosis that reduced the diameter of the artery by at least one-third. Only 10% of patients had tandem extracranial carotid stenosis > 50%. During a mean follow-up of 30 months, 17 patients (29%) had a stroke (11 of which were ipsilateral to the siphon stenosis) and 25 patients (43%) died (11 from CAD, 9 from stroke, 5 from other causes). The annual ipsilateral stroke rate was 7.6% per year, and there were no apparent differences in stroke rates in patients whose siphon lesions were asymptomatic at entry versus patients whose siphon lesions were symptomatic. Additionally, the degree of siphon stenosis had no effect on outcome. These subgroup analyses, however, need to be interpreted cautiously because of the low power of this study.

The only prospective estimate of stroke risk in patients with carotid siphon stenosis comes from the extracranial-intracranial (EC-IC) bypass study.[29] One of the subgroups enrolled in this study was patients with stenosis of the internal carotid artery at or above the C-2 vertebral body. It is likely that most of these patients had carotid siphon stenosis, given the typical distribution of atherosclerosis in the distal internal carotid artery. Of 72 patients with ICA stenosis > 70% at or distal to C-2 who were treated with aspirin (325 mg qid), 26 (36%) had a nonfatal or fatal stroke in any vascular distribution (ipsilateral stroke rate not provided). The follow-up period for this subgroup of patients was not specified, but the mean follow-up for all patients in the study was 55.8 months. Overall, these studies suggest that the annual rate of stroke in patients with high-grade carotid siphon stenosis is 4% to 12% in any vascular territory and approximately 8% in the territory supplied by the diseased carotid siphon (Table 1).

The EC-IC bypass study also provides the most reliable data on risk of stroke in patients with symptomatic *MCA stenosis*. Studies prior to the EC-IC bypass study suggested that the long-term risk of stroke was low, however, these studies were retrospective and included small numbers of patients.[30,31] In the medical arm of the EC-IC bypass study, 85 patients with TIA or nondisabling stroke caused by MCA stenosis were treated with aspirin (1,300 mg/day) and followed for a mean of 43.3 months. During follow-up, 18 patients (21%) had a stroke and 10 patients (12%) died (3 from stroke, 2 from coronary disease, and 5 from other causes). The rate of stroke in any vascular territory was 9.5% per patient-year and the rate of ipsilateral stroke was 7.8% per patient-year. The mortality rate was 3.3% per year. There were no apparent differences in the rates of stroke or death in patients with < 70% stenosis versus patients with > 70% stenosis of the MCA.

The long-term prognosis of atherosclerotic *anterior cerebral artery stenosis* has not been studied systematically. In our limited experience with these patients, stroke in the ACA territory is uncommon during follow-up, but stroke in other territories or myocardial infarction has occurred, suggesting that these patients have widespread atherosclerosis.

There are only a few studies on the prognosis of patients with symptomatic *intracranial vertebral artery stenosis*. In the largest study, 31 patients with TIA or stroke caused by > 50% vertebral artery stenosis were treated with warfarin or aspirin and followed for a mean of 20 months. Seven (23%) patients had a recurrent stroke (four in the territory of the stenotic vertebral artery, three in a different territory) and two patients (6%) died.[32] In another study of 25 patients with > 50% stenosis of an intracranial vertebral artery (asymptomatic and symp-

Table 1 Risk of Stroke in Patients with Stenosis of the Major Intracranial Arteries

Intracranial artery	Annual risk of stroke
Carotid siphon	4–12% in any territory, 8% in same territory
Middle cerebral artery	10% in any territory, 8% in same territory
Vertebral artery	4–13% in any territory, 3%–8% in same territory
Basilar artery	3–15% in any territory, 2.5%–11% in same territory

tomatic patients included), five patients (25%) had a stroke (three in the vertebrobasilar distribution) during a mean follow-up of 6.1 years.[33] These studies suggest that the annual rates of recurrent stroke in patients with > 50% vertebral artery stenosis are 4% to 13% in any vascular territory and 2.5% to 7.6% in the vertebral artery territory (Table 1).

The long-term risk of stroke in patients with symptomatic *basilar artery stenosis* appears to be worse than in patients with vertebral artery stenosis.[32–34] In the largest study to date, 28 patients with TIA or stroke related to > 50% basilar artery stenosis were treated with warfarin or aspirin and followed for a mean of 20 months. Seven patients (25%) had a recurrent stroke (five in the territory of the stenotic basilar artery, two in a different territory), and four patients (14%) died. The annual rates of stroke were 15% in any vascular territory and 11% in the basilar artery territory.[32] In two other, smaller studies of patients with basilar artery stenosis, the rates of stroke were substantially lower. In one study of 19 patients with > 50% stenosis of the basilar artery followed for a mean period of 6.1 years, three patients (16%) had a stroke (one brainstem, one occiptal lobe, one uncertain territory). In another study of nine patients with symptomatic stenosis (40% to 90%) of the middle or distal segments of the basilar artery, most of whom were treated with warfarin, only one patient (11%) had a stroke during a median follow-up of 2 years. This patient had a fatal brainstem stroke.[34] Overall, these studies suggest that the rates of stroke in patients with basilar artery stenosis are 3% to 15% in any vascular territory, and 2.5% to 11% in the basilar artery territory (table 1).

ESTABLISHING THE DIAGNOSIS OF INTRACRANIAL STENOSIS

Several diagnostic procedures are currently used to identify intracranial stenosis. These include conventional angiography, transcranial Doppler ultrsaound (TCD), magnetic resonance angiography (MRA), and computerized CT angiography (CTA). The gold standard for establishing the diagnosis of intracranial large artery disease is conventional cerebral angiography. Angiography enables an accurate measurement of the degree of stenosis of the diseased artery, diagnosis of arterial occlusion, evaluation of collateral flow patterns, and evaluation of other intracranial and extracranial arteries. The major drawback of angiography is the risk of stroke, which is approximately 1.2%.[24,35,36]

The other procedures offer nonivasive and less expensive methods for evaluating the intracranial circulation, but there have been no prospective multicenter studies to evaluate the sensitivity and specificity of these procedures for diagnosing intracranial stenosis. Available data from single-center studies suggest that TCD may have a sensitivity as low as 75% and a specificity as low as 80% for detecting intracranial stenosis,[37,38] and that MRA may have a sensitivity as low as 86% and a specificity as low as 67%[39–41] when compared to conventional angiography. As such, MRA and TCD are currently not sufficiently reliable to diagnose or rule out intracranial arterial stenosis. Moreover, methods have not been established using TCD, MRA, or CTA to accurately measure the percent stenosis of an intracranial artery,[42] whereas conventional angiography does permit such measurements.

TREATMENT OPTIONS FOR SYMPTOMATIC INTRACRANIAL STENOSIS

Despite the importance of intracranial stenosis as a cause of ischemic stroke, there have been no prospective trials evaluating antithrombotic therapy in patients with this disease.

Antiplatelet agents (aspirin or ticlopidine) are frequently used in this setting based on studies that have shown a benefit of these agents for lowering the risk of stroke in patients with noncardioembolic TIA or minor stroke.[43] However, the efficacy of antiplatelet agents has not been established in patients with symptomatic intracranial large-artery disease. In fact, the high rate of stroke in patients with carotid siphon or MCA stenosis who were treated with high-dose aspirin (1,300 mg/day) in the medical arm of the EC-IC bypass study (7.7% to 9.5% per patient-year) raises a question about the efficacy of aspirin in this setting.[29,44]

Ticlopidine, another antiplatelet agent, has been shown to be slightly more effective than aspirin for secondary stroke prevention in patients with noncardioembolic TIA or minor stroke.[45] However, the efficacy of ticlopidine in patients with symptomatic intracranial stenosis has not been established either. A post hoc analysis of the Ticlopidine Aspirin Stroke Study (TASS) suggests that ticlopidine may be more effective in blacks than in whites.[46] Since blacks are at higher risk of intracranial large-artery stenosis, it might be inferred that ticlopidine is effective therapy for this disease. However, blacks are also at higher risk of intracranial small-vessel disease, for which ticlopidine may be effective. If cerebral angiography had been performed routinely in TASS, clarification of the role of ticlopidine in patients with intracranial large-artery stenosis may have been possible. However, angiography was only performed in approximately half the patients in this study, most of whom had carotid territory symptoms. Of note is that in the subgroup of patients with extracranial carotid stenosis >70%, ticlopidine was significantly less effective than aspirin for preventing stroke.[47] This finding raises a question about the efficacy of ticlopidine for the treatment of intracranial large-artery stenosis.

Warfarin is frequently used for the treatment of intracranial stenosis based on the results of nonrandomized, retrospective studies of patients with symptoms suggestive of vertebrobasilar disease.[48,49] In a retrospective, nonangiographic study of patients with vertebrobasilar symptoms, Whisnant et al. found that patients treated with anticoagulation had a lower risk of stroke in the first 6 months of treatment than untreated patients; however, the rates of stroke beyond six months were similar in the two groups.[49]

In a recent retrospective, nonrandomized, multicenter study, warfarin was compared with aspirin for prevention of major vascular events (stroke, myocardial infarction, or vascular death) in patients with symptomatic, angiographically proven stenosis (50% to 99%) of a major intracranial artery. Qualifying criteria for the study were: (1) 50% to 99% stenosis of one of the major intracranial arteries; (2) a TIA or stroke in the distribution of the stenotic artery; and (3) therapy with aspirin or warfarin. Treatment with aspirin or warfarin was based on local physician preference. The most common dose of aspirin prescribed was 325 mg/day, and the dose of warfarin was typically adjusted to maintain prothrombin times (PT) in the range of 1.2 to 1.6 × control. Primary endpoints in this study were stroke in any vascular territory, MI, or sudden death. Safety of warfarin and aspirin was assessed by recording hemorrhagic complications. Hemorrhages were classified as major (fatal hemorrhage, any intracranial hemorrhage, bleeding requiring hospitalization, bleeding requiring transfusion) or minor (any other bleeding complication).

Of the 151 patients who qualified for the study, 96 (64%) were male, and 55 (36%) were female; 100 (66%) were white, 42 (28%) were black, five (3%) were Hispanic, and four (3%) were Asian or Arabic. Stroke was the qualifying event in 89 patients (59%) and TIAs were the qualifying events in 62 patients (41%). The stenotic lesions at angiography involved the anterior circulation in 83 patients (55%) and the posterior circulation in 68 patients (45%). The percent stenosis of the symptomatic intracranial artery was 50% to 69% in 62 patients (41%) and 70% to 99% in 89 patients (59%).

Of the 151 patients in the study, 88 patients (58%) were treated with warfarin and 63 patients (42%) were treated with aspirin. There were no significant differences in the frequency of risk factors for stroke between the two groups. The rates of endpoints and hemorrhagic complications in the two treatment groups are shown in Table 2. Major ischemic events (ischemic stroke, MI, or sudden death) occurred in 26 patients on aspirin during 143 patient-years of follow-up, and in 14 patients on warfarin during 166 patient-years of follow-up ($P < .01$, log rank test). Hemorrhagic complications occurred in 13 patients on warfarin (3 major, 10 minor) during 166 patient-years of follow-up, and in two patients on aspirin (both minor) during 143 patient-years of follow-up ($P < .01$, log rank test).

Cox proportional hazards analysis showed that the relative risk of stroke, MI, or sudden death in patients treated with warfarin was 0.45 (95% CI 0.23 to 0.86) compared with patients treated with aspirin. The major effect of warfarin

Table 2 Rates of Endpoints and Hemorrhagic Complications in a Retrospective Study Comparing Warfarin vs. Aspirin in Patients with Symptomatic Intracranial Arterial Stenosis

	Warfarin (n = 88)	Aspirin (n = 63)
Median follow-up	14.7 months	19.3 months
Stroke	6 (7%)	15 (24%)
Fatal	1 (1%)	3 (5%)
Nonfatal	5 (6%)	12 (19%)
Fatal MI or SD	5 (6%)	6 (10%)
Nonfatal MI	3 (3%)	5 (8%)
Stroke/100 pt-years	3.6	10.4
Fatal MI or SD/100 pt-yrs	3.0	4.2
Nonfatal MI/100 pt-yrs	1.8	3.5
Major hem/100 pt-yrs	1.8	0
Minor hem/100 pt-yrs	5.9	1.4

was in preventing stroke (Table 2). A Kaplan Meier analysis that included hemorrhagic deaths as a primary endpoint (i.e., in addition to ischemic stroke, MI or sudden death) showed that a significantly higher proportion of patients treated with warfarin survived free of these endpoints compared with patients treated with aspirin ($P = .03$, log rank test).

Patients with moderate intracranial stenosis (50% to 69%) had a lower risk of stroke in the same vascular territory than patients with a severe intracranial stenosis (70% to 99%). Of 62 patients with 50% to 69% intracranial stenosis, five patients (6%) had a stroke in the same territory as the stenotic artery during a median follow-up of 20 months (4 of 28 [14%] on aspirin, 1 of 34 [3%] on warfarin). In comparison, of 89 patients with 70% to 99% intracranial stenosis, nine patients (10%) had a stroke in the same territory as the stenotic artery during a median follow-up of 14 months (5 of 35 [14%] on aspirin, 4 of 54 [7%] on warfarin). Patients with stenosis of the vertebral or basilar arteries had a higher rate of stroke in the same vascular territory than patients with carotid siphon or MCA stenosis (basilar artery 11%/year, vertebral artery 8%/year, carotid siphon 2%/year, MCA 3%/year).[50]

In summary, the major findings in this retrospective study[32] were the following.

1. Warfarin lowered the combined endpoint of stroke, MI, or sudden death by nearly 50% compared with aspirin (325 mg/day), and the major benefit of warfarin was for preventing stroke;

2. The rate of major hemorrhagic complications in patients with symptomatic intracranial stenosis treated with warfarin (PT 1.2–1.6 × control) was approximately 1.8/100 patient-years, which is similar to the rate of major hemor-

rhagic complications in patients treated with warfarin in the stroke prevention in atrial fibrillation trials.[51] Despite the increased risk of major hemorrhagic complications in patients on warfarin, the overall risk/benefit strongly favored warfarin.

3. Patients with 70% to 99% stenosis of a major intracranial artery had the highest risk of stroke in the territory of the stenotic artery.

Although warfarin appears to be more effective than aspirin in patients with 70% to 99% intracranial stenosis, the risk of ipsilateral stroke on warfarin is still high (>5% per year) in these patients. While this retrospective study strongly suggests that warfarin is more efficacious than low-dose aspirin (325 mg/day) for the treatment of smptomatic intracranial arterial stenosis, definite recommendations regarding the use of warfarin vs. antiplatelet agents in this setting must await confirmation of these findings in a prospective, randomized trial.

Intracranial bypass surgery is also a therapeutic option for patients with intracranial arterial stenosis; however, enthusiasm for bypass has waned since the EC-IC bypass study results were reported.[29] In that study, patients with extracranial carotid occlusion, distal carotid occlusive disease, or MCA stenosis were randomized to medical therapy alone (risk factor management and antithrombotic therapy—usually aspirin 325 mg qid) versus medical therapy and EC-IC bypass. The results demonstrated that EC-IC bypass was ineffective for preventing stroke in these patients. Subgroup analyses of patients with distal carotid or MCA stenosis showed that EC-IC bypass was also ineffective in these groups.[29] In patients with carotid siphon stenosis > 70%, 26 of 72 patients (36%) treated medically and 29 of 77 patients (38%) who underwent EC-IC bypass had a stroke during a mean follow-up of 55.8 months. In patients with MCA stenosis > 70%, those undergoing EC-IC bypass actually had a poorer outcome than medically treated patients: 14 of 59 (24%) patients treated medically and 22 of 50 (44%) patients treated surgically had a stroke during follow up ($P < .05$).[29] Bypass surgery or endarterectomy has also been used occasionally for the treatment of intracranial vertebral artery occlusive disease,[52,53] but the efficacy of these procedures has not been evaluated systematically.

Transluminal angioplasty is another therapeutic option for the treatment of intracranial stenosis. Early experience suggested that intracranial angioplasty was associated with an unacceptably high risk of stroke or death, and the procedure was largely abandoned.[54,55] However, advances in microcatheter and balloon technology have led to renewed interest in intracranial angioplast. [54–62]

Recent studies have shown that intracranial angioplasty is technically feasible and may be performed relatively safely. In one study of 27 patients with stenosis of a major intracranial artery (carotid, MCA, vertebral, or basilar) who had recurrent cerebral ischemic symptoms on anticoagulation, angioplasty was technically successful in 82% of cases. The average preangioplasty stenosis was 72% and the average postangioplasty stenosis was 46%. There were three strokes during angioplasty for a 30-day morbidity rate of 11%. [57,59] During an average follow-up of 28 months, one patient (4%) had a fatal stroke referable to the treated vessel, and three patients (11%) had TIA. In another study of 19 patients with TIA or stroke caused by stenosis of an intracranial artery, angioplasty was performed because of "unstable neurological symptoms" on antiplatelet therapy. Angioplasty was technically successful in 13 of 19 (68%) patients, with the average preangioplasty stenosis = 83% and the average postangioplasty stenosis = 36%. None of the patients had a stroke during angioplasty, though two had transient hemiparesis and one had an asymptomatic dissection. Moreover, none of the 13 patients who had successful angioplasty had recurrent stroke during follow-up ranging from 6 to 12 months, whereas two of the six patients whose angioplasty was unsuccessful had "neurological deterioration" 2 months later.[60] In a Japanese study, Hyodo et al.[61] recently reported 36 patients who had angioplasty for symptomatic > 70% stenosis of a major intracranial artery. Three patients (8%) had a stroke during the procedure. During a mean follow-up of 35 months none of the patients had TIA or stroke and angiography in 28 patients showed restenosis in five patients (18%) and occlusion in one patient. The long-term clinical outcome in 21 patients undergoing intracranial angioplasty has also been evaluated by Marks et al.[62] Angioplasty was technically successful in 91% of cases. One patient (4.5%) died during the procedure from rupture of the vessel, and another patient (4.5%) had ischemic symptoms immediately after angioplasty that resolved following thrombolytic therapy. During a mean follow-up of 31.3 months, one patient had a stroke in the territory of the treated artery and another patient had a stroke in a different territory. The annual stroke rates were 3.8% in the territory of the treated artery and 5.8% for all strokes.[62] These recent studies suggest that angioplasty is a promising therapy that is increasingly being used to treat symptomatic intracranial stenosis. However, more data on safety, long-term outcome, and restenosis rates in patients undergoing intracranial angioplasty are needed before this therapy should be evaluated in a controlled, multicenter clinical trial. Moreover, best medical therapy for intracranial stenosis, which will serve as the proven control group in such a trial, has yet to be determined.

REFERENCES

1. Hass WK, Fields WS, North RR, Kricheff II, Chase NE, Bauer RB. Joint Study of Extracranial Arterial Occlusion. II. Arteriography, techniques, sites, and complications. JAMA 1968; 203(11):961–968.
2. McGarry P, Solberg LA, Guzman MA, Strong JP. Cerebral atherosclerosis in New Orleans. Comparisons of lesions by age, sex, and race. Lab Invest 1985; 52:533–539.

3. Moosy J. Cerebral infarction and intracranial arterial thrombosis. Arch Neurol 1966; 14:119–123.
4. Kieffer SA, Takeya Y, Resch JA, Amplatz K. Racial differences in cerebrovascular disease. Angiographic evaluation of Japanese and American populations. AJR 1967; 101:94–99.
5. Gorelick PB. Distribution of atherosclerotic cerebrovascular lesions. Effects of age, race, and sex. Stroke 1993; 24(suppl):16–19.
6. Sacco RL, Kargman D, Gu Q, Zamanillo MC. Race-ethnicity and determinants of intracranial atherosclerotic cerebral infarction. The Northern Manhattan Stroke Study. Stroke 1995; 26:14–20.
7. Qureshi AI, Safdar K, Patel M, Janssen RS, Frankel MR. Stroke in young black patients. Risk factors, subtypes, and prognosis. Stroke 1995; 26:1995–1998.
8. Weisberg LA. Clinical characteristics of transient ischemic attacks in black patients. Neurology 1991; 41:1410–1414.
9. Bauer RB, Sheehan S, Wechsler N, Meyer JS. Arteriographic study of sites, incidence, and treatment of arteriosclerotic cerebrovascular lesions. Neurology 1962; 12:698–711.
10. Naylor AR, Sandercock PAG, Sellar RJ, Warlow CP. Patterns of vascular pathology in acute, first-ever cerebral infarction. Scott Med J 1993; 38:41–44.
11. Passero S, Rossi G, Nardini M, Bonelli G, D'Ettore M, Martini A, et al Italian multicenter study of reversible cerebral ischemic attacks. Part 5. Risk factors and cerebral atherosclerosis. Atherosclerosis 1987; 63:211–224.
12. Wityk R, Lehman D, Klag M, Coresh J, Ahn H, Litt B, et al. Racial differences in extracranial and intracranial atherosclerosis. Neurology 1995; suppl 4:A461.
13. Bogousslavsky J, Van Melle G, Regli F. The Lausanne Stroke Registry: analysis of 1,000 consecutive patients with first stroke. Stroke 1988; 19:1083–1092.
14. Gorelick PB, Caplan LR, Hier DB, et al. Racial differences in the distribution of anterior circulation occlusive disease. Neurology 1984; 34:54–59.
15. Inzitari D, Hachinski VC, Taylor DW, Barnett HJM. Racial differences in the anterior circulation in cerebrovascular disease. How much can be explained by risk factors? Arch Neurol 1990; 47:1080–1084.
16. Heyden S, Heyman A, Goree JA. Nonembolic occlusion of the middle cerebral artery and carotid arteries—a comparison of predisposing factors. Stroke 1970; 1:363–369.
17. Gorelick PB, Caplan LR, Hier DB, Patel D, Langenberg P, Pessin MS, et al. Racial differences in the distribution of posterior circulation occlusive disease. Stroke 1985; 16:785–790.
18. Nishimaru K, McHenry LC, Toole JF. Cerebral angiographic and clinical differences in carotid system transient ischemic attacks between American Caucasian and Japanese patients. Stroke 1984; 15:56–59.
19. Feldmann E, Daneault N, Kwan E, Ho KJ, Pessin MS, Langenberg P, et al. Chinese-white differences in the distribution of occlusive cerebrovascular disease. Neurology 1990; 40:1541–1545.
20. Gorelick PB, Caplan LR, Langenberg P, Hier DB, Pessin MS, Patel D, et al. Clinical and angiographic comparison of asymptomatic occlusive cerebrovascular disease. Neurology 1988; 38:852–858.

21. Williams AO, Resch JA, Loewenson RB. Cerebral atherosclerosis—a comparative autopsy study between Nigerian Negroes and American Negroes and Caucasians. Neurology 1969; 19:205–210.
22. American Heart Association. Heart and Stroke Facts: 1996 Statistical Supplement. AHA, 1995.
23. National Stroke Association. Brain Attack Statistics. NSA., 1995.
24. Executive Committee for the Asymptomatic Carotid Atherosclerosis Study. Endarterectomy for asymptomatic carotid artery stenosis. JAMA 1995; 273:1421–1428.
25. Stroke Prevention in Atrial Fibrillation Study Group. Preliminary report of the stroke prevention in atrial fibrillation study. N Engl J Med 1990; 322:863–868.
26. Marzewski DJ, Furlan AJ, St Louis P, et al. Intracranial internal carotid artery stenosis: long-term prognosis. Stroke 1982; 13:821–824.
27. Wechsler LR, Kistler JP, Davis KR, Kaminski MJ. The prognosis of carotid siphon stenosis. Stroke 1986; 17:714–718.
28. Craig DR, Meguro K, Watridge C, Robertson JT, Barnett HJM, Fox AJ. Intracranial internal carotid artery stenosis. Stroke 1982; 13:825–828.
29. EC/IC Bypass Study Group. Failure of extracranial-intracranial arterial bypass to reduce the risk of ischemic stroke. Results of an international randomized trial. N Engl J Med 1985; 313:1191–1200.
30. Hinton RC, Mohr JP, Ackerman RH, Adair LB, Fisher CM. Symptomatic middle cerbral artery stenosis. Ann Neurol 1979; 5:152–157.
31. Corston RN, Kendall BE, Marshall J. Prognosis in middle cerebral artery stenosis. Stroke 1984; 15:237–241.
32. Chimowitz MI, Kokkinos J, Strong J, Brown MB, Levine SR, Silliman S, et al. The warfarin-aspirin symptomatic intracranial disease study. Neurology 1995; 45:1488–1493.
33. Moufarrij NA, Little JR, Furlan AJ, Leatherman JR, Williams GW. Basilar and distal vertebral artery stenosis: long term follow-up. Stroke 1986; 17:938–942.
34. Pessin MS, Gorelick PB, Kwan ES, et al. Basilar artery stenosis: middle and distal segments. Neurology 1987; 37:1742–1746.
35. North American Symptomatic Carotid Endarterectomy Trial Collaborators. Beneficial effect of carotid endarterectomy in symptomatic patients with high grade carotid stenosis. N Engl J Med 1991; 325:445–453.
36. Dion JE, Gates PC, Fox AJ, Barnett HJM, Blom RJ. Clinical events following neuroangiography: a prospective study. Stroke 1987; 18:997–1004.
37. deBray JM, Joseph PA, Jeanvoine H, Maugin D, Dauzat M, Plassard F. Transcranial Doppler evaluation of middle cerebral artery stenosis. J Ultrasound Med 1988; 7:611–616.
38. Rorick MB, Nichols FT, Adams RJ. Transcranial Doppler correlations with angiography in detection of intracranial stenosis. Stroke 1994; 25:1931–1934.
39. Dagirmanjian A, Ross JS, Obuchowski N, et al. High resolution, magnetization transfer saturation, variable flip angle, time-of-flight MRA in the detection of intracranial vascular stenoses. J Comp Assist Tomogr 1995; 19:700–706.
40. Katz DA, Marks MP, Napel SA, Bracci PM, Roberts SL. Circle of Willis: evaluation with spiral CT angiography, MR angiography, and conventional angiography. Radiology 1995; 195:445–449.

41. Stock KW, Radue EW, Jacob AL, Bao XS, Steinbrich W. Intracranial arteries: prospective blinded comparative study of MR angiography and DSA in 50 patients. Radiology 1995; 195:451–456.
42. Rother J, Wentz K-U, Rautenberg W, Schwartz A, Hennerici M. Magnetic resonance angiography in vertebrobasilar ischemia. Stroke 1993; 24:1310–1315.
43. Antiplatelet Trialists' Collaboration. Secondary prevention of vascular disease by prolonged antiplatelet treatment. Br Med J 1988; 296:320–331.
44. Bogousslavsky J, Barnett HJM, Fox AJ, Hachinski VC, Taylor W, EC/IC Bypass Study Group. Atherosclerotic disease of the middle cerbral artery. Stroke 1986; 17:1112–1120.
45. Hass WK, Easton JD, Adams HP Jr, Pryse-Phillips W, Molony BA, Anderson S, et al. A randomized trial comparing ticlopidine hydrochloride with aspirin for the prevention of stroke in high risk patients. N Engl J Med 1989; 321:501–507.
46. Weisberg LA, Ticlopidine Aspirin Stroke Study Group. The efficacy and safety of ticlopidine in non-whites: analysis of a patient subgroup from the Ticlopidine Aspirin Stroke Study. Neurology 1993; 43:27–31.
47. Grotta JC, Norris JW, Kamm B, TASS Baseline and Angiographic Data Subgroup. Prevention of stroke with ticlopidine: who benefits most? Neurology 1992; 42:111–115.
48. Millikan CH, Siekert RG, Shick RM. Studies in cerebrovascular disease. III. The use of anticoagulant drugs in the treatment of insufficiency or thrombosis within the basilar arterial system. Mayo Clin Proc 1955; 30:116–126.
49. Whisnant JP, Cartlidge NEF, Elveback LR. Carotid and vertebral-basilar transient ischemic attacks: effect of anticoagulants, hypertension, and cardiac disorders on survival and stroke occurrence—a population study. Ann Neurol 1978; 3:107–115.
50. Warfarin-Aspirin Symptomatic Intracranial Disease (WASID) Study Group. Prognosis of patients with symptomatic vertebral or basilar artery stenosis. Stroke 1995; 26:162 (abstract).
51. Albers GW. Laboratory monitoring of oral anticoagulant therapy: are we being misled? Neurology 1993; 43:468–470.
52. Sundt TM, Whisnant JP, Piepgras DG, Campbell JK, Holman CB. Intracranial bypass grafts for vertebral-basilar ischemia. Mayo Clin Proc 1978; 53:12–18.
53. Ausman JI, Diaz FG, de los Reyes RA, Pak H, Patel S, Boulos R. Anastomosis of occipital artery to anterior inferior cerebellar artery for vertebrobasilar stenosis. Surg Neurol 1981; 16:99–102:
54. Piepgras DG, Sundt TM, Forbes GS. Balloon catheter transluminal angioplasty for vertebral basilar ischemia. In: Berguer R, Bauer R, eds. Vertebrobasilar Arterial Occlusive Disease. New York: Raven Press, 1984:215–224.
55. Sundt TM Jr, Smith HC, Campbell JK, Vlietstra RE, Cucchiara RF, Stanson AW. Transluminal angioplasty for basilar artery stenosis. Mayo Clin Proc 1980; 55:673–680.
56. Jensen ME, Mathis JM, DeNardo AJ, Dion JE. Angioplasty of brachiocephalic and cerebral vessels in atherosclerotic disease. Stroke 1994; 25:273 (abstract).
57. Clark WM, Barnwell SL, Nesbit G, O'Neill OR, Wynn ML, Coull BM. Safety and efficacy of percutaneous transluminal angioplasty for intracranial atherosclerotic stenosis. Stroke 1995; 26:1200–1204.

58. Higashida RT, Tsai FY, Halbach V, et al. Transluminal angioplasty for atherosclerotic disease of the vertebral and basilar arteries. J Neurosurg 1993; 78:192–198.
59. Kellog J, Nesbit GM, Clark W, Barnwell SL. Percutaneous transluminal angioplasty for intracranial atherosclerotic stenosis: long term follow-up. Intervent Neuroradiol 1997; 3(suppl 1):39 (abstract).
60. Touho H. Percutaneous transluminal angioplasty in the treatment of atherosclerotic disease of the anterior cerebral circulation and hemodynamic evaluation. J Neurosurg 1997; 82:953–960.
61. Hyodo A, Matsumaru Y, Anno I, Sato H, Kato T, Nakai Y, et al. Percutaneous transluminal angioplasty for atherosclerotic stenosis of the intracranial cerebral arteries. Results with more than one year follow-up. Intervent Neuroradiol 1997; 3(suppl 1):38 (abstract).
62. Marks MP, Marcellus ML, Norbash AN, Steinberg GK, Albers GW. Evaluation of long term clinical outcome in patients undergoing intracranial angioplasty. Intervent Neuroradiol 1997; 3(suppl 1):38–39 (abstract).

25

Anticoagulation and Extracranial Arterial Disease

Ashfag Shuaib
University of Alberta Hospital, Edmonton, Alberta, Canada

INTRODUCTION

Because of the prominent role of thrombosis in stroke, the use of anticoagulation has been the focus of much attention and controversy.[1] Secondary prevention strategies are effective in stroke prevention in patients with atrial fibrillation,[2–6] asymptomatic bruits,[7–9] transient ischemic attacks (TIAs), and completed stroke.[10,11] Antiplatelets or anticoagulants have been shown to reduce the risk of further stroke. Antiplatelet medications (ASA[12–18] and ticlopidine[19,20]) are particularly useful in patients in whom an arterial source is suspected as a possible etiology. Anticoagulation therapy is indicated in patients with a cardiac source (e.g., atrial fibrillation or acute anterior wall myocardial infarction[2,3]) or a hypercoagulable state [21]. Anticoagulant therapy is also frequently used in patients with artery-to-artery emboli, arterial thrombosis or when the patient continues to have symptoms while on antiplatelet therapy. Risk factor management remains a pivotal cornerstone in any comprehensive plan. Excellent reviews have recently been published on the subject.[22–29]

This chapter will briefly review the mechanisms producing ischemic stroke in patients with extracranial disease and discuss relevant publications on the usefulness of anticoagulant therapy in preventing stroke recurrence in patients with atherosclerosis in the neck vessels. Indications for use of anticoagulation therapy in patients with cardiac disease and intra-cranial atherosclerosis is discussed elsewhere.

MECHANISM OF STROKE IN PATIENTS WITH EXTRACRANIAL ATHEROSCLEROSIS

The mechanism of stroke in most patients with atherosclerosis in the extracranial circulation is artery-to-artery emboli. The risk of thrombus formation increases with progressive narrowing of the arterial lumen and is particularly common in over 70% to 80% stenosis of the carotid artery.[1] In many such patients the endothelial surface is damaged and the resulting ulceration becomes a perfect focus for thrombus formation. In most cases, a small platelet-fibrin "white" thrombus may be evident over the plaque on direct inspection. White thrombi form in areas of high flow and are composed of platelets and fibrin. In areas where blood flow is slow, a large number of red blood cells are trapped within the fibrin clot and a red thrombus may form. However, large "red" thrombi are not frequently seen in carotid arteries.[30,31] Thrombi with artery-to-artery emboli may be seen in both the carotid and vertebrobasilar circulations.[32] The aorta is also becoming recognized as a site where larger thrombi may form over atherosclerotic plaques and potentially embolize to the brain.[33]

In patients with an acute ischemic stroke, if cerebral angiography is done early, arterial occlusion may be detected in the majority of patients. These are likely a result of artery-to-artery emboli. The frequency of occlusion is related to the timing of the angiogram from the onset of symptoms. If the angiogram is done within 6 hours of the onset of symptoms, arterial occlusions are seen in 71% to 80% of patients.[34] However, if angiography is delayed for more than 24 hours, arterial occlusion is evident in only about 25% of patients.[35] The decrease in the frequency of demonstrated arterial occlusion is likely due to spontaneous thrombolysis.[35] While most strokes are secondary to fibrin-platelet emboli, a significant proportion may be secondary to dislodgement of a thrombus from the neck arteries. In the coronary arteries of patients with symptomatic stenosis, two types of thrombi are recognized with different presentations. Angioscopic examination has revealed gray-white (fibrin-platelet) thrombi in patients with angina, and red clots in patients with a completed myocardial infarction.[36] It is not clear if similar mechanisms are at play in patients with TIAs and completed ischemic strokes.

ANTICOAGULATION

Mechanism of Action of Warfarin and Pharmacology[37]

Warfarin acts as an anticoagulant by antagonizing the action of vitamin K. This effect is within the liver where the medication directly inhibits the synthesis of coagulation Factors II, VII, IX, and X. It also inhibits the formation of the anticoagulant proteins—protein C and protein S. The anticoagulant effect of warfarin begins as soon as the circulating coagulation factors begin to decrease. Factor VII is depressed very rapidly and disappears within 24 hours of initiation of therapy. Other factors may take up to 72 hours or longer to significantly decrease because of longer half-lives. The long half-life of coagulation factors makes warfarin a poor choice when rapid anticoagulation is needed. If urgent anticoagulation is required, the patient should be treated with heparin for the initial 4 to 5 days. During this time, the warfarin therapy is started and heparin stopped when therapeutic prolongation of prothrombin time (or International Normalized Ratio [INR]) is achieved.

Warfarin has a long half-life. The mean half-life may be >40 hours and this is affected by a variety of factors including drugs, diet, and liver or kidney damage. The unbound fraction of the plasma warfarin is chemically active. As >95% of the drug is bound to protein, medications that may increase the unbound fraction can result in prolongation of the prothrombin time. The amount of medications needed to maintain a therapeutic level is not constant and may vary from 3.0 mg to over 10.0 mg per patient. The precise dose may vary over time in the same subject. Warfarin is metabolized in the liver and its metabolism may be slowed or enhanced by a variety of medications and liver diseases. It is therefore important to regularly follow prothrombin time in an individual patient on warfarin therapy.

Therapy in Stroke Prevention

There are several clinical situations in which anticoagulation therapy is used in prevention of or recurrence of cerebral infarction. The use of such medication is clearly indicated in patients with cardioembolic disease. There are, however, only a limited number of studies where anticoagulant therapy has been tested in patients with TIAs or completed stroke. Most of the studies are from the 1960s and a comparison with antiplatelet agents had not been done in the earlier studies.

Prevention of Ischemic Stroke in Patients with TIAs

There are four small randomized trials where the efficacy of anticoagulation was tested against placebo in patients with TIAs.[38–41] The studies were done in the 1960s and the number of patients in each trial was very small. The medication was tested against placebo in all four studies. These studies showed that while the rate of subsequent events was decreased, there was also an unexpected increase in the risk of hemorrhage in the anticoagulated patients (see Table 1). The very small number of patients and the lack of proper methodology of clinical trials make judgment on all of these studies impossible. The combined total of patients in the four studies was 178 (85 placebo and 93 in the active group), and the mean follow-up was 19 to 21 months. During this time a total of eight strokes occurred in the warfarin group and 10 in the placebo group. Death was, however, more

Table 1 The use of Anticoagulants in Stroke Prevention in TIA Patients

	Follow-up (months)		Stroke	Hemorrhage
1. VA (1961)[41]				
Controls	15	13	0	Not reported
Anticoagulated	22	9	4.6%	Not reported
2. Baker (1962)[38]				
Controls	20	20	25%	0
Treated	24	18′	5.6%	11%
3. Pearce (1965)[40]				
Controls	20	11	10%	Not reported
Treated	17	11	5.9%	
4. Baker (1966)[39]				
Controls	30	41	23	None
Treated	30	38	6.7	None
Total				
Control	85	21	16.5	
Anticoagulated	93	19	5.4	Date not sufficient

common in the active treatment group. Fifteen patients in the warfarin group versus 10 in the placebo group died during follow-up. Most of the deaths in the active group were secondary to brain hemorrhage. These early studies were done before the era of CT scans. Most studies lacked information on etiology of the stroke, monitoring of prothrombin time was not rigorous, and patient compliance to therapy was not well documented. While it is true that anticoagulation has not been shown to prevent stroke in noncardiac disease, the lack of its effectiveness has also not been proven.

Prevention of Recurrent Stroke

There are seven randomized studies where anticoagulation was tested in patients with acute completed stroke.[38,41,42] In six of the seven studies, therapy was ineffective.[38,41–43] Once again, similar to the studies with TIAs, the numbers of subjects in the studies were small and comparison with antiplatelet agents was not done. Therefore no definite conclusions can be drawn from the published data. The study published by Enger and Boyesen suggested that anticoagulation therapy decreased the risk of recurrent stroke.[44] This was, however, offset by an increase in intracerebral hemorrhage.

Two ongoing studies may provide useful information in the near future. The Warfarin Aspirin Recurrent Stroke study (WARS) is evaluating the efficacy of warfarin compared to ASA in patients with a completed ischemic stroke. In the Stroke Warfarin Aspirin Trial (SWAT), warfarin is being tested against ASA or a combination of ASA+warfarin. Both are prospective studies and are excluding patients with cardioembolic stroke and patients with critical carotid stenosis requiring surgery.

A number of nonrandomized studies have also compared the efficacy of warfarin to ASA. Similar to all the studies mentioned above, the data have to be viewed with caution as the studies have a small number of patients and the follow-up has been very brief. In an early study, Olssen reported on the efficacy of anticoagulation in patients with TIAs and completed stroke. A total of 178 patients were followed and many patients had to be excluded because medications were discontinued. Only one stroke was reported in the patients on therapy. Once medication was stopped, six additional strokes occurred amongst the 104 patients who completed the study.[45] Buren et al. compared the warfarin (60 patients) to ASA+dipyridamole (65 patients). Patients were followed for a mean of 24 months. The number of strokes were too few in the two groups to make any meaningful conclusions (two and four, respectively). Minor complications were seen in four patients in the anticoagulated group (transient hematuria). This did not require the medication to be stopped.[46] Eriksson showed that the rate of stroke was lower in a comparative study between warfarin (92 patients) versus ASA (500 mg/d) plus dipyridamole (75 mg/d) (96 patients). During follow-up, significantly fewer patients treated with anticoagulant treatment had TIA. Stroke was seen in six patients treated with warfarin and 12 patients treated with antiplatelet agents. Death occurred in 11 anticoagulated patients and in 17 patients treated with antiplatelet therapy. The differences were not statistically significant. Bleeding complications occurred in 20 patients. Two of these were serious events (one fatality with a cerebellar hematoma and one major bleed into a duodenal ulcer).[47] Finally, in a study by Garde et al., 241 patients were treated with ASA (127) or anticoagulation (114). Cerebral infarction developed in four patients in each group during a mean follow-up of 20 months. While bleeding complications were more common in the anticoagulated group, other side effects, especially gastrointestinal upset, were more common in the ASA-treated group.[48] In total, 409 patients treated with aspirin were compared to 384 patients treated with warfarin. The rate of stroke was 13% in the aspirin-treated group compared to 10% in the anticoagulated groups. Stroke or death was also not significantly different in the two groups.

CLINICAL PRACTICE WITH ANTICOAGULANT THERAPY

Lacking definitive data, anticoagulation is being used empirically in patients who develop ischemic symptoms which may be secondary to atherosclerotic disease in the neck arteries. In many patients with ischemic symptoms, the etiology is not evident despite extensive investigations. While a clear cardiac source may not be apparent in many such patients, an embolic event is suspected on clinical grounds and the patient is anticoagulated. This is especially common when the cranial CT or MRI shows multiple ischemic infarctions.

In patients with severe carotid stenosis and recent or frequent TIAs, anticoagulation therapy is often offered. This is particularly common in patients in whom angiography reveals an associated ulcer on the stenotic plaque. Such patients are usually admitted to hospital for heparin therapy followed by oral anticoagulation until the carotid endarterectomy. There is no proof that this course is superior to using antiplatelet therapy while waiting for carotid endarterectomy. In most large randomized studies on endarterectomy, patients with tight stenosis were treated with ASA or ticlopidine during the time preceding surgery. This has been our practice. It avoids unnecessary hospitalization. Surprisingly, anticoagulation is also often used in patients with asymptomatic carotid stenosis by internists.[49] There are no data that this is of any benefit to the patient. We would strongly recommend against this practice until such time as efficacy is shown with prospective clinical trials. To our knowledge, no such trial is under way.

There are a few clinical situations where anticoagulation therapy is recommended as the risk of recurrent stroke may be high. Dissection in the carotid or vertebral arteries is a common cause of stroke in the young. Most dissections occur with little trauma and can often be multiple. In most patients with such dissections, the neurological symptoms are believed to be secondary to distal emboli from thrombi forming at the site of the lesion.

The rationale of the anticoagulation is to prevent recurrences.[50] Treatment is initiated with heparin and followed with warfarin therapy. Antiplatelet medications are recommended after an initial 3 to 6 months of warfarin therapy. Repeated angiography may be necessary to show healing of the vascular defect. The primary use of ASA without anticoagulation has not been tested. We have found the symptoms to subside once anticoagulation is initiated.[51] Bleeding complications are rarely seen with dissection in the extracranial arteries. Bleeding may, however, be seen with dissection in intracranial vessels.[52] Anticoagulants should be avoided in patients with intracranial arterial dissection.

Patients in whom angiography shows a thrombus in the carotid artery over a plaque are at an increased risk of stroke.[31] Emergency carotid endarterectomy may carry a significant risk of complications. In such patients a brief course of anticoagulant therapy followed by repeated angiography is suggested. If the second angiogram shows resolution of the carotid thrombus, the patient should be switched to antiplatelet therapy and considered for surgery, provided the carotid stenosis is >70%. Patients with a completely occluded carotid artery may on occasion have thrombi form at the stump, which may be a source of distal emboli.[53]

These may travel via collateral vessels that supply blood to the brain. In such patients anticoagulation may be required for 4 to 6 months before switching to long-term antiplatelet therapy.[53]

From 10% to 15% of patients with TIAs or acute stroke may have evidence of carotid disease and also a potential cardiac source of emboli.[54] The incidence of such combined lesions may be higher in the elderly population. If the suspicion is high for a potential cardiac (for example, atrial fibrillation) source despite significant carotid stenosis, the patient should be treated with anticoagulation. However, no clinical trials in these situations have been done to compare anticoagulation to antiplatelet therapy or placebo.

Transesophegeal echocardiography (TEE) is used increasingly in stroke patients. Identification of atherosclerotic lesions in the aorta is possible with TEE. Such lesions have been shown to increase the risk of recurrent stroke. The proper therapy for such lesions remains to be better defined. In the absence of proper trials, anticoagulation is often used to prevent thrombus formation and subsequent stroke recurrence.

Risk of Cerebral Hemorrhage

Intracranial hemorrhage can occur in approximately 1% (range 0% to 3.3%) of patients treated with anticoagulation therapy with careful attention to maintaining the INRs in the range of between 2 and 4. Whereas the bleeding can occur anywhere in the cranial cavity, most large hematomas develop within the cerebral hemispheres. The risk of hemorrhage increases in patients with preexisting cerebrovascular disease (including leukoariosis), advancing age, the presence of hypertension, and the intensity of anticoagulation.[55]

Combination Therapy of Antiplatelets and Anticoagulation in Stroke Prevention

Anticoagulant therapy has been used successfully to prevent emboli in patients with valvular disease and other conditions that increase thrombi formation in the heart. Unfortunately, despite adequate anticoagulation, some patients continue to have symptoms. Small asymptomatic emboli can be often be detected on transcranial Doppler in such patients. There is evidence that the addition of aspirin to warfarin may reduce the risk of subsequent stroke significantly in patients with mechanical cardiac valves.[56] While bleeding complications may increase a little, the benefits outweigh the risks.[56] Combination therapy with ASA or ticlopidine and warfarin may be recommended in the occasional patient who continues to have symptoms while on either therapy alone. In our experience, symptomatic patients on single therapy may have silent emboli on TCD. These may disappear with the combination therapy. More experience is, however, needed before the therapy can be recommended for general use. An interesting report in 1985 looked at the effects of combination therapy with ASA and anticoagulation in patients with severe atherosclerosis and repeated events while on antiplatelet therapy. Thirteen of the 20 patients had symptoms referable to the brain. Twenty patients were followed for an average of 5.8 years and none developed new symptoms. Complications to therapy were seen in seven of the 20 patients.[57]

SUMMARY

A recent survey of neurologists, neurovascular surgeons, and primary care physicians polled regarding the use of antiplatelet and anticoagulation therapy revealed important findings.[49] The physicians were questioned about the use of antiplatelet agents and warfarin in symptomatic and asymptomatic patients with moderate (50% to 70% stenosis) and severe carotid disease (>70% stenosis). While most physicians were using antiplatelet agents for stroke prophylaxis, a significant proportion reported the use of anticoagulant therapy as the primary therapy in both symptomatic and asymptomatic patients with carotid disease. Physicians were more likely to use anticoagulation if there was severe carotid stenosis, especially if the patient had contraindications to surgery. Of a total of 1,007 physicians who responded to the survey, 15% responded that they would always or often treat asymptomatic stenosis of 50% to 70% with anticoagulation. If the stenosis was >70% in asymptomatic patients, 43% of respondents reported the use of anticoagulant therapy. In symptomatic patients, 28% would treat 50-70% stenosis with anticoagulation. This increased to 49% if the stenosis was >70%. Anticoagulant therapy was preferred to antiplatelet agents by a significantly larger number of primary care physicians and internists compared to neurologists. The frequent use of anticoagulant therapy in asymptomatic individuals with carotid stenosis is alarming. The use of anticoagulation as primary therapy in symptomatic patients is worrisome. Figure 1 shows details of the various subspecialties with the percent responses from the survey.

Anticoagulation is essential in stroke prevention in most patients with a cardiac source of embolus. Indications for anticoagulant therapy in noncardioembolic disease are not clear. Please refer to Table 2. Clinical trials are urgently needed for the appropriate indication in patients with extracranial disease. Current ongoing trials would hopefully provide answers in the next few years. Heparin therapy followed by warfarin is probably indicated in patients with carotid dissection, in patients where angiography shows a thrombus on a carotid plaque or the carotid stump syndrome. In such patients, warfarin should be stopped in 3 to 6 months and patients maintained on long-term antiplatelet treatment. It may also be indicated in patients with evidence of artery-to artery emboli in the pos-

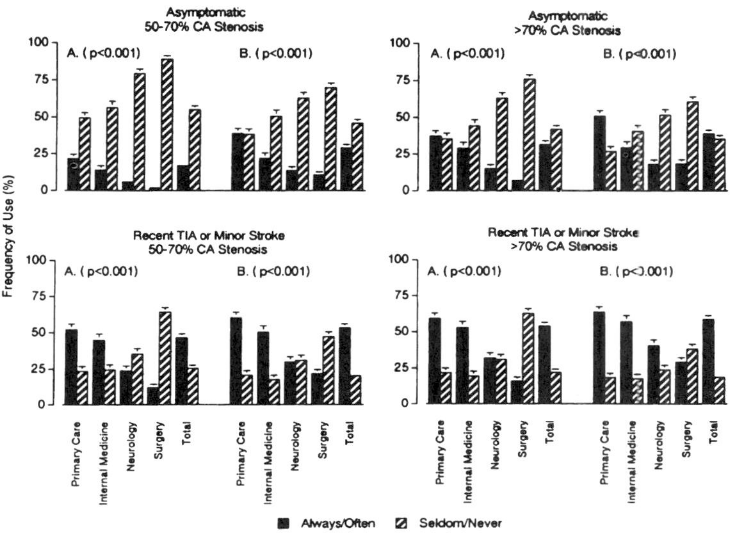

Figure 1 Reported frequency of use (always or often vs seldom or never) of anticoagulants by physician specialty (noninternist primary care physicians, internists, neurologists, or surgeons) in patients without (A) or with (B) contraindications for carotid endarterectomy and who are asymptomatic and have 50% to 70% stenosis of the extracranial carotid artery (CA) (top left); are asymptomatic and have more than 70% CA stenosis (top right); had a recent (within the last month) transient ischemic attack (TIA) or minor stroke and have 50% to 70% CA stenosis (bottom left); or had a recent TIA or minor stroke and mroe than 70% CA stenosis (bottom right). The reported frequency of use of anticoagulants varied significantly with physician specialty, symptom status, degree of stenosis, and presence of surgical contraindications. Error bars indicate 1 SEE. (From Ref. 49.)

Table 2 Indication for long-term anticoagulation in extracranial non-cardioembolic disease.

Asymptomatic carotid stenosis	Not-indicated
Symptomatic carotid stenosis	Recommended only if antiplatelet therapy ineffective in preventing recurrence (not sufficient proof of efficacy). Antiplatelet and anticoagulants are in addition to surgery.
Symptomatic vertebrobasilar disease	Frequently used with little proof of efficacy
Crescendo TIAs	Often used (no data of efficacy)
Carotid stenosis with thrombus	Short-term anticoagulant therapy
Carotid stump syndrome	Short-term anticoagulant therapy
Carotid/vertebral dissection	Short-term anticoagulant therapy

terior circulation. It is often used in patients who "fail" antiplatelet therapy.[58] While there is no proof that this course is superior to maintaining antiplatelet therapy, the practice is common and unlikely to change. Anticoagulation therapy should not be used as primary therapy in patients with carotid stenosis with or without contraindications to surgery, as antiplatelet therapy has been shown to reduce the risk of subsequent stroke whereas such an effect has not been shown with warfarin. Finally, we would strongly advise against the use of anticoagulation in patients with asymptomatic carotid stenosis.

REFERENCES

1. Hillered L, Persson H. Microdialysis for neurochemical monitoring in human brain injuries. In: Tsubokawa T, Marmarou A, Robertson C, eds. Neurochemical Monitoring in the Intensive Care Unit. Microdialysis, Jugular Venous Oximetry and Near-Infrared Spectroscopy. Tokyo: Springer-Vertag, 1995:59–63.
2. Petersen P, Boysen G, Godtfredsen J, Andersen E, D., Andersen B. Placebo-controlled randomized trial of warfarin and aspirin for prevention of thromboembolic complications in atrial fibrillation. Lancet 1989; 1:175–179.
3. Anonymous. Preliminary report of the stroke prevention in atrial fibrillation study. N Engl J Med 1990; 322:863–868.
4. Wolf PA, Abott RD, Kannel WB. Atrial fibrillation: a major contributor to stroke in the elderly. Arch Intern Med 1987; 147:1561–1564.
5. Anonymous. The effect of low-dose warfarin on the risk of stroke in patients with nonrheumatic atrial fibrillation. N Engl J Med 1990; 323:1505–1511.
6. Boston Area Anticoagulation Trial for Atrial Fibrillation Investigations. The effect of low-dose warfarin on the risk of stroke in patients with nonrheumatic atrial fibrillation. N Engl J Med 1990; 323:1505–1511.
7. Executive committee for the Asymptomatic Carotid Atherosclerosis Study. Endarterectomy for asymptomatic carotid artery stenosis. JAMA 1995; 273:1421–1428.
8. Barnett H, Eliasziw M, Meldrum BS, Taylor DW. Do the facts and figures warrant a 10-fold increase in the performance of carotid endarterectomy on asymptomatic patients. Neurology 1996; 46:603–608.
9. Hobson RW, Weiss DG, Fields WS, et al. Efficacy of carotid endarterectomy for asymptomatic carotid stenosis. N Engl J Med 1993; 328:221–227.
10. North American Symptomatic Carotid Endarterectomy Trial Collaborators. Beneficial effects of carotid endarterectomy in symptomatic patients with high-grade stenosis. N Engl J Med 1991; 325:445–453.
11. Meissner I, Meyer FB. Carotid stenosis and carotid endarterectomy. Cerebrovasc Brain Metab Rev 1994; 6:163–179.
12. Anonymous. Secondary prevention of vascular disease by prolonged antiplatelet treatment. Br Med J 1988; 296:320–331.
13. Anonymous. United Kingdom transient ischemic attack (UK-TIA) aspirin trial: interim report. Br Med J 1988; 296:316–320.

14. Gijn J. Results of the Dutch aspirin trial: 30 versus 300 mg in 3150 patients. Conference report at the 16th international joint conference on stroke and cerebral circulation. Stroke 1991; 22:149.
15. Easton JD. Antiplatelet therapy for the prevention of ischemic stroke. Cerebrovasc Dis 1992; 2(suppl. 1):6–13.
16. SALT Collaborative Group. Swedish Aspirin Low-dose Trial (SALT) of 75 mg aspirin as secondary prophylaxis after cerebrovascular ischemic events. Lancet 1991; 338:1345–1349.
17. Dyken ML, Barnett H, Easton JD, et al. Low-dose aspirin and stroke: "it ain't necessarily so." Stroke 1992; 23:1395–1399.
18. Jonas S, Zeleniuch-Jacquotte A. Effect of aspirin on risk of stroke or death in women who have suffered cerebral ischemia. Cerebrovasc Dis 1994; 4:157–162.
19. Hershey LA. Stroke prevention in women: role of aspirin versus ticlopidine. Am J Med 1991; 91:288–292.
20. Hass WK, Easton JD, Adams JP. A randomized trial comparing ticlopidine with aspirin for the prevention of stroke in high-risk patients. N Engl J Med 1989; 321:501–507.
21. Tatlisumak T, Fisher M. Hematologic disorders associated with ischemic stroke. J Neurol Sci 1996; 1–11.
22. Whisnant JP, Homer D, Ingall TJ, Baker HL, O'Fallon WM, Wiebers DO. Duration of smoking is the strongest predictor of severe extracranial carotid artery atherosclerosis. Stroke 1990; 21:707–714.
23. Donnan GA, McNeil JJ, Adena MA, O'Malley HM, Neill GC. Smoking as a risk factor for cerebral ischemia. Lancet 1989; 2:643–647.
24. Farquhar JW, Fortmann SP, Flora JA, et al. Effects of community wide education on cardiovascular disease risk factors. JAMA 1990; 264:359–365.
25. Mas JL, Zuber M. Epidemiology of ischemic stroke. Cerebrovasc Dis 1991; 1(suppl. 1):36–44.
26. Dutch TIA Trial Study Group. Predictors of major vascular events in patients with a transient ischemic attack or nondisabling stroke. Stroke 1993; 24:527–531.
27. Psaty BM, Koepsell TD, Monolio TA. Risk ratios and risk differences in estimating the effect of risk factors for cardiovascular disease in the elderly. J Clin Epidemiol 1990; 43:961–970.
28. Gorelick PB. Stroke prevention. An opportunity for efficient utilization of health care resources during the coming decade. Stroke 1994; 25:220–224.
29. Goode GK, Miller JP, Heagerty AM. Hyperlipidemia, hypertension, and coronary heart disease. Lancet 1995; 345:362–364.
30. Fisher CM, Ojemann RG. A clinico-pathological study of carotid artery plaques. Rev Neurol 1986; 142:573–589.
31. Buchan AM, Gates PC, Pelz D, Barnett H. Intraluminal thrombus in the cerebral circulation. Stroke 1988; 19:681–687.
32. Caplan LR, Amarenco P, Rosengart A, et al. Embolism from vertebral artery disease. Neurology 1992; 42:1505–1512.
33. Amarenco P, Cohen A, Tzourio C, et al. Atherosclerotic disease of the aortic arch and the risk of ischemic stroke. N Engl J Med 1994; 331:1474–1479.

34. Fieschi C, Argentino C, Lenzi GL, Sacchetti ML, Toni D, Bozzao L. Clinical and instrumental evaluation of patients with ischemic stroke within the first six hours. J Neurol Sci 1989; 91:311–322.
35. Delal PM, Shah PM, Aiyar RR. Angiographic study of cerebral embolism. Lancet 1965; II:258–261.
36. Mitzuno K, Satumora K, Miyatomo A. Angiographic evaluation of coronary artery thrombi in acute coronary arteries. N Engl J Med 1992; 326:287–291.
37. Majerus PW, Broze GJ, Melitich JP, Tollefsen DM. Anticoagulant, thrombolytic and antiplatelet drugs. Goodmans and Gilman's The Pharmacological Basis of Therapeutics 8th ed. 1991:1311–1332.
38. Baker RN, Broward JA, Fang HC. Anticoagulant therapy in cerebral infarction. Neurology 1962; 12:823–835.
39. Baker RN, Schwartz W, Rose AS. Transient ischemic attacks—a report of a study of anticoagulant treatment. Neurology 1966; 16:841–846.
40. Pearce JMS, Gubbay SS., Walton J, N. Long term anticoagulant therapy in transient ischemic attacks. Lancet 1965; i:6–9.
41. Veterans Administration. An evaluation of anticoagulation therapy in the treatment of cerebrovascular disease. Neurology 1961; 11:132–138.
42. McDowell F, McDevitt E. Treatment of completed stroke with anticoagulation. Six and one-half year experience. In: Siekert R, G., Whisnant J, P. eds. Cerebrovascular Disease. New York: Grune & Stratton, 1965:185–199.
43. Howard FA, Cohen P, Hicker RB. Survival following stroke. JAMA 1963; 183:921–925.
44. Enger E, Ammar AD. Long term anticoagulant therapy in patients with cerebral infarction. Acta Med Scand 1965; 178(suppl 438):1–61.
45. Olsson J, Muller R, Berneli S. Long term anticoagulant therapy in patients with TIAs and minor stroke with minimum residuum. Stroke 1976; 7:444–451.
46. Buren A, Ygge J. Treatment program and comparison between anticoagulants and platelet aggregation inhibitors in transient ischemic attacks. Stroke 1981; 12:578–580.
47. Eriksson SE. Enteric coated acetylsalicylic acid plus dipyridamole compared with anticoagulants in the prevention of ischemic events in patients with transient ischemic attacks. Acta Neurol Scand 1985; 71:485–493.
48. Grade A, Samuelsson K, Falhgren A. Treatment after transient ischemic attacks: a comparison between anticoagulants and inhibitors of platelet aggregation. Stroke 1983; 14:677–681.
49. Goldstein LB, Bonito AJ. Matchar DB, Duncan GW, Samsa GP. U.S. national survey of physician practices for the secondary prevention of ischemic stroke. Medical therapy for patients with carotid artery stenosis. Stroke 1996; 27:1473–1478.
50. Saver JL, Easton JD, Hart RG. Dissections and trauma of cervicocerebral arteries. In: Barnett HJ, Mohr JP, Stein BM, Yatsu FM. eds. Stroke: Pathophysiology, Diagnosis and Management. 2d ed. New York: Churchill Livingstone, 1992:671–689.
51. Shuaib A. Stroke from other etiologies masquerading as migraine-stroke. Stroke 1991; 22:1068–1074.
52. Adams HP, Aschenbrener CA, Kassell NF. Intracranial hemorrhage produced by spontaneous dissecting intracranial aneurysm. Arch Neurol 1982; 39:773–776.

53. Barnett H, Pearless SJ, Kaufmann JC. "Stump" of internal carotid artery—a source of further cerebral embolic ischemia. Stroke 1978; 9:48–53.
54. Bogousslavsky J, Hachinski, V, Boughner D,R., Fox AJ., Vinuela F, Barnett HJ. Cardiac and arterial lesions in carotid transient ischemic attacks. Arch Neurol 1986; 43:223–228.
55. Hart RG. Oral anticoagulation for secondary prevention of stroke. Stroke 1997; 7 (suppl 6):24–29.
56. Turpie AG, Gent M, Laupacis A, et al. A comparison of aspirin with placebo in patients treated with warfarin after heart-valve replacement. N Engl J Med 1993; 329:524–529.
57. Miller A, Lees RS. Simultaneous therapy with antiplatelet and anticoagulant drugs in symptomatic cardiovascular disease. Stroke 1985; 16:668–675.
58. Feinberg W, Albers GW., Barnett H, et al. Guidelines for the management of transient ischemic attacks. Stroke 1994; 25:1320–1335.

26

Surgical Stratification and Management of Carotid Atherosclerosis

Zachary T. Levine and Laligam Sekhar
George Washington University, Washington, D.C.

INTRODUCTION

The association between carotid artery insult and neurologic sequelae dates back to ancient Greece. Carotid compression was known to cause a deep sleep or coma.[35] However, the cause of the "sleep," namely ischemia, was not known until the 17th century with the work of Thomas Willis and Johann Wepfer.[35] Apoplexy, as it was then called, was still a confounding disease with protean manifestations. It was not until 19th century, when surgery on the carotid artery and the results from occlusion, both fortunate and not so fortunate, that the documentation of stroke from carotid disease was formalized. Scattered reports of elective carotid occlusion for tumor or trauma revealed the capricious nature of the carotid arteries. Some patients tolerated occlusion without neurologic deficit while others died shortly after surgery or never awakened.[35]

In 1905, Chiari first described carotid artery disease. In pathologic notes he recorded the typical plaques at the carotid bifurcation and their contribution to stroke. He even deduced and designed a model to explain how embolic stroke may evolve from these plaques.[1] From the time of this observation, knowledge of cerebrovascular disease and its causes have grown rapidly. The most important modern contribution to our current knowledge of stroke is that of C. Miller Fischer, in two important papers from 1951 and 1954. In addition to describing the evolution of cerebrovascular disease he projected the need for surgical intervention: "Some day vascular surgery will find a way to bypass the occluded portion of the artery."[12,13] Carotid artery bypass had been done prior to Fischer's publications; however, at about the same time, William Spence submitted to the

Journal of Neurosurgery the first report of successful carotid endarterectomy. It was rejected.[35] The first published account of carotid endarterectomy was by Cooley et al. in 1958.[35] The elegance of the procedure and the presumed benefit from return of flow allowed rapid spread of its use in cerebrovascular disease. The search for more specific indications was needed as the frequency of surgery increased. The goal was to prevent the devastation of stroke much the way coronary artery bypass prevented myocardial infarction.

The treatment of stroke is highly dependent on the ability of the diagnostician to stratify the patients appropriately. Using radiographs and a well-focused neurologic exam, patients can be directed toward suited therapy. In this chapter we will focus on the stratification and surgical treatment of cerebrovascular disease. Our attention will be aimed on the anterior circulation (carotid arteries) since the most common surgical intervention for stroke is carotid endarterectomy.

Stroke can be described geographically, etiologically, and temporally. The symptoms and radiographs can define a specific stroke geographically to known vascular territories. These are grossly broken down to either anterior (carotid) distribution or posterior (vertobrobasilar) distribution. More precise localization to specific arteries and regions of the brain is important; however, this discussion is reserved for a more in-depth look at stroke syndromes. Briefly, strokes can be divided etiologically into embolic strokes and ischemic strokes (low flow states as well as hypertensive ischemic syndromes). The time course of the stroke can help define the nature of the stroke. Reversible neurological deficits associated with cerebral vascular disease are transient ischemic attacks (TIAs). TIAs are thought to be due to emboli from atherosclerotic disease of the carotid arteries. Usually occurring ipsilateral to the diseased vessel, emboli transiently occlude smaller, distal vessels, resulting in neurologic deficit. Symptomatic TIAs precede approximately 15% of all full-blown strokes.[1] As the stenosis increases in a given vessel, the rate of TIAs and stroke increases, putting those people with the highest grade of stenosis at greatest risk.[1]

The majority (85%) of strokes in adults are due to thromboembolism or atherothrombosis.[1] The origin of emboli may be extracranial vessels (most commonly the carotids), other diseased intracranial vessels, or the heart. Embolus from the heart is associated with cardiac abnormality: atrial fibrillation, valvular abnormality including endocarditis. Also, an infrequent but important cause of stroke can be emboli from giant intracranial aneurysms.

Medical therapies including antiplatelet drugs and anticoagulation have effectively decreased the risk of stroke. However, they do not reverse the atherosclerotic disease ultimately responsible for stroke. The side effects of medical therapy can be problematic. In an attempt to treat the disease, not just the symptoms, a number of studies have been conducted to identify those patients who would benefit the most from surgical intervention opposed to medical therapy, realizing the risks inherent in both treatments.

TRIALS FOR SYMPTOMATIC CAROTID STENOSIS

NASCET

The North American Symptomatic Carotid Endarterectomy Trial (NASCET) was formed to establish guidelines for carotid endarterectomy. With a sevenfold increase in carotid artery surgery from 1971 to 1985 coupled with a decrease in initial and fatal strokes, a more detailed examination was required to assess the utility of carotid artery endarterectomy.[28] NASCET was a prospective randomized controlled study. Enrollment began on Jan. 1, 1988. The study focused on patients with symptomatic carotid disease and ipsilateral carotid stenosis ranging from 30% to 99% (30% to 69%: low-grade stenosis; 70% to 99%: high-grade stenosis) stenosis. The study was designed to compare carotid artery endarterectomy to the best medical care.[28]

Prior to randomization each patient was evaluated both clinically and radiographically. Enrollees were < 80 years old and "had a hemispheric TIA or monocular blindness persisting less than 24 hours or a nondisabling stroke with persistence of symptoms or signs for more than 24 hours with 120 days" prior to entrance into the study. Each potential enrollee received an angiogram and was excluded from the study if each did not have ipsilateral carotid artery stenosis that was surgically accessible or had received carotid artery endarterectomy to the ipsilateral vessel. Additional exclusion criteria included lack of visualization of carotid arteries and intracranial branches by angiogram; another, more severe lesion of the intracranial vessels; organ failure (renal, hepatic, or pulmonary) or cancer that was potentially fatal (within the following 5 years); "symptoms . . . attributed to non-atherosclerotic disease," or cardioembolic symptoms associated with known valvular disease.[28]

Each enrolled patient was randomized as to his/her treatment after eligibility was established. Treatment included antiplatelet therapy (approximately 1,300 mg acetylsalicylic acid [ASA] per day) in addition to management of hypertension, hyperlipidemia, and diabetes when indicated for both surgical and medical arms of the study. Those randomized for surgery underwent carotid artery endarterectomy. Fifty centers that had sufficient experience with carotid artery endarterectomy were chosen as the study sites. The acceptable complication rate was <6% int he 30-day postoperative period.[28]

On Feb. 1, 1991, the study was halted for patients with high-grade stenosis because the review of the data was conclusive. After the enrollment of 662 patients with high-grade stenosis, the determination of carotid artery endarterectomy vs. medical therapy was made. Patients with high-grade, symptomatic carotid artery stenosis are good candidates and benefited from carotid artery endarterectomy in addition to receiving maximal medical therapy over medical therapy alone. The data were reviewed and the two groups were evenly matched (Table 1). The rate of stroke was lower for the surgically managed group. The

Table 1 Comparison of Medical and Surgical Arms of NASCET

Characteristic	Medical group (n=331)	Surgical group (n=328)
	% of group	
Male	69	68
Female	31	32
Transient ischemic attack at entry	69	67
Stroke at entry	31	33
Ipsilateral stenosis		
70–79%	43	40
80–89%	33	38
90–99%	24	22
Contralateral stenosis (70–99%)	9	8
Race		
White	89	93
Black	4	2
Other	7	5
Prior myocardial infarction	18	18
Stable angina pectoris	25	22
Hypertension	61	60
Diabetes	21	17
Intermittent claudication	16	15
Current cigarette smoking	33	37
Antithrombotic medication	85	85

Source: Ref. 28

life table comparisons graphically demonstrate the long-term benefit for carotid artery endarterectomy in this select group of patients (Fig. 1).[28]

A statistical comparison included the 622 patients that were randomized with high-grade stenosis (70% to 99%) as evaluated by two views on a standard internal carotid angiogram. The surgical arm contained 328 patients, and the medical arm 331 patients. Three patients failed to meet study criteria and were excluded. No patients were lost to follow-up. The relative risk reduction in the surgical group after 24-month follow-up was 65%. The ipsilateral stroke rate of the patents managed medically was 26%, compared to 9% for those who underwent carotid artery endarterectomy (P<.001). However, examination of the survival curves reveals that early in the study there was increased risk for the surgically treated patients.[28]

During the first month of the study the risk of major stroke or death is higher for the surgical group (2.1%) than for the medical group (0.9%). With longer follow-up the risk for the surgical group becomes lower than the medically man-

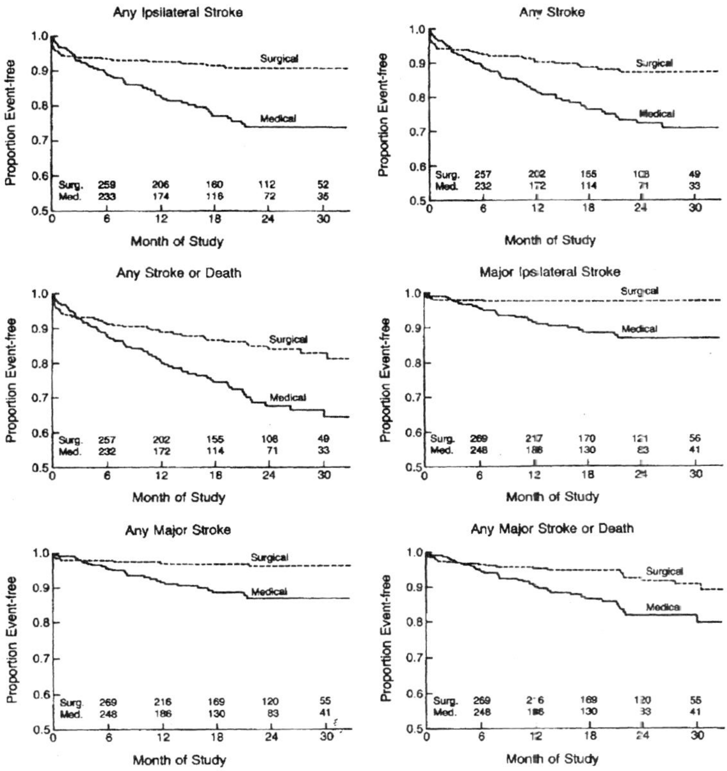

Figure 1 These Kaplan-Meier survival curves show the probability of surviving six events indicating treatment failure after randomization. The number of patients who remained event-free in each treatment group is shown at the six-mont intervals at the bottom of each graph; the numbers at time zero are 328 in the surgical group and 331 in the medical group. The curves of the groups differed significantly (by Mantel-Haenszel chi-squared test P<0.001 for all events except "any major stroke or death" for which $P<0.01$). (From Ref. 28.)

aged patients; crossover occurs at 3 months. More importantly, this risk reduction continues to persist with time, imparting some long-term benefit to patients with high-grade stenosis who received carotid artery endarterectomy.[28]

This study also elucidated the acceptable postoperative complication rate. In order for the surgery to be an acceptable option, the surgeon must not operate with a complication rate >3%. Further analysis also revealed that patients with the highest degree of stenosis benefited the most from surgery. The risk reduction improved as percent stenosis increased: 26%±8.1% for patients with 90% to 99% stenosis, 18%±6.2% for patients with 80% to 89% stenosis, and 12%

± 4.8% for patients with 70% to 79% stenosis. Therefore, carotid artery endarterectomy imparts the greatest benefit to those with the highest degree of stenosis. These numbers are convincing for high-grade, symptomatic, carotid artery stenosis; however, the results for lower grades of symptomatic stenosis are not so promising for surgery.[28]

ECST

The European Carotid Surgery Trial (ECST) began in 1981. The study randomized 2,518 patients in 10 years. In May 1991 the data were presented for 2,200 of the patients with a mean follow-up of 3 years. Analyzed data available at that time show significant results for this patient with 0% to 29% ("mild") stenosis and 70% to 99% ("severe") stenosis. However, at the time of publication of these data, there were no significant results for patients with 30% to 69% ("moderate") stenosis.[9]

In June 1996 a rapid communication of early, yet significant data for patients with moderate stenosis was published from the same group.[8] The ECST was designed to examine the efficacy of carotid artery endarterectomy versus the best medical treatment for patients with symptomatic carotid stenosis.[8,9] Paramount to the study was stratification of patients into one of three groups and analyzing the data for each separately.[8,9]

ECST enrolled "patients with a carotid territory non-disabling [ischemic] stroke, transient ischemic attack, or retinal infarction during the previous 6 months." However, eligibility was also determined by the treating physicians. If physicians were "substantially uncertain" whether to recommend surgery for the involved artery after angiogram, the patient was then considered a candidate for enrollment. Candidates were considered ineligible if the treating physicians were reasonably certain that surgery was or was not indicated.[9] (See Fig. 2.)

Once enrolled, the patients were tracked as a mild, moderate, or severe stenosis based on the angiogram. Patients in each category were followed and treated appropriately. The focus of ECST was the application of three questions to each category: (1) What was the 30-day postoperative risk of death or disabling stroke, (2) What is the long-term effect of surgery on further disabling strokes or death after surviving the initial 30-day period, and (3) How long does the benefit (if any) from surgery last?[9]

Data from the initial report in 1991 were similar to those reported in NASCET. When the data were analyzed at this midpoint there was an asymmetrical representation of patients among the 2,200 available.[9] The surgical arm enrolled 1,321 patients and the medical arm 888. Of those enrolled, 52% (1,152 patients) had either mild or severe stenosis. Patients with mild stenosis were randomized: 219 to surgery, and 155 to medical therapy alone. The patients with severe stenosis totaled 778, with 455 receiving surgery and the remaining 323

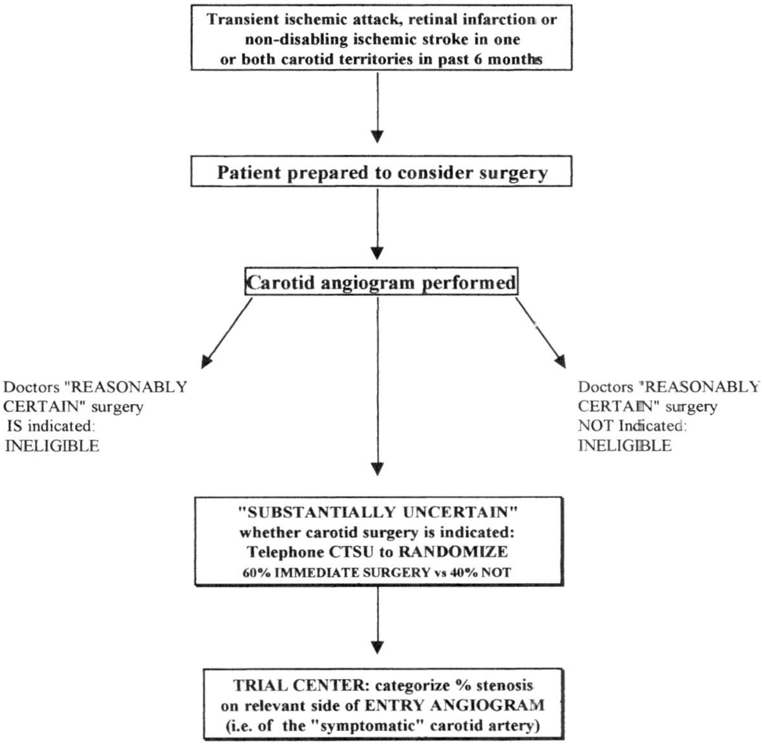

Figure 2 Trial eligibility, based on the uncertainty principle. (From Ref. 9.)

treated medically (Table 2). In the rapid communication from 1996, 1,590 patients had been randomized into the moderate-stenosis group, with at least a 4-month follow-up period. Carotid artery endarterectomy was performed on 959 of the moderate-stenosis patients, and 631 received medical therapy alone.[8]

Adverse events during the study were tracked for all three groups. In the immediate postoperative period (30 days), 3.7% of those with severe stenosis either had a disabling stroke or died.[8,9] For patients with mild stenosis, only 2.3% suffered from the same perioperative complications. The moderate stenosis group had a higher rate of perioperative complications: 7.9%. Although these data are easily compared among the groups, we will consider the remainder of results from the mild and severe groups separately from the moderate-stenosis group.[8,9]

As was seen in the NASCET data previously presented, ECST data supported carotid artery endarterectomy for symptomatic, severe carotid stenosis. Of the 455 patients allocated to surgery, 14 suffered any type of ipsilateral ischemic

Table 2 Baseline Characteristics of Randomized Patients (ECST study)

	Severe stenosis (70–79%)	Mild stenosis (0–29%)
No. with data in computer	788	374
Mean age (years)	62.2	59.7
Male (%)	70	72
Previous transient ischemic attack/ amaurosis fugax (%)	78	59
Previous stroke, residual neuro signs, or infarct on pre-randomization CT	50	61
Mean delay (days from last ischemic event to randomization	57	56
Previous myocardial infarction and/or angina (%)	27	13
Diabetic (%)	9	9
Mean systolic blood pressure (mm Hg)	151	148
Mean diastolic blood pressure (mm Hg)	86	87
Mean cholesterol (mmol/l)	6.5	6.3
Current cigarette smokers (%)	56	55
Mean obesity index (kg/m^2)	24.8	25.1

Source: Ref. 9

stroke, compared to 71 of the 323 treated medically. This breaks down to an eight-fold risk reduction for the surgical group ($P<.0001$).[9] (See Figs. 3 and 4.)

ECST went further and specifically analyzed the mild-stenosis group, and although there was no significant difference in the perioperative complication rate between the two groups, there was a significant difference in the risk for stroke between mild and high-grade stenosis in the surgical candidates. It is dangerous to operate on those patients with mild stenosis. Data collected on the 374 patients with mild stenosis were informative. Those patients with 0% to 29% stenosis have such a small risk of stroke that surgery imparted no long-term benefit over standard medical therapy, and in fact, the increased risk of stroke associated with surgery made surgical intervention undesirable for these patients.[9]

The first data set analyzed by ECST was useful in determining whether symptomatic high-grade or low-grade stenosis was surgically treatable; the more difficult question, for moderate stenosis, remained. ECST continued to enroll patients after releasing the data for "mild" and "severe" stenosis; however, the enrollees were those patients with 30% to 69% stenosis with symptomatic cerebral ischemia. The data for the "moderate" stenosis group were the first of their kind published.[8] Again, to demonstrate its results more graphically, ECST divided the "moderate" stenosis group in two. The first had 30% to 49% stenosis with a

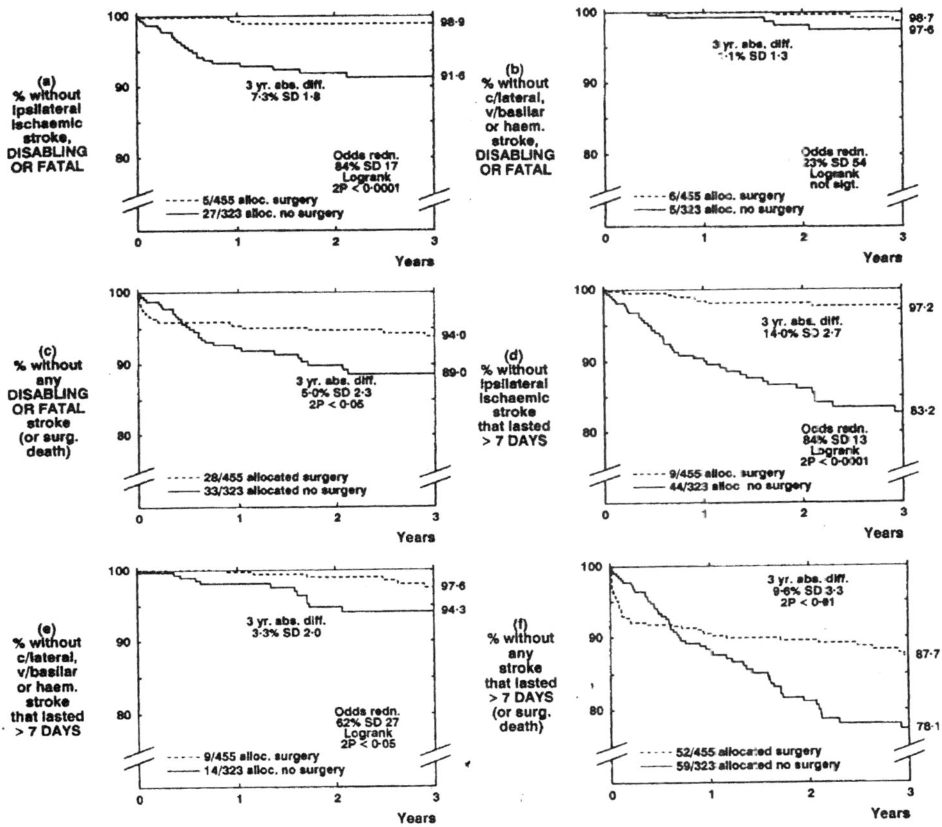

Figure 3 Main analysis of strokes (a-c disabling-fatal; d-f, lasting more than 7 days) or of surgery-associated mortality of patients with severe stenosis (70–99%) on the pre-randomization angiogram. Key(# with this as first event)/(# with some follow-up). (From Ref. 9.)

mean follow-up of 4.5 years for both surgical and medical arms. The second group (50% to 69% stenosis) had a mean follow-up of 4.3 years for the medically managed patients and 3.9 years for surgically treated patients. The percentage of strokes of any kind or at any location, after randomization, was not statistically significant for any subgroup. However, the stroke rates were significantly different between the surgical group and medical group for both degrees of moderate stenosis. There was an "adverse effect" on stroke-free survival attributed to surgery for both the 30% to 49% and 50% to 69% stenosis groups. Up to 2.3 years after randomization there was a significantly ($P<.05$) increased risk of stroke in operated subjects in the 50% to 69% stenosis group. In the 30% to 49% stenosis there was also a significantly increased risk of stroke until 3.4 years after ran-

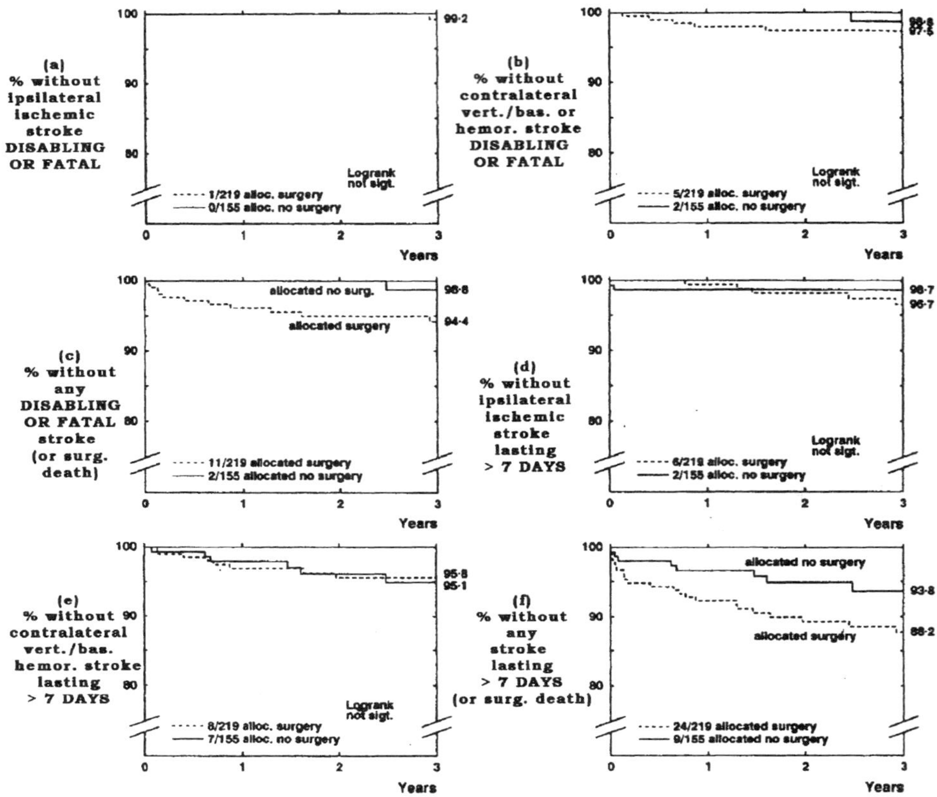

Figure 4 Main analysis of strokes (a-c disabling-fatal; d-f, lasting more than 7 days) or of surgery-associated mortality of patients with mild stenosis (0–29%) on the pre-randomization angiogram. Key(# with this as first event)/(# with some follow-up). (From Ref. 9.)

domization. After these points the risks for the surgical and medical groups were not statistically different.[8] (See Figs. 5 and 6.)

In summary, the ECST and NASCET both support carotid artery endarterectomy in the setting of symptomatic, severe carotid stenosis.[8,9,28] However, for patients with < 70% stenosis, the risk of surgery may outweigh the risk of standard medical therapy. All of this must be analyzed in the appropriate setting of experienced surgeons and adequate radiographic studies. In both of these studies surgical morbidity was kept to a minimum (2.1%). Radiographic studies consisted of standard x-ray angiogram with analysis of two views of the carotid. These two studies are the most complete to date on surgical indications for symptomatic carotid stenosis.

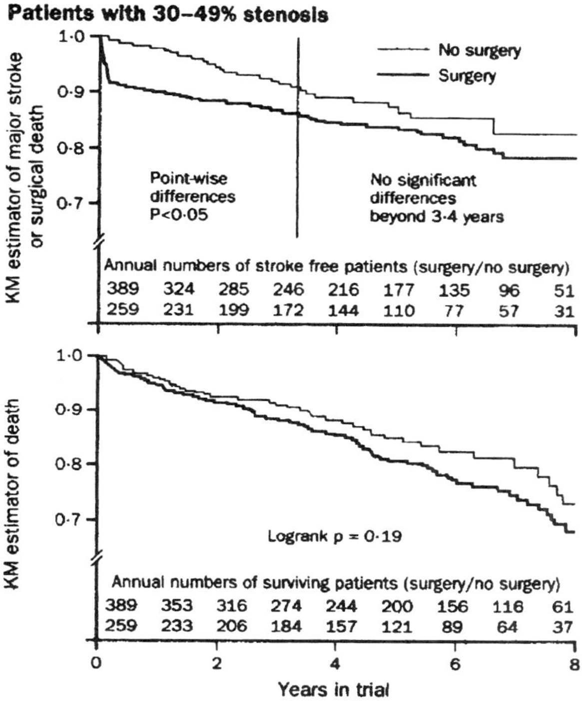

Figure 5 Kaplan-Meier estimates of major stroke or surgical death, and of death from any cause, within 30–49% stenosis ranges of symptomatic carotid stenosis. (From Ref. 8.)

TRIALS FOR ASYMPTOMATIC CAROTID STENOSIS

Carotid stenosis is strongly tied to cerebral ischemia and strokes. People with higher degrees of symptomatic carotid stenosis benefit more from surgery. Therapies available for carotid stenosis include medical regimens (antiplatelet drugs and anticoagulation) as well as surgical intervention (carotid endarterectomy). Medical therapy can prevent carotid plaques from forming dangerous emboli or prevent thrombosis of stenotic vessels; however, it cannot reverse the athersclerotic changes responsible for plaque formation. Surgeons can remove the plaques and therefore the source of emboli with endarterectomy. However, the surgery itself is risky, as temporary occlusion or at least manipulation of the affected vessel is necessary to achieve adequate results. And even in the best of

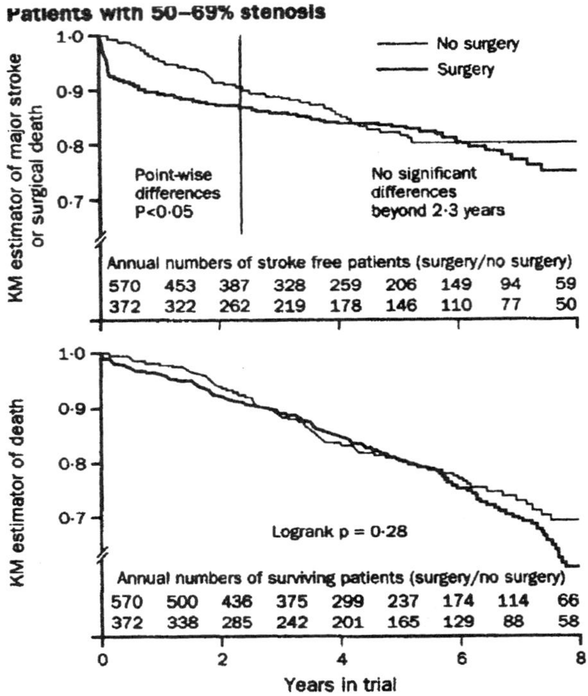

Figure 6 Kaplan-Meier estimates of major stroke or surgical death, and of death from any cause, within 50–69% stenosis ranges of symptomatic carotid stenosis. (From Ref. 8.)

hands there is an approximately 2% risk of stroke associated with surgery.[7] In order to discern which therapy is indicated for which patients, prospective studies were designed to examine the effect of each in a population. The studies were also designed to examine at which degree of stenosis is surgical intervention effective, if at all.[6,10,18,21,24]

Two of these well-designed randomized, controlled trials yielded similar information. Carotid artery endarterectomy not only decreases the risk of stroke in high-grade (>70%), symptomatic carotid artery stenosis, but imparts a long-term protection against future stroke.[8,9,28] The European trial went further to investigate those patients with the least amount of stenosis, with less than surprising but equally important information.[8,9] Surgery not only was ineffective in reducing the long-term risk for stroke, but actually imparted an increased risk of acute stroke due to perioperative morbidity. The indications for surgical management of symptomatic carotid stenosis is clear. Those patients with stenosis >

70% with ipsilateral symptoms are good candidates for endarterectomy. Taking this into consideration, if we can stratify those patients with symptomatic disease who present after transient ischemic attack or major stroke, can we identify and treat those people with "silent" stenosis? Is there a population of patients who have carotid artery stenosis, without any overt symptoms, who may benefit from surgery?

Mayo

Over a 30-month period, 158 patients with a symptomatic carotid stenosis were studied at the Mayo Clinic. The study randomized 71 patients. The remaining 87 patients were eligible but not randomized.[21] Admission criteria included carotid artery stenosis > 50% without history of cerebral or retinal ischemia. Carotid stenosis was measured by either Doppler (diameter reduction method), angiography (linear stenosis measurements), or ocular pneumoplethysmography. Only those patients entering the surgical arm were required to have carotid angiography. Patients with carotid occlusion were excluded. The study looked at patients from 18 years old to 79, excluding any women of childbearing age. Patients with known medical conditions that precluded the use of aspirin were also excluded. Other medical conditions such as unstable angina, myocardial infarction in the past 6 months, or cardiac sources of embolus also invalidated eligibility.[21]

Once enrolled, each of the 71 randomized patients was assigned to the medical or surgical arm. Medical therapy included 80 mg/day aspirin, and additional doses were discouraged. The surgical group was discouraged from taking aspirin unless it was previously prescribed for other medical reasons. The endpoints of the study included any TIA, ischemic or hemorrhagic stroke, or death. Myocardial infarction and coronary bypass surgery were considered secondary endpoints. Analysis of data included review of primary and secondary endpoints. Internal review of data was performed to delineate any significant difference in treatment. Early termination of the study was to be instituted if the safety of the patients was jeopardized by the protocol.[21]

Of the 158 patients, 68 were tracked in the surgical arm (36 randomized) and 90 were treated with aspirin alone (35 randomized). In the eligible but nonrandomized group a significantly higher percentage of men (45%) received surgery than women (19%). Two patients randomized to aspirin therapy received carotid endarterectomy prior to reaching any endpoint. Nine patients in the randomized, surgical arm did not undergo surgery.[21]

The outcome data from this study did not show any significant difference in stroke rates between the randomized groups. In the aspirin therapy group there were four ischemic events: three ischemic strokes, one TIA. Three ischemic events occurred in the surgical group: two occurred after randomization but prior to surgery, and the third occurred in the right posterior cerebral artery distribution, 4 days after left carotid endarterectomy. In addition there, were eight myocardial infarctions (MIs) in the randomized surgical group, and none in the aspirin therapy group. If MI and stroke are evaluated together there is a slightly decreased risk for poor outcome in the medical therapy group (*P*=.0363). The nonrandomized but eligible groups were subject to the same analysis. The statistics revealed a slightly significant difference in primary and/or secondary endpoint occurrence in favor of the group receiving aspirin therapy (*P*=.0412). However, the most significant data were the rates of MI in the surgical group compared to the medically treated group. The surgical group (both randomized and nonrandomized) had 18 MIs (26%). Sixteen of these 18 patients were not taking aspirin, per the protocol. In the medical group there were eight MIs (9%), and two of these patients had discontinued aspirin therapy temporarily. The rate of MI in the surgical group associated with lack of aspirin therapy was significant (*P*=.0011). Due to the high incidence of secondary endpoint occurrence in the surgical group, the study was halted. The role of antiplatelet therapy and coronary artery disease was supported by the findings of the study. In the final analysis no conclusions could be drawn concerning the value of carotid endarterectomy for asymptomatic stenosis.[21]

CASANOVA

In 1981 the CASANOVA committee was formed to evaluate carotid artery endarterectomy and best medical therapy versus medical therapy alone for asymptomatic carotid artery stenosis. Enrollment was begun with Doppler studies of patients and confirmation of stenosis with angiography. The goal of the study was to evaluate asymptomatic patients with carotid stenosis and stratify them for appropriate therapy in order to decrease the number strokes. Unfortunately, this study was begun prior to the result from the previously mentioned reports for symptomatic disease and the investigators did not have the privilege of this information. Due to the climate for carotid endarterectomy, and with the patients' best interests in mind, the investigators immediately excluded those patients with > 90% carotid artery stenosis. During evaluation for enrollment, those patients who were found to have > 90% stenosis on angiogram, as evaluated by an experienced neuroradiologist, were advised to undergo carotid artery endarterectomy. This protocol mad statistical evaluation of this important group of patients impossible.[6]

The remainder of the data from the study are important and will be reviewed. CASANOVA was a European-based protocol that enrolled all patients with < 90% but > 50% stenosis of the carotid artery either unilaterally or bilaterally. Degrees of stenosis were labeled mild (50% to 70% stenosis), moderate (70%

to 90% stenosis), and severe (>90%). These measurements were made using linear diameters of the narrowest point in comparison with the normal artery distal to the carotid bulb. Also, flow characteristics were used to measure stenosis. Enrollees were excluded if angiography revealed stenosis > 90% or < 50% of the surgically accessible cervical carotid, significant stenosis of other cervical vessels or intracranial carotid. In addition, patients who had prior endarterectomy (within 3 months of enrollment) or myocardial infarction within 6 months were also excluded. Any patient who was unable to take ASA, had renal failure (creatinine >1.5 mg/dL), dementia, or other systemic disease that shortened life expectancy significantly was also excluded from the study.[6]

The study design randomized patients into two categories: group A, who received unilateral or bilateral endarterectomy as indicated; and group B, who received no surgery in the case of unilateral stenosis or unilateral endarterectomy of the more stenotic side in the case of bilateral stenosis. All patients were placed on a regimen of 990 mg ASA per day and 225 mg dipyridamole per day. Patients were followed closely and received endarterectomy midstudy if: stenosis of the vessel in question progressed to > 90%, bilateral stenosis ensued > 50% on either side, TIA occurred ipsilateral to the stenotic carotid (>50%), or if one of the group A subjects developed contralateral stenosis or restenosis of >50%. As in all the previously mentioned studies, endpoints included stroke and death. Also, an interruption of the study was allowed if trends pointed toward significant benefit in either of the therapies or excessive morbidity associated with surgery or angiography.[6]

The results from randomized patients included statistically insignificant differences in the number of patients who reached an "endpoint" in the study (stroke, not including TIA, or death). Including TIAs as an endpoint, surgery imparted no significant benefit over medical therapy for the groups studied (Fig. 7). The investigators further analyzed the data accumulated, and discovered that 42% of the ischemic events that occurred in follow-up were in "an area that could not be protected by carotid surgery."[6]

Although the data showed no significant difference in medical therapy and surgery versus medical therapy alone, a crucial population was excluded from the protocol. Those patients with the worst degree of stenosis (>90%) were not analyzed. As mentioned earlier, the higher degree of stenosis is associated with increased risk of stroke for symptomatic patients, and one might infer the same for asymptomatic patients. Unfortunately, this study failed to examine this population. In addition, the investigators admit there are too few enrolled patients to make conclusions about the difference in therapy and that "there were several patients who did not comply with the protocol."[6] Study design also required that nearly half of the patients in the medically managed group undergo carotid endarterectomy. In their final conclusions they could not recommend carotid ar-

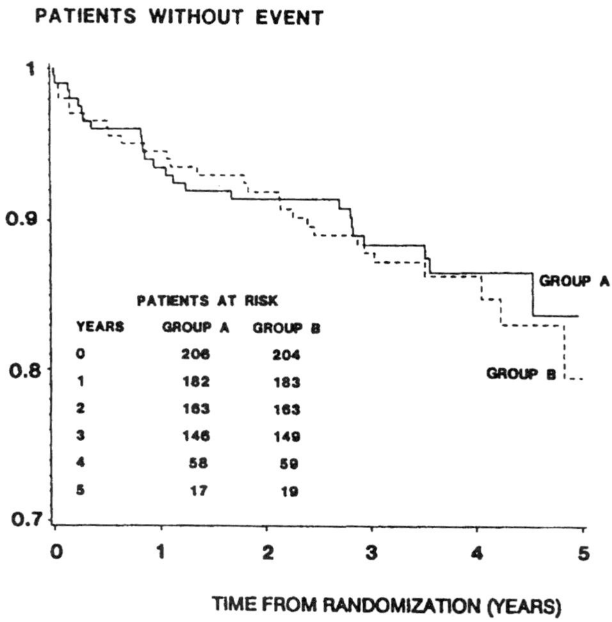

Figure 7 Kaplan-Meier plot of patients without event in group A (solid line) and group B (broken line). Number of patients "at risk" at a defined point in time after randomization is shown in the lower left. (CASANOVA study group, Ref. 6.)

tery endarterectomy (CAE) for asymptomatic patients with < 90% stenosis unless surgery was being done as part of a controlled clinical trial.[6]

CASANOVA therefore did not answer the question posed for treatment of asymptomatic carotid stenosis. The study failed to examine patients with the most critical stenoses. Also, the number of patients studied was inadequate to make any meaningful conclusions regarding surgery or medical therapy.[6]

VA

The Veterans Affairs Cooperative enlisted 11 centers within the VA system to reanalyze the effect of CAE on asymptomatic carotid stenosis. A comparison of surgery and aspirin therapy versus medical therapy (aspirin and optimized medical treatment of concomitant disease) was used to evaluate the effect of CAE on TIA, stroke, or death for patients with at least 50% carotid stenosis. Unlike CASANOVA, patients were not excluded based on the degree of stenosis, except for documented carotid occlusion.[6]

Enrollment began on April 1, 1983, and continued until Sept. 30, 1987. In that time 1,935 adult males were screened for randomization. Inclusion criteria required each enrollee to be asymptomatic, adult, male, and have carotid stenosis suspected on noninvasive studies (Doppler, or ocular pneumoplethysmography). Carotid stenosis was confirmed by angiogram; only those with ≥ 50% stenosis were included. Excluded from the study were any patients with previous ipsilateral cerebral infarction, previous endarterectomy with restenosis, previous extracranial to intracranial bypass, high surgical risk from other medical processes, long-term anticoagulation, intolerance to aspirin therapy, long-term aspirin therapy, or life expectancy of < 5 years. With these criteria, 444 of the screened patients were enrolled in the VA cooperative study. Of these, 211 were randomized to surgery and 233 to medical management. After randomization, every patient enrolled received an angiogram to document stenosis and was placed on aspirin therapy (650 mg bid or 325 mg qd if higher dose was not tolerated).[18]

In the surgical arm of the study, 211 endarterectomies were performed on 203 patients. Eight patients refused surgery after randomization, and eight patients required bilateral carotid endarterectomies. The eight patients that refused surgery were included in the data analysis. The perioperative complication rate was 4.7% for stroke or death; however, the investigators also reported transient cranial nerve dysfunction, postoperative hematoma, hemodynamic instability (pharmacologically treated), and nonfatal MI. With the addition of nonfatal MI, their significant complication rate was 6.6% in the 30-day postoperative period. In the comparable period there were only one death (due to suicide), one stroke, and one TIA in the medical arm of the study (1.3% event rate).[18]

Statistical analysis of the two groups produced meaningful data. There was a statistically significant risk reduction for the surgical group if all neurologic endpoints were considered jointly (Fig. 8). However, when considering death or stroke alone, there was no significant difference between the two groups (Fig. 9). Although the VA study group did find that CAE significantly reduces the rate of TIAs and strokes together, and TIAs alone in men with asymptomatic carotid stenosis, no conclusions could be drawn concerning the more important endpoints of stroke alone and death.[18]

ACAS

A fourth study was designed to evaluate the surgical management of asymptomatic carotid artery stenosis. The Asymptomatic Carotid Atherosclerosis Study (ACAS) investigators began enrolling patients in 1987 at 39 centers. Subjects were identified by carotid bruit or if cerebral angiogram for peripheral vascular disease (i.e., contralateral symptomatic carotid stenosis) revealed a stenotic carotid artery irrigating an asymptomatic hemisphere or retina. Enrollment depended on "hemodynamically significant carotid stenosis." This was defined by either (1) 60% diameter reduction by arteriogram; (2) Doppler studies "showing a frequency or velocity greater than the instrument-specific cut point with 95% posi-

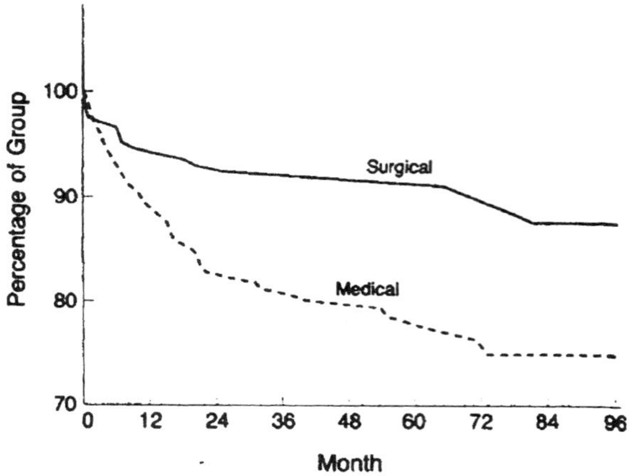

Surgical	211	181	163	150	122	88	45	18
Medical	233	194	166	148	121	85	58	32

Figure 8 The analysis shows the time to the first event in the surgical and medical groups. The number of patients remaining event free and in the study at the beginning of each 12-month period is shown below the graph. Comparisons between treatment groups by the log-rank test demonstrated significant differences favoring the surgical group ($P<0.001$). The relative risk in the surgical group as compared with the medical group was 0.38 (95 percent confidence interval, 0.22 to 0.67). (From Ref. 18.)

tive predictive value (PPV)"; or (3) Doppler studies demonstrating frequency or velocity greater than the instrument-specific cut point with 90% PPV and confirmation by ocular pneumoplethysmography. The investigators used the diameter reduction method of calculating carotid stenosis. It is important to note that not all angiograms were done as part of the study (postrandomization). Only those patients enrolled in the surgical arm via Doppler studies had postrandomization angiograms for surgical planning. Patients with bilaterally hemodynamically significant carotid stenosis were only enrolled unilaterally. The more stenotic artery was the chosen for the study. In the case of bilaterally equally significant carotid stenosis, the left artery was randomized and studied. The remaining artery was medically managed unless symptoms developed; at that point surgery was allowed.[10]

The surgical arm of the study required preoperative angiogram and computed tomography (CT) of the brain. CAE was performed within 2 weeks after randomization. If radiographs revealed any other vascular pathology, CAE was not performed but the patients were retained in the surgical arm of the study. Asymptomatic infarctions found on head CT did not preclude surgery or entrance in the study. The 30 days after surgery were considered the "postoperative pe-

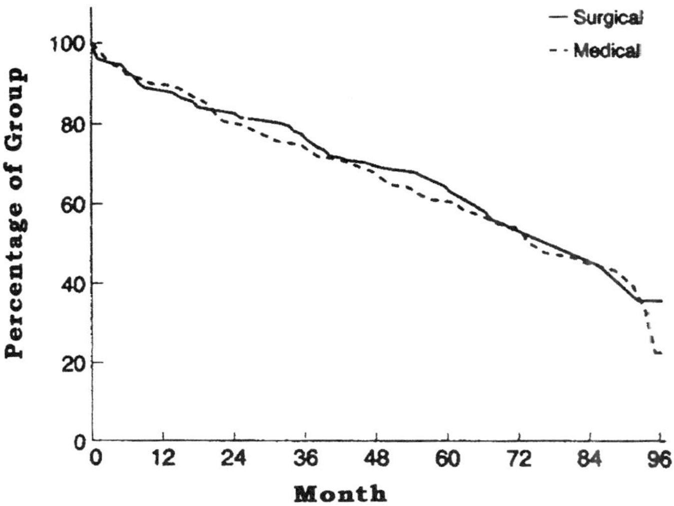

Surgical 211	**181**	**163**	**150**	**122**	**88**	**45**	**18**
Medical 233	**184**	**166**	**148**	**121**	**85**	**58**	**32**

Figure 9 The number of patients remaining event-free and in the study at the beginning of each 12-month period is shown below the graph. Comparisons between treatment groups by the log-rank test demonstrated no significant differences The relative risk in the surgical group as compared with the medical group was 0.92 (95 percent confidence interval, 0.66 to 1.22). (From Ref. 18.)

riod" and all events occurring in this period were assigned to surgical morbidity or mortality, respectively.[10]

Patients in the medical and surgical arms of the study received daily enteric-coated aspirin (325 mg). Also, both groups were counseled on risk reduction. They were advised to lower serum lipid levels and to control diabetes and hypertension when appropriate. Investigators gave advice to reduce alcohol and tobacco use, as well.[10]

The study design required follow-up at regular intervals, decreasing in frequency over time. Doppler studies were done routinely as part of follow-up, and head CT was done when either a potential endpoint was reached or at exit from the study. Patients were required to fill out forms at clinic visits for record keeping and to report any potential events to their enrolling physician.[10]

ACAS initial endpoints included TIAs (defined as "focal ischemic neurologic deficit or abrupt onset lasting at least 30 seconds and resolving completely in 24 hours"), stroke (any deficit that lasted > 24 hours), and death. Endpoints were broken down to include primary and secondary analysis. Primary analysis changed to examine only ipsilateral stroke or death during the perioperative and follow-up period.[10] This analysis was predicated on the results of the VA asymptomatic carotid stenosis trial and the NASCET trial. The former had already established that CAE reduced the risk of TIAs in asymptomatic carotid stenosis, and the latter established the role of CAE in symptomatic disease.

The two cohorts studied were well matched (see Table 3). The power of the study required only 750 participants in each arm of the study to evaluate the 5-year difference between treatments. The study persisted for 6 years (ending 1993). At that time 1,662 patients were randomized. Three of the patients in the surgical arm were lost to follow-up, leaving 825 in the surgical arm and 834 in the medical arm. As can be seen in Table 3, the vast majority of participants were white males in their mid-60s. This does bear significantly in the data.[10]

The results of the data include the 101 patients from the surgical arm who did not undergo CAE and the 45 patients in the medical arm who underwent CAE. Nineteen of the surgical patients reached primary endpoint of either death or stroke in the perioperative period (2.3%). Of these, five were directly related to angiography (one of whom died). Ten patients had strokes and one patient suffered a fatal myocardial infarction. In the medical arm during the perioperative period there were only three patients that reached a primary endpoint (two strokes, one death) for risk of 0.4%.[10]

Angiographic complications played a role in surgically managed patients. As stated previously, all surgical patients were required to have a carotid angiogram prior to CAE; however, only 414 had angiography postrandomization. If all surgical candidates received angiography as part of study protocol, with the current angiographic complication rate the overall rate of stroke or death would be 2.7% (not significantly higher, and acceptable).[10]

Although the initial complication rate and survival seemed dismal for the surgical arm, as follow-up ensued, the survival curves of the medically managed and surgically managed groups converged. At 2.7 years into the study significant statistics on 5-year risk reduction were apparent. The overall 5-year risk reduction for ipsilateral stroke or perioperative stroke or death was 53% (P=.004). The risk for those patients who received only aspirin therapy was 11% over a 5-year period. Surgically treated patients had a 5.1% risk of ipsilateral stroke or perioperative stroke or death over the same period. In addition, in the surgical arm, risk reduction for overall or perioperative ipsilateral TIA, stroke, or perioperative death was 57% (P<.05). Statistical analysis yielded insignificant results in regard to any stroke or death. The Kaplan-Meier tables show a trend in risk reduction for the surgical arm (20%), but this was not statistically significant. Risk reduction in regard to perioperative death or any stroke was insignificant, but again showed a trend in favor of carotid endarterectomy (Fig. 10).

Table 3 Baseline Characteristics of Randomized Patients by Treatment Assignment, in Percentages[a] from ACAS

Baseline characteristic	Surgical (n=825)	Medical (n=834)
Age. Y		
40–49	2	2
50–59	13	15
60–69	50	46
70–79	36	38
Race		
White	94	95
Black	3	3
Other	3	2
Sex		
M	66	66
F	34	34
History		
Coronary artery disease[b]	69	69
Hypertension[c]	64	64
Cancer	12	10
Diabetes mellitus	25	21
Lung disease at entry	6	5
Current cigarette smoker	28	24
Bilaterally eligible arteries	10	9
Previous contralateral		
Endarterectomy	20	19
TIA or stroke[d]	22	27
EC-IC bypass	<1	0
Subclavian bypass	<1	<1
Bruits in neck[e]		
Ipsilateral	76	74
Contralateral	44	42
Infarct on CT scan[f]		
Any location	22	24
Ipsilateral silent	8	9
Contralateral occlusion by Doppler	10	9

[a]TIA indicates transient ischmeic attack; EC~IC, external carotid-internal carotid; and CT, computed tomography.
[b]Defined as previous history of angina, coronary artery bypass, previous myocardial infarction, or abnormal electrocardiogram.
[c]Positive response to "Has your doctor ever told you that you had high blood pressure or were hypertensive?"
[d]Significant difference between groups at .05 level (unadjusted for multiple comparisons).
[e]Bruit question not evaluated for 51 surgical and 52 medical patients. Ipsilateral/Contralateral refers to randomized artery.
[f]CT scan was not available on 71 surgical and 60 medical patients.

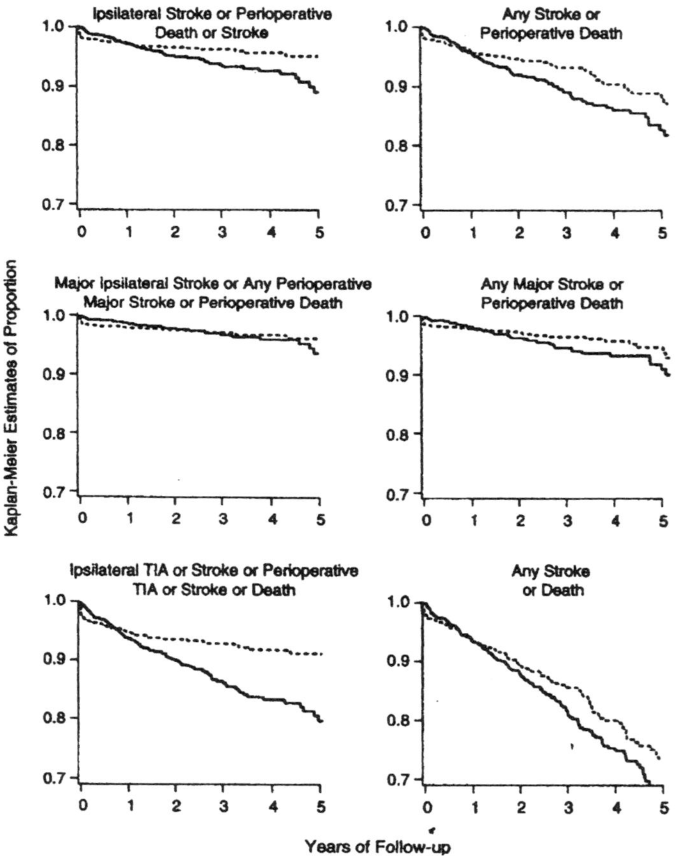

Figure 10 Proportion of patients without end point at a given time during follow-up, by treatment group, using Kaplan-Meier estimations. Solid line indicates medical patients, broken line, surgical patients and TIA, transient ischemic attack. (From Ref. 10.)

In order to better understand who would benefit from endarterectomy for asymptomatic disease, the ACAS group analyzed groups of patients based on sex, race, age, and degree of stenosis. With this meta-analysis men received significant benefit from CAE for asymptomatic carotid stenosis regardless of the degree of stenosis beyond a 60% diameter reduction. There was a significant risk reduction over a 5-year period. The study failed to show a significant risk reduction for women. If all subgroups are included, the rate of stroke or death for patients with asymptomatic carotid stenosis (>60%) is 11% if treated medically and 5.1% if treated surgically. This difference is statistically significant.[10]

STRATEGIES IN SURGICAL CANDIDATES

After presenting the data in support of CAE in the appropriate circumstance, we will discuss the assessment of patients for surgery. When evaluating a patient with carotid stenosis for potential surgery a number of factors have been shown to be of importance: presence/absence of symptomatic disease; medical fitness of the patient (concurrent disease); radiographic evidence of stenosis; and willingness of the patient to undergo surgery.

Patient Assessment

Candidates for surgery require a vigorous preoperative assessment prior to surgical decision making. As always, a complete history and physical are of paramount importance. The history records timing of events and characterization of symptoms. The presence of a transient neurologic deficit (TIA) apposed to a permanent one will help determine treatment guidelines. The quantity and quality of events can also assist in decision making. Those patients who report repeated transient neurologic episodes of increasing frequency (stuttering or crescendo TIAs) may be at a greater risk for future events or stroke. Permanent deficit weighs heavily in surgically planning as well.[15,25,29,38]

Asymptomatic patients who have carotic artery stenosis diagnosed incidentally may be surgical candidates. Strict interpretation of the ACAS study would suggest only males < 80 years old with >60% diameter reduction are appropriate candidates for surgery.[10] However, there have been studies that have shown that octogenarians are not at increased risk for stroke from CAE in symptomatic disease.[29] The sex bias of ACAS is borne out in its numbers. There were too few women enrolled at ACAS to make any statistically significant conclusions.[10] It is safe to assume that at least a 60% diameter reduction as measured on angiogram must be present for surgery to be presented as an option. Otherwise careful follow-up and patient education in regard to TIAs including amaurosis fugax are indicated.

Completed stroke represents the proverbial cow out of the barn. Unfortunately, only 15% of strokes are preceded by TIA.[1] If there were other more obvious warnings that embolic stroke was imminent, stratifying high-risk patients would be easier. Routine physicals with auscultation for carotid bruits can serve as a rough screen for asymptomatic patients, but largely this population represents a diagnostic and therapeutic quandary, as evidenced by the multitude of clinical investigations in this area.[10,16,18,21,24,26] If a patient presents with a completed stroke, the work-up and eventual surgical treatment are different from the patient who is diagnosed with carotid stenosis with TIAs or by routine physical exam (a suspicion of carotid bruit). In all circumstances, even though initial screening radiographically might include Doppler studies or magnetic resonance angiography, we recommend standard (preferably digital subtraction) angiography. (Fig. 11A, B, C) Angiography is the gold standard for measurement of stenosis and diagnosis of carotid occlusion. In addition, an experienced angiographer can demonstrate if and where collateral flow has been established, the presence of steal phenomena, and concurrent cerebral atherosclerosis or tandem lesions.

Patients with carotid stenosis often have concurrent disease. The risk factors for carotid atherosclerosis and stroke also contribute to coronary artery disease and increased risk for MI. Carotid stenosis represents only one form of atherosclerosis. A vigorous preoperative workup to evaluate coronary disease and cardiac performance prior to surgery is often warranted. These patients should also be followed by a cardiologist and treated appropriately. The discussion of

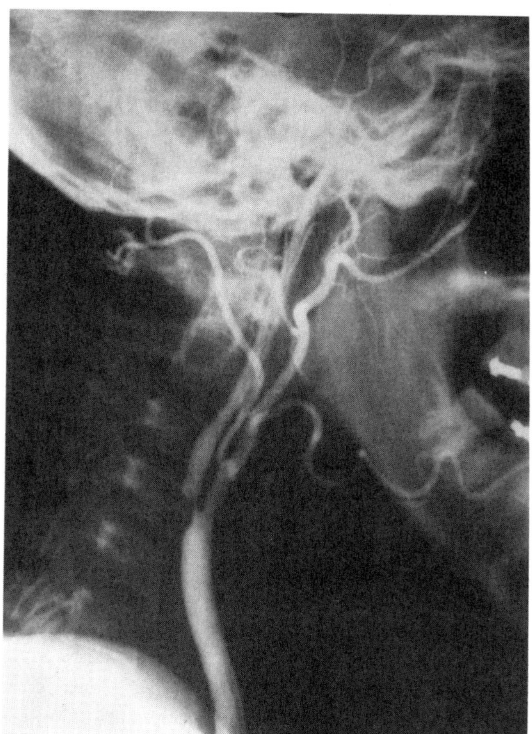

A

Figure 11 A. Digital subtraction angiogram of right carotid artery demonstrating a high-grade stenosis of the internal carotid artery at its origin. B. Digitial subtraction angiogram of left carotid artery demonstrating a high-grade stenosis of the internal carotid artery at its origin. C. Magnetic resonance angiogram of the left carotid artery of the same patient.

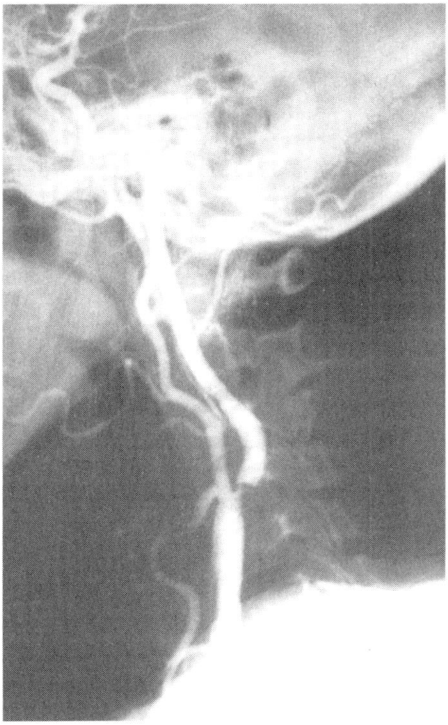

B

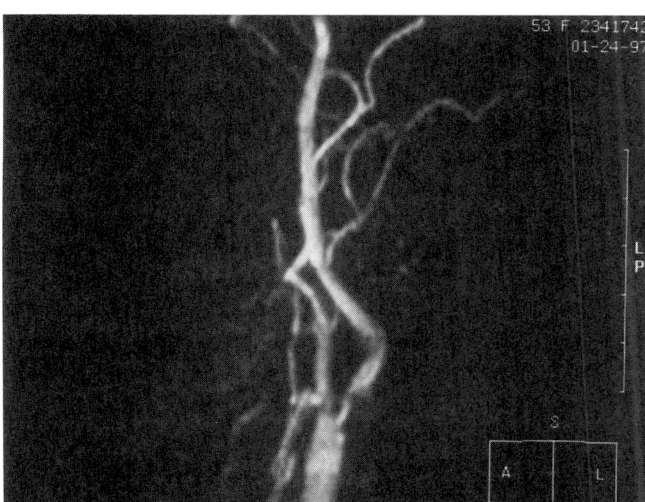

C

coronary bypass and carotid artery endarterectomy is a topic debated in the literature, and is not the focus of this chapter.[38]

It is not unusual to find patients with bilateral carotid stenosis with symptoms only referable to one side. Carotid occlusion can be found opposite symptomatic carotid stenosis. In addition, angiography might uncover more severe stenosis opposite a symptomatic lesion, or a "tandem lesion" might be found ipsilaterally and distal to the lesion being evaluated. All of these anatomic factors play an important role in surgical decision making. Angiography is the best way to adequately delineate the anatomy as well as the degree of stenosis.

Patients who present with simple unilateral carotid stenosis diagnosed on angiography and a history of transient neurologic deficits are good candidates for surgery, provided the stenosis is > 70%.[28] If the same patient presents with a permanent neurologic deficit or stroke, the management changes.[15,36]

A number of studies have evaluated the danger of CAE in the face of recent cerebral infarction (Fig. 12)[15,36] previously, a 4- to 6-week recovery period was arbitrarily recommended after completed stroke to carotid endarterectomy. Anecdotal and retrospective analysis implicated an increased risk of cerebral hemorrhage with early surgery after completed stroke.[15] In 1990 a prospective study was done and found that there was no significant difference in the rate of cere-

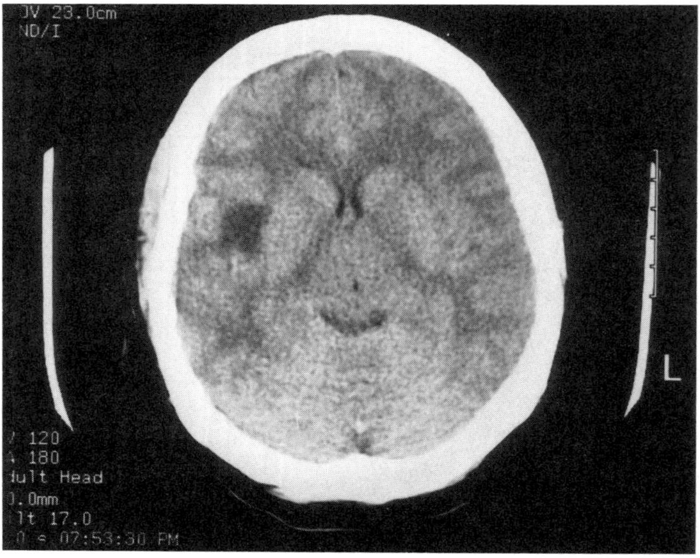

Figure 12 Computed tomography of the patient from figure 11 with right sided carotid-middle cerebral distribution, subcortical infarct.

brovascular events for patients operated on prior to or after the 6-week window.[29] The recommendation from this group was to wait for the neurologic deficits to plateau prior to attempting angiography and surgery.[29]

Patients may present with carotid stenosis unilaterally by history or exam but are diagnosed with bilateral stenosis after radiologic studies. Additional noninvasive techniques, such as Doppler, or cerebral blood flow studies help define which lesion is more hemodynamically significant.[17] The general principle is to operate on the most stenotic and hemodynamically compromised vessel first, regardless of symptomotology. Following recovery from surgery, the other vessel is pursued. Interceding anticoagulation may be required if both vessels are significantly stenotic.

Bilateral or unilateral symptoms may lead to the diagnosis of bilateral carotid stenosis or unilateral stenosis and carotid occlusion contralaterally. In this circumstance the evaluation and treatment of the stenotic lesion should not be delayed. There is no contraindication to CAE in this circumstance. There are surgical techniques and intraoperative monitoring that can be used to assist surgeon and ensure adequate cerebral perfusion during surgery.

Shunts, catheters that divert flow around the stenotic artery during surgery, allow ipsilateral cerebral perfusion during endarterectomy. Somatosensory-evoked potentials (SSEP) and intraoperative electroencephalography (EEG) give real time physiologic measurements of brain activity.[38,39] These monitoring techniques can assist the surgeon by giving information confirming brain viability at crucial points.

The importance of angiography is highlighted by those patients with so-called tandem lesions and with steal syndromes. These patients may be managed in a number of ways. Usually, the second stenosis is intracranial and inaccessible from standard surgical approaches. Some surgeons advocate CAE on the proximal lesion of stenosis is severe (2 mm lumenal diameter) with close follow-up and anticoagulation or antiplatelet therapy.[37] Although small extracranial to intracranial bypass (EC-IC bypass) using the superficial temporal (STA) or occipital arteries to a distal middle cerebral artery (MCA) branch has not been shown to be of value in preventing further neurologic events in patients with inaccessible stenotic lesions, no one has adequately evaluated the use of long, large-caliber bypasses.[19,20,30,31,33] In our institution we more frequently use long, saphenous vein or radial artery bypass (ICA or ECA to MCA) for intracranial tumor compression of the cavernous carotid; however, we have used this technique for patients with intractable cerebral ischemia.[40] Recently, some reports show there is a small population of patents who actually demonstrate decreased cerebral blood flow with carotid and cerebral artery stenoses.[33,40] These patients may be amenable to long bypass. The traditional approach of CAE and antiplatelet therapy has not been adequately studied either. Even conservative surgeons might advocate bypass if symptoms persist after CAE and adequate anticoagulation or antiplatelet therapy. The evaluation of EC-IC bypass was abandoned over a decade ago after the last study revealed little utility for such an elegant procedure.[18,19,20,31] The technology to quantify cerebral perfusion was not available, and also the bypass evaluated (STA-MCA) is not the only technique used for cerebral reperfusion. With the current radiologic tests (xenon blood flow and acetazolamide challenge) as well as more popular surgical techniques (carotid bypass), there may be a role for EC-IC bypass in intractable cerebral ischemia and stroke prevention.

COMPLICATIONS

Every surgery is a controlled injury, and thus there are always risks of complications. These are kept to a minimum with knowledge of the anatomy, sufficient preoperative workup, and careful surgical planning for each individual patient. The complications specifically associated with carotid artery surgery include vascular insults and cranial nerve injury.

Cerebral ischemia or, worse, infarction can result from carotid artery surgery. SSEP and EEG preoperatively and intraoperatively can help the surgeon avoid dangerous, prolonged ischemia during surgery.[38,41] However, the danger is not only immediate, during the operation. Intimal injury during surgery or kinking of the artery after dissection might result in postoperative ischemia and stroke. We often obtain an intraoperative angiogram to evaluate the vessel after repair. Bypass procedures always include an intraoperative angiogram with careful attention to the anastamosis sights. This allows revision of the repair or anastamosis while the wound is still open. However, if an intraoperative angiogram is not obtained, postoperative imaging is always done—either three-dimensional computed tomographic angiogram (3DCT) (Fig. 13) or digital subtraction angiogram. If the patient still has evidence of TIAs or ischemia, anticoagulation may be instituted.

In addition to cerebral infarction, hemorrhage can be problematic. Large series in 1963 reported six out of 900 patients who received CAE.[36] Although this can be devastating or lethal, it is quite rare. Careful blood pressure management and awareness of preoperative areas of infarction may help in preventing hemorrhage or guiding therapy.

Cranial nerve injury associated with carotid artery surgery might affect the 12th, 10th, and, rarely seventh nerves. The 12th nerve crosses the bifurcation of the common carotid artery and may be injured during dissection.[41] As long as the nerve is not transected, only transient ipsilateral tongue deviation will result. Injury to the vagus nerve is usually due to retraction. This nerve may cross anterior to the ICA and may be adherent to it. This may result in hoarseness from unilateral vocal cord paresis. Lower-lip palsy may result from injury to a branch of the seventh nerve while obtaining access to a high lesion of the cervical ICA.

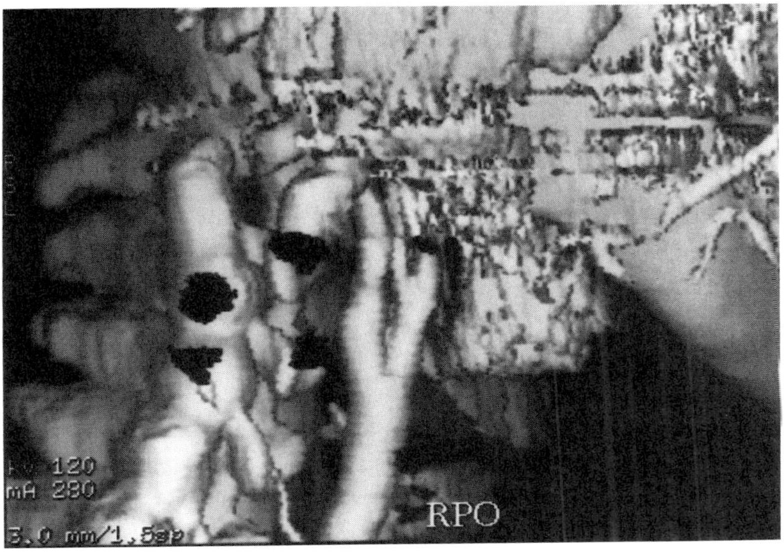

Figure 13 3D-computed tomographic angiogram of right internal carotid artery after endarterectomy on the patient shown in figures 11 and 12.

Making the incision away from the angle of the mandible, facial palsy can be avoided. Lastly, the sympathetic fibers that form a plexus around the ICA may be injured as well. This usually results in a peripheral Horner's syndrome and will heal with time.[37]

CONCLUSIONS

The role for surgery in carotid stenosis becomes increasingly clear with time and experience. The importance of defining the disease of the patient and then appropriately stratifying that patient is the cornerstone to proper surgical management. The role of medical therapy can never be over looked in these cases. As experience with new surgical techniques and imaging enhances, we will find ways of predicting who is at greatest risk for stroke and who will benefit the most from surgical intervention—either endarterectomy or perhaps bypass when indicated.

At present, the firmest data in favor of surgical intervention for carotid stenosis are in the symptomatic patient.[8,9,28] Those patients with > 70% stenosis and TIAs or stroke will benefit the most from surgery.[8,9,28] Their benefit is realized on a long-term basis, as their rate of future neurologic events decreases after surgery. Data also support surgery for asymptomatic patients with carotid stenosis.[10]

However, there are still unanswered questions concerning inaccessible lesions of the intracranial circulation and management of those patients who continue to have symptoms despite maximal medical and surgical therapy. Future controlled, prospective studies are needed to more finely define the disease and stratify patients to the correct therapy.

REFERENCES

1. Adams RD, Victor M. Principles of Neurology. 4th ed. Cerebrovascular Diseases. New York: McGraw-Hill, Inc.
2. Barnet HM. The dilemma of surgical treatment for patients with asymptomatic carotid disease. Ann Intern Med 1995; 123:723–725.
3. Boop F, et al. Cerebral revascularization with artificial graft: long term follow-up and discussion of the role of graft pretreatment with modified host endothelial cells. Surg Neurol 1993; 40:155–159.
4. Brott, T Toole, JF Medical compared with surgical treatment of symptomatic carotid artery stenosis. Ann Intern Med 1995; 123:720-722.
5. Bruetman ME, Fields WS, et al. Cerebral hemorrhage in carotid artery surgery. Arch Neur 1963; 9:458–467.
6. CASANOVA Study Group. Carotid surgery versus medical therapy in asymptomatic carotid stenosis. Stroke 1991; 22:1229–1235.
7. Crowell RM, Ogilvy, CS, Ojemann RG. Extracranial carotid artery atherosclerosis; carotid endarterectomy. In: Wilkins RH, Rengachary SS, eds. Neurosurgery. Vol. II. 2d ed. New York, McGraw-Hill.
8. European Carotid Surgery Trialists' Collaborative Group. Endarterectomy for moderate symptomatic stenosis: interim results from MRC European Carotid Surgery Trial. Lancet 1996; 347:1591–1593.
9. European Carotid Surgery Trialists' Collaborative Group. MRC European Carotid Surgery Trial: interim results for symptomatic patients with severe (70–99%) or with mild (0–29%) carotid stenosis. Lancet 1991; 347:1235–1243.
10. Executive Committee for ACAS. Endarterectomy for asymptomatic carotid artery stenosis. JAMA 1995; 273:1421–1428.
11. Fields WS, et al. Joint study of extracranial arterial occlusion. JAMA 1970; 211:1993–2003.
12. Fisher CM. Occlusion of the internal carotid artery. Arch Neurol Psychol 1951; 65:364–377.
13. Fisher CM. Occlusion of the carotid arteries. Arch Neurol Psychol 1954; 72:187–204.
14. Fitzpatrick BC, et al. Cervical to petrous internal carotid artery bypass procedure. J Neurosurg 1993; 79:138–141.
15. Giordano JM, Trout HH, et al. Timing of carotid artery endarterectomy after stroke. J Vasc Surg 1985; 2:250–254.

16. Hankey GJ. Asymptomatic carotid stenosis: how should it be managed? Med J Aust 1995; 163:197–200.
17. Hartl WH, Janssen I, Furst H. Effect of carotid endarterectomy on patterns of cerebrovascular reactivity in patients with unilateral carotid stenosis. Stroke 1994; 25:1952–1957.
18. Hobson RW, et al. Efficacy of carotid endarterectomy for asymptomatic carotid stenosis. NEJM 1993; 328:221–227.
19. Holohan TV. Extracranial-intracranial bypass to reduce the risk of ischemic stroke. Can Med Assoc J 1991; 144:1457–1465.
20. Ishikawa T. Cerebral haemodynamics and long term prognosis after extracranial-intracranial bypass surgery. J Neurol Neurosurg Psychiatry 1995; 59:625–628.
21. MACE Study Group. Results of a randomized controlled trial of carotid endarterectomy for asymptomatic carotid stenosis. Mayo Clin Proc 1992; 67:513–518.
22. McCormick P, et al. Disabling cerebral ischemic attacks. J Neurosurg 1991; 75:891–901.
23. McNamara JO, et al. The value of carotid endarterectomy in treating transient ischemia of the posterior circulation. Neurology 1977; 27:682–684.
24. Mayberg, Winn. Endarterectomy for asymptomatic carotid artery stenosis. JAMA 1995; 273:1459–1461.
25. Meyer FB, Piepgras DG. Emergency arotid endarterectomy for patients with acute carotid occlusion and profound neurological deficits. Ann Surg 1986; 203:82–89.
26. Moneta, et al. Operative versus nonoperative management of asymptomatic high-grade internal carotid artery stenosis: improved results with surgery. Stroke 1987; 18:1005–1010.
27. Moore, et al. Guidelines for carotid endarterectomy. Stroke 26:188–201.
28. NASCET Collaborators. Beneficial effect of carotid endarterectomy in symptomatic patients with high grade carotid stenosis. NEJM 1991; 325:445–453.
29. Piotrowski JJ, Bernhard VM, et al. Timing of carotid endarterectomy after acute stroke. J Vasc Surg 1990; 11:45–52.
30. Regali L, Piepgras DG. The late patency of long saphenous vein bypass to the anterior and posterior cerebral circulation. J Neurosurg 83:806–811.
31. Samson D, Boone S. Extracranial-intracranial (EC-IC) arterial bypass: past performance and current concepts. Neurosurgery 1978; 3:79–86.
32. Samson D. Saphenous vein interposition grafts in the microsurgical treatment of cerebral ischemia. Arch Surg 1981; 116:1578–1582.
33. Schmiedek P, et al. Improvement of cerebrovascular reserve capacity by EC-IC arterial bypass surgery in patients with ICA occlusion and hemodynamic cerebral ischemia. J Neurosurg 1994; 81:236–244.
34. Sen C, Sekhar LN. Direct vein graft reconstruction of the cavernous, petrous and upper cervical internal carotid artery: lesions learned from 30 cases. Neurosurgery 1992; 30:732–743.
35. Thompson JE. The evolution of surgery for the treatment of stroke. The Willis Lecture. Stroke 27:1427–1433.
36. Wylie EJ, Hein MF, et al. Intracranial hemorrhage following surgical revascularization for treatment of acute strokes. 1963; 212–216.

37. Zambraski JM, Greene KA, et al. Carotid endarterectomy. In: Carter LP, Spetzler RF, eds. In: Neurovascular Surgery. New York: McGraw-Hill Inc.
38. Sundt TM, Sandok BA, Hishant PJ. Carotid endarterectomy: complications and preoperative assessment of risk. Mayo Clin Proc 1975; 50:301–306.
39. Sundt TM, Sharbrough FW, et al. Correlation of cerebral blood flow and electroencephaographic changes during carotid endarterectomy. Mayo Clin Proc 1981; 56:533–543.
40. Levine ZT, Sekhar LN. Carotid artery bypass for cerebral ischemia intractable ischemia. Data presented January 1997. Neurosurgery Society of the Virginias White Sulfur Springs, WV.
41. Imparato Am Bracco A, et al. The hypoglossal nerve in carotid arterial reconstructions. Stroke 1972; 3:576–578.

Index

About the Editors

ASHFAQ SHUAIB is Professor of Medicine and Director of Neurology at the University of Alberta Hospital, Edmonton, Canada. The author or coauthor of over 130 peer reviewed publications on cerebral vascular disease, Dr. Shuaib is a Fellow of the American Academy of Neurology, the Heart and Stroke Foundation of Canada, the American Heart Association, and the Royal College of Physicians and Surgeons of Canada. He received the M.D. degree (1980) from Khyber Medical College, Pakistan.

LARRY B. GOLDSTEIN is Associate Professor of Medicine (Neurology) and Director of the Duke Center for Cerebrovascular Disease at the Center for Clinical Health Policy Research, Duke University Medical Center, Durham, North Carolina, and attending neurologist at the Durham VA Medical Center, North Carolina. The author or coauthor of more than 90 professional papers, book chapters, and editorials, and over 50 abstracts, Dr. Goldstein is a Fellow of the American Academy of Neurology and the Stroke Council of the American Heart Association, and a member of the American Neurological Association. He received the A.B. degree (1977) from Brandeis University, Waltham, Massachusetts, and the M.D. degree (1981) from the Mt. Sinai School of Medicine, New York City.